70¢

# Laboratory Handbook
# of Medical Mycology

# Laboratory Handbook of Medical Mycology

## Michael R. McGinnis

*Clinical Microbiology Laboratories
North Carolina Memorial Hospital*

*and*

*Department of Bacteriology
and Immunology
University of North Carolina
Chapel Hill, North Carolina*

1980

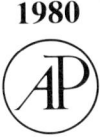

**ACADEMIC PRESS**

*A Subsidiary of Harcourt Brace Jovanovich, Publishers*

New York   London   Toronto   Sydney   San Francisco

COPYRIGHT © 1980, BY ACADEMIC PRESS, INC.
ALL RIGHTS RESERVED.
NO PART OF THIS PUBLICATION MAY BE REPRODUCED OR
TRANSMITTED IN ANY FORM OR BY ANY MEANS, ELECTRONIC
OR MECHANICAL, INCLUDING PHOTOCOPY, RECORDING, OR ANY
INFORMATION STORAGE AND RETRIEVAL SYSTEM, WITHOUT
PERMISSION IN WRITING FROM THE PUBLISHER.


ACADEMIC PRESS, INC.
111 Fifth Avenue, New York, New York 10003


*United Kingdom Edition published by*
ACADEMIC PRESS, INC. (LONDON) LTD.
24/28 Oval Road, London NW1 7DX


**Library of Congress Cataloging in Publication Data**

McGinnis, Michael R
    Laboratory handbook of medical mycology.

    Includes index.
    1. Medical mycology--Laboratory manuals.
I. Title. [DNLM: 1. Mycology--Laboratory manuals.
QW25.3. M145L]
RC117.M3    616.9'69'0028    79–15297
ISBN 0-12-482850-7


PRINTED IN THE UNITED STATES OF AMERICA

80 81 82 83   9 8 7 6 5 4 3 2 1

# Contents

| | |
|---|---|
| **Preface** | xi |
| **Acknowledgments** | xiii |

**Chapter 1  Basic Terminology and Classification**
| | |
|---|---|
| Vegetative Growth | 3 |
| Asexual Reproduction | 7 |
| Sexual Reproduction | 34 |
| Classification | 46 |
| Selected References | 55 |

**Chapter 2  Laboratory Safety**
| | |
|---|---|
| General Recommendations | 57 |
| Disinfection and Sterilization | 59 |
| Biological Hazards | 60 |
| Fire Hazards | 64 |
| Chemical Hazards | 66 |
| Flammable Liquid Hazards | 67 |
| Waste Disposal | 68 |
| Safety Equipment | 70 |
| Gas Cylinder Storage, Transport, and Use | 70 |
| Grounding of Electrical Equipment | 71 |
| Selected References | 72 |

**Chapter 3  Clinical Specimens**
| | |
|---|---|
| *Part 1.  General Information* | 73 |
| Selected References | 87 |

| | |
|---|---:|
| **Part 2. Techniques** | 88 |
| Abscess Specimens | 88 |
| Blood Specimens | 89 |
| Bone Marrow Specimens | 91 |
| Cerebrospinal Fluid | 91 |
| Fluids | 92 |
| Hair | 92 |
| Nails | 93 |
| Skin Scrapings (Stratum Corneum) | 94 |
| Sputum | 95 |
| Tissue Specimens | 96 |
| Urine Specimens | 98 |
| Selected References | 99 |
| **Part 3. Direct Examination of Clinical Specimens** | 100 |
| Giemsa Stain | 100 |
| Periodic Acid–Schiff Stain | 100 |
| Potassium Hydroxide Preparation | 101 |
| Selected References | 102 |

# Chapter 4 Mould Identification

| | |
|---|---:|
| **Part 1. Concepts** | 103 |
| Hughes's Experimental Classification System | 106 |
| Barron's Classification System | 109 |
| General References | 120 |
| **Part 2. Techniques** | 121 |
| Colony Characteristics | 121 |
| Confirmation of Dimorphic Fungi | 121 |
| Cycloheximide Resistance | 124 |
| Forcibly Discharged Conidia or Spores | 125 |
| *In Vitro* Hair Test | 125 |
| Mixed Cultures | 127 |
| Nutritional Studies | 130 |
| Proteolytic Activity | 132 |
| Rice Grain Test | 133 |
| Slide Culture Technique | 133 |
| Sporulation and Sterile Isolates | 136 |
| Subculturing Isolates | 137 |
| Tease Mount | 138 |
| Temperature Studies | 139 |

Contents

|  |  |
|---|---|
| Urea Hydrolysis | 141 |
| Selected References | 142 |
| **Part 3. *Taxonomy*** | **144** |
| Ascomycetes | 162 |
| Coelomycetes | 175 |
| Hyphomycetes | 179 |
| Zygomycetes | 304 |
| General Identification References | 326 |
| References Cited | 327 |

## Chapter 5  Yeast Identification

|  |  |
|---|---|
| **Part 1. *Basic Concepts*** | **337** |
| Selected References | 350 |
| **Part 2. *Techniques*** | **350** |
| Asci and Ascospores | 350 |
| Assimilation | 352 |
| Chlamydospore Development (Dalmau Plate) | 357 |
| Demonstration of Capsules | 359 |
| Direct Mounts | 361 |
| Fermentation | 362 |
| Forcibly Discharged Conidia | 364 |
| Germ Tube Test | 364 |
| Mixed Cultures | 367 |
| Nitrate Utilization | 369 |
| Pigment Formation by *Cryptococcus neoformans* | 371 |
| Temperature Studies | 372 |
| Urea Hydrolysis | 373 |
| Selected References | 373 |
| **Part 3. *Taxonomy*** | **375** |
| Ascomycetous Yeasts | 375 |
| Basidiomycetous Yeasts | 381 |
| Imperfect Yeasts | 387 |
| Characteristics of Medically Imported Yeasts | 401 |
| References Cited | 410 |

## Chapter 6  Susceptibility Testing and Bioassay Procedures

|  |  |
|---|---|
| *In Vitro* Susceptibility Testing | 412 |

|  |  |  |
|---|---|---|
| | Bioassay to Determine Drug Levels in Body Fluids | **432** |
| | Synergism Studies | **442** |
| | Selected References | **446** |

## Chapter 7  Culture Collection

| | |
|---|---|
| Culture Records | **447** |
| Receiving New Isolates | **448** |
| Reconstituting Lyophilized Cultures | **450** |
| Storage Techniques | **451** |
| Difficult-to-Revive Cultures | **454** |
| Mites | **454** |
| Mailing Cultures | **456** |
| Depositing Unusual Isolates in Major Culture Collections | **457** |
| Killed Cultures for Study or Teaching | **457** |
| Selected References | **458** |

## Chapter 8  Quality Control

| | |
|---|---|
| General Recommendations | **459** |
| Media Control | **461** |
| Equipment Control | **461** |
| Proficiency Evaluations | **472** |
| Selected References | **472** |

## Chapter 9  Synopsis of the Mycoses

| | |
|---|---|
| Aspergillosis | **475** |
| Blastomycosis | **477** |
| Candidiasis | **480** |
| Chromoblastomycosis | **482** |
| Coccidioidomycosis | **484** |
| Cryptococcosis | **486** |
| Eye Infections | **488** |
| Hair, Nail, and Skin | **491** |
| Histoplasmosis Capsulati | **500** |
| Histoplasmosis Duboisii | **502** |
| Lobomycosis | **504** |
| Mycetoma | **505** |
| Otomycosis | **508** |

| | | |
|---|---|---|
| | Paracoccidioidomycosis | 509 |
| | Phaeohyphomycosis | 511 |
| | Rhinosporidiosis | 512 |
| | Sporotrichosis | 514 |
| | Zygomycosis | 516 |
| | Selected References | 522 |

**Chapter 10  Media and Reagents**
Text  523

**Glossary**  589

**Appendix A  Some Simple Symmetrical Shapes**  612

**Appendix B  Commonly Encountered Synonyms and Other Obsolete Names**  614

**Appendix C  Reported Fungal Pathogens of Man**  619
References Cited  627

**Taxonomic Index**  645

**Subject Index**  655

# Preface

This laboratory handbook summarizes the concepts dealing with the laboratory aspects of medical mycology. Owing to the increased importance of fungi in medicine, there is a pressing need to discuss important topics such as laboratory safety and emergency procedures, quality control of media and equipment, new isolation techniques, susceptibility testing, and modern concepts for the identification of fungi. The information included in this handbook is intended to assist laboratory technologists, microbiologists, and mycologists in safely isolating and accurately identifying fungi of medical importance.

In contrast to other mycological works dealing with medically important fungi, the laboratory aspects of mycoserology and the identification of the actinomycetes have been excluded. The actinomycetes were omitted because they are bacteria, not fungi. Study of the actinomycetes is rapidly becoming a highly specialized field of study. To include them as a minor component of this handbook would be an injustice to this important and intriguing group of organisms. The techniques used for the serodiagnosis of the mycoses have been omitted because any attempt to include these techniques would be a duplication of what is available in other books.

The approach that I have taken in writing this book is to utilize as much contemporary mycological thought as possible. The key to understanding any field of science necessitates a thorough understanding of its language. It is, therefore, extremely important that the first chapter of this book be read first. Each of the terms, concepts and techniques of special interest to medical mycologists is clearly and concisely defined. These descriptions are supplemented with a large glossary, as well as a large number of photomicrographs. Many of the newer terms and concepts, especially those associated with conidiogenesis, may at first be difficult to grasp totally; however once they are clearly understood, most laboratorians will find medical mycology much easier.

The emphasis of this handbook is directed toward the identification of fungi that are commonly encountered in the medical mycology laboratory. This emphasis on identification is important since the ultimate function of each diagnostic and reference mycology laboratory is to identify fungi rapidly and accurately. This handbook will be a valuable asset in achieving this goal.

# Acknowledgments

Dr. Barry Katz, a good friend and colleague, is responsible for most of the photomicrographs of the various fungi included in this handbook. I am indebted to Dr. Katz and wish to express my sincere appreciation for his contribution.

I would like to thank Mrs. Lynne Sigler and Drs. Libero Ajello, J. W. Carmichael, Leanor Haley, Barry Katz, George Kobayashi, C. P. Kurtzman, John Richardson, Michael Rinaldi, Donald P. Rogers, Smith Shadomy, and G. A. de Vries for their generous cooperation in reviewing various portions of this laboratory handbook. Their valuable comments and suggestions have significantly enhanced the quality of the text. I am indebted to Mrs. Lynne Sigler and Drs. Mary English, Donald Greer, S. J. Hughes, G. F. Orr, E. Punithalingam, Emory Simmons, and Phyllis Stockdale for cultures that were used in the preparation of some of the photomicrographs; Ms. Christine Pinello and Drs. Libero Ajello, George Barron, Richard Benjamin, Garry Cole, A. S. El-Ani, Bryce Kendrick, and Lindsay Olive for the use of their photomicrographs; and Drs. G. C. Ainsworth, Libero Ajello, S. J. Hughes, Christine Philpot, and K. B. Raper for permission to reproduce some of their published work.

# Laboratory Handbook
of Medical Mycology

Chapter 1

# Basic Terminology and Classification

Ultrastructural, genetic and biochemical studies of many different types of living organisms have revealed that the prokaryote–eukaryote dichotomy is far more basic than the traditional animal–plant dichotomy. This new understanding of living organisms and their relationships to each other has stimulated a reevaluation of our current phylogenetic concepts. As a result, it is now realized by some that at least five kingdoms are necessary to accommodate all living things (Table 1.1). In this new classification scheme, the fungi are placed in the Kingdom Fungi, which contains the Chytridiomycetes (chytrids), Zygomycetes, Ascomycetes, Basidiomycetes, Fungi Imperfecti (Deuteromycetes) and lichens. Organisms previously considered to be fungi, that is, mycetozoans, labyrinthulids, thraustochytrids, plasmodiophorids, and oomycetes are now classified by many in the Kingdom Protista.

Mycology is that branch of biology which deals with the study of fungi. Medical mycology is a specialized area concerned with the study of fungi that are able to incite disease in man and animals. Fungi (sing. fungus) are eukaryotic organisms that usually grow in a filamentous, or yeastlike form, or both. Their nucleus, like that of other eukaryotic organisms, contains a nucleolus and several chromosomes that are bound by a nuclear membrane. The latter usually persists during nuclear division. The term coenocytic is used to describe the condition of a cell, nonseptate hypha or other structural unit when it contains many nuclei. Hyphal cells in septate hyphae may be uninucleate, binucleate, or multinucleate. For the most part, cellular and nuclear division are independent events, especially with respect to vegetative growth. As in other eukaryotic organisms, fungi have mitochondria, 80 S ribosomes, and centrioles. Flagellate cells are produced only by the chytrids. These motile, 1-celled, asexual spores called zoospores, have a single whiplash-type posterior flagellum, which is of the 9 + 2 fibril construction.

The cell wall of fungi primarily consists of chitin, chitosan, glucan and mannan, and rarely cellulose, in various combinations. Fungi are carbon heterotrophs and therefore require preformed organic compounds as a carbon source. Unlike plants, fungi cannot use carbon dioxide as a sole carbon source because they do not have chlorophyll. When supplied a carbon source such as glucose, fungi can synthesize their own proteins and usually most amino acids and vitamins if nitrogen and the essential minerals are available. Many fungi must have some vitamins, amino acids, or both supplied, or at least their precursors. They all synthesize lysine by the L-$\alpha$-adipic acid pathway.

**Table 1.1.** The Five Kingdoms of Organisms[a]

| Kingdoms | Principal features | Representative members |
|---|---|---|
| Monera | Prokaryotic; absorptive nutrition; mitotic apparatus absent; asexual reproduction by binary fission | Bacteria and blue-green algae; 14 phyla |
| Protista | Eukaryotic; ingestive, absorptive or photoautotrophic nutrition; mitotic reproduction; DNA and RNA; unicellular or multicellular; flagella or cilia with microtubules in 9 + 2 pattern | Protozoans, plasmodiophorids, labyrinthulids, hyphochytrids, mycetozoans, oomycetes, etc.; 30 phyla |
| Fungi | Eukaryotic; absorptive nutrition; zygotic meiosis; unicellular or filamentous; posterior whiplash-type flagella present (chytrids), cilia absent; cell walls chitinous; lysine synthesis by the L-$\alpha$-adipic acid biosynthetic pathway | Chytridiomycetes, zygomycetes, ascomycetes, basidiomycetes, fungi imperfecti, lichens; 5 divisions |
| Plantae | Eukaryotic; photoautotrophic nutrition; tissue highly differentiated; diploid phase arising from embryophyte | Liverworts, mosses, vascular plants; 9 divisions |
| Animalia | Eukaryotic; heterotrophic nutrition; gametic meiosis; multicellular; develop from diploid blastula, gastrulation occurs | Sponges, coelenterates, worms, arthropods, echinoderms, mammals, etc.; 32 phyla |

[a] Modified from Margulis (1974).

Actinomycetes (Kingdom Monera) superficially resemble fungi because of their filamentous nature. The actinomycetes are prokaryotic, Gram-positive, filamentous bacteria. Their nucleus consists of a continuous single chromosome that is not enveloped by a nuclear membrane. The cell wall of the actinomycetes consists of a glycosaminopeptide complex. The actinomycetes can serve as hosts to bacteriophages, whereas the fungi cannot serve as their hosts. These organisms are sensitive to antibacterial agents, such as penicillin, but not to antimycotic agents such as amphotericin B. The converse holds true for the fungi. As a more practical method to distinguish actinomycetes and fungi, medical mycologists usually consider an organism with Gram-positive filaments 0.5–1.0 $\mu$m in diameter to be an actinomycete. Care must be exercised in using size, since fungi may also be Gram-positive and some fungi, such as members of the genus *Fusidium,* are morphologically similar to the actinomycetes.

## VEGETATIVE GROWTH

Fungi pathogenic to man can be conveniently separated into two basic groups, moulds and yeasts. Moulds consist of those fungi that grow in a filamentous form, whereas yeasts are characterized by a unicellular morphology that reproduces by budding. Some mycologists prefer to restrict the term yeast to unicellular budding fungi that have the ability to reproduce by sexual means, and the term "yeastlike" to similar fungi that reproduce only asexually. In this handbook, the term yeast will be used to encompass all unicellular budding fungi, regardless of how they reproduce. A number of fungi (*Blastomyces dermatitidis, Coccidioides immitis, Histoplasma capsulatum, Sporothrix schenckii,* and *Paracoccidioides brasiliensis*) are dimorphic. That is, except for *C. immitis,* they can grow as a mould at room temperature and as a yeast at 37°C or in tissue. *Coccidioides immitis* grows as a mould at room temperature and as spherules producing endospores in tissue or on specialized media at 37°C.

Each vegetative filament or element of a fungus is called a hypha. A number of these filaments are referred to as hyphae, and a large amount of hyphae is known as mycelium. Since mycelium can be either single or collective, there is no need to use the expression mycelia. Hyphae are the actively growing assimilative phase of fungi. New growth occurs as linear elongation originating in a zone immediately behind the growing tip of the hypha. As a result of this linear elongation, the walls of hyphae tend to be parallel. As the hypha develops, it becomes divided into compartments or cells by the development of cross walls called septa (sing. septum). Such hyphae are referred to as being septate. The septa may either be partial,

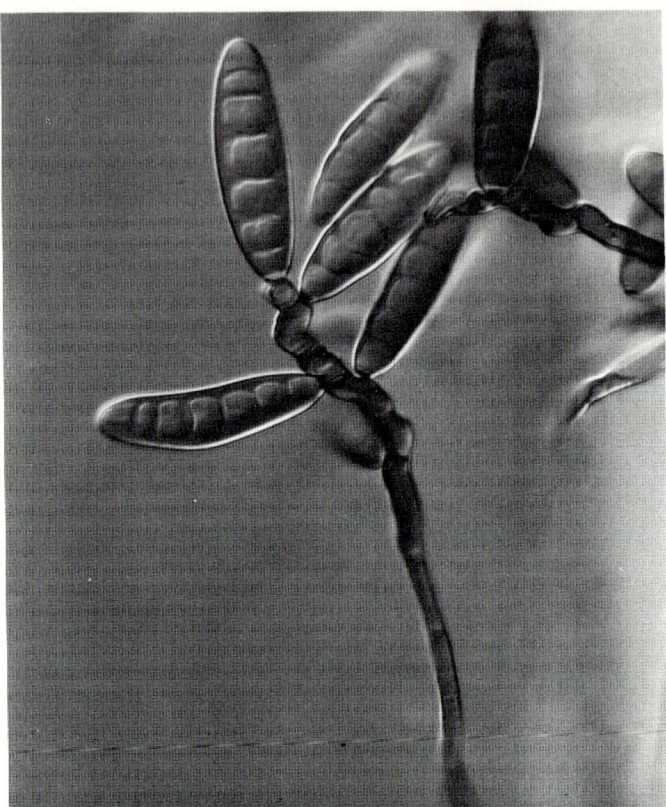

**Fig. 1.1** *Drechslera* sp. The conidia have pseudosepta.

complete, or perforated. Partial septa (pseudosepta) result as thickenings of the lateral walls of the hyphae. They may be abortive cross walls. Complete septa result from centripetal growth of the lateral walls until the ingrowing septal walls meet each other, usually leaving a minute pore(s). Perforated septa, which may be uniperforate or multiperforate, develop in the same manner as complete septa, but have a wider central pore. This type of septum is typically seen in the Ascomycetes and Fungi Imperfecti. If pores are present, then nuclei have the potential to move from one cell to the next. Pores may be plugged in a numbers of manners. Woronin bodies are organelles that commonly plug septal pores in some fungi. In some hyphae, septa are rarely formed. For example, in the Zygomycetes septa are formed to wall off empty cells and to separate asexual and sexual structures from the rest of the hypha. The septa in this group of fungi are variable; nuclei do not migrate from one cell to the next. For hyphae that contain occasional septa, the expression sparsely septate is preferred to the terms aseptate or nonseptate. Some fungi, such as species of *Drechslera*, develop pseudosepta (partial septa) in their conidia. Pseudosepta are thick outgrowths from the inner cell wall layer that grow toward the center of the conidium (asexual propagule), but do not completely wall off each compartment (Fig. 1.1).

The diameter of the hyphae is a useful characteristic in distinguishing hyphae of the Zygomycetes from other fungi. The Zygomycetes typically develop hyphae that can be characterized as being sparsely septate, branching irregularly, and having a diameter of approximately 10–15 $\mu$m. In general, excluding the Zygomycetes and fungi like *Fusidium*, most hyphae are approximately 1.5–3.5 $\mu$m in diameter.

Hyphal cells may be quite variable in shape and size. Many fungi when grown under unfavorable conditions develop swollen hyphal cells called vesicles (Fig. 1.2). Vesicles, unlike chlamydospores (Fig. 1.3), do not function as reproductive propagules but as cells for the storage of food substrates or materials toxic to the fungus. They may be thick-walled; this can result in a superficial resemblance to chlamydospores. The dermatophytes, as well as many other fungi, occasionally develop hyphae that

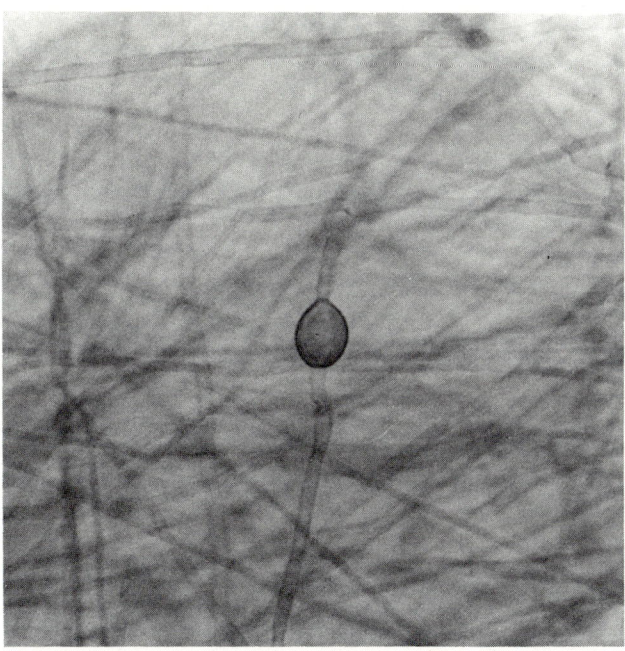

**Fig. 1.2** A vesicle is a swollen vegetative cell.

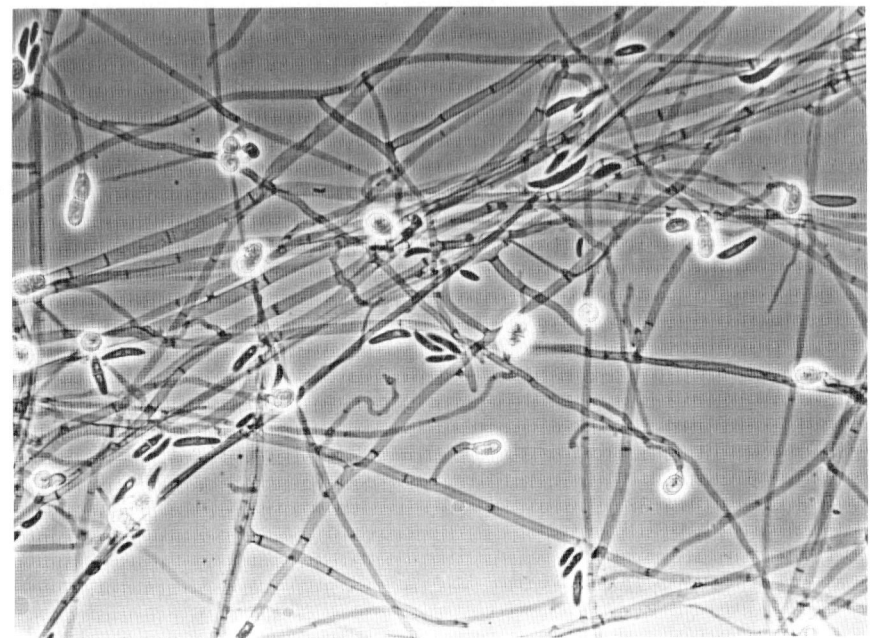

**Fig. 1.3** Chlamydospores are usually thick-walled because they serve the function of survival during adverse conditions. A. *Fusarium solani*. B. *Chlamydoabsidia padenu*.

contain cells having one end swollen at the distal portion. Such hyphae, or racquet hyphae (Fig. 1.4), are not unique to any one particular genus or species. Another form of swollen hyphae produced by fungi, such as *Trichophyton schoenleinii*, are favic chandeliers. A favic chandelier (Fig. 1.5) is a cluster of repeatedly branching, swollen hyphae that have the overall appearance of a chandelier. These various types of swollen hyphae have no real taxonomic value, but they do occasionally aid in identifying a fungus. A classic example is the terminal vesicles of *Microsporum audouinii*, which may have a very distinctive spinelike terminal appendage (Fig. 1.6).

When harsh environmental conditions occur, some fungi form a sclerotium. A sclerotium (pl. sclerotia) is a complex mass of hyphae or cells that is organized into a rounded resistant structure that contains reserve food materials. Sclerotia may be either large, that is, approaching several millimeters in diameter (Fig. 4.8), or relatively small. Some species of *Aspergillus* (especially *A. flavus*), *Fusarium, Rhizoctonia*, and similar fungi commonly develop these structures.

One final vegetative structure that must be discussed is the pseudohypha (pl. pseudohyphae, pseudomycelium). A pseudohypha represents, in essence, a series of blastoconidia that have remained attached to each other,

# Asexual Reproduction

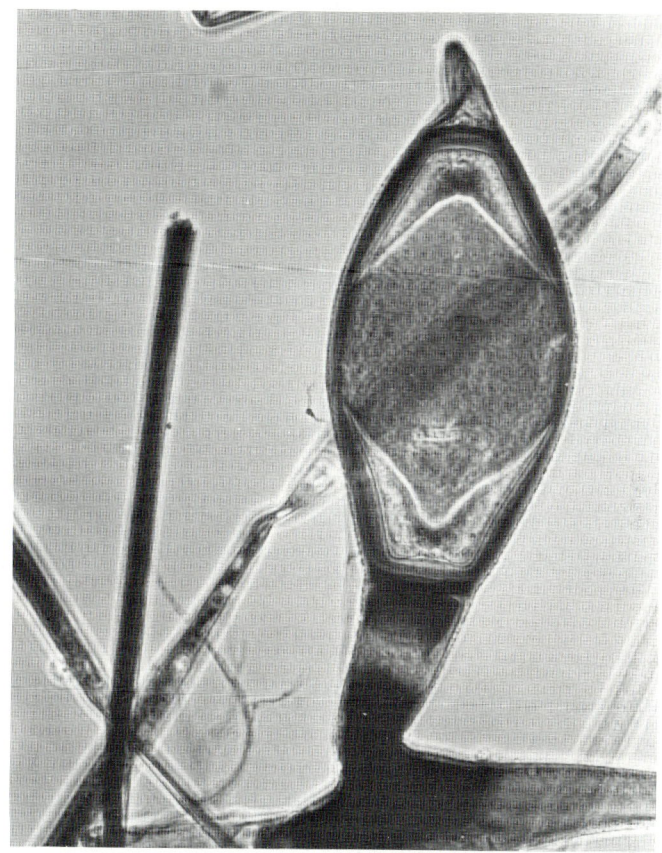

**B**

**Fig. 1.3** Continued

forming a hyphalike filament. The confusion between true hyphae and pseudohyphae (Fig. 1.7) becomes most apparent when the cells of pseudohyphae are extremely elongated. The major differences between hyphae and pseudohyphae are set forth in Table 1.2.

## ASEXUAL REPRODUCTION

Fungi reproduce by asexual means, sexual means, or both. Asexual reproduction is either an increase in the vegetative phase of the fungus or the development of asexual propagules. In either case, such reproduction does not involve the union of nuclei or gametes. The vegetative phase is commonly referred to as the thallus and usually consists of hyphae being aggregated into a colony.

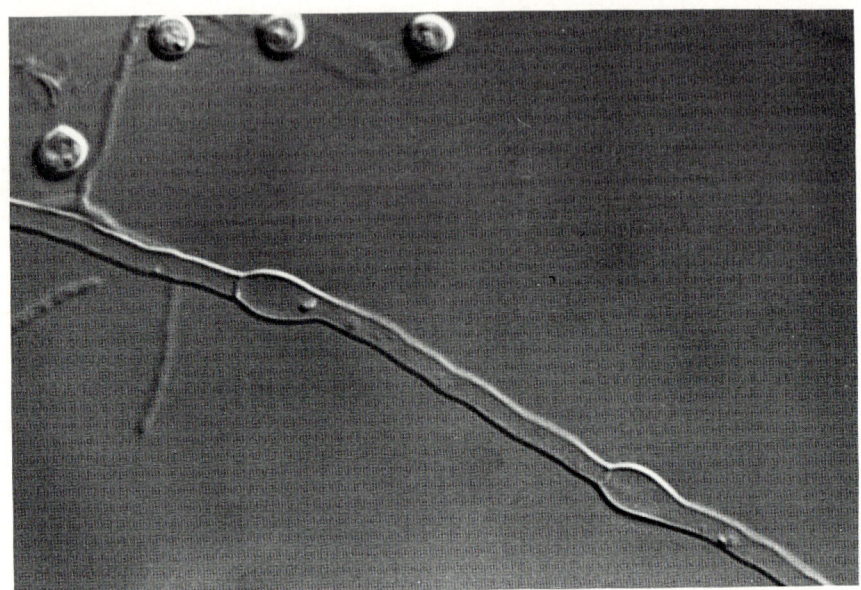

Fig. 1.4  *Blastomyces dermatitidis*. Racquet hypha.

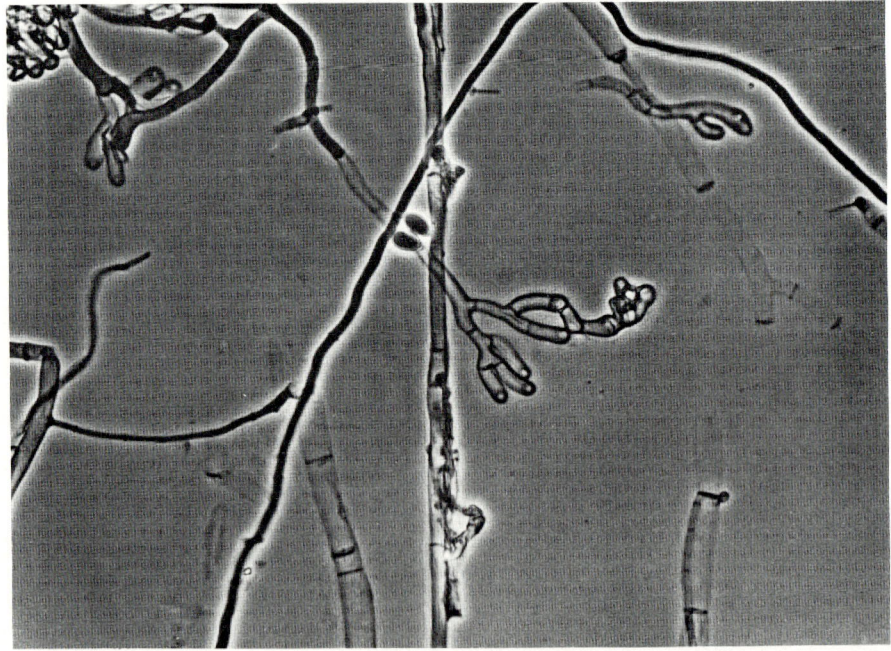

Fig. 1.5  *Botrytis cinerea*. Favic chandeliers.

# Asexual Reproduction

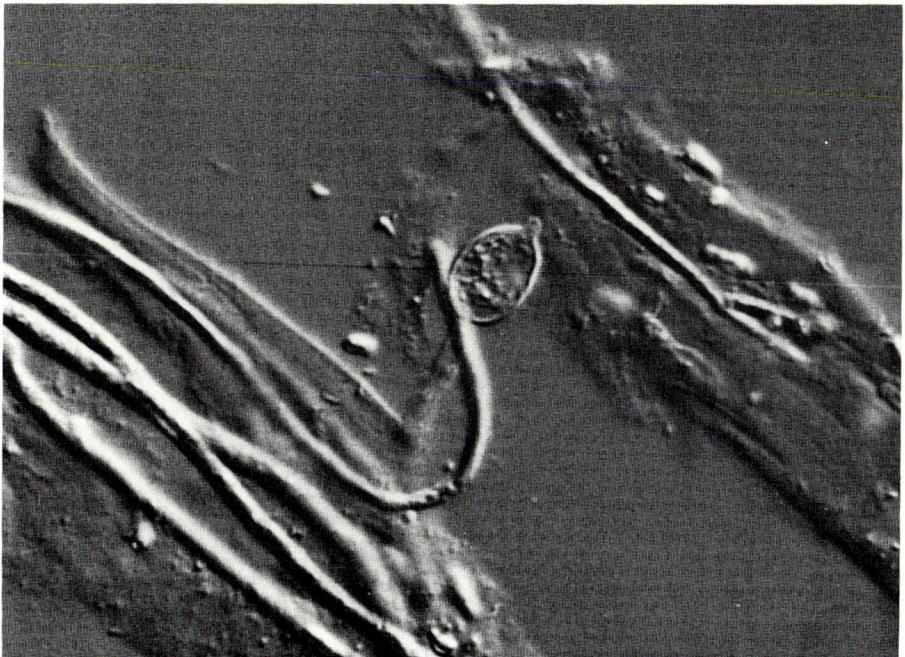

**Fig. 1.6** *Microsporum audouinii.* A short spinelike appendage is often seen at the apices of the vesicles produced by this dermatophyte.

Asexual reproduction in the Zygomycetes is typified by a structure called a sporangium. A sporangium (pl. sporangia) is a saclike cell in which the entire internal contents are cleaved into spores (Fig. 1.8). Each spore is called a sporangiospore and may have from one to several nuclei. Sporangiospores may be either randomly distributed in the sporangium or in a row. A sporangium having its sporangiospores in a row, such as in the genus *Syncephalastrum,* is referred to as a merosporangium (Fig. 1.9). In other Zygomycetes, like *Cunninghamella,* the sporangium is reduced in size to the point that only one sporangiospore occurs within each sporangium (Fig. 1.10) or, in the case of species of *Circinella,* where only a few sporangiospores are formed within each sporangium (Fig. 1.11). Such reduced sporangia are referred to as sporangiola (sing. sporangiolum). A sporangiolum consisting of one spore is often incorrectly called a "conidium." In general, sporangiola have persistent sporangial walls. Because of their small size, sporangiola do not usually have a columella. A columella (pl. columellae) is a small, sterile domelike area at the apex of the sporangiophore that resulted from the membranes of the vesicles in the protoplasm coalescing along a cleavage furrow and then being covered with cell wall material (Fig. 1.12). The term apophysis is applied to any

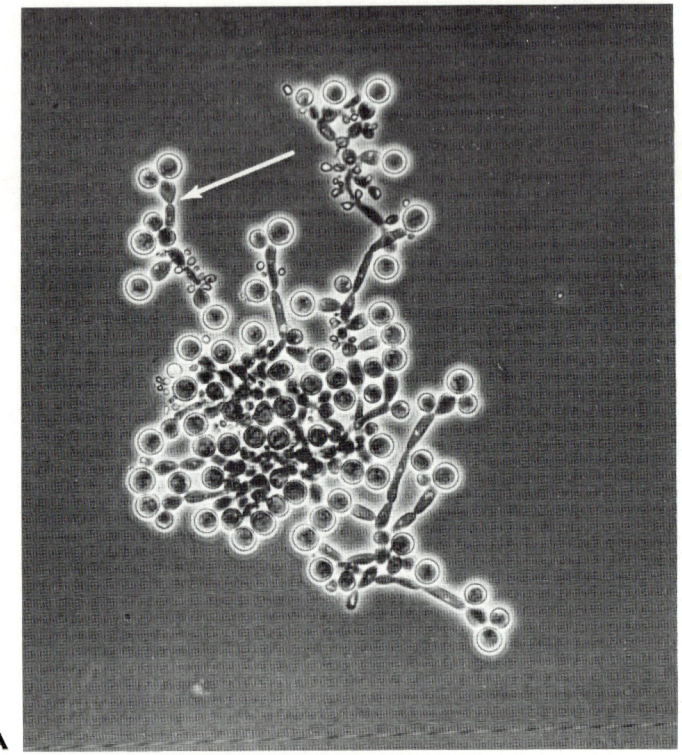

**Fig. 1.7** A. *Candida albicans*. Pseudohyphae are typically constricted at each septum (arrow). They are in essence a series of elongated blastoconidia. B. *Botrytis cinerea*. True hyphae have parallel walls, are not constricted at the septa, and grow by linear elongation at their apices.

swelling in the sporangiophore that is immediately below the columella. The protoplasm and nuclei in the young developing sporangium are concentrated toward the periphery of the cell, the central area becoming highly vacuolated. The protoplasm containing nuclei divides into portions by progressive cleavage, thereby forming the sporangiospores. In this process, the spore protoplasts are separated by cleavage, through which the entire content of the sporangium is distributed among the sporangiospores. When the wall of the sporangium ruptures or dissolves, the sporangiospores are released into the environment and then germinate via a germ tube. If remnants of the sporangial wall remain attached as a small collar at the junction of the columella and sporangiophore, this is referred to as a collarette. A sporangium usually develops on a specialized hypha called a sporangiophore.

# Asexual Reproduction

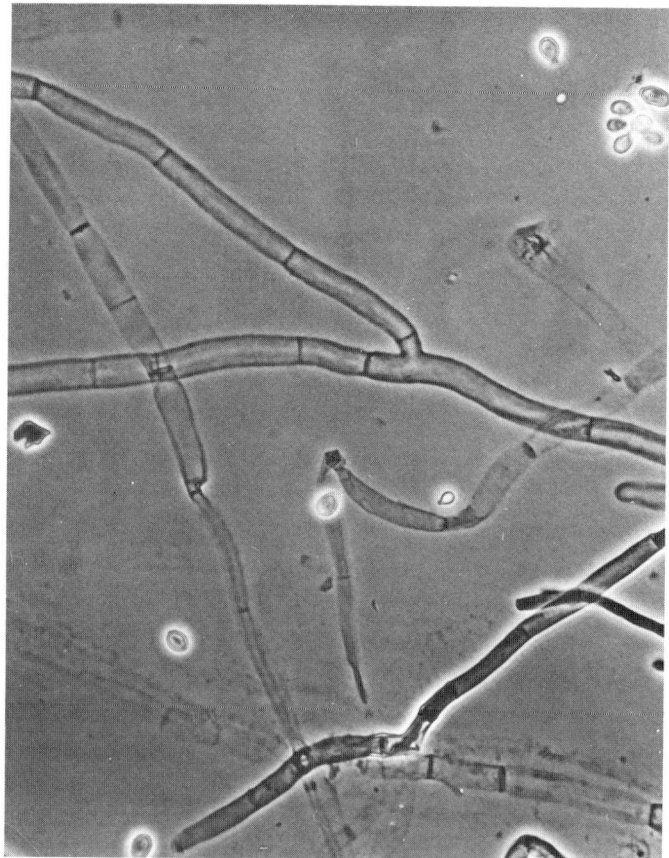

**Fig. 1.7** Continued

Some Zygomycetes form vegetative hyphae that are similar to the runners of higher plants. These runners or stolons become important features in delineating several of the genera of Zygomycetes. The origin of the sporangiophore and the location of the rhizoids with respect to the stolon is very important. A node is where a stolon touches the substrate, and the arch formed between it and the next node is the internode. Some sporangiophores arise only at the node, whereas others arise only from the internode. When rhizoids develop, that is, rootlike hyphal structures, they may do so at a node. These structures are best seen by focusing at the edge of the Petri dish or test tube with a dissecting microscope (Fig. 1.13).

Most fungi of medical interest do not produce sporangia, but form conidia upon specialized hyphae called conidiophores. A conidium (pl.

Table 1.2. Differentiation between Hyphae and Pseudohyphae

| Hyphae | Pseudohyphae |
|---|---|
| Growth results from the hyphal apex by linear elongation with subsequent formation of septa | Growth results from a blowing-out process and subsequent-appearing basal constriction of each new blastoconidium, without the separation of each blastoconidium from its parent cell |
| The terminal cell of a hypha is typically longer than the preceding cell just behind the first septum | The terminal cell of a pseudohypha is typically shorter or equal to the preceding cell just behind the first septum |
| The terminal cell is usually cylindrical | The terminal cell is usually rounded |
| The walls are typically parallel with no invaginations at the septa | The walls typically contain marked constrictions at the septa |
| The septa are refractive and straight | The septa are often difficult to discern and are usually curved |
| Side branches are not constricted at their point of origin, and the first septum is some distance from the main hypha | Side branches are constricted at their point of origin and there is a septum at the origin of the branch |

conidia) is a nonmotile, usually deciduous propagule that resulted from asexual reproduction, that is, mitosis. It is therefore genetically like its parent cell. The current trend in mycology is to restrict the term spore to those propagules that develop within a sporangium or via sexual reproduction (ascospore, basidiospore, and zygospore). In contrast, the term conidia is used for propagules that originate by asexual means other than in a sporangium.

The cell that gives rise to the conidium is known as the conidiogenous cell, and the process or sequence of events that resulted in the new conidium is referred to as its mode of conidiogenesis. Under some circumstances, the conidiophore and conidiogenous cell may actually be one and the same (Fig.1.14). In the case of *Acremonium* species, the distinctive hypha arising laterally from the vegetative hyphae with a ball of conidia at its tip is considered to be a conidiophore. This conidiophore also produces the conidia, hence it is a conidiogenous cell too. In contrast, the conidiogenous cells of the genus *Aspergillus* are distinctively different from the

## Asexual Reproduction

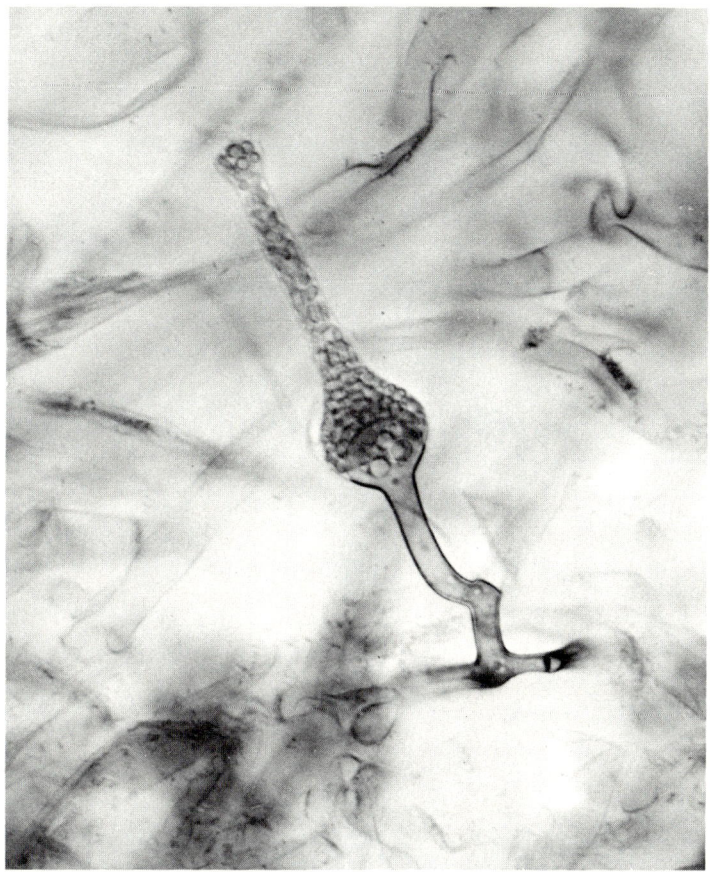

**Fig. 1.8** *Saksenaea vasiformis*. The sporangiospores are formed in a sporangium that has a necklike extension. (Reproduced by permission of L. Ajello and Mycologia from *Mycologia* **58**:52–62, 1976.)

conidiophore (Fig 1.15). In this case, the conidiogenous cells and the conidiophore are two entirely different structures. Micronematous is a useful term to describe conidiophores that are morphologically similar to the vegetative hyphae; semimacronematous for conidiophores that are slightly different from the vegetative hyphae; and macronematous for conidiophores that are morphologically distinct from the vegetative hyphae. Conidiophores may be either free, that is, they are randomly dispersed, or they may be united together to form a large upright macroscopic structure called a synnema (pl. synnemata) (Fig. 1.16). The conidia may develop along the sides, at the apex, or both, from the synnema. The terms

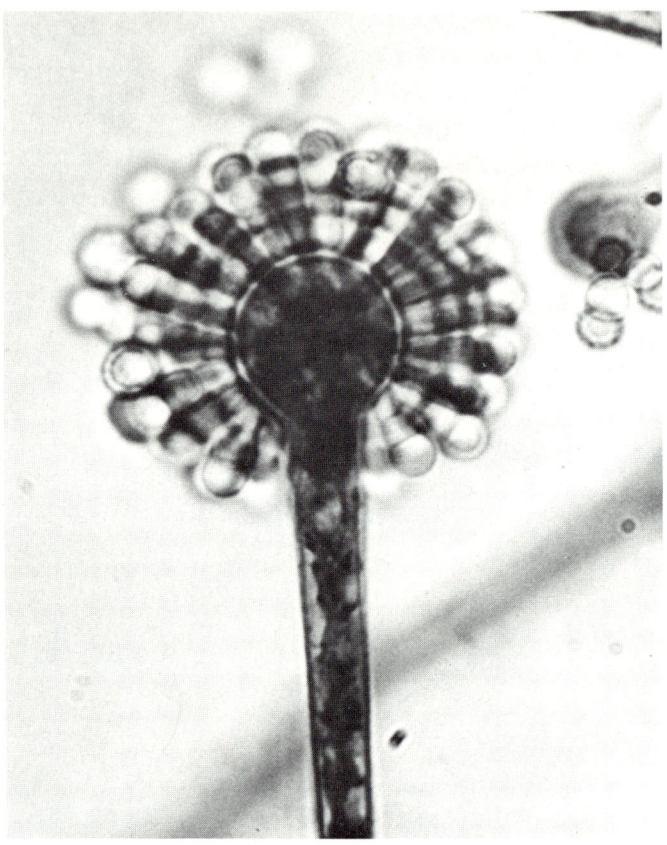

**Fig. 1.9** *Syncephalastrum racemosum.* The merosporangia develop from a vesicle at the apex of the sporangiophore. The sporangiospores occur in a row within each merosporangium (arrow).

coremium (pl. coremia) and synnema are synonymous. Some mycologists use coremium to describe a synnema that is loosely formed, but it is not meant to be used in lieu of fascicles for the rope- or cordlike hyphal bundles produced by some fungi. Synnemata and free conidiophores may occur together in the same culture. When conidiophores occur as a covering over a cushion-shaped mycelial mat, the entire structure is called a sporodochium (pl. sporodochia). In contrast to a cushion-shaped mass, some fungi develop their conidiophores on a tightly bound flat mat of mycelium, an acervulus (pl. acervuli). From a practical point of view, since acervuli usually form under the cuticle or epidermis of plants, they are rarely found in culture. A pycnidium (pl. pycnidia) is a large, round to

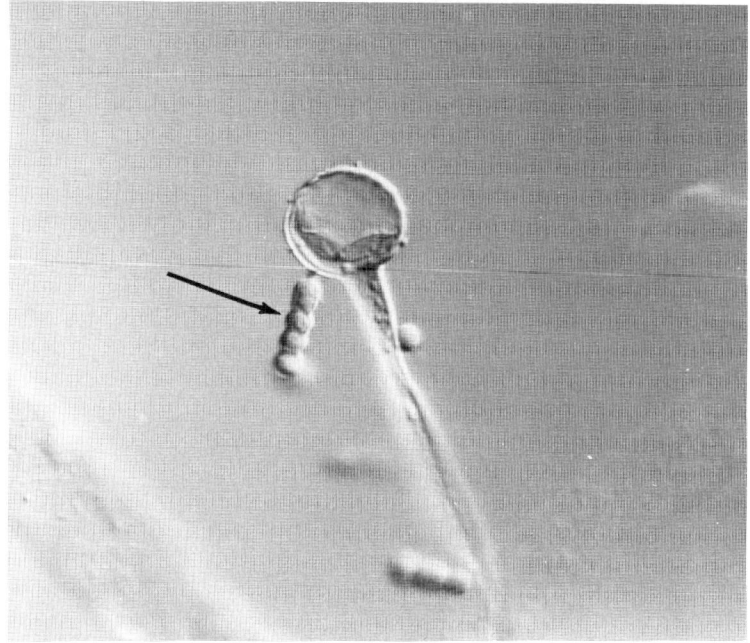

**Fig. 1.9** Continued

flask-shaped fruiting body (Fig. 1.17). The center of the pycnidium is usually a lysed cavity with conidiophores developing from the lining of the cavity. If the pycnidium has an opening (ostiole), it is referred to as being ostiolate. From ostiolate pycnidia, the conidia usually ooze from the ostiole. Sterile spinelike structures called setae may be present (Fig. 1.17).

Conidium development has become increasingly important for the rapid and accurate identification of fungi. The major components of conidium development having the greatest diagnostic value include the origin of the conidium, origin of the conidial wall, type of conidiogenous cell, arrangement of conidia, and site or area that gives rise to the conidium (Table 1.3).

Conidia originate in one of two principal manners. In the first method, the young conidium initially begins to enlarge and is then differentiated from its parent cell by the development of a septum. The conidium originates from part of its parent cell, since only a portion of the parent cell gives rise to the conidium. Such development is called blastic (Fig. 1.18). This type of development can be recognized with the light micro-

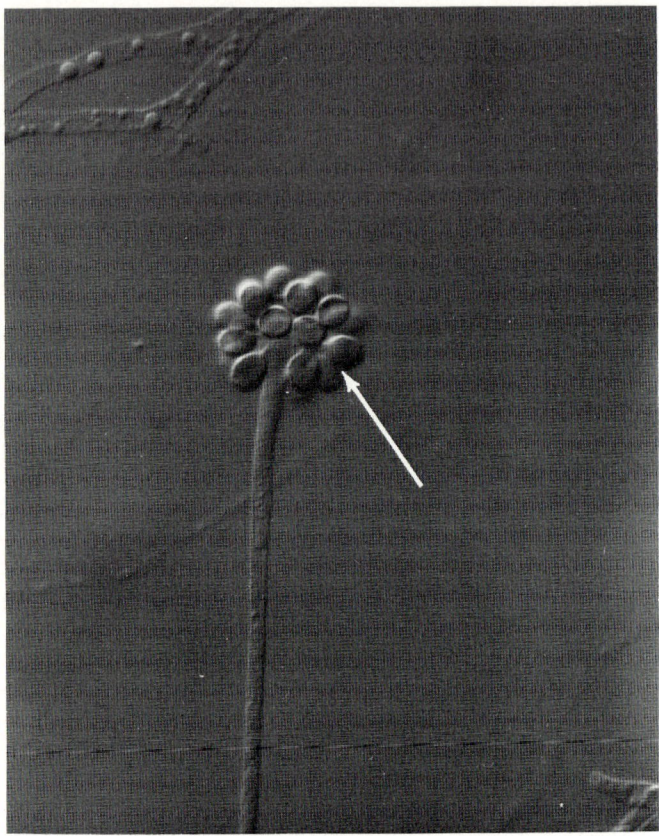

**Fig. 1.10** *Cunninghamella bertholletiae*. Each of the spores is a reduced sporangium called a sporangiolum (arrow).

scope by seeing a limited amount of apical growth, or a dome. In the second mode of conidiogenesis, the young conidium does not begin to develop until after it has become differentiated by a septum. The conidium originates from the entire parent cell, since all of it becomes the conidium. This manner of development is called thallic and is typified by fungi such as *Geotrichum candidum* (Fig. 1.19). It can be recognized by the presence of elongated, hyphalike growth. The cell walls of conidia and hyphae are composed of several layers of material. When all the wall layers actively participate in the formation of the conidium, the origin of the conidial wall is either holoblastic or holothallic, depending upon whether the conidium is blastic or thallic in origin. The prefix "holo" simply denotes that all the wall layer(s) were involved. In holoblastic development, the outer cell wall

## Asexual Reproduction

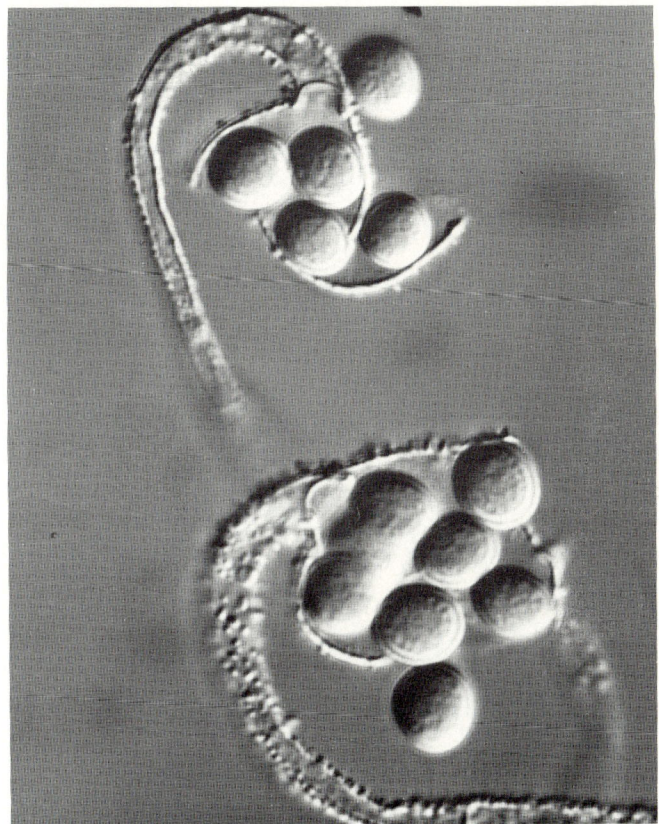

**Fig. 1.11** *Circinella* sp. Each sporangium contains only a few sporangiospores.

layer(s) remain intact, whereas they break in enteroblastic development. Some conidia may develop through a channel or pore in the outer cell wall layer(s). Such porogeneous development results in poroconidia. The budded cells produced by the genus *Candida* and the conidia of *Drechslera* (Fig. 1.20) are holoblastic. The conidia produced by *Drechslera* are poroconidia. The area, point, or zone of the conidiogenous cell that gives rise to the conidium is called the conidiogenous locus (pl. loci).

In thallic conidiogenesis, if the propagules fragment and then disarticulate from the parent hypha, this is referred to as arthric development (Fig. 1.19). Holoarthric development is characterized by having all of the cell wall layers involved in the formation of the conidial wall. The term enteroarthric is used when the outer cell wall layer(s) usually separates from the newly formed cell wall of the conidium. *Geotrichum candidum* is

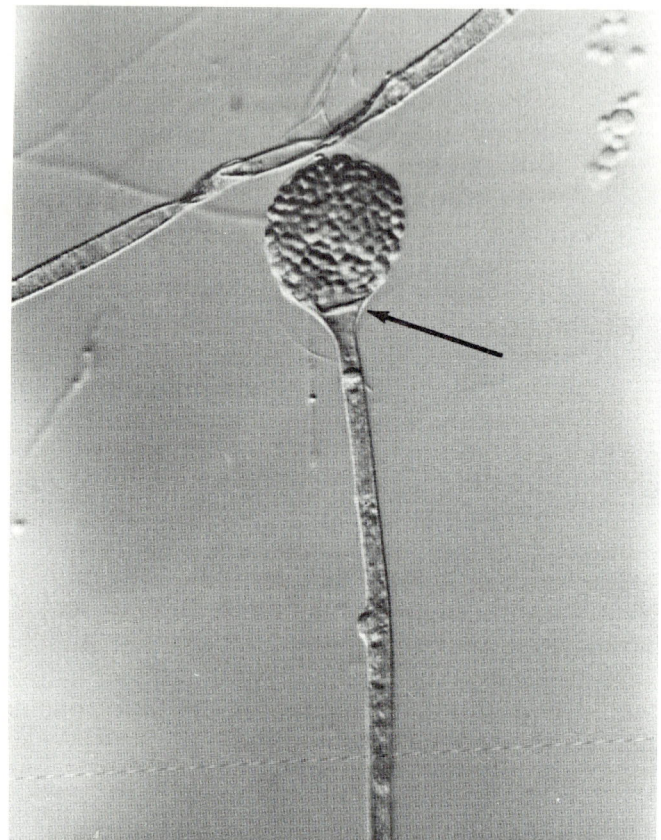

**Fig. 1.12** *Absidia* sp. The apophysis (arrow) is the swelling in the sporangiophore where it merges with the columella.

an excellent example of holoarthric development, whereas *Coccidioides immitis* is typical of enteroarthric development. In contrast to arthric conidia, dermatophytes such as *Microsporum gypseum* produce holothallic conidia.

Conidiogenous cells may cease to grow in length just before or at the onset of conidium formation. These conidiogenous cells or conidiophores are determinate because no further elongation will occur, regardless of the number of conidia produced (Fig. 1.21). In contrast to determinate development, some fungi produce conidiogenous cells or conidiophores that continue to increase in length prior to, during, or just after each new conidium is formed. Such conidiogenous cells or conidiophores are inde-

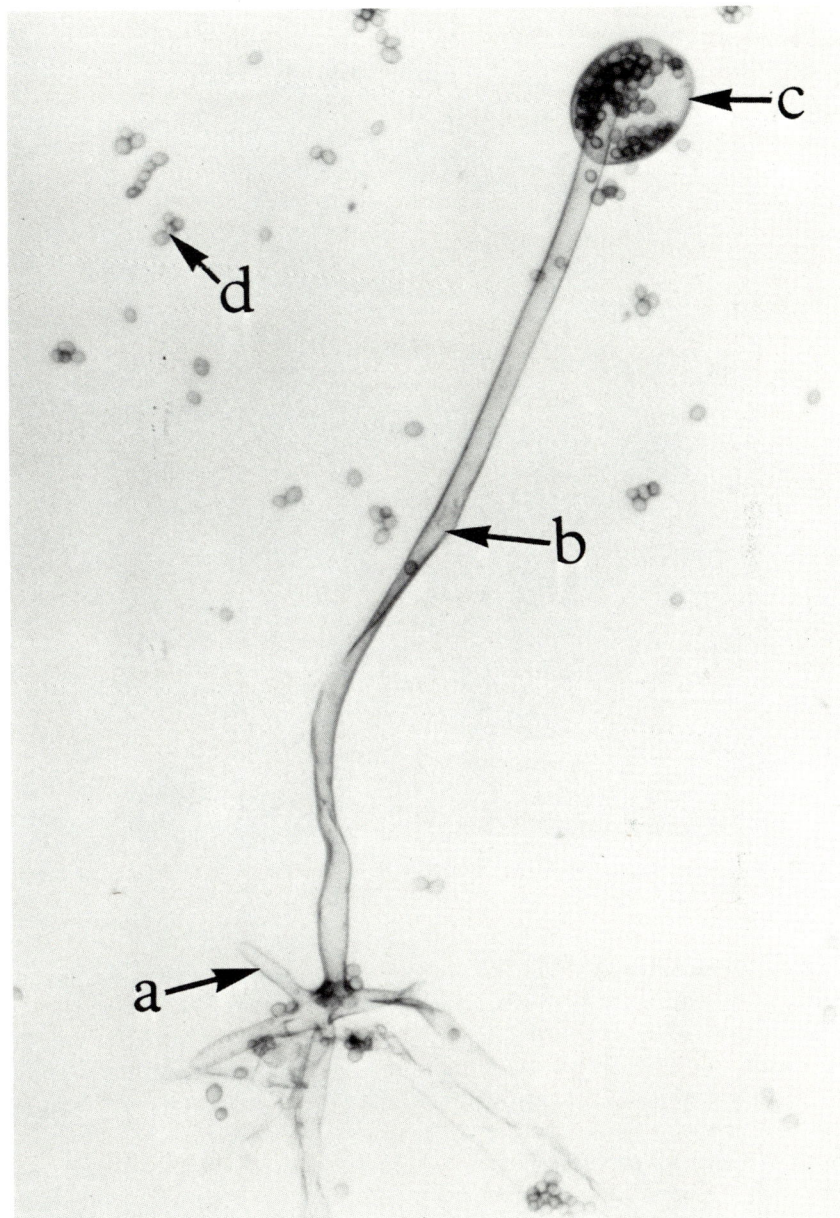

**Fig. 1.13** *Rhizopus stolonifer*. The rhizoids (a) are opposite the sporangiophore (b). The columella (c) and the sporangiospores (d) have become more evident after the sporangial wall dissolved.

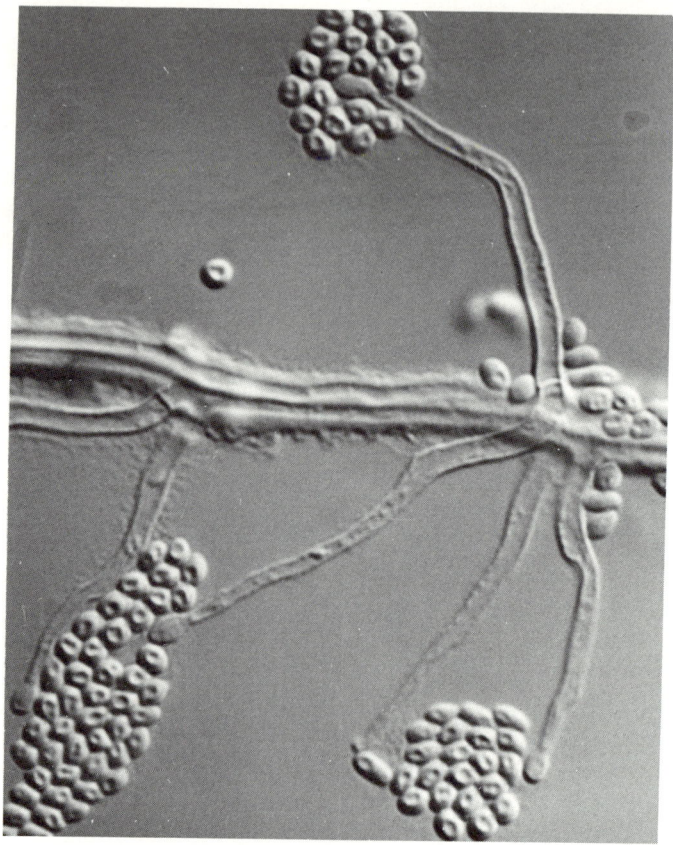

**Fig. 1.14** *Acremonium kiliense.* The conidia are accumulating at the apices of the conidiophores. The conidiophores and the conidiogenous cells are one in the same in this fungus.

terminate or proliferous (Fig. 1.22). The term retrogressive is applied to determinate conidiogenous cells or conidiophores that become shorter as they are converted into conidia. (Fig. 1.23). In contrast to retrogressive, the term stable refers to determinate conidiogenous cells that do not produce conidia retrogressively. In this instance, the conidiophores do not become shorter as new conidia are formed.

With respect to proliferous conidiogenous cells or conidiophores, the growth of the conidiophore may occur at the base (basauxic) or at the apical region (acroauxic). In medical mycology, we are primarily concerned with fungi that produce acroauxic conidiophores. The sympodial conidiogenous cell represents a classic example of proliferous acroauxic growth. The conidiogenous cell grows vegetatively and then forms a

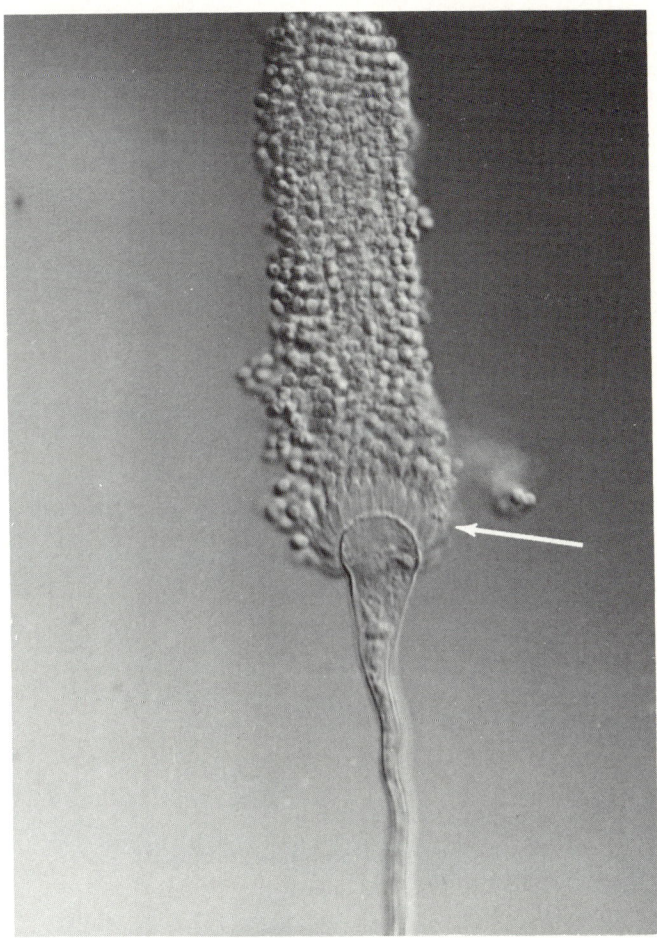

Fig. 1.15 *Aspergillus fumigatus*. The hyphalike conidiophore has expanded to form a vesicle at its apex. Upon the vesicle, a row of flask-shaped conidiogenous cells (arrow) are producing chains of conidia. The conidiophore and the conidiogenous cells are different. (Reproduced by permission from *Southern Medical Journal* **70**:886–888, 1977.)

conidium at its apex. A new growing point develops below and to one side of the developing conidium. This new subterminal growing point begins to grow and increases in length. After the new apex has grown, a second conidium then begins to form at the new apex. The net effect of this type of growth, conidium development, new subterminal growth, and subsequent new conidium development, is an increase in the length (Figs. 1.24 and 1.25) and usually an accompanying swelling of the conidiogenous cell

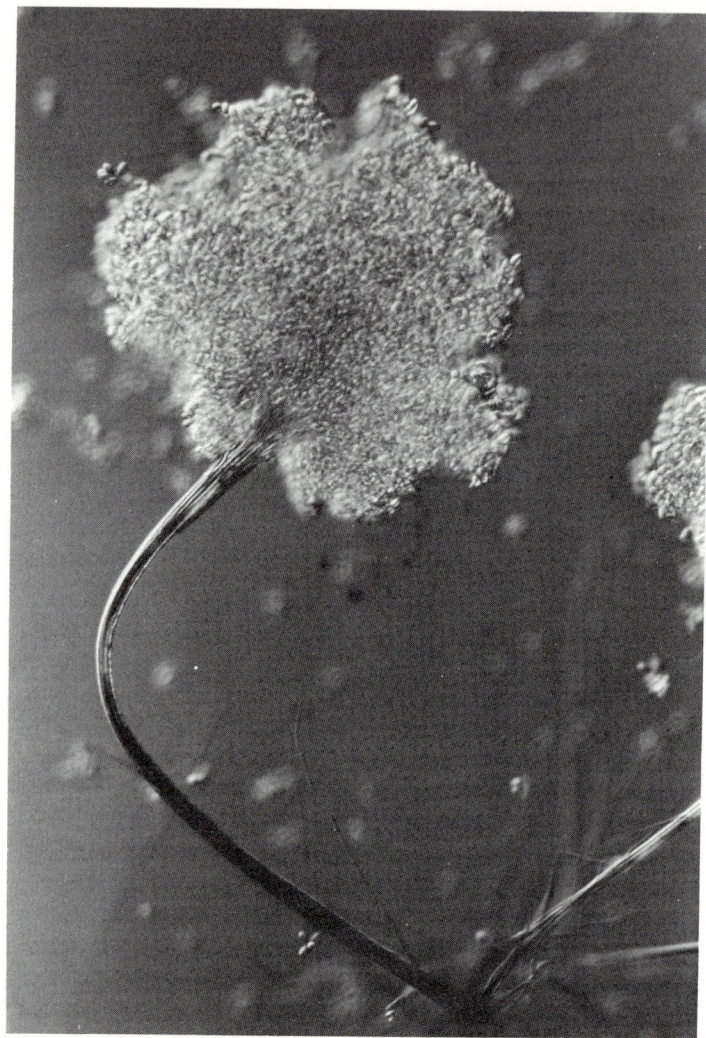

**Fig. 1.16** *Graphium* sp. The synnema is an upright macroscopic structure composed of fused conidiophores. In this fungus, the conidia accumulate as a ball at the apex of the synnema.

## Asexual Reproduction

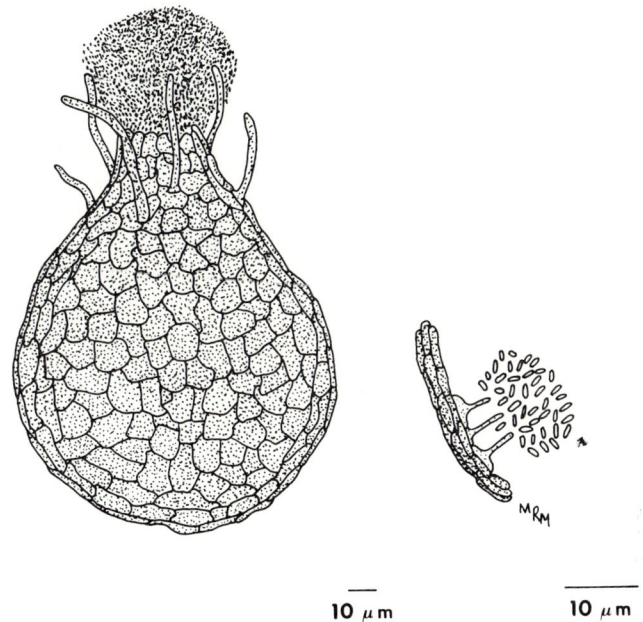

10 μm    10 μm

**Fig. 1.17** *Pyrenochaeta unguis-hominis.* The pycnidium is a saclike fruiting body in which conidia are formed. Setae are present near the ostiole, through which the conidia escape.

or conidiophore. This type of conidiophore often has a characteristic appearance, like a series of bent knees, that is, geniculate (Fig. 1.20). The conidia that are produced by a sympodial conidiogenous cell have been referred to as sympodioconidia in the past. This term should not be used because it defines the conidium on the basis of how the conidiogenous cell developed, not on the basis of how the conidium developed. The conidia may be holoblastic or enteroblastic, depending upon which cell wall layer(s) was involved in the formation of the conidia. Fungi with sympodial conidiogenous cells include species of *Curvularia, Drechslera, Tritirachium, Ulocladium,* and others.

A second type of conidiogenous cell that is of interest to medical mycologists is the annellide. The first conidium produced by an annellide is holoblastic in origin. This terminal conidium then breaks free from the conidiogenous cell. Once the conidium is no longer attached, there is a proliferation of new growth through the area where the conidium was attached. At the apex of this new growth, a second conidium develops enteroblastically. Using the light microscope, this appears to be holoblastic with all the cell wall layers involved, which, of course, is not the situation.

**Table 1.3.** Ontogeny and Arrangement of Conidia Produced by Fungi of Medical Interest

```
                                                                  ┌─ asynchronous
                                                     ┌─ botryose ─┤
                                                     │            └─ synchronous
                                                     │
                                 ┌─ arrangement of ──┤            ┌─ acropetal
                                 │     conidia       ├─ catenulate┤
                                 │                   │            └─ basipetal
                                 │                   │
                                 │                   │            ┌─ acropleurogenous
                                 │                   └─ solitary ─┤  balls
                                 │                                └─ single
                      ┌─ blastic ┤
                      │          │  origin of conidium  ┌─ holoblastic
                      │          ├─   wall           ───┤
                      │          │                      └─ enteroblastic
                      │          │
                      │          │                         ┌─ determinate   ┌─ basauxic
                      │          │  growth of conidiogenous┤─ proliferous ──┤─ percurrent
                      │          ├─        cell            └─ retrogressive └─ sympodial
                      │          │
                      │          │                         ┌─ annellide
                      │          └─ special conidiogenous ─┤  phialide
 Origin of ──────────┤                    cells            └─ porogenous
  conidia             │
                      │                                    ┌─ solitary
                      │          ┌─ arrangement of ────────┤
                      │          │      conidia            └─ catenulate
                      │          │
                      │          │                         ┌─ holothallic
                      └─ thallic ┤  origin of conidium ────┤  holoarthric
                                 ├─     wall               └─ enteroarthric
                                 │
                                 │                         ┌─ determinate
                                 └─ growth of conidiogenous┤
                                          cell             └─ proliferous ── sympodial
```

Once the second conidium is released, the entire process is repeated. Such continued growth through subsequent apices is referred to as percurrent. Thus, there are a number of new conidiogenous loci formed by an annellide. When each conidium breaks free from the tip of the annellide, a ring of outer cell wall material is left behind. These rings or annellations (Fig. 1.26) may be regular or irregular around the tip of the annellide. In addition to proliferous growth, basipetal succession, and annellations, the diameter of the apex of the annellide becomes smaller as each new

# Asexual Reproduction

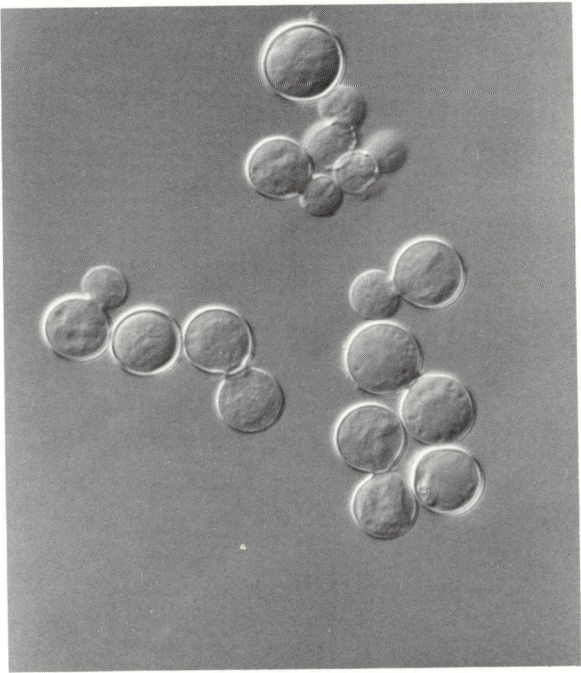

**Fig. 1.18** *Blastomyces dermatitidis*. Each blastoconidium originates from part of its parent cell. After the conidium initial has begun to enlarge, a septum is formed between the parent and daughter cells. This type of development is blastic.

proliferation occurs through the area where the previous conidium developed (Fig. 1.27). The septal pore at the base of each conidium is sealed by a Woronin body. *Exophiala* and *Scopulariopsis* species are two well known groups of fungi of medical importance that produce annellides. The conidia produced from annellides are called annelloconidia.

The phialide is a conidiogenous cell found in many fungi. It is usually elongate to flask-shaped. The first conidium produced is holoblastic in origin. After the conidium is released by the rupture or dissolution of the upper wall area of the phialide, there is no additional elongation of the conidiogenous cell. Additional phialides may develop in a percurrent manner in some species of fungi. In the genus *Phialophora*, a cuplike extension of outer cell wall material remains at the apex of the phialide when the first conidium is released. This collar of cell wall material is known as a collarette (Fig. 1.28). The collarette includes the cell wall material distal from the conidiogenous locus, that is, the zone that is manufacturing the conidia. All the subsequent conidia after the first one

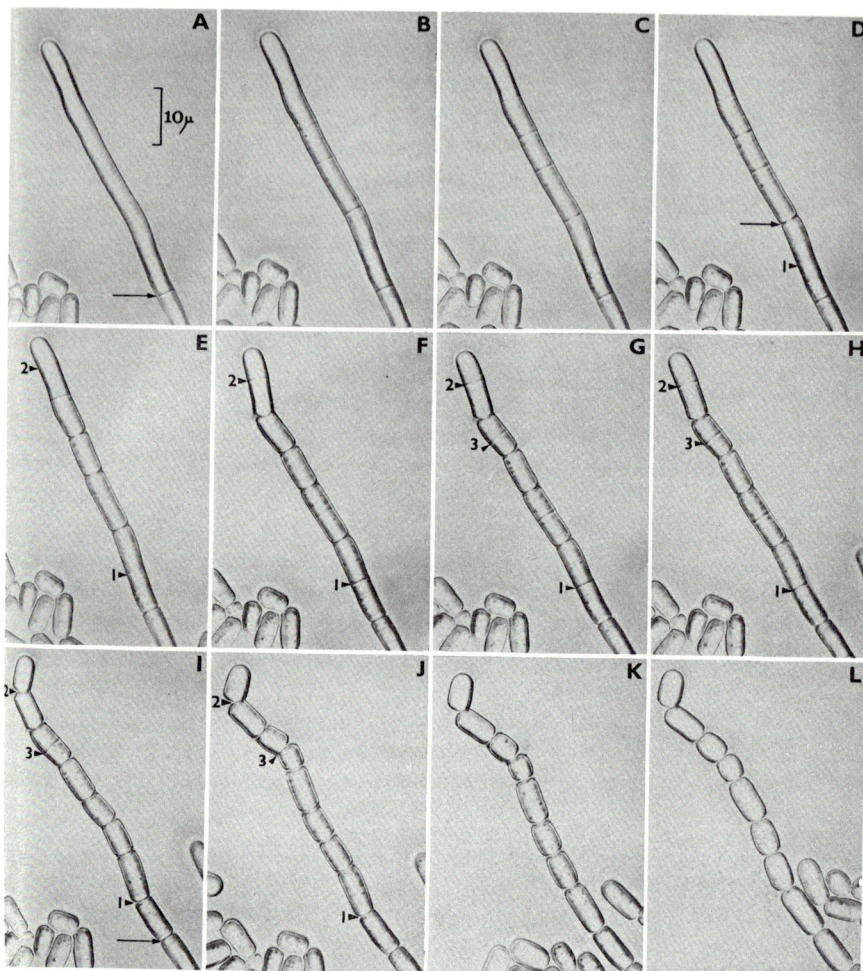

**Fig. 1.19** *Geotrichum candidum.* A time-lapse sequence of arthroconidium development. The arrows in A, D, I, and L indicate a common reference point. The arrowheads in D–J indicate the order of septation and separation. A–L are at 0, 15, 25, 35, 45, 60, 75, 85, 105, 170, 420, and 1140 min, respectively. This type of development is thallic (holoarthric). (Reproduced by permission of G. Cole and the National Research Council of Canada from *Canadian Journal of Botany* **47**:1773–1780, 1969.)

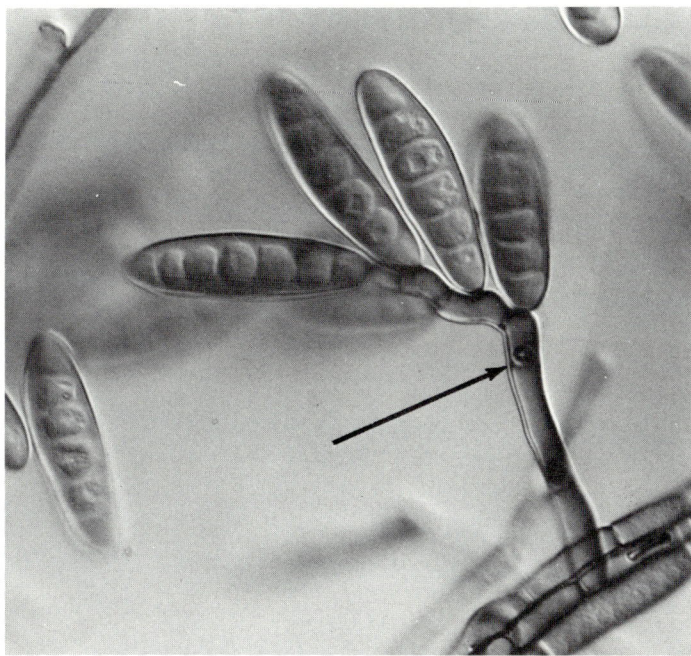

**Fig. 1.20** *Drechslera* sp. Poroconidia develop through channels (arrow) in the cell wall of the conidiophore.

are produced enteroblastically. In some phialides, there is an accumulation of cell wall material as rings (abstriction scars from the conidia) or simply a thickening of the cell wall inside the collarette. This results in a thick and dark appearing apex when viewed with the light microscope. Phialoconidia develop in a basipetal manner from a fixed conidiogenous locus with the youngest conidium at the base of the chain (or ball in some genera) and the oldest conidium at the tip. In contrast to basipetal development, acropetal development is characterized by having the youngest conidium at the tip of the chain and the oldest conidium at the base. Phialides in contrast to annellides, typically have collarettes or apical thickenings, do not increase in length with phialoconidium production, have a complete septum at the base of each conidium (Woronin bodies absent), and have one conidiogenous locus that gives rise to many conidia (Fig. 1.29). Annellides do not have collarettes; they increase in length, have annellations at their apices, and form each new conidium from a new conidiogenous locus. There is a continuum between annellides and phialides.

A conidium may be either sessile, that is, arising directly from the conidiophore, or formed on a small toothlike projection known as a

28                                                      1   Basic Terminology and Classification

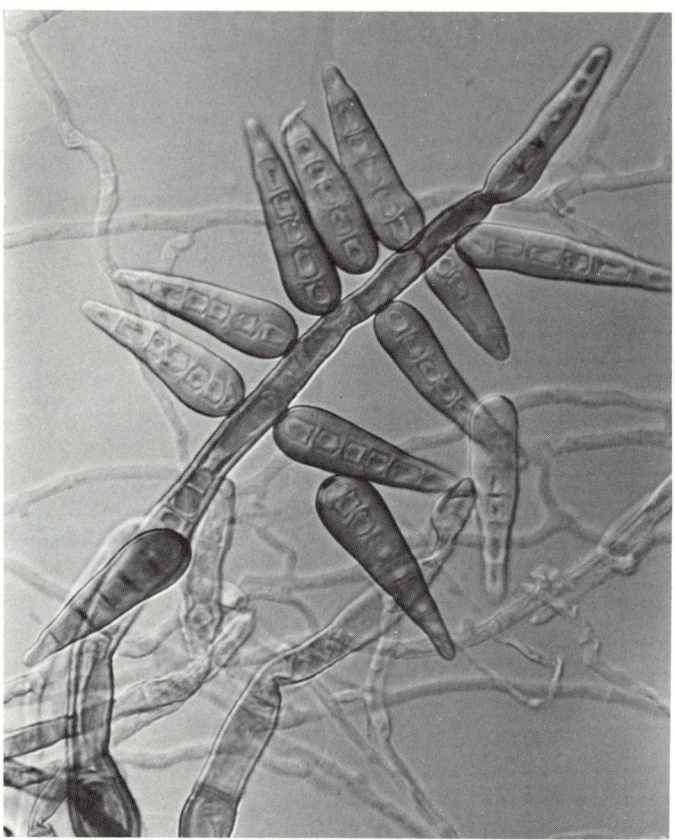

**Fig. 1.21** *Helminthosporium solani*. The determinate conidiophore ceases to grow in length after the terminal conidium is produced.

denticle, or on a swollen conidiogenous cell called an ampulla (pl. ampullae) (Fig. 1.30). Conidia may form in either an asynchronized or synchronized manner. A synchronized manner is characterized by all the conidia developing more or less at one time. Some fungi produce macro- and microconidia, which are conidia of two different sizes produced by one fungus in the same manner. Macro- and micro- refer to large and small conidia, respectively. Botryose is a term used to describe conidia that are formed in clusters. Acropleurogenous is used to describe conidia that are arranged at the apex and around the fertile hypha.

The differentiation between blastoconidia and aleuriospores has often plagued medical mycologists. In the development of blastoconidia (holoblastic), there is a softening of the cell wall of the conidiogenous cell

## Asexual Reproduction

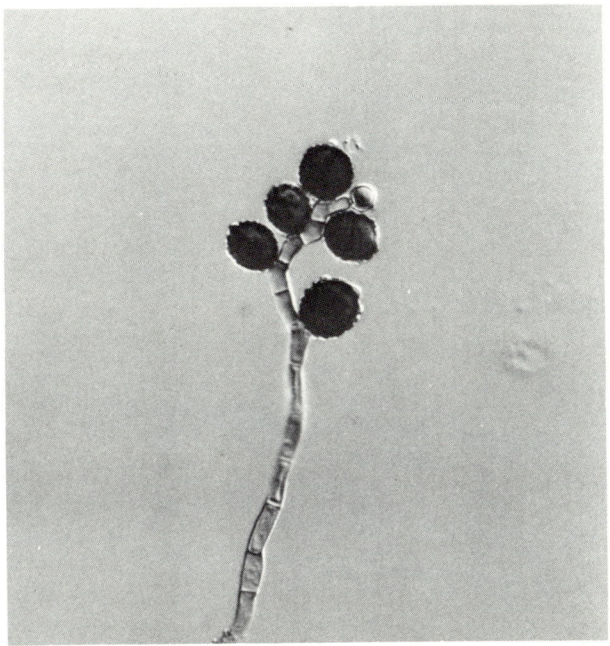

**Fig. 1.22** *Ulocladium atrum*. The proliferous conidiophore continues to grow in length prior to, during, or just after each new conidium is formed. A young developing conidium can be seen at the apex of the conidiophore.

followed by an expansion process that results in a new conidium. After being blown out, the blastoconidium usually appears to be constricted or pinched in at its base (Fig. 1.31). It is typically separated from the parent cell by a double septum. A double septum is a special septum that is thicker than a normal vegetative septum and has a weak zone in its middle. The middle zone breaks or splits, thereby separating the two cells. Some blastoconidia, such as those produced by *Sporotrichum aureum*, are released by the fracture or lysis of the supporting cell, leaving an annular frill. An annular frill is a skirt or remnant of cell wall material remaining at the base of the conidium. Aleuriospore is an obsolete term that was used primarily for terminal, swollen, thallic conidia that are released by the fracture or lysis of the supporting parent cell below the basal septum of the conidium. If one looked very carefully at the base of an aleuriospore, an annular frill was usually visible (Fig. 1.32). Many mycologists prefer not to use the term aleuriospore because it has been used to describe so many different types of conidia.

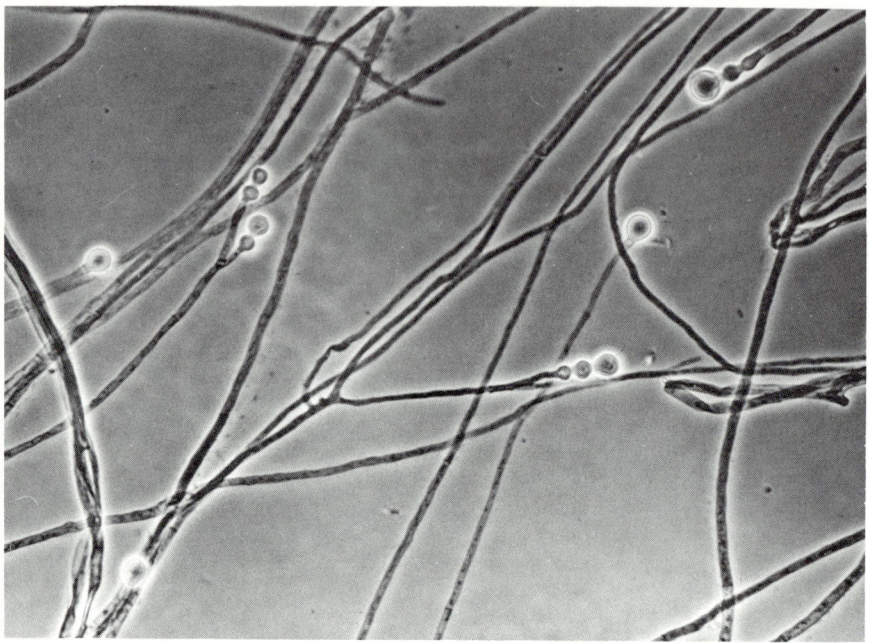

**Fig. 1.23** *Basipetospora rubra*. The conidiophores are retrogressive because they become shorter as each new conidium is produced.

The genera *Coccidioides, Geotrichum, Malbranchea,* and a number of other fungi produce arthroconidia. Arthroconidia are arthric conidia that resulted from the fragmentation of a hypha (Fig. 1.19). These conidia may be randomly dispersed within the hypha or separated from each other by a sterile cell called a disjunctor cell (Fig. 1.33). Arthroconidia are released either by fission through a double septum (schizolytic) or by the fracture or lysis of the supporting cell(s) (rhexolytic). This definition of arthroconidia includes many conidia that would previously have been called chlamydospores. Like the aleuriospore, the chlamydospore has been very poorly defined in the past. A chlamydospore is a holothallic conidium with a thickened cell wall that may be terminal or intercalary (within a hypha), and serves the function of survival. The chlamydospore is released either by fracture or lysis of the surrounding vegetative cell(s). Chlamydospores (Fig. 1.3) may be one-celled, multicelled, dematiaceous, or hyaline.

Mature conidia and spores may either germinate and produce a germ tube or develop a secondary conidium, which in turn may germinate via a germ tube or develop another conidium. The development of secondary

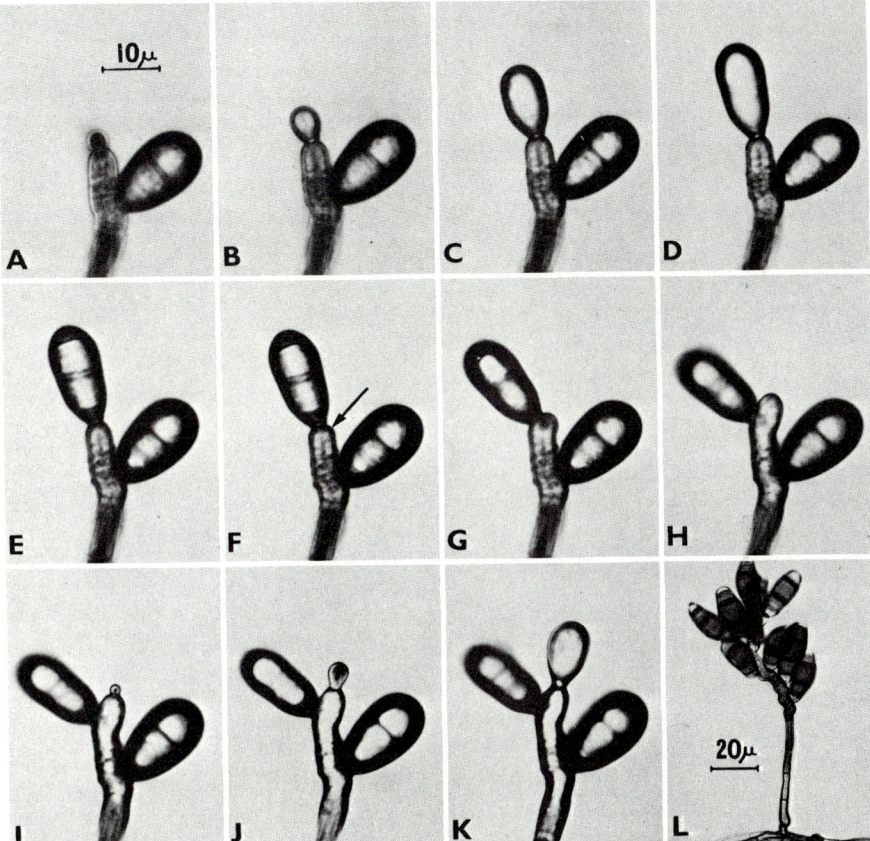

**Fig. 1.24** *Curvularia inaequalis.* A time-lapse sequence of sympodial development. The arrow in F indicates the location of a new growing point. L shows a mature conidiogenous cell. A–L are 0, 15, 60, 75, 240, 285, 315, 375, 435, 465, 480, and 525 min, respectively. (Reproduced by permission of G. Cole and the University of Toronto Press from "Taxonomy of Fungi Imperfecti," p. 145, 1971.)

conidia instead of germ tubes frequently occurs in genera such as *Aureobasidium.* Prior to producing a germ tube, the conidium swells by absorbing water. Germ tubes typically develop at a predetermined point or through preformed germ pores or germ slits. Most mycologists consider the process of germination to be complete when the germ tube has developed its first septum. At this stage, it is a young hypha. The term pseudo-germ-tube has been used in the past by some medical mycologists to describe the germ tube produced by the yeast cells of *Candida albicans,* because

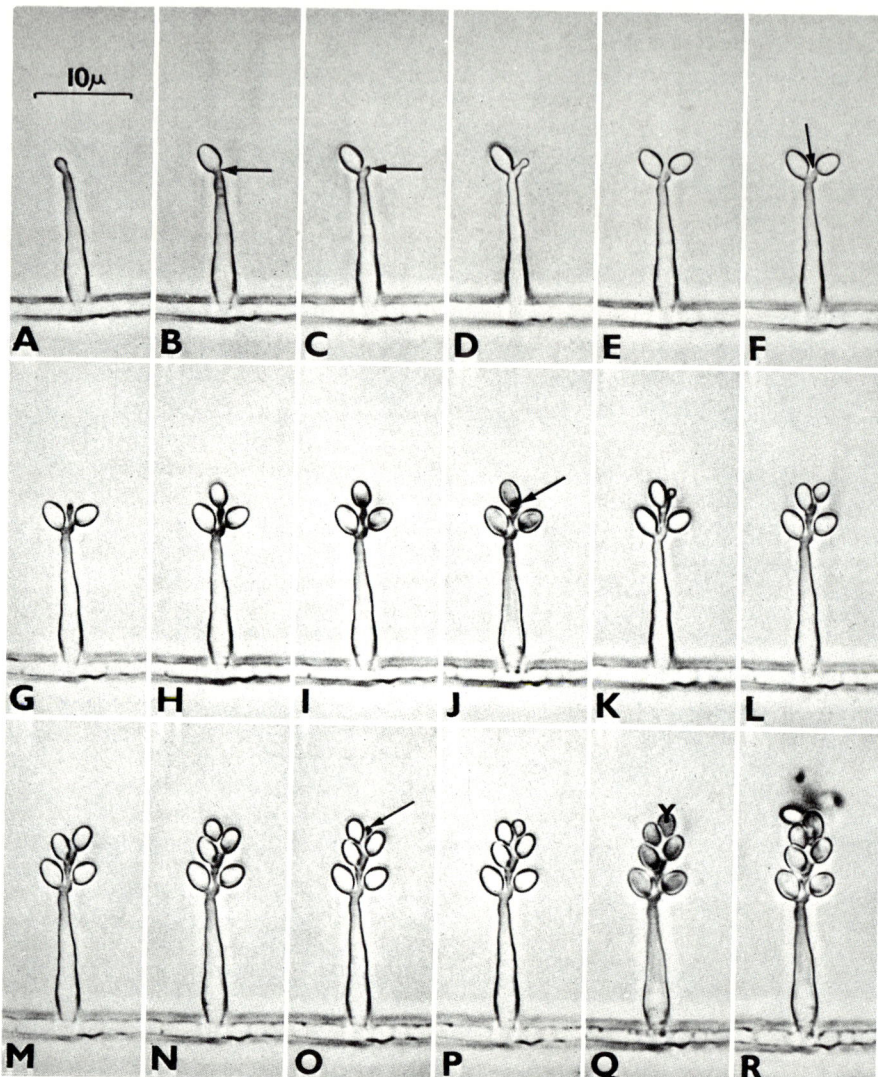

**Fig. 1.25** *Tritirachium album.* A time-lapse sequence of sympodial development. The arrows in B, C, F, J, and O indicate the location of new growing points. The letter Y in Q indicates the location of the youngest conidium at that particular stage of development. A–R are at 0, 0.75, 1.25, 1.75, 2, 2.75, 3.25, 4, 4.25, 5.25, 5.5, 5.75, 7.25, 9.75, 11.5, 11.75, 12.25, and 28.5 hr, respectively. (Reproduced by permission of G. Cole and the University of Toronto Press from "Taxonomy of Fungi Imperfecti," p. 144, 1971.)

# Asexual Reproduction

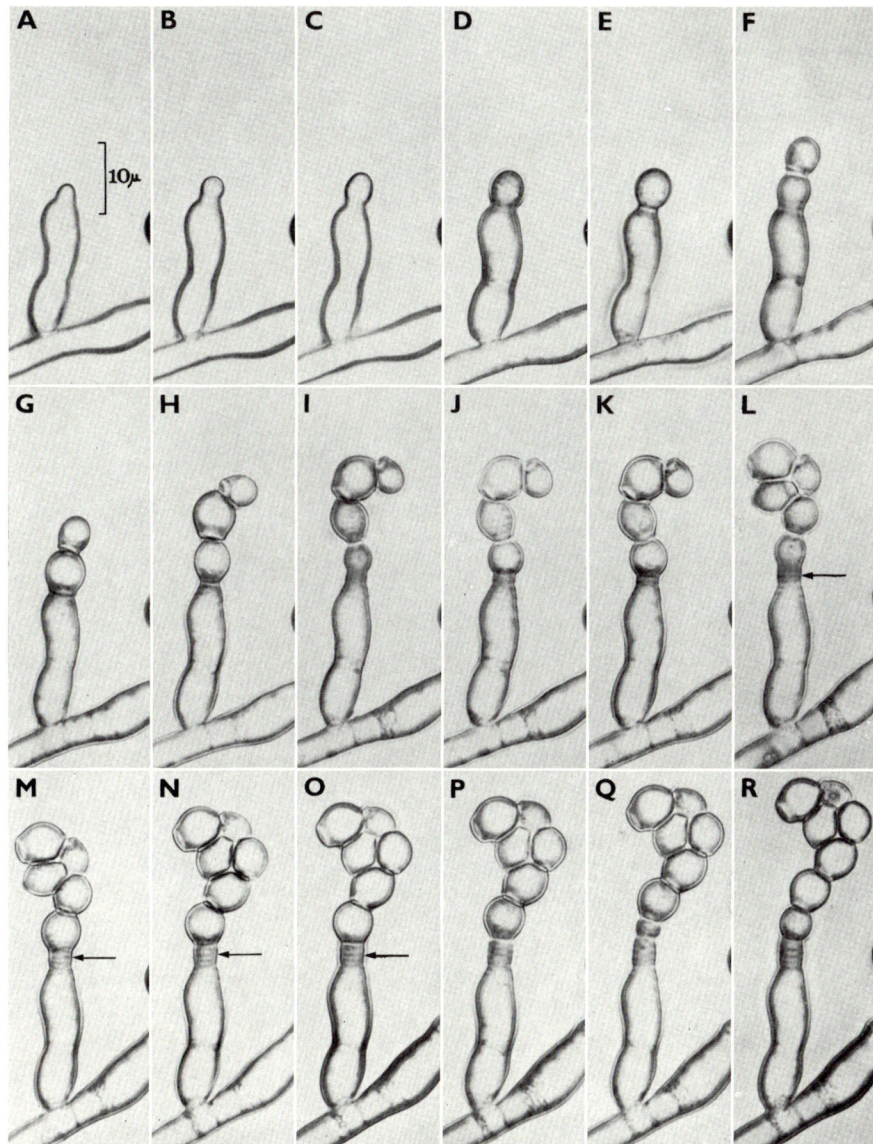

**Fig. 1.26** *Scopulariopsis brevicaulis.* A time-lapse sequence of annelloconidia development. The arrows in L–O indicate a common reference point. A–R are at 0, 0.75, 1.25, 2, 3.75, 6, 8.25, 19, 23, 24, 25, 31, 33, 45.25, 49, 50.25, 53, and 58 hr, respectively. (Reproduced by permission of G. Cole and the National Research Council of Canada from *Canadian Journal of Botany* **47**:925–929, 1969.)

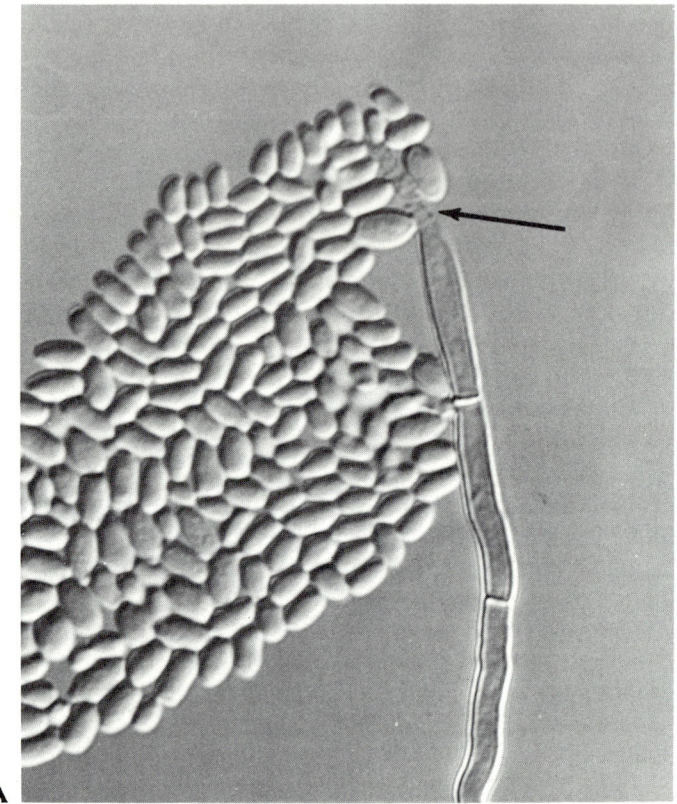

**Fig. 1.27** Annellides are characterized in part by the development of annellations (arrows) or rings at their apices. A. *Exophiala spinifera*. B. *Scopulariopsis brevicaulis*.

apparently the cells did not swell prior to the development of the germ tube. Since this seems to be splitting hairs, the term germ tube in this handbook will refer to the initial hypha developing from a conidium or spore. The germ tube represents an immature hypha that can be distinguished from an elongated blastoconidium by its parallel walls at its point of origin from the parent conidium.

## SEXUAL REPRODUCTION

Sexual reproduction involves the union of two compatible nuclei. Plasmogamy, the fusion of two protoplasts but not their nuclei, is the first step in sexual reproduction. The purpose of plasmogamy is to bring two nuclei

# Sexual Reproduction

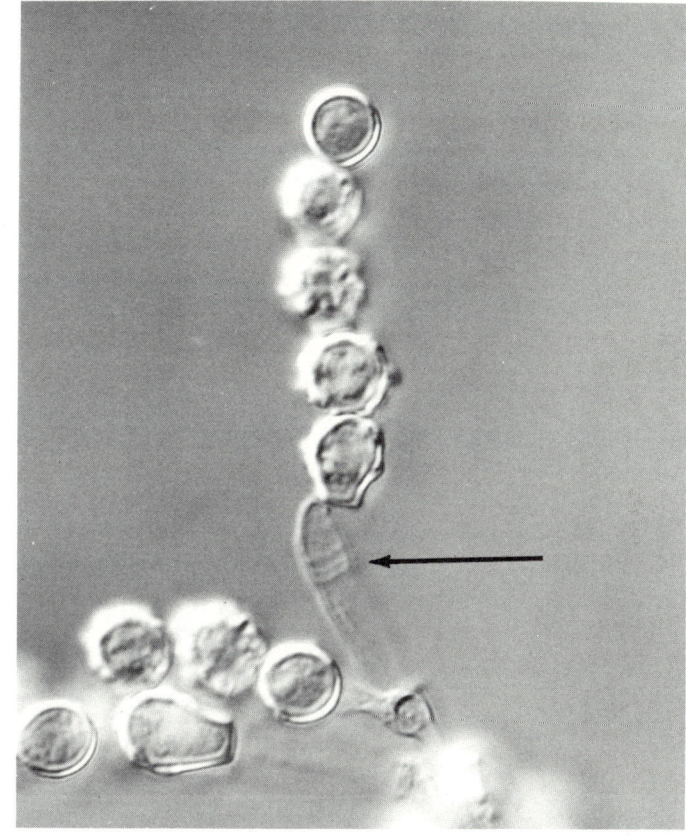

**Fig. 1.27** Continued

close to each other so that karyogamy can occur. Karyogamy is the actual fusion of the two compatible nuclei. The product of karyogamy is a diploid (2*n*) or zygote nucleus. Once plasmogamy and karyogamy have taken place, meiosis can occur, resulting in four haploid (*n*) nuclei. In the majority of fungi, meiosis immediately follows karyogamy; however, in some fungi, such as *Saccharomyces cerevisiae,* there may be a long intervening diploid state. In the Basidiomycetes and higher Ascomycetes, plasmogamy usually occurs early in their development, but not karyogamy, which occurs some time later. The two haploid nuclei do not fuse, but behave as though they were one nucleus. Such a nuclear condition is called dikaryotic (*n* + *n*). Unlike asexual reproduction, sexual reproduction does not occur at a high frequency. Sexual reproduction and its accompanying structures are used to determine phylogenetic relationships among the fungi.

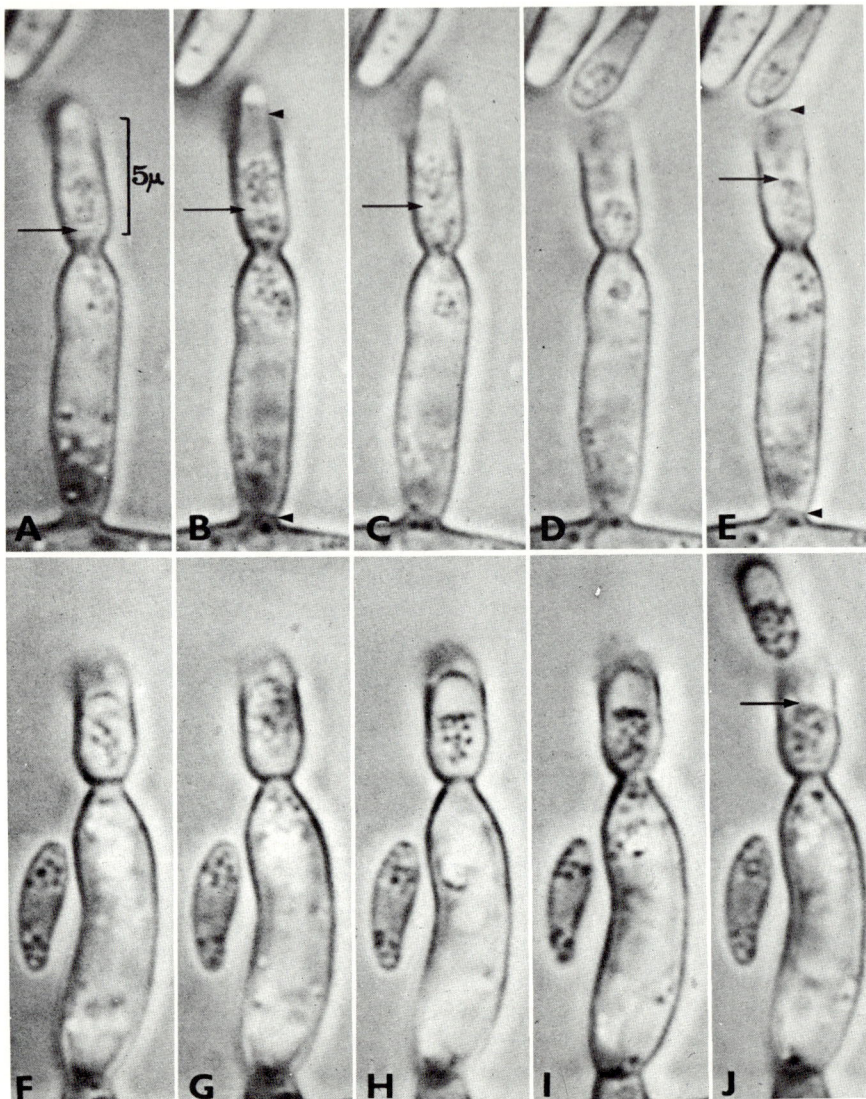

**Fig. 1.28** *Phialophora lagerbergii*. A time-lapse sequence of phialoconidia development. The arrows in A–C, E, and J indicate the apex of a developing conidium. The arrowheads in B and E indicate common reference points for the basal septum and upper limit of the collarette. A–E are at 0, 7, 8, 13, and 50 min, respectively; F–J are at 0, 23, 63, 90, and 165 min, respectively. (Reproduced by permission of G. Cole and the National Research Council of Canada from *Canadian Journal of Botany* **47**:779–789, 1969.)

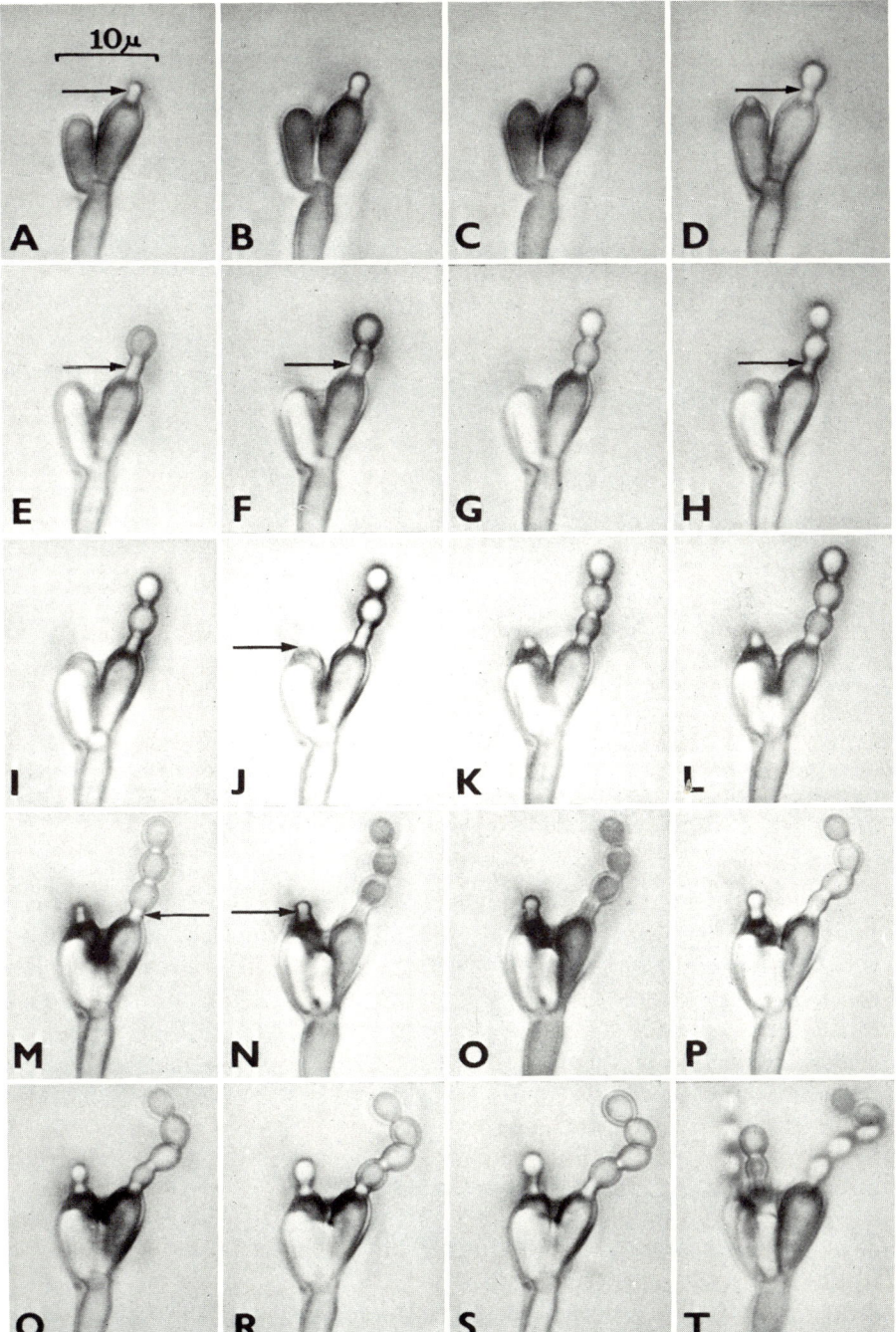

**Fig. 1.29** *Penicillium corylophilum*. A time-lapse sequence of phialoconidia development. The arrows in A, D–F, H, J, M, and N indicate the apex of the phialides. A–T are at 0, 15, 25, 35, 60, 75, 85, 100, 110, 120, 135, 145, 155, 165, 170, 180, 185, 205, 215, and 250 min, respectively. (Reproduced by permission of G. Cole and the National Research Council of Canada from *Canadian Journal of Botany* **47**:779–789, 1969.)

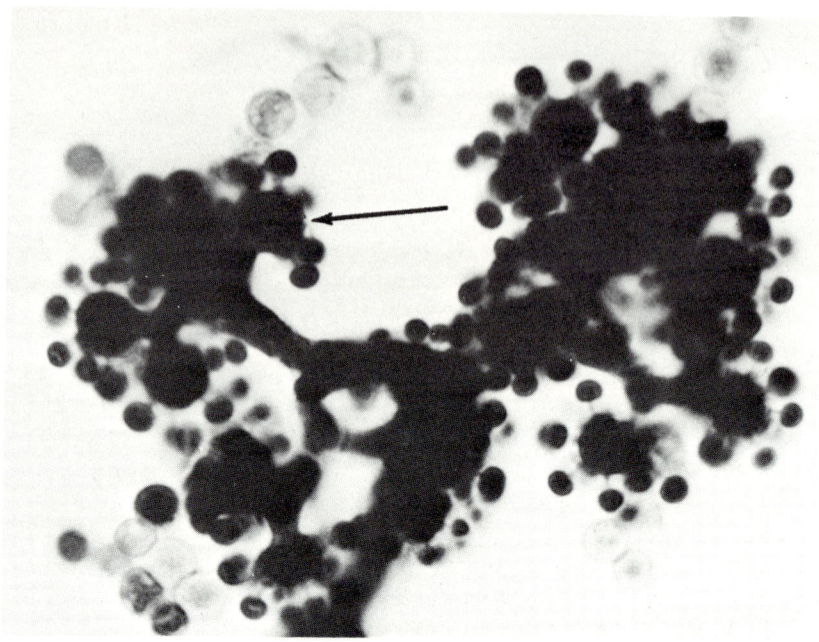

**Fig. 1.30** *Botrytis cinerea*. The ampullae are swollen cells (arrow) from which conidia develop. In *Botrytis*, the botryose conidia are formed in a synchronized manner.

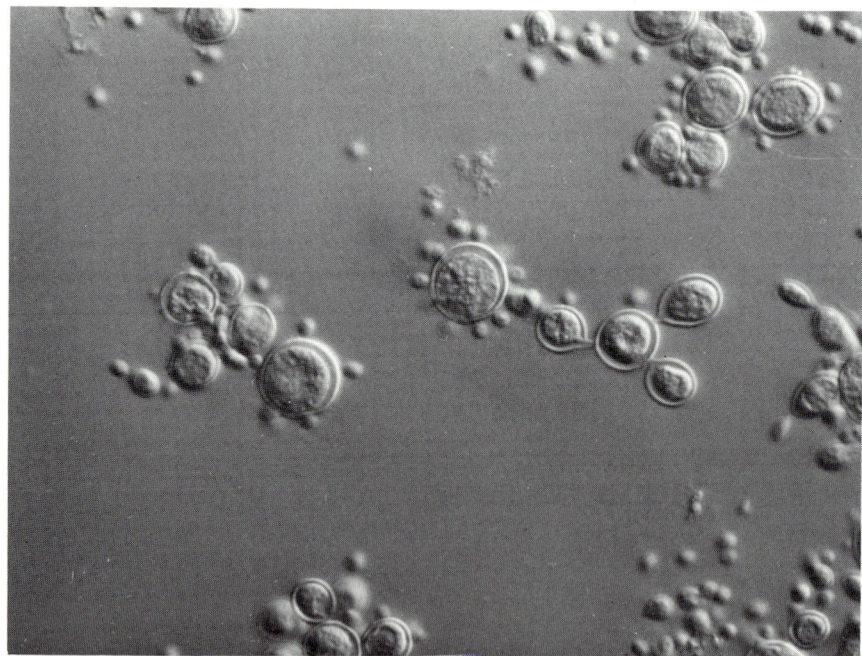

**Fig. 1.31** *Paracoccidioides brasiliensis*. The blastoconidia are constricted at their bases.

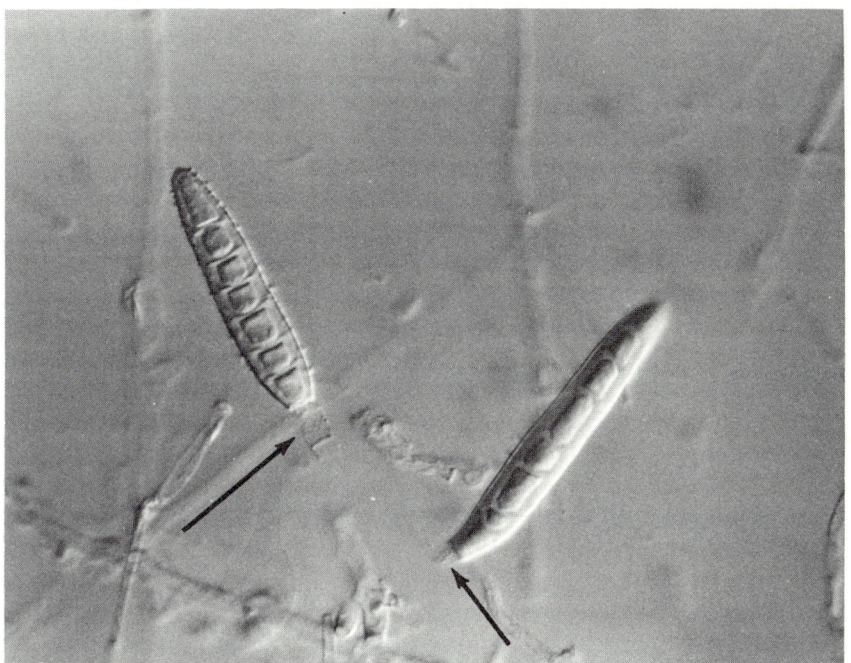

**Fig. 1.32** *Microsporum cookei*. Holothallic conidia often have an annular frill (arrows) at their bases.

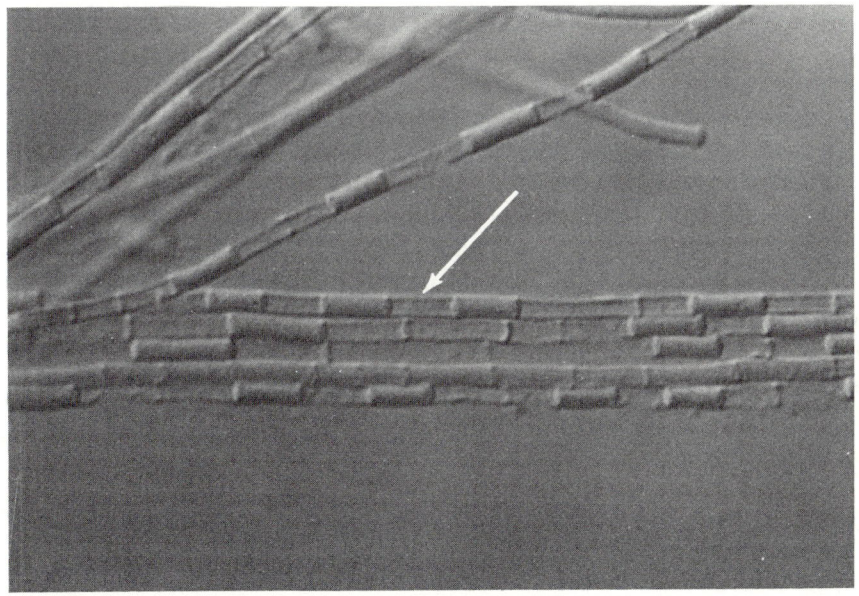

**Fig. 1.33** *Malbranchea albolutea*. Disjunctor cells (arrow) are between each of the arthroconidia. The arthroconidia are released when the disjunctor cells break.

The sexual organs of the fungi are known as gametangia (sing. gametangium). Gametangia may either form gametes (sex cells) or may simply contain one or more nuclei that will function as gamete nuclei. The gametangia may either be heterogametangia or isogametangia. Heterogametangia are gametangia and gametes that morphologically differ from each other, whereas isogametangia are morphologically identical to each other.

Sexual reproduction is infrequently seen in the medical mycology laboratory primarily because of sexual compatibility systems. Sexual compatibility may be either homothallic or heterothallic. Homothallic simply means that each individual is sexually self-fertile and that mating types are not necessary in order for sexual reproduction to occur. In contrast, heterothallic fungi require the union of gametes from two different isolates, since each isolate is sexually self-sterile. Each isolate is commonly referred to as a mating type. Heterothallic fungi may have either a bipolar or tetrapolar compatibility system. Bipolar compatibility means that two mating types, usually designated "+ and −" or "A and a," are necessary for sexual reproduction to take place. Tetrapolar compatibility involves complementary mating types at two locations on the chromosomes, "A, a" and "B, b." Since heterothallism is more common than homothallism, sexual structures are fairly uncommon because isolates usually consist of only one mating type. Occasionally, some fungi with secondary homothallism are found. In this case, each cell contains a nucleus of each of the compatible mating types that originated when the sexual spores were being formed. Such an isolate appears homothallic.

Zygospores, which are characteristic of the Zygomycetes, are rounded thick-walled spores that resulted from the union of gametangia. Meiosis usually occurs during the germination process. These spores may require a long dormancy period prior to germination. Zygospore size, cell wall sculpturing, suspensor cells, and presence or absence of appendages are used in part to differentiate the various zygomycete genera (Fig. 1.34). Zygospores form following the contact of two hyphal tips, which may originate either from homothallic or heterothallic isolates. These hyphal branches bear at their tips the progametangia (sing. progametangium). At the point of contact, there is an enlargement due to the flowing of protoplasm and associated nuclei into this area. As this body increases in size, it is separated from the two progametangia by septa. The enlarged body area becomes the gametangium, and the remaining portions of the progametangia result in suspensor cells. Most of the nuclei fuse in the gametangium, resulting in many diploid nuclei. If nuclei are not fused, they apparently disintegrate. Meiosis occurs at the time of germination, and the zygospores may then either produce a germ tube or form a sporangium, depending upon the genus and species.

## Sexual Reproduction

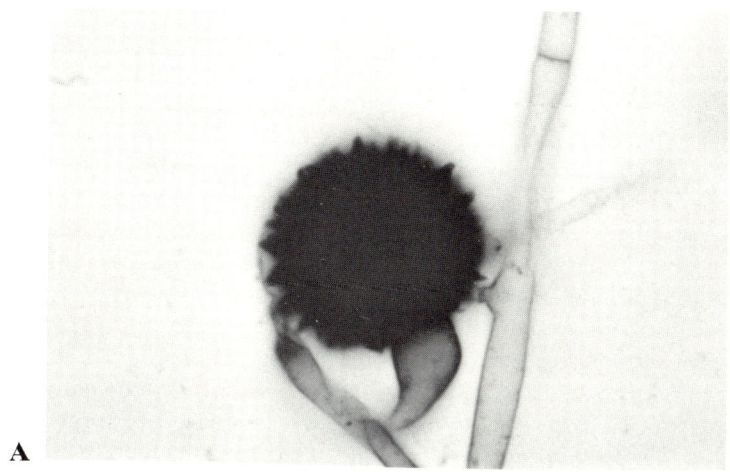

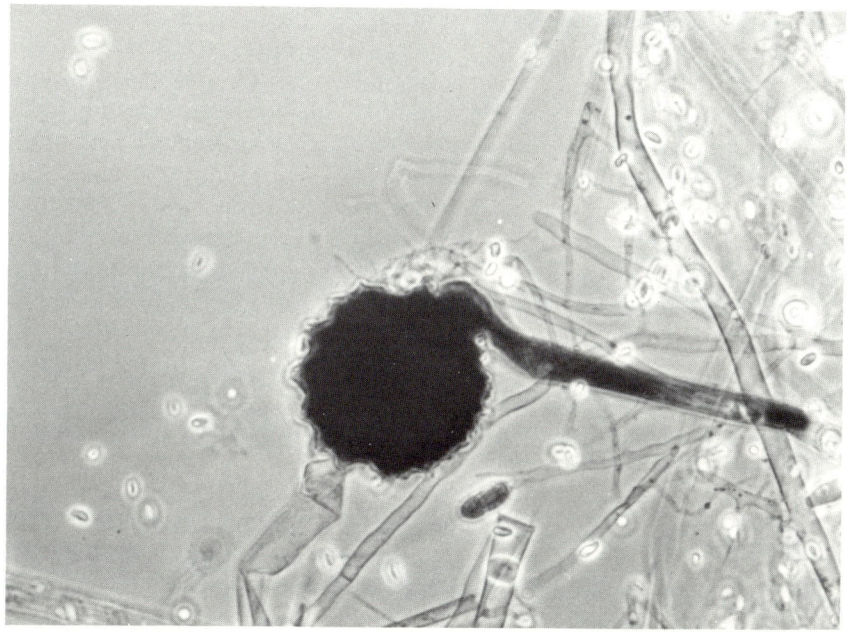

**Fig. 1.34** Zygospores are sexual spores in which the process of meiosis occurs. A. *Zygorhynchus* sp. B. *Mucor bainieri*.

Ascomycetes are characterized by the development of saclike cells called asci (sing. ascus), which usually contain eight ascospores. Sexual reproduction in the Ascomycetes may involve several different methods. The ones of greatest interest to medical mycologists are gametangial copulation and gametangial contact. Gametangial copulation is typically found in the yeasts and is characterized by the contact of two compatible gametangia, fusion at the point of contact, and then development of an ascus. This is very similar to the events resulting in a zygospore. Gametangial contact usually involves heterogametangia, which are referred to as antheridia (male) and ascogonia (female). The male gamete is simply passed from the antheridium into the ascogonium through a pore at the point of contact between the two heterogametangia. Some ascogonia may have a trichogyne, which is a specialized hyphalike filament designed to receive the male gamete during plasmogamy. From the ascogonium, ascogenous hyphae develop. They contain pairs of nuclei ($n + n$) from which the asci will eventually form. The top of each ascogenous hypha may bend over and form a hooklike structure called a crozier (many higher Ascomycetes do not form croziers). The apical cell that is separated from the remaining portion of the crozier becomes the ascus mother cell. In the ascus mother cell, karyogamy occurs, resulting in a zygote nucleus ($2n$). It is important to remember that the young ascus is first dikaryotic ($n + n$) and then later becomes diploid ($2n$). As the ascus mother cell becomes a young ascus, meiosis occurs, resulting in four haploid ($n$) nuclei. By free cell formation, the protoplasm is cleaved into ascospores, each one usually containing one haploid nucleus. In this process, the nuclei are provided with a sheath of cytoplasm by free-cell formation, through which a portion of the content of the ascus remains outside the ascospores. If mitosis occurs prior to free cell formation, then more than four ascospores will result. The occurrence of mitosis prior to free cell formation is characteristic of many genera and species of Ascomycetes. The asci may be either unitunicate or bitunicate, depending whether they have a single wall or two walls, respectively. The arrangement of the ascospores within the ascus may be either biseriate (two rows), fasciculate (in a cluster or bundle), inordinate (random), or uniseriate (one row). Asci usually release their ascospores either by dissolving, or rupturing, or by a plug, pore or operculum mechanism. If an ascocarp is formed, it develops as an indirect result of the $n + n$ condition.

Asci may form in a specialized fruiting body called an ascocarp. A fruiting body is a complex structure giving rise to conidia or spores. An ascocarp is a special type of fruiting body that gives rise to asci and ascospores. The development of the centrum (central area of the ascocarp) is very important in distinguishing ascocarp types. The five major types of ascocarps are as follows:

1. Gymnothecium (pl. gymnothecia). A gymnothecium (Fig. 1.35) is a round ascocarp with a loosely organized network of hyphae (peridium) enclosing randomly dispersed asci. There is no natural opening or ostiole in gymnothecia. The ascospores are usually small, globose and hyaline. Appendages in the form of setae, conidia, etc., may be present or absent, depending upon the species. Gymnothecia are so simple that usually one can see through them with a microscope. This type of ascocarp is characteristic of the Gymnoascaceae.

2. Cleistothecium (pl. cleistothecia). A cleistothecium (Fig. 1.36) is a round, nonostiolate ascocarp with a peridium consisting of a well organized membranelike layer of cells that enclose randomly dispersed asci, a hymenium (flat layer of asci), or a basal bush of asci. With this definition in mind, any round, nonostiolate ascocarp would be called a cleistothecium. A cleistothecium can also be defined as a round, nonostiolate ascocarp containing only randomly dispersed asci. This latter concept is better because it restricts the term to a more closely related group of Ascomycetes. This concept is based upon centrum development, not just upon the gross morphology of the ascocarp. In the former definition, many nonrelated Ascomycetes could be characterized as forming cleistothecia. Hülle cells, that is, enlarged thick-walled cells with a small lumen, are occasionally associated with or make up part of the peridial hyphae, especially in genera like *Emericella*.

3. Perithecium (pl. perithecia). A perithecium (Fig. 1.37) is a round to flask-shaped ascocarp with a distinct ostiole from which ascospores can escape. The asci are either arranged in a hymenium or in a basal bush. Paraphyses, which are sterile hyphae, are often found inside the centrum. They originate from the wall of the ascocarp. Periphyses are sterile hyphae that develop inside the ascocarp neck. If a cleistothecium is defined as containing only randomly dispersed asci, then the concept of a perithecium must be expanded to include ascocarps without ostioles.

4. Apothecium (pl. apothecia). An apothecium is an open, disk- to cup-shaped ascocarp that may be sessile or stalked, with asci developing on the exposed hymenium (Fig. 1.38).

5. Ascostroma (pl. ascostromata). An ascostroma (Fig. 1.39) is an ascocarp in which a cavity is either dissolved or formed via compression in a stroma (mass of hyphae), after which the asci are formed within the cavity (locule). This is quite different from the other types of ascocarps, since the ascogenous hyphae are initiated at the same time as the ascocarp. The asci in an ascostroma are bitunicate.

Basidiomycetes are unique in that their vegetative cells are normally dikaryotic ($n + n$). Theoretically, any one of these cells could give rise to sexual spores. Most Basidiomycetes maintain the dikaryotic state via

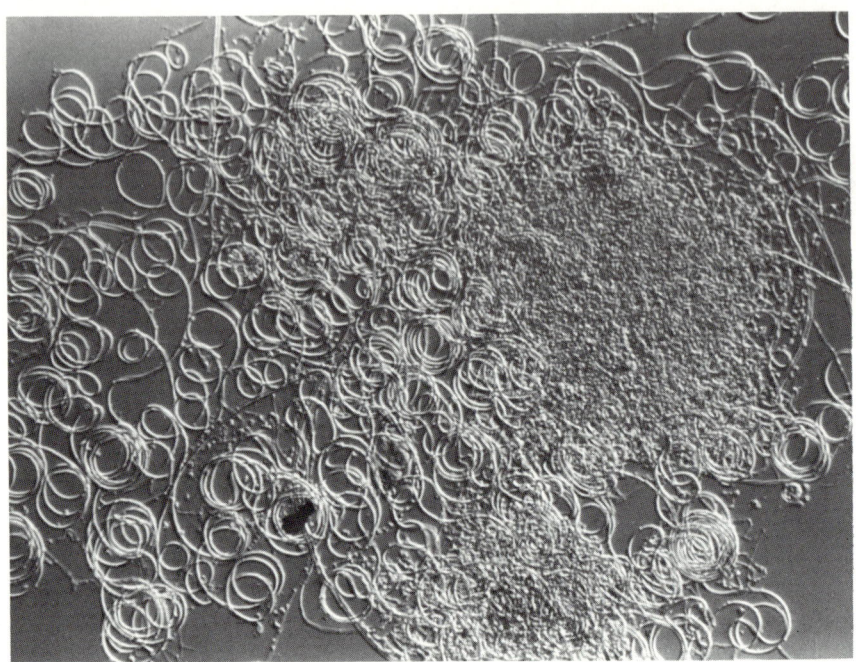

**Fig. 1.35** *Ajellomyces dermatitidis*. The gymnothecium is composed of spirals and a loosely organized peridium. Asci and ascospores develop within the gymnothecium.

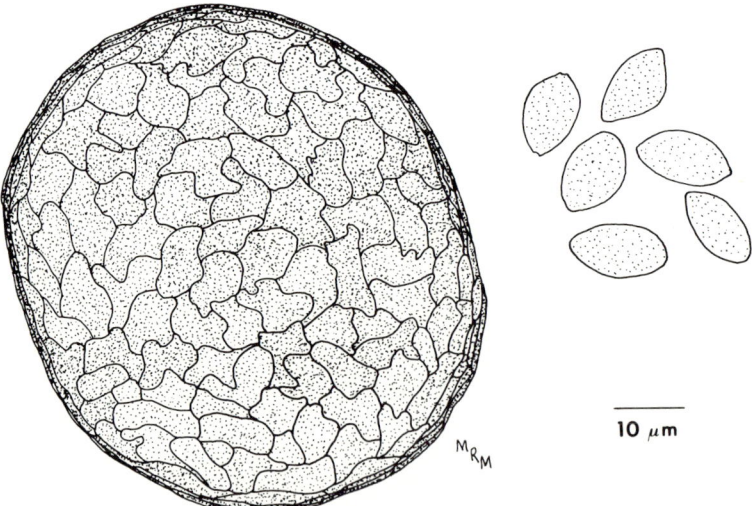

**Fig. 1.36** *Thielavia* sp. The cleistothecium is an enclosed ascocarp in which random asci develop.

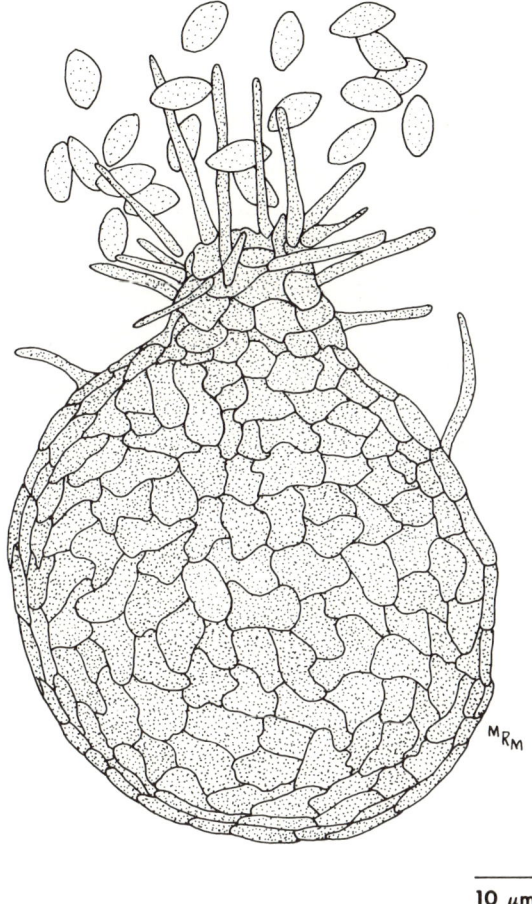

**Fig. 1.37** *Petriella* sp. The perithecium is a flask-shaped ascocarp with an ostiole. The ascospores escape through the ostiole to the outside. Setae are present around the neck of the perithecium in this genus.

connections and special septa called dolipore septa, which at times prevent the migration of nuclei from one cell to the next. A clamp connection (Fig. 1.40) is a specialized hypha-bridge that permits the simultaneous mitosis of two nuclei in such a position that the $n + n$ compatible nuclei are duplicated. The terminal cell of a dikaryotic hypha typically becomes the basidium (pl. basidia). As the basidium enlarges, karyogamy occurs, resulting in a zygote nucleus ($2n$). The diploid nucleus undergoes meiosis and forms four haploid nuclei. While these events are occurring, four short stalks or sterigmata (sing. sterigma) begin to develop from the top of the

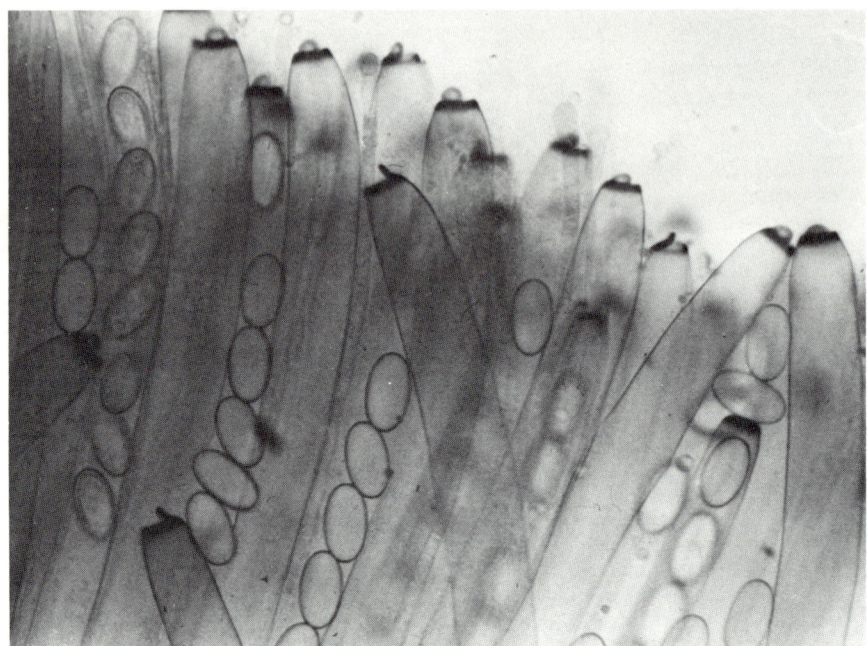

**Fig. 1.38** *Peziza* sp. The asci containing ascospores formed as a hymenium on the surface of the apothecium. Each ascus has a lid or operculum at its apex.

basidium. The tips of the sterigmata enlarge, forming the basidiospore initials. A haploid nucleus then migrates through each sterigma into the young developing basidiospore. The spores become sealed at their bases, and, as they mature, a droplet of water accumulates at their bases. Once the droplet reaches a certain size, each basidiospore is forcibly discharged from its sterigma. It is important to mention that not all Basidiomycetes produce propelled basidiospores or sterigmata. Except for poisonous mushrooms, fungi of medical importance rarely produce basidia and basidiospores in basidiocarps (that is, mushrooms, puff balls, etc.).

## CLASSIFICATION

It has been estimated that there are approximately 100,000–200,000 species of fungi. Of these, approximately 175 or so species have proved to be agents of disease in man (Appendix C). The primary objective of a sound medical mycology laboratory is to identify the fungi recovered from clinical materials.

# Classification

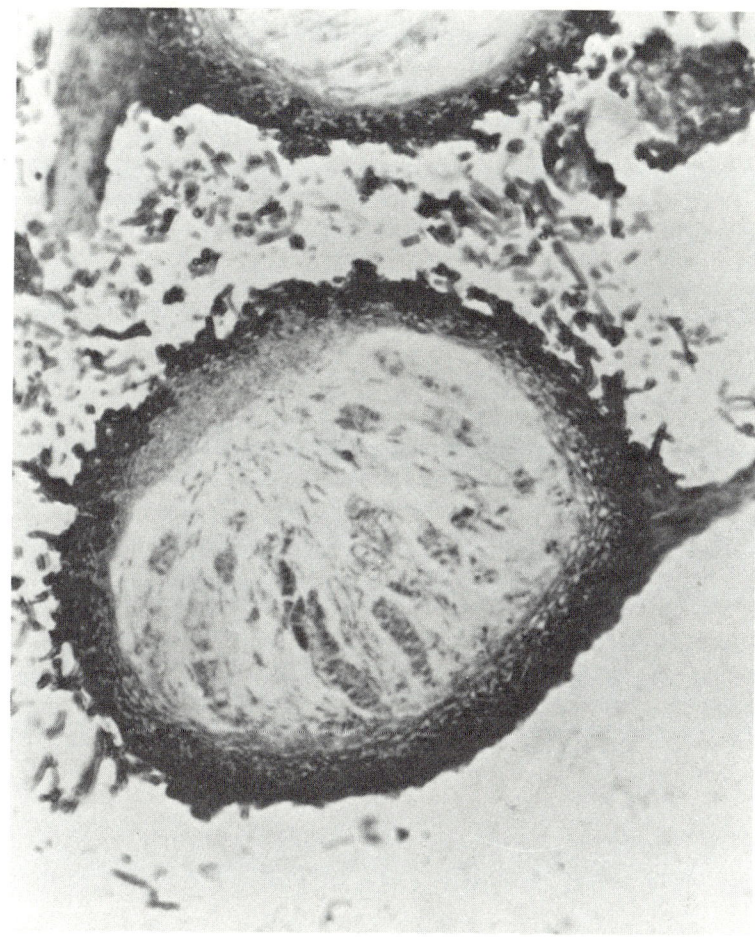

A

**Fig. 1.39** *Leptosphaeria tompkinsii.* A and B. The asci and ascospores are produced within an ascostroma. The cavity is formed prior to the initiation of the asci. (Reproduced by permission of A. El-Ani and Mycologia from *Mycologia* **58**:406–411, 1966.)

Many medical mycologists use the terms taxonomy and nomenclature interchangeably. Taxonomy deals with the classification of fungi and the characteristics that are considered to be important in distinguishing one fungus from the next. The purpose of taxonomy is to permit one mycologist to readily communicate with another. The name given to each fungus in essence represents the sum of the knowledge of that fungus. As new information is discovered, it must be incorporated into our classification systems. Nomenclature on the other hand deals with the principles and

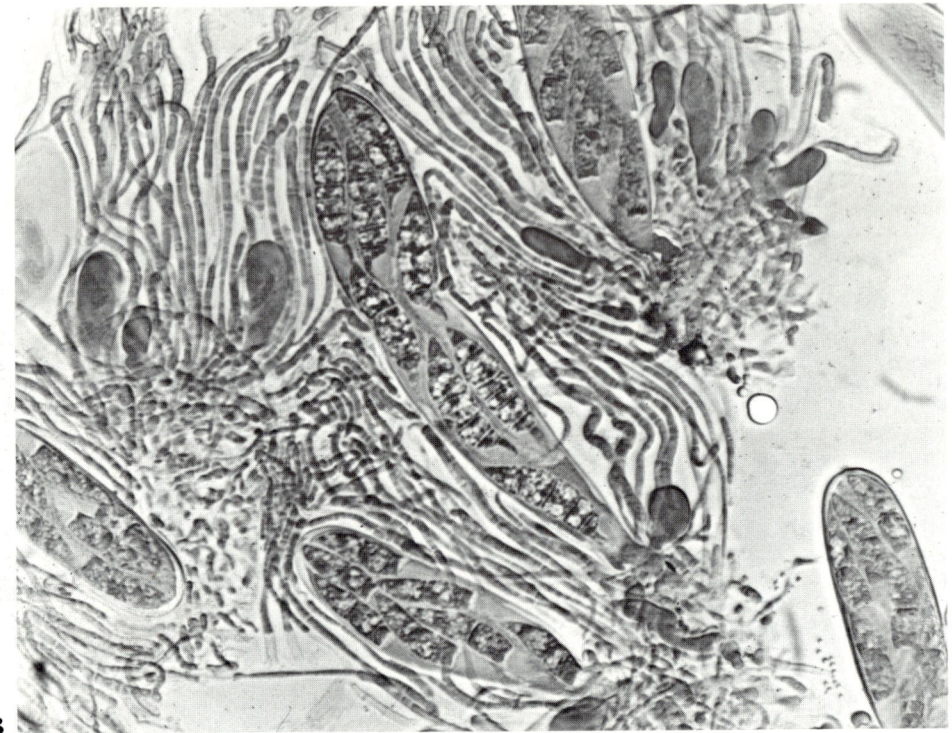

B

**Fig. 1.39** Continued

rules for naming fungi. Nomenclature ensures that each fungus is named in a uniform and proper manner. There is much less flexibility in nomenclature than in taxonomy.

When first described, each different fungus is given a Latin or Latinized scientific name. Latin was selected because it is a "dead" language and is no longer subject to change as are our contemporary languages. The scientific name consists of two words, which are always underlined or italicized. The scientific name or binomial consists of a genus (pl. genera) name and a species epithet. Following the binomial. some mycologists write the name of the person who first named the fungus. Frequently, the year in which the new name was proposed is placed directly after the author's name. If a name is present in parentheses between the scientific name and the author's name, this name refers to the person who originally described the fungus. The name following the parenthesis is the person who is responsible for its present name. This style of listing author names and dates makes it easier for other mycologists to trace the history of the fungus.

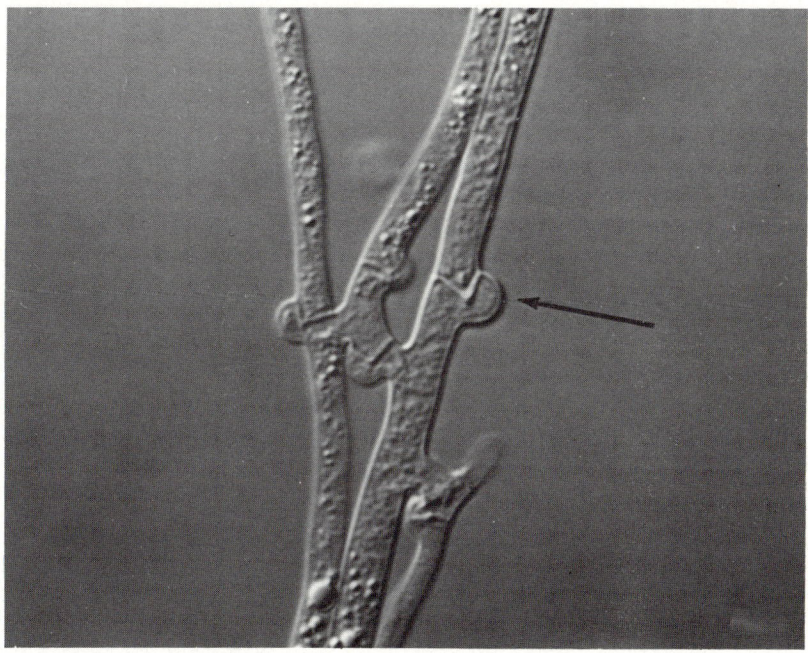

**Fig. 1.40** Clamp connections (arrow) are hypha-bridges that permit the simultaneous mitosis of two nuclei. They are characteristic of the Basidiomycetes.

**Table 1.4.** Classification Scheme for the Kingdom Fungi

| Group | Group ending |
|---|---|
| Kingdom | No specific ending |
| Division | -mycota |
| Subdivision | -mycotina |
| Class | -mycetes |
| Subclass | -mycetidae |
| Order | -ales |
| Family | -aceae |
| Genus | No specific ending |
| Species | No specific ending |

The classification scheme used in this handbook is modified from that of Dr. Ainsworth in "The Fungi, An Advanced Treatise" (Ainsworth *et al.*, 1973, Vol. 4A). The major group endings and keys to the major groups of fungi are included in Tables 1.4 and 1.5. In reality, the average clinical mycology laboratory will encounter the more common Ascomycetes, Fungi Imperfecti, and Zygomycetes. Occasionally, Basidiomycetes will be

**Table 1.5.** Keys to the Higher Groups of the Kingdom of Fungi[a]

---

**Key to the Divisions of the Fungi**

1. Zoospores posteriorly uniflagellate (flagella whiplash type) . . . . . . Chytridiomycota
1'. Zoospores absent . . . . . . . . . . . . . . . . . . . . . . . . . . . . . . . . . . 2
   2. Zygospores or sporangia present . . . . . . . . . . . . . . . . . . . Zygomycota
   2'. Zygospores or sporangia absent . . . . . . . . . . . . . . . . . . . . . . 3
3. Perfect state present . . . . . . . . . . . . . . . . . . . . . . . . . . . . . . . 4
3'. Perfect state absent . . . . . . . . . . . . . . . . . . . . . . . . . . . Fungi Imperfecti
   4. Ascospores present . . . . . . . . . . . . . . . . . . . . . . . . . . . Ascomycota
   4'. Basidiospores present . . . . . . . . . . . . . . . . . . . . . . . . Basidiomycota

I. Chytridiomycota
**Key to the Classes of Chytridiomycota**

1. Thallus variously constructed, always penetrating substratum by means of rhizoids or hyphae, or entirely within it . . . . . . . . . . . . . . . . . . . . . . . . . . . . . . . . . 2
1'. Thallus uniaxial, eucarpic with proximal basal or subbasal disklike holdfast on surface only of substratum, that is, epiphytic or epizooic; distal part composed of upper sporogenous and lower nucleated vegetative region, which persists after sporulation and is capable of sporulation . . . . . . . . . . . . . . . . . . . Harpochytridiomycetes
   2. Thallus holocarpic, eucarpic, monocentric, or polycentric, variously developed; zoospores often with a conspicuous globule, germination monopolar . . . . . . . . . . . . . . . . . . . . . . . . . . . . . . . . . . . . . . . . . . . . . . . . . . . . . . . Chytridiomycetes
   2'. Thallus nearly always differentiated into a well-developed hyphalike vegetative system bearing numerous reproductive bodies, occasionally monocentric; zoospores without a conspicuous globule, germination bipolar . . . . . . . . . . . 3
3. Thallus usually bearing a thick-walled, usually punctate or ornamented, asexually formed resting spore at some stage of its life history; sexuality varied by iso- or anisoplanogametes; not oogamous . . . . . . . . . . . . . . . Blastocladiomycetes
3'. Thallus without above type of resting spore; oogamous, with motile sperms and encysted oospores . . . . . . . . . . . . . . . . . . . . . . . . . . . . . . . Monoblepharidiomycetes

II. Zygomycota
**Key to the Classes of Zygomycota**

1. Saprobic or, if parasitic or predacious having mycelium immersed in host tissue . . . . . . . . . . . . . . . . . . . . . . . . . . . . . . . . . . . . . . . . . . . . . . . . . Zygomycetes
1'. Associated with arthropods and attached to the cuticle or digestive tract by a holdfast and not immersed in host tissue . . . . . . . . . . . . . . . . . . . . . . Trichomycetes

**Table 1.5.** *Continued*

### III. Ascomycota
#### Key to the Classes of Ascomycota

1. Ascocarps and ascogenous hyphae absent; thallus mycelial or yeastlike
   . . . . . . . . . . . . . . . . . . . . . . . . . . . . . . . . . . Hemiascomycetes
1'. Ascocarps and ascogenous hyphae present; mycelial. . . . . . . . . . . . . . . .2
   2. Asci bitunicate; ascocarp an ascostroma. . . . . . . . . . .Loculoascomycetes
   2'. Asci typically unitunicate; if bitunicate, ascocarp an apothecium . . . . . . .3
3. Asci evanescent, randomly scattered within the ascocarp; ascocarp cleistothecium or gymnothecium; ascospores aseptate · . . . . . . . . . . . . . . . . Plectomycetes
3'. Asci in hymenium or basal tuft . . . . . . . . . . . . . . . . . . . . . . . . 4
   4. Exoparasites of arthropods; thallus reduced; ascocarp a perithecium; asci inoperculate. . . . . . . . . . . . . . . . . . . . . . . . . . Laboulbeniomycetes
   4'. Not exoparasites of arthropods . . . . . . . . . . . . . . . . . . . . . . .5
5. Ascocarp typically a perithecium, usually ostiolate; asci inoperculate with an apical pore or slit . . . . . . . . . . . . . . . . . . . . . . . . . . . . . Pyrenomycetes
5'. Ascocarp an apothecium; asci inoperculate or operculate . . . . . . . . Discomycetes

### IV. Basidiomycota
#### Key to the Classes of Basidiomycota

1. Basidiocarp absent; teliospores present, parasites of vascular plants . . . . Teliomycetes
1'. Basidiocarp well developed; basidia usually forming a hymenium; saprobic or rarely parasitic. . . . . . . . . . . . . . . . . . . . . . . . . . . . . . . . . . . 2
   2. Basidiocarp typically gymnocarpous or semiangiocarpous; basidia holobasidia or phragmobasidia; basidiospores ballistospores . . . . . . . . . Hymenomycetes
   2'. Basidiocarp typically angiocarpous; basidia holobasidia; basidiospores not ballistospores · . . . . . . . . . . . . . . . . . . . . . . . . . . . Gasteromycetes

### V. Fungi Imperfecti (Deuteromycota)
#### Key to the Classes of Fungi Imperfecti

1. Yeast with or without pseudomycelium; true mycelium absent or rudimentary
   . . . . . . . . . . . . . . . . . . . . . . . . . . . . . . . . . . . Blastomycetes
1'. Mycelium well developed, yeast typically absent . . . . . . . . . . . . . . . .2
   2. Pycnidium or acervulus present . . . . . . . . . . . . . . . Coelomycetes
   2'. Pycnidium or acervulus absent . . . . . . . . . . . . . . . . Hyphomycetes

---

[a] Reproduced and modified by permission of G. Ainsworth and Academic Press from "The Fungi, An Advanced Treatise," 1973.

recovered, which are usually recognized by the presence of clamp connections, sclerotia and rarely by basidiospores. One of the best indications of a potential basidiomycete in the clinical laboratory is a sterile fungus with clamp connections. The characteristics and procedures for the identification of the fungi will be discussed in Chapters 4 and 5.

Many medical mycologists and laboratory technologists find the system used in mycology of giving the sexual stage of a fungus one name and the asexual stage a second name perplexing. Occasionally, a more confusing dilemma involves deciding which name should be used when a fungus is forming more than one type of asexual stage. And finally, deciding when a fungus should be referred to by its sexual name instead of its asexual name can be bewildering.

In mycology, there are in essence two independent classification systems, one for sexual stages or teleomorphs and a second for asexual forms or anamorphs. A teleomorph is any reproductive structure that is morphologically, karyologically, or both, specialized for the production of sexual spores or their homologs, whether by normal sexual means or parthenogenesis. An anamorph is any asexual or somatic reproductive structure, whether specialized or generalized, that is neither karyologically nor morphologically sexual. The entire fungus, which includes all of its anamorphs, its teleomorph, or both, is referred to as the holomorph. Like other eukaryotic organisms, the fungi are classified according to their sexual forms, even when asexual forms are present too. This permits mycologists to study the phylogeny of fungi and to determine relatedness of different groups. The confusion arises when fungi are isolated that apparently reproduce solely by asexual means. Since the classification of fungi is primarily based upon sexual structures, the presence of asexual structures only must be treated differently.

To avoid confusion in using these two different concepts, a form-division, form-classes, form-orders, form-families, form-genera and form-species are commonly used for the various anamorphs or conidial states. The prefix form- is usually used to denote that these groups are neither intended to show nor imply phylogenetic (natural) relationships, but only to serve as groupings for similar imperfect fungi so that one mycologist can effectively communicate with another. Even though the prefix form- was established for fossils, it is used by many mycologists for the Fungi Imperfecti. Imperfect fungi are "imperfect" only in the sense that their perfect stages (teleomorphs) are yet unknown. In essence, the concept of Fungi Imperfecti is like a file cabinet in which everything is in an organized format, but the individual components are not necessarily meant to be related to each other. The term Fungi Imperfecti is preferred for these asexual fungi instead of the term Deuteromycota. The term Deuteromycota implies that these fungi have equal taxonomic status to the other fungi classified upon their teleomorphs. By tradition, the asexual forms of the rust fungi and the Zygomycetes are treated with the Uredinales and Zygomycota, respectively.

Many of the imperfect fungi can produce sexual structures under appropriate conditions. When the teleomorph is present, the proper name for the fungus is the name based upon the sexual stage. If one wishes to refer to the asexual form, it is referred to as the "anamorph of," "state of" or by its mode of conidiogenesis. For example, the ascomycete *Ajellomyces dermatitidis* forms an asexual form called *Blastomyces dermatitidis,* which was known several years before the sexual form was discovered. The name *A. dermatitidis* is the correct name for the whole fungus (holomorph). To refer to the asexual form, expressions such as "*Blastomyces* anamorph of *A. dermatitidis*" or the "*Blastomyces* state of *A. dermatitidis*" would be appropriate. The most ideal expression would be "anamorph of." In the clinical laboratory, only the *B. dermatitidis* anamorph of this fungus is seen. Since *B. dermatitidis* is apparently the only anamorph of *A. dermatitidis,* clinical isolates could also be referred to as the "*Blastomyces* state of *A. dermatitidis*," even though gymnothecia are absent. The use of "anamorph of" is a convenient and concise way of referring to a particular morphological part, to avoid using two species names, and to tie an asexual form to its corresponding sexual state.

A number of fungi with sexual stages may form more than one type of anamorph. In this instance, it would be nearly impossible to associate a particular anamorph occurring by itself with a specific teleomorph. The converse may also hold true, as one anamorph may be associated with several different teleomorphs. For example, the anamorph *Microsporum gypseum* is produced by more than one species of *Nannizzia.*

Polymorphic fungi, that is, those fungi that form more than one kind of conidium, cause a special problem. There are three basic approaches that can be taken in deciding what to call a polymorphic fungus. The first is to give each different anamorph its own name. If a particular fungus has three different types of conidia, it would have three different binomials. For obvious reasons, this is entirely impractical and unsatisfactory. The second approach is to have one name for the entire fungus (holomorph), which is based on all the different conidial states. Each different combination of anamorphs would have its own name. This approach is typified by the old concept of *Fonsecaea,* which was based upon the presence of *Rhinocladiella*-like, *Cladosporium*-like and *Phialophora*-like forms of conidiogenesis. If one of these anamorphs were absent, then the fungus would be called something different. In essence, *Fonsecaea* would not be a genus. It would be a group of genera since it would consist of a combination of anamorphs. The third approach, which is the most reasonable, is to base the name upon the most distinctive, conspicuous, often encountered, and stable anamorph. Each genus would therefore be based on one anamorph. Other forms that were present would simply be referred to as "anamorph of" or by their mode of conidiogenesis. For example, the genus *Fusarium* is characterized by large, multiseptate, sickle-shaped macrophialoconidia. The absence or the presence of one-celled microphialoconidia does not affect the identification of *Fusarium.* This second type of asexual form is referred to as the "*Acremonium* anamorph of *Fusarium.*" Since the sickle-shaped macroconidia are more distinctive than the smaller one-celled microconidia, they are used for the basis of the name. Regardless of the approach taken, the rules of priority apply to the name that is selected for the fungus.

In mycology, there are no universal characteristics that can be applied to all groups of fungi. Each group of fungi has its own particular characteristics. For example, the hyphae of the filamentous fungi have no real taxonomic value, but in the yeast fungi the presence or the absence of hyphae could be a key characteristic in separating two genera. Some characteristics may be valuable in many groups, but not necessarily equally. Phialides with collarettes are a key characteristic of the dematiaceous hyphomycete genus *Phialophora.* Yet identical phialides in *Fonsecaea* species have only a secondary importance. The relative value of different characteristics depends upon the group being studied and the taxonomists studying that group. Without doubt, there are few characteristics that hold true 100% of the time. The most ideal characteristics are ones that hold true most of the time. For this reason, a combination of characteristics is mandatory and no one characteristic should be used alone in identifying or describing a fungus.

To summarize the major characteristics used to distinguish and identify the various fungi, mycologists traditionally prepare dichotomous keys and flow charts. The dichotomous key is designed to give the user sets of two opposing groups of characteristics. By selecting the one choice that most closely fits the unknown fungus, the user is led through a series of elimination steps to a tentative identification of the unknown fungus. The characteristics in each series of choices are listed from the most important to the least important. Thus, the first characteristic is more important than the others. A decision as to which choice should be made is not always clear. In this event, the fungus should be keyed out as if both choices were correct. If the key does not lead to a reasonable identification, the fungus may not have been meant to be keyed out with that particular key. A fungus should never be "force fitted" into a particular name or group.

## Selected References

1. Ainsworth, G. C., F. K. Sparrow, and A. S. Sussman, (eds.) (1965-1973). "The Fungi: An Advanced Treatise," Vols. I-IVB. Academic Press, New York.
2. Alexopoulos, C. J., and C. W. Mims (1979). "Introductory Mycology," 3rd. ed. Wiley, New York.
3. Bessey, E. A. (1950). "Morphology and Taxonomy of Fungi." McGraw-Hill (Blakiston), New York.
4. Cole, G., and R. A. Samson (1979). "Patterns of Development in Conidial Fungi." Pitman, London.
5. Kendrick, B., ed. (1971). "Taxonomy of Fungi Imperfecti." Univ. of Toronto Press, Toronto.
6. Kendrick, B., ed. (1979). "The Whole Fungus." Vols. I-II. Univ. of Waterloo Press, Waterloo.
7. Margulis, L. (1974). The classification and evolution of prokaryotes and eukaryotes. *In* "Handbook of Genetics" (R. C. King, ed.), Vol. I, pp. 1-41. Plenum, New York.
8. McGinnis, M. R. (1977). Human pathogenic species of *Exophiala, Phialophora,* and *Wangiella. Proc. Int. Conf. Mycoses, 4th, PAHO Sci. Publ. No.* 356, pp. 37-59.
9. Müller, E., and W. Loeffler (1976). "Mycology: An Outline for Science and Medical Students." Thieme, Stuttgart.
10. Smith, J. E., and D. R. Berry (1974). An Introduction to the Biochemistry of Fungal Development." Academic Press, New York.
11. Whittaker, R. H. (1969). New concepts of kingdoms of organisms. *Science* **163**:150-160.

*Chapter 2*

## Laboratory Safety

Laboratory safety in medical mycology requires continuous attention and training. It should never be assumed that laboratory personnel have adequate knowledge or skill in laboratory safety practices. Safety skills and knowledge must be developed through a well designed and thorough training program if accidents are to be prevented—and accidents can be prevented.

Safety is the responsibility of every individual, supervisor, and institution. The individual must be familiar with the potential hazards in his laboratory and the safeguards that must be exercised to prevent accidents. The primary responsibility of each supervisor is to develop, implement, monitor, and evaluate laboratory practices and policies on a daily basis. The supervisor provides supervision, arranges for training when indicated, and plans for emergency situations. The ultimate success of the safety program rests upon the institution's administration and its willingness to support laboratory safety with ample facilities, funds, and equipment and a sincere belief that safety is an integral component of good laboratory practice.

### GENERAL RECOMMENDATIONS

Emergency phone numbers (a single emergency number if possible), and a list of emergency personnel must be immediately accessible to everyone in the laboratory in the event of an accident. Phone numbers and personnel are subject to frequent change; therefore, these lists must be reviewed and updated on a regular basis. If the medical mycology laboratory is not located within a hospital, explicit directions to the laboratory (planned in advance) must be given to emergency rescue personnel (rescue squad, police, fire department) to ensure that they can reach the site of the emergency promptly. It is important to acquaint them in advance with the nature of the emergency. Under no circumstances should accident victims be permitted to go to an emergency room by themselves, regardless of how they feel. If safety equipment, such as fire extinguishers, eye wash stations, safety showers, and first aid kits, has been used, the items used must be recharged or replaced as soon as possible.

Each new employee should receive a written (procedural manual) and oral safety orientation that includes the practices and standards expected. The orientation is recorded in the individual's personnel file. The supervisor can then determine how and when to present refresher courses and updatings.

A current chest X-ray and a tine or PPD skin test should be given to each person annually. These tests are important because most specimens for mycological evaluation originate from a pulmonary site. In addition to the tine test, it is also a good practice to have each new employee skin tested with coccidioidin and histoplasmin. These two tests are done only once, since the value of the fungal skin test lies in the conversion of a negative to a positive test. The time interval between the negative and positive tests allows the physician to determine when the infection probably occurred. A positive skin test means that the individual has or has had an infection. It does not necessarily imply the existence of an active infection.

Serum from each new employee should be obtained and kept for future reference. Many serological procedures require the demonstration of a fourfold change in titer before the diagnosis of a fungal infection can be made. This reference serum obtained at the time of initial employment can serve as a base line specimen. A serum sample should always be obtained prior to skin testing to ensure that the skin test does not incite false-positive reactions in subsequent serological studies. If it is discovered that the skin test(s) or chest X-ray convert to positive during a later check-up, or if an accident occurs, the following steps must be taken immediately.

a. The individual must be given a complete medical evaluation, including appropriate cultural and serological tests.
b. All safety practices and procedures in the laboratory must be reevaluated. Determine what happened, whether the procedures were followed, were appropriate, should be changed.
c. The personal work habits of the individual must be reevaluated. This evaluation is in addition to the constant evaluation of each individual on a regular basis by the supervisor.

All accidents must be reported to the supervisor, regardless of whether the accident seems insignificant. This will point out problem areas and serve as a basis for prevention or corrective measures to prevent it from reoccurring with a potentially grave outcome. Smoking should not be permitted in any area of the laboratory because

a. It increases the risk of bringing potentially dangerous organisms and chemicals to the mouth.
b. It may result in a fire.
c. Smoking is annoying to others.

Eating and drinking in the laboratory should not be permitted since food and drinks may become contaminated with pathogenic organisms. Food and drink, to be consumed outside the laboratory, should not be kept in the laboratory refrigerators.

If possible, contact lenses should not be worn by members of the laboratory staff. Contact lenses, especially soft ones, can absorb some of the solvents and other reagents used in the laboratory. In the event of an accident involving the eyes, contact lenses may also prevent prompt treatment by simply being in the way. Chemicals can become trapped in the capillary space between the contact lenses and the cornea. If the contact lens is displaced or the eye becomes painful, muscle spasms may prevent the removal of the lens. Contact lenses do not provide eye protection. If contact lenses are worn, the individual must wear safety goggles when doing procedures involving potential eye hazards.

Laboratory coats are worn at all times to protect the clothing. They should always be removed prior to leaving the laboratory for any reason. The material of these coats should not contain large amounts of acetate because this material is extremely flammable. Owing to the continuous handling of clinical materials and cultures, the hands should be washed frequently. Gloves are always worn when handling specimens. All pipetting should be done with an automatic pipetting device, never by mouth.

## DISINFECTION AND STERILIZATION

The ultimate purpose of the various decontaminants and techniques of sterilization are the destruction of potentially dangerous organisms. Potentially infectious materials and equipment should always be sterilized prior to being washed or discarded. If sterilization is to be accomplished by autoclaving, hazardous materials are never left in the autoclave in anticipation of someone else autoclaving them. All floors, benches, equipment, and other surfaces where biohazardous materials are handled should be disinfected on a regular basis. The principal decontaminants available include alcohol (concentrations of 70–95%), formaldehyde (8% formalin or 8% formalin in 70% alcohol), quaternary ammonium compounds, 5% phenol, 5% Wescodyne, or 5% hyphochlorite (50,000 ppm available chlorine).

Most sterilizations are accomplished in the steam autoclave. Dry heat and ethylene oxide sterilization have limited value in medical mycology. Sixteen hours of exposure to paraformaldehyde at 1 gm/ft$^3$, 40–60% relative humidity at 25°C is an effective sterilization technique. Steam sterilization of laundry in the autoclave should be for 30 minutes at 15 psi and 121°C; 1 hour at 15 psi and 121°C for trash and glassware; and 1 hour for each gallon at 15 psi and 121°C for liquids. Timing is started once the autoclave has reached its proper temperature and pressure. Autoclaving should be monitored with biological indicators (Killet ampoules) to verify the efficacy of the treatment.

## BIOLOGICAL HAZARDS

In the event of a serious accident involving living fungi, the following must be done immediately:

a. Hold your breath and leave the room immediately, closing the door behind you.
b. Warn all the other people in the laboratory of the type of danger and *do not* permit anyone to enter the contaminated area.
c. Decontaminate the exposed person(s).

A minor accident can be taken care of by immediately covering the spill with a towel and then flooding it with disinfectant and waiting approximately 1 hour before picking it up. Wherever cultures are being worked with, bottles containing a disinfectant must be readily available. To prevent accidents, all specimens and cultures are carried in baskets or racks.

Exposure to fungi can occur in several ways in the laboratory. The major routes involve inhalation of airborne particles following spills, breakage of containers, and removal of caps or cotton test tube plugs; ingestion by mouth pipetting or failure to wash hands after handling cultures or clinical specimens; direct inoculation as a result of accidents involving needles, scalpels, and broken glassware; and skin contact and subsequent entrance through cuts and scratches.

Dangerous fungi, such as *Blastomyces dermatitidis, Coccidioides immitis, Cryptococcus neoformans, Histoplasma capsulatum, Paracoccidioides brasiliensis,* and *Sporothrix schenckii,* must be worked with in a Class II or

III biological safety cabinet. Two of the more commonly used laminar-flow devices are the laminar-flow clean bench, which protects supplies from airborne contamination, but not the mycologist, and the vertical laminar-flow biological safety cabinet (Table 2.1) which protects the mycologist. Only vertical laminar-flow biological safety cabinets should be used in medical mycology. For especially hazardous fungi, a gastight Class III biological safety cabinet should be used in lieu of the other types of safety cabinets.

High-efficiency particulate air (HEPA) filters in safety cabinets must be tested and certified to be at least 99.97% efficient in removing particles 0.3 $\mu$m or larger in size by the dioctyl phthalate (DOP) test. The HEPA filter housing must be sealed properly around the edges to ensure that unfiltered air does not bypass the HEPA filter. The air flow across the front of the safety cabinet should be approximately 90–100 linear feet per minute. Depending upon the opening size, a minimum of 75 linear feet per minute is recommended by the National Sanitary Foundation (NSF) for Class II safety cabinets. The prefilter must be periodically cleaned and replaced. Under no circumstances should equipment or supplies be placed on the grid panels in any safety cabinet, because these can disturb the air flow pattern of the cabinet. Safety cabinets should be recertified every 6 months, or at least once a year.

Safety cabinets usually contain ultraviolet (UV) lights that are designed to reduce the number of fungi on the cabinet surfaces and in the air. Ultraviolet radiation is not an effective sterilizing procedure. Current recommendations by NSF are that UV lights should not be used. If they are present, they must be changed when they emit 70% or less of their initial rated output. The lamps are cleaned twice a month with an alcohol moistened cloth to remove dust and dirt, which reduces the effectiveness of the UV lamps. No one should ever be permitted to work in a biological safety cabinet while the UV lamps are turned on. In fact, they must be turned off when entering the area.

Eye and skin protection is necessary when determining the output of the UV lamps (see Chapter 8). Eye overexposure results in painful inflammation of the conjunctiva, cornea, and iris within 3–12 hours, a foreign body sensation, lacrimation, with symptoms disappearing in 1–2 days. Erythema in 1–8 hours characterizes skin overexposure. Eye protection against overexposure consists of wearing safety glasses with side shields or goggles with solid side pieces to protect the eyes from reflected and direct radiation. Face shields, caps, and gloves can be worn to protect the skin.

Accidents involving clinical specimens and fungi may occur either within a safety cabinet or outside the cabinet. An accident outside the safety cabinet is by far the most difficult to manage.

**Table 2.1.** Classes of Biological Safety Cabinets

| | |
|---|---|
| Class I. | An open-front, ventilated safety cabinet with an uncirculated (within the cabinet) inward flow of air from the operator. The cabinet protects the operator from low- to moderate-risk biological hazards. There is no product protection within the cabinet. The exhaust air is usually filtered through high-efficiency particulate air (HEPA) filters prior to being discharged to the outside atmosphere. |
| Class II. | An open-front, ventilated safety cabinet with recirculated (within the cabinet) inward flow of air from the operator. The cabinet protects the operator from low- to moderate-risk biological hazards. Owing to the recirculated air, products within the cabinet are also protected. The exhaust air is filtered through HEPA filters. These cabinets are not meant to be used as chemical fume hoods. |
| Class III. | A closed-front, ventilated safety cabinet with negative air pressure. The gastight construction provides total protection for the operator and products within it. The supply and exhaust air is treated to protect the atmosphere. When Class III cabinets are fitted with rubber gloves, they can be used for high-risk agents. |

a. Accidents outside the safety cabinet involving clinical specimens and cultures of fungi that are not potentially dangerous should be handled as follows:
   (1) Shut down the ventilation to the area and wait for approximately 1 hour before reentering the room so that aerosols created can settle.
   (2) Wearing a long-sleeve gown, mask, and rubber gloves, cover the clinical material, broken cultures, or spills with 5% phenol, 5% Wescodyne, 5% hypochlorite, or similar agent. These will kill the fungi and prevent the dried particles from becoming airborne.
   (3) Keep the area wet with the disinfectant for approximately 1 hour before cleaning up the spill.
   (4) All the contaminated and potentially contaminated equipment must be disinfected.
   (5) After disinfection of the accident site, autoclave and discard all the waste. Never use bare hands to clean up waste material. If the hands should contact this material, wash them with soap and water, 70% isopropyl alcohol, or both.

## Biological Hazards

b.  Accidents outside the safety cabinet involving dangerous fungi must be handled as follows:
   (1) Shut down the ventilation to the area and wait for approximately 1 hour before entering the room to permit any aerosols present to settle.
   (2) Wearing a jumpsuit with tight-fitting wrists, respirator, and shoe covers, cover the accident area with 5% phenol, 5% Wescodyne, 5% hypochlorite, or similar agent. Pour the disinfectant around the accident site, but not directly onto the spill. The disinfectant will flow into the spill without causing a serious re-aerosolizing of the hazardous material.
   (3) Place paper towels soaked with the disinfectant over the spill and permit it to stand for at least 1 hour. Space decontamination with paraformaldehyde may be necessary.
   (4) Using an autoclavable dust pan and squeeze, transfer all the contaminated material to a deep discard pan and then autoclave.
   (5) Clean the laboratory equipment and furniture with disinfectant.

If the accident involves *Blastomyces dermatitidis, Coccidioides immitis,* or *Histoplasma capsulatum*, the entire area should be gassed with paraformaldehyde (1 gm/ft$^3$). In reality, the average medical mycology laboratory has neither the equipment nor trained personnel to handle accidents outside of a biological safety cabinet when dangerous fungi are involved. The most ideal solution is to establish an agreement with a university safety department or commercial company to handle such an emergency situation.

c.  Accidents occurring in a centrifuge should be handled as follows:
   (1) Holding your breath, turn off the centrifuge and immediately leave the area shutting the door behind you.
   (2) Warn the other personnel in the laboratory of the problem and shut down the ventilation to the area.
   (3) Wait approximately 1 hour before reentering the room.
   (4) Wearing protective clothing, enter the area and disinfect the centrifuge with a disinfectant such as 5% Wescodyne or 5% phenol.
   (5) Clean the equipment and room with disinfectant.
   (6) Autoclave and discard all the cleaning materials.

Centrifuges represent a special potential source of laboratory accidents. If the instrument is not used properly, aerosols can result. Safety carriers that are sealed shut must be used whenever clinical specimens or known etiologic agents of disease are centrifuged. If living potentially infectious fungi are being centrifuged, the sealed safety cups should be opened only in a biological safety cabinet.

- d. If an accident should occur within a biological safety cabinet, the following should be done:
  - (1) Leave the cabinet on to prevent the escape of any hazardous material into the room.
  - (2) Wearing gloves, spray or wipe all the walls, work surfaces, and equipment with 5% Wescodyne, 5% phenol, or similar disinfectant. A disinfectant-detergent such as Wescodyne has the advantage of preventing organic substances from interfering with the reaction between the fungus and the antimicrobial agent.
  - (3) If the biological safety cabinet has a top tray, drain pans and catch basins below the work surface, flood them with the disinfectant and allow to stand for 10–15 minutes.
  - (4) Excess disinfectant from the tray, surface, and drain pans should be dumped into the cabinet base. After this has been done, lift out the tray and remove the exhaust grill work and then wipe off the top and bottom surfaces.
  - (5) Replace the parts, collect the gloves and sponges, and autoclave them.
  - (6) Drain the disinfectant from the cabinet base, autoclave and then discard.

## FIRE HAZARDS

Each laboratory must have an up-to-date fire plan, and all the emergency exits must be clearly marked and free of obstructions (carts, equipment, buckets, etc.) that could delay immediate evacuation. Simply because an emergency has never arisen, it cannot be assumed that one will not occur. In the event of a fire, prompt action to evacuate the laboratory is mandatory. Planning and preparation are the most important factors to ensure that the response of the laboratory people is prompt, correct, and effective in order to minimize damage and injury. In the event of a fire, the following steps should be taken.

- a. Alert everyone in the immediate vicinity and tell them the nature and extent of the emergency. Emergency fire fighting personnel should be concurrently notified. This can be accomplished by calling an emergency number, the operator, or the fire department. Be sure to tell them what, when, where and an estimate of the problem and hazards that are involved.

**Fire Hazards** 65

    b. Each individual in the laboratory should have the following preassigned responsibilities:
       (1) Close all doors, vents, and windows to confine the fire so that others will have time to reduce the amount of damage.
       (2) Turn off all gas burners, disconnect electrical equipment by tripping the circuit breakers, and shut off all gas cylinders.
    c. If the fire is small, try to extinguish it. The first few minutes are vital, so move as fast as possible. Use the appropriate fire extinguisher for the type of fire. When using a fire extinguisher, always stay low to the ground to avoid heat and smoke, and stay between a door and the fire so that you can escape. Ventilate the area only after the fire is out.
    d. If the fire is too large, evacuate the laboratory, following the evacuation plan, and then await professional help. If members of the laboratory staff have been trained in the use of self contained breathing equipment, these individuals can provide valuable assistance to the emergency personnel by showing them potentially dangerous situations.

All employees in the laboratory should be familiar with the location, description, and operation of the laboratory fire extinguishers. Water should never be used to extinguish electrical or chemical fires because it tends to splash and spread burning chemicals. It is also a good conductor of electricity and can potentially result in serious shock. The most common type of extinguisher used for the control of flammable liquid or electrical fires is the carbon dioxide extinguisher. To use an extinguisher properly the following procedures are essential:

    a. Read the instructions on the extinguisher before a fire occurs.
    b. To operate the extinguisher, pull the locking pin out and squeeze the handle. Do not invert $CO_2$ and dry chemical extinguishers.
    c. Do not touch the discharge nozzle, because it becomes extremely cold.
    d. Carbon dioxide extinguishers have a limited range. Therefore, you must get close to the fire.
    e. For flammable-liquid fires, apply the carbon dioxide near the edge of the fire and sweep slowly from side to side.
    f. For electrical fires, apply the carbon dioxide directly to the source of the fire.
    g. Continue to discharge carbon dioxide on the area after the fire is extinguished to prevent reflash.

If someone is on fire, place the individual under the safety shower or smother the fire with the fire blanket, a laboratory coat, or towel. Each employee must be familiar with the location and use of the safety shower and fire blanket to ensure that valuable time is not wasted. The burned area should be cooled immediately. The safety shower can both extinguish the fire as well as cool the burn area. Ice water should not be used for a large burned area because it can result in shock. The burn victim should be immediately taken to an emergency room for medical care.

When you hear the fire alarm sound, you must assume that there is a fire and everyone in the laboratory must leave the area via the nearest exit or corridor. If handicapped people are present, emergency personnel should be notified immediately of their location. In the event of an immediate threat to life, the handicapped personnel should be carried to an area of safety. It is therefore important that at least two persons remain with each handicapped person during the emergency.

Should you encounter a closed door between you and the emergency route of exit, feel the door before opening it. If it feels warm or hot, there is a good chance that there is a fire behind it. Open the door slowly, and only slightly, to determine whether the corridor is safe to enter. If it is safe, then quickly proceed to the nearest exit or exit stairwell. Never attempt to use an elevator since you could become trapped within it. After exiting the building, count noses to be sure that everyone in the laboratory is safe. If someone is missing, immediately tell the emergency people, but do not go back into the building. Re-enter the building only when advised to do so by the emergency personnel.

## CHEMICAL HAZARDS

Dangerous chemicals consist of caustic, corrosive, poisonous, flammable, and explosive reagents. The most frequent accidents involve acid or base spills. For this reason, whenever acids or bases are being handled, a protective face shield, goggles, and chemically resistant gloves and apron must be worn. Under no circumstances should acids or bases be stored or placed on high shelves. These chemicals can be accidentally spilled into the eyes or onto exposed skin areas, resulting in severe burns.

Acid or base spills can be neutralized with sodium bicarbonate or zinc sulfate, respectively. Plastic containers containing these chemicals or similar reagents should be available wherever acids and bases are handled. A quantity of the solid greater than the volume of the spilled liquid is used to neutralize the spill, regardless of whether it is a concentrated reagent or not. The neutralizing chemical is mixed into the spill, and some water is added to provide the necessary solvent. After the spill has been neutralized, it is mopped up and rinsed with water. Commercially available spill kits are also effective and convenient.

If chemicals are splashed into the eyes, wash the eyes immediately at the eye wash station or at a sink with copious amounts of water. Be sure to wash both the upper and lower eye lids. After washing the eyes, neutralize the acid or base burns with a 5% solution of sodium bicarbonate or 3% boric acid, respectively. Take the victim to the emergency room at once. Eyewash bottles are only slightly better than nothing. They tend to be universally contaminated, inadequate in volume, difficult to use, and hard to find when needed.

If chemicals are spilled onto the body, they must be washed off with copious amounts of water under the safety shower or in a sink. Be careful that chemicals on the face are not washed into the eyes. Chemically soaked clothing must be removed immediately either by cutting or tearing.

Most laboratory thermometers contain mercury, and occasionally they are accidentally broken. Mercury is a poison that is cumulative, producing its effect via inhalation of vapors and absorption through the skin. The spilled mercury should be collected into a pool on a smooth surface by raking it with the side of a $3 \times 5$ inch card. Since mercury is very mobile, the raking is done slowly. If on a table top, the droplets of mercury can be pushed off the edge of the table into a beaker. If on the floor, the pool can be picked up with note cards or a suction flask with a trap. Once the spill has been picked up, the surface should be wiped with a damp sponge (droplets do not adhere to wet or dry sponges). The strokes should be slow and in one direction. As the droplets are collected, the sponge is washed off with water into a pan. The water is discarded and the remaining mercury is discarded as chemical waste. Excellent commercial spill kits for mercury are available.

## FLAMMABLE LIQUID HAZARDS

A flammable solvent is a liquid having a flash point below 60°C and a vapor pressure not exceeding 40 psi at 38°C. The quantity of flammable liquids in the laboratory must be kept to a minimum, stored safely, and used in a safe manner. Flammable fluids should be stored in nonflammable storage cabinets or in smaller nonflammable storage cans when the container size is one-half gallon or larger, or when the cumulative amount is greater than 2 gallons in one room. If storage cans are to be purchased, make sure before purchasing the container that the fluid can be easily poured from the can. Flammable fluids are not to be stored in a refrigerator, except if the laboratory procedure requires "cold extraction" with chilled solvents. Storage units must be of an explosion-proof design and clearly marked as such on the outside door. Be sure to mark refrigerators not meant to store flammables with a warning sign. Flammable fluids as well as acids and similar hazardous chemicals should be transported on carts only, not carried by hand. If a small quantity (single bottle) is going to be hand carried, it should be carried in a rubber bucket with both hands. Smoking is never permitted in elevators used to transport flammable solvents or in the areas where these reagents are located. After flammable solvents are used, they are discarded as chemical waste, and never flushed down the drain or thrown in the trash can. When working with flammable solvents, use the smallest container compatible with the test; keep a minimum supply in the laboratory; and anticipate accidents by removing ignition sources (turn off burners).

## WASTE DISPOSAL

### a. Chemical Waste

Chemical waste that is dangerous or potentially dangerous is usually decomposed, decontaminated, or buried in a landfill or other designated area. Arrangements should be made with a safety department for the pickup and burial of these materials. Flammable fluids and other chemicals are placed in their original containers and then properly sealed and labeled as to what they contain. These materials should never be washed down the drain, since chemical reactions can occur producing potentially dangerous fumes. In addition, these materials may inactivate sewage treatment facilities as well as destroy the plumbing system of the laboratory.

If the waste is not dangerous, is miscible in water, and the volume is less than a pint, these solvents can usually be flushed down the drain using large amounts of water. If the solvents are not miscible in water, or if the amount is greater than 1 pint, these materials should be discarded in a solvent waste can for later pickup and disposal.

### b. Solid Waste

Solid waste generally consists of needles and syringes, broken or chipped glassware, plastics and noncontaminated items, such as paper and packaging materials. For the protection of the laboratorian and the housekeeping staff, these basic types of materials should be disposed of in the proper manner.

Needles, syringes, and scalpels are especially dangerous because of the possibility of accidental puncture wounds or cuts. The range of possible infective agents encompasses hepatitis viruses from blood specimens to systemic pathogens in tissues. If these instruments are simply thrown in the trash can, housekeeping personnel become prime candidates for an accident, and possibly a subsequent mycotic infection. Needles, syringes, and scalpels should be discarded in a strong, leakproof, puncture proof container clearly labeled as containing contaminated waste. Caps should not be replaced over the needle once it is used. Commerically available wax-coated cardboard containers specifically manufactured for needle discard are ideal. In no instance should these items be discarded into the trash prior to autoclaving. Some states require that syringes be made inoperable prior to discard. By autoclaving these discard boxes prior to discard, the instruments are without doubt made inoperable.

Broken and chipped glassware is dangerous. Like needles, syringes, and scalpels, these glass items are never discarded into trash cans. Glassware to be discarded is placed into a strong cardboard box that is clearly labeled as containing broken glassware. Arrangements with the housekeeping department can be made for the safe disposal of this dangerous material. If there is any possibility of the glassware being contaminated, it must be autoclaved prior to discard. Empty bottles can simply be washed with water and then discarded.

Noncontaminated waste items, such as paper towels, packaging materials, and some plastics, are discarded directly into the trash. The trash cans in the laboratory should either be metal or UL approved in order to comply with Federal regulations.

Biologically contaminated waste is in many respects the most dangerous material dealt with in the medical mycology laboratory. There is always the possibility of infection if biologically contaminated waste is not dealt with properly. Biologically contaminated waste, that is, clinical specimens, materials contaminated with blood, plasma, or serum, inoculated media, cultures, glassware, slides, pipettes, and other potentially dangerous materials should be placed directly into discard pans containing 5% hyphochlorite or 5% aqueous phenol or a similar disinfectant (to prevent the formation of aerosols), or placed directly into autoclave bags that are clearly marked "contaminated." Autoclave bags are never sealed during autoclaving since sealed bags hamper the penetration of the steam. Lids on discard pans containing contaminated materials should be marked with autoclave tape. Prior to discarding contaminated items, they must be autoclaved to ensure that there are no viable organisms remaining. Discard noncontaminated disposable items in the trash, and wash and reuse nondisposable supplies. Disposable and nondisposable items should not be placed in the same discard pan; use separate pans or containers.

When handling cultures in Petri dishes, care must be exercised to ensure that the cover does not fly off, creating an aerosol. Since plastic Petri dishes are often difficult to handle in large numbers, use care when discarding them.

## SAFETY EQUIPMENT

Every medical mycology laboratory must have safety equipment readily available and each employee must be able to use it promptly and correctly. Training in the use of this equipment should be given with regular follow-up training. The basic equipment for the laboratory should include the following items.

a. Fire extinguisher, type A (for paper, wood, and similar materials)
b. Fire extinguisher, type B-C (flammable fluids or electrical)
c. First aid kit
d. Eye wash station, either mechanical or a squeeze bottle containing tap water (with 0.1% methyl paraben). If the latter is used, the water must be changed weekly. Tap water should be used in lieu of distilled water, since it contains residual chlorine.
e. Fire blanket
f. Emergency shower. Check it every 6 months.
g. Automatic pipetting devices
h. Splash proof face shield and safety goggles
i. Chemically resistant gloves and apron
j. Biological safety cabinet and chemical fume hood

## GAS CYLINDER STORAGE, TRANSPORT, AND USE

Gas cylinders may act like a rocket with enough force to penetrate a concrete wall if the tank falls and the valve is knocked off. Gas cylinders must always be secured to a wall or solid bench by tank straps or chains, and the valve safety cover must be kept on the valve until the pressure regulators or needle valves are ready to be attached. In addition to the possible rocket effect, the size and weight of gas cylinders can easily cause a serious injury if an employee is hit by a falling cylinder. Whenever a cylinder is moved, it is done so with a tank-carrying dolly or cart, the tank being strapped to the cart. Before a tank is moved, it is important to ensure that the protective valve cover is screwed over the valve to prevent the valve from being broken off in the event of an accident. Gas cylinders should always be stored in a cool location. One should never attempt to adapt valves, gauges, or fittings made for one type of gas (oxygen) with another type of gas. Never lubricate valves, regulators, or fittings, and be sure to mark empty tanks.

A gas cylinder that is not clearly marked or color coded as to its contents should neither be used nor be accepted from the vendor. To prevent damage and possible leaks, the regulators or needle valves should be tightened only with a nonadjustable wrench of the proper size. Pliers and adjustable wrenches can easily damage the fittings. Each cylinder should be tested for leaks with a soap solution or "Snoop$^R$" before the regulator or needle valve is attached in order to ensure that there are no leaks at the junction of the cylinder and the cylinder valve and in the valve. After the regulator is attached and the cylinder valve is opened, the valve stem packing, connecting fittings, regulator or needle valve, and the transfer lines should be tested for leaks too. If a cylinder leaks, it should be returned to the loading dock for pickup by the vendor. If the contents of the cylinder are hazardous, the safety department, local fire department, or military installation should be contacted immediately for instructions, disposal of the cylinder, or both.

## GROUNDING OF ELECTRICAL EQUIPMENT

All equipment in the medical mycology laboratory with three-prong plugs must be properly grounded. The third prong is the ground prong and should be connected to the metal frame of the piece of equipment and to the ground of the electrical circuit into which it plugs. The ground prong is never cut off in order to make the plug fit a two prong outlet. If the wall socket will not accept a three-prong plug, an adaptor can be used. This can be done only if the receptacle itself is properly grounded and when local building codes are followed. The adaptor will have a wire that must be attached to the ground of the outlet.

Proper grounding will prevent:
   a. Electrical shocks and burns
   b. Fires
   c. Faulty operation of the equipment
   d. Disruption of the laboratory routine and procedures

## Selected References

1. Center for Disease Control (1971). "Biological Safety Cabinet." Center for Disease Control, Atlanta, Georgia.
2. Center for Disease Control (1977). "Laboratory Safety at the Center for Disease Control," DHEW Publ. No. CDC 77-8118. Center for Disease Control, Atlanta, Georgia.
3. Environmental Services Branch (1974). "National Institutes of Health Biohazard Safety Guide," GPO stock No. 1740-00383. National Institutes of Health, Bethesda, Maryland.
4. Federal Supply Service (1973). "Federal Standard Clean Room and Work Station Requirements, Controlled Environment," Federal Standard No. 209B, April 24, 1973. General Services Administration, Washington, D.C.
5. Hanel, E., and R. H. Kruse (1967). "Laboratory-Acquired Mycoses," Misc. Publ. 18, Department of the Army, Fort Detrick, Maryland.
6. National Institutes of Health (1978). "National Institutes of Health Laboratory Safety Monograph. A Supplement to the NIH Guidelines for Recombinant DNA Research." National Institutes of Health, Bethesda, Maryland.
7. National Sanitation Foundation Advisory Committee (1976). "National Sanitation Foundation Standard No. 49 for Class II (Laminar Flow) Biohazard Cabinetry." National Sanitation Foundation, Ann Arbor, Michigan.
8. Steere, N. V., ed. (1976). "Handbook of Laboratory Safety," 2nd ed. Chemical Rubber Publ. Co., Cleveland, Ohio.

*Chapter 3*

# Clinical Specimens

### Part 1.  General Information

The principal goals of a sound clinical mycology laboratory are to isolate efficiently and identify accurately the suspected etiologic agents of fungal infections. Success in achieving these goals is, in part, dependent upon the quality of the clinical specimens sent to the mycology laboratory for study. Without appropriately collected, promptly transported, and correctly processed specimens, the results obtained may be of marginal value, or even meaningless.

Mycologists must always insist that clinical specimens be collected properly. If the specimens are unacceptable (Table 3.1), they should not be processed for mycological study. Poor quality specimens often result in incorrect information, which can adversely affect the patient concerned. If specimens of poor quality must be accepted, the attending physician should be required to assume all responsibility in writing for the specimens and their results. Such a requirement often results in a new clinical specimen being submitted for examination. All specimens that are sent to the laboratory for study, must be clearly labeled with the patient's name and unit number, date and time of collection, source of the specimen, and the name of the attending physician. Tables 3.1 and 3.2 summarize the major types of specimens usually submitted for mycological study and the principal genera of fungi they may contain.

There are approximately 30 different formulations and types of media routinely used in clinical laboratories for the recovery of medically important fungi. The more commonly used media are listed in Table 3.3. The selection of media to be used is based upon the experience of the mycologist and the fungi that are typically recovered in that particular geographical region. Before new procedures or media are introduced, they should always be compared to the current procedures and media utilized in the laboratory. What works well for one mycologist may not necessarily be ideal for another.

Table 3.1. Frequently Received Clinical Specimens for Mycological Study

| Specimens | Collection[a] | Unacceptable specimens | Direct mount | Processing[b] | Media[c] | Discard as negative |
|---|---|---|---|---|---|---|
| Abscess | Aseptically with needle and syringe from undrained abscesses; pus expressed from military abscesses opened with a scalpel | Swabs, material from open wounds | 10% KOH or PAS | Direct inoculation or centrifugation; process within 2 hours; refrigerate specimen prior to processing | 1 Tube each SAB agar, SAB+C+C, BHIA; 30°C | 4 Weeks |
| Biopsy (see Tissue) | | | | | | |
| Blood | 8.0 ml in yellow vacutainer containing Liquoid | Clotted blood | PAS, Giemsa, or Gram stain | Membrane filter or vented biphasic blood bottles; within 1 hour; maintain specimen at 37°C prior to processing | 1 Plate SAB agar, if blood bottles used; subculture each 48 hours to 1 tube each SAB agar and BHIA; 30°C | 2 Weeks; 4 weeks if blood bottles are used |
| Bone marrow | 0.2–0.3 ml in a heparinized syringe | Clotted bone marrow | PAS or Giemsa | Direct inoculation; process within 2 hours; maintain specimen at 37°C prior to processing | 1 Tube each SAB agar, Sabhi with blood, SAB+C+C; 30°C | 4 Weeks, 12 weeks if *Histoplasma* is suspected |
| Bronchial brush | Brush for mycological study in sterile container | Dried specimen | 10% KOH or PAS | Direct inoculation of tissue fragments to media, brush placed in broth; within 2 hours; refrigerate specimen prior to processing | 1 Tube each SAB agar, SAB+C+C, BHIA; brush in a tube of BHI broth; 30°C | 4 Weeks |
| Bronchial washing (See Sputum) | | | | | | |

| | | | | | |
|---|---|---|---|---|---|
| Cerebrospinal fluid | 3.0 ml in a sterile tube | Insufficient quantity | India ink; at least 3 smears are necessary before considering specimen negative | Membrane filter or direct inoculation; process within 2 hours; refrigerate specimen prior to processing | 1 Plate SAB agar; if direct plating is used, 1 tube each SAB agar, BHIA; 30°C | 2 Weeks |
| Fluids | Sterile tube, or heparinized syringe | Swabs | 10% KOH or PAS | Direct inoculation or centrifugation; process within 2 hours; refrigerate specimen prior to processing | 1 Tube each SAB agar, SAB+C+C, BHIA; 30°C | 4 Weeks |
| Hair | Hair and base of shaft; sterile Petri dish, between 2 clean glass microscope slides, or in paper envelope | Hair clippings | 10% KOH or PAS | Direct inoculation; specimen may be kept up to several days prior to processing at 25°C | 1 Tube each SAB agar, SAB+C+C; 30°C | 4 Weeks |
| Nails | Clean site with 70% ethanol; collect shavings and material under the nail plate; discard first 4 or 5 scrapings; sterile Petri dish or in paper envelope | Swabs and random nail clipping | 10% KOH, KOH-DMSO, or PAS | Pulverize nails; direct inoculation; specimens may be kept up to several days prior to processing at 25°C | 1 Tube each SAB agar, SAB+C+C; 30°C | 4 Weeks |
| Serology | Serum, 1.0–2.0 ml, 1 : 1000 parts merthiolate/ml of serum final concentration; remove serum aseptically; 3.0–5.0 ml of spinal fluid with same concentration merthiolate, paired sera | Specimens collected after skin testing with histoplasmin; nonpaired specimens; contaminated specimens | None | None | None | None |

*(continued)*

Table 3.1. (Continued)

| Specimens | Collection[a] | Unacceptable specimens | Direct mount | Processing[b] | Media[c] | Discard as negative |
|---|---|---|---|---|---|---|
| Skin scrapings | Clean site with 70% ethanol; center and edge of lesion, any exudate; sterile Petri dish, between 2 clean microscope slides, or in paper envelope | Swabs | 10% KOH or PAS | Direct inoculation, except pityriasis versicolor, which is not cultured | 1 Tube each SAB agar, SAB+C+C; 30°C | 4 Weeks |
| Sputum | 5.0–10.0 ml; early morning, prior to eating, use mouth rinse and brush teeth; sterile sputum cup | Saliva, nasal secretions, throat swabs, and specimens in fecal cups, 24-hour collections | 10% KOH or PAS | Direct inoculation of suspicious material, NALC digestion, process within 2–4 hours; refrigerate specimen prior to processing | 1 Tube each SAB, agar, SAB+C+C, 1 plate of yeast-extract phosphate medium; 30°C | 4 Weeks, 12 weeks if *Histoplasma* is suspected |
| Tissue | Between 2 sterile gauze pads, sterile Petri dish or tube; if latter, add 2.0–3.0 ml of sterile water or broth (SAB, BHI), but not thioglycolate; center, edge, and normal tissue of lesion | Swabs | 10% KOH or PAS | Direct inoculation of suspicious material, homogenize tissue, process within 2–4 hours; refrigerate prior to processing. If a zygomycete is suspected, use a tube containing sterile bread without preservatives or malt extract agar with chloramphenicol | 1 Tube each SAB agar, SAB+C+C, 1 plate of yeast-extract phosphate medium; 30°C | 4 Weeks; 12 weeks if *Histoplasma* is suspected |

| | | | | |
|---|---|---|---|---|
| Urine | 25.0–50.0 ml; suprapubic aspirate, catheterized, or clean catch specimen, first morning specimen, in sterile container | 24-hour collection; specimens other than clean catch, suprapubic aspirate, or catheterized specimens | 10% KOH, PAS or Gram stain | Centrifugation; process within 2–4 hours; refrigerate prior to processing | 1 Tube each SAB agar, SAB+C+C, BHIA: 30°C | 2 Weeks |
| Vaginal | Moist swabs from vagina, in sterile container | In transport medium, dry swabs | 10% KOH | Direct inoculation | 1 Tube SAB agar with chloramphenicol; 30°C | 2 Weeks |

---

[a] Specimens should be kept moist with sterile distilled water or saline, except dermatological specimens.

[b] NALC, N-acetyl-L-cysteine.

[c] SAB agar, Sabouraud dextrose agar, 2% glucose; SAB+C+C, Sabouraud dextrose agar with cycloheximide and chloramphenicol, Mycosel or Mycobiotic agar; BHIA, brain heart infusion agar.

Table 3.2. Clinical Specimens and Commonly Suspected Fungi

| Clinical specimens | Principal genera of pathogenic fungi frequently encountered (alphabetical order) |
| --- | --- |
| Blood | *Candida, Cryptococcus, Histoplasma, Torulopsis* |
| Bone and bone marrow | *Blastomyces, Cryptococcus, Histoplasma* |
| Cerebrospinal fluid | *Candida, Coccidioides, Cryptococcus, Histoplasma* |
| Corneal scrapings | *Aspergillus, Candida, Fusarium* |
| External auditory canal debris | *Aspergillus, Candida* |
| Hair | *Microsporum, Piedraia, Trichophyton, Trichosporon* |
| Joint fluids | *Blastomyces, Coccidioides, Sporothrix* |
| Mucocutaneous tissue | *Candida, Paracoccidioides* |
| Nails | *Aspergillus, Candida, Epidermophyton, Microsporum, Scopulariopsis, Trichophyton* |
| Nasal tissue | *Absidia, Aspergillus, Mucor, Rhinosporidium, Rhizopus* |
| Prostate fluid | *Blastomyces, Coccidioides* |
| Skin | *Candida, Blastomyces,* Chromoblastomycosis (*Cladosporium, Fonsecaea, Phialophora*), *Coccidioides, Cryptococcus* (rare), *Epidermophyton, Histoplasma, Malassezia* (in direct mounts only), *Microsporum,* Mycetoma (*Acremonium, Scedosporium*), *Trichophyton* |
| Sputum and bronchial washings | *Aspergillus, Blastomyces, Candida, Coccidioides, Cryptococcus, Geotrichum, Histoplasma, Mucor, Paracoccidioides, Rhizopus, Sporothrix* |
| Subcutaneous tissue and abscesses | *Blastomyces, Cladosporium, Coccidioides, Cryptococcus, Exophiala, Fonsecaea, Histoplasma, Loboa, Phialophora, Sporothrix* |
| Urine | *Candida, Cryptococcus, Histoplasma, Torulopsis* |
| Vaginal specimens | *Candida* |

Whenever a medium containing antimicrobial agents is used, a second medium without these agents is necessary. It cannot be assumed that the fungi present in a particular clinical specimen are resistant to the antimicrobial agents in the isolation medium. Under no circumstances should media containing antimicrobial agents be incubated at elevated temperatures, specifically, 37°C. At an elevated temperature, many fungi that are not normally sensitive to these agents may become so. As an example, the yeast form of *Histoplasma capsulatum* is sensitive to the antibacterial agent chloramphenicol at 37°C.

An ideal combination of media for the primary recovery of pathogenic fungi includes Sabouraud dextrose agar (SAB agar), Mycosel or Mycobiotic agar, and brain heart infusion agar (BHIA) with or without sheep blood. Sheep blood is used in lieu of human blood because human blood often contains inhibitory substances. C. W. Emmons' modification of SAB agar is recommended. This modification contains 2% glucose and has a pH reaction that is near neutral. Fungi grow much better on media with low concentrations of glucose and a slightly acid pH reaction. Standard SAB agar, which contains 4% glucose and has an acidic pH reaction, is primarily used for studying the colonial morphology of the dermatophytes. Mycosel or Mycobiotic agar, which are commercially available media, is included as a selective medium for the recovery of dimorphic fungi and dermatophytes. The cycloheximide in these media inhibit the growth of many moulds and yeast, whereas the chloramphenicol suppresses bacterial contamination. Since a number of opportunistic pathogens such as species of *Scopulariopsis, Aspergillus, Candida, Cryptococcus neoformans,* and others are sensitive to cycloheximide, care must be exercised when using a medium that contains this material. As a complement to the SAB agar and a medium containing cycloheximide and chloramphenicol, an enriched medium, such as BHIA, is occasionally necessary. Enriched media are helpful in recovering the dimorphic fungi. Sabhi with blood is especially suited for the recovery of *H. capsulatum.* For contaminated clinical specimens, yeast-extract phosphate medium is ideal for the recovery of *H. capsulatum, Blastomyces dermatitidis,* and *Coccidioides immitis.*

Medically important fungi can be extremely dangerous. Care must always be exercised in selecting the containers for the isolation media. The most dangerous container is the Petri dish. Petri dishes are not recommended (except yeast-extract phosphate medium) because when they are opened a dangerous aerosol is created; the media rapidly dehydrate; and dishes are easily contaminated. The large surface area and the ease in reaching colonies represents a distinct advantage of Petri dishes. The greater the amount of the clinical specimen that is touching the medium surface, the greater is the opportunity of recovering fungi present in the specimen. If dishes are used, they should be sealed with parafilm or placed in plastic bags for safety and to retard the dehydration process. Many mycologists prefer to use screw-cap bottles in lieu of Petri dishes. Bottles offer a great deal of safety and a reasonable surface area. Bottles, however, have one distinct disadvantage, that is, they have a narrow neck which makes it nearly impossible to reach colonies that are just beneath the opening. Standard 16 × 125 mm test tubes are not recommended because of the tremendously reduced surface area. Test tubes are extremely safe

Table 3.3. Principal Media for the Recovery of Fungi

| Medium | Comments |
| --- | --- |
| Blood agar | This medium is used for the recovery of opportunistic and dimorphic pathogens. Antimicrobial agents, such as penicillin and streptomycin, are usually incorporated into the medium. Blood agar is not used for hair, nail, or skin specimens. |
| Blood heart infusion agar (BHIA) | Blood heart infusion agar is used for the recovery of opportunistic and dimorphic pathogens. Antimicrobial agents, such as penicillin and streptomycin, may be incorporated into the medium. BHIA is commonly used as a complement to SAB agar and a medium containing cycloheximide. Many dimorphic fungi will develop their tissue form at 37°C on this medium. BHIA is not used for hair, nail, or skin specimens. |
| Brain heart infusion biphasic blood culture medium | This medium is used only for the recovery of fungi from blood specimens. It is recommended when the filtration technique is not being used for the recovery of fungi from blood specimens. Trypticase soy biphasic medium is equivalent to BHI biphasic medium. |
| Bread | Sterile bread (without preservatives) in cotton-plugged test tubes is recommended for the recovery of Zygomycetes from clinical specimens. Bread is often superior to other media used in the clinical mycology laboratory for recovering this group of opportunistic pathogens. |
| Caffeic acid agar | Caffeic acid agar is employed when *Cryptococcus neoformans* is suspected. The distinctive black colonies aid in recognizing this opportunistic pathogen. This medium is not used for definitive identifications. |
| Dermatophyte test medium (DTM) | Dermatophyte test medium was designed to recover dermatophytes from patients in the tropics. The medium is supplemented with cycloheximide, gentamicin, and chlortetracycline. The medium is not recommended, except when hair, nail, or skin specimens are heavily contaminated with bacteria. Many nondermatrophytes will turn this medium red. Fungi on DTM exhibit atypical colonial and microscopic morphology. If DTM is used, only hair, nail, or skin is inoculated onto it. |

Table 3.3. *Continued*

| Medium | Comments |
| --- | --- |
| Media with cycloheximide | Mycosel (BBL) and Mycobiotic agar (Difco) are two excellent commercially prepared media. One of these media is used as a complement to SAB agar and BHIA. They both contain 1% glucose and cycloheximide and chloramphenicol. The two brands differ in their peptones and concentrations of antimicrobial agents. These media are used for the selective recovery of dimorphic fungi and dermatophytes. |
| Sabhi | Sabhi, especially Sabhi with sheep blood, was designed for the recovery of *Histoplasma capsulatum* and *Blastomyces dermatitidis*. The medium consists of one-half SAB agar and one-half BHIA that is supplemented with chloromycetin. Sabhi is useful as a complement to SAB agar and a medium containing cycloheximide. It is not used for hair, nail, or skin specimens. |
| Sabouraud dextrose agar (SAB agar) | A number of formulations of Sabouraud dextrose agar are utilized by different mycologists. The original formulation contains 4% glucose (pH 5.6), which is ideal for studying dermatophyte colony morphology. C. W. Emmons' modification contains 2% glucose (pH 6.5) and is the medium of choice for recovery of opportunistic and dimorphic fungi from clinical specimens. Various antimicrobials, such as cycloheximide, chloramphenicol, gentamicin, penicillin, streptomycin, or tellurite, have been added to SAB agar by various microbiologists. |
| Yeast extract–phosphate medium | A yeast extract–phosphate medium supplemented with chloramphenicol and ammonium hydroxide has been developed for the enhanced recovery of *Blastomyces dermatitidis* and *Histoplasma capsulatum* from contaminated clinical specimens. The medium is used in Petri dishes. |

and there is no difficulty in reaching colonies. The 25 × 125 mm test tube makes an ideal container because it is safe and has adequate surface area. When screw-cap containers are used, they should never be tightly screwed since this inhibits gas exchange, which may suppress growth and sporulation.

The inoculated media should be incubated at 30°C; if a 30°C incubator is not available, then the media should be incubated at 25°C. A temperature of 30°C is ideal for the recovery of fungi because most of the medically important fungi will grow optimally at this temperature. That a fungus can cause disease at 37°C does not necessarily mean that the fungus will grow well at 37°C in the laboratory. The incubation of media at 37°C is unnecessary and wasteful. If *Aspergillus fumigatus* is suspected, an additional set of media can be incubated at 46–48°C since this mould is thermotolerant and will rapidly grow at that temperature.

Cultures are usually kept for 4–6 weeks, depending upon the specimen and the suspected etiologic agents before they are discarded as negative. If *H. capsulatum* is suspected, the cultures should be held for 12 weeks before being discarded. A significant number of *H. capsulatum* isolates are not seen until 10–12 weeks of incubation. Each culture should be examined every 2–3 days for the presence of new growth. Cultures should not be discarded as soon as a fungus is isolated. Instead, they should be kept for the entire period of incubation to ensure that other more slowly growing fungi are not overlooked.

Once the properly labeled clinical specimen has been received, it should be grossly examined for the presence of particles, caseous, purulent, bloody areas, and necrotic material. These materials are selectively examined microscopically (Tables 3.4 and 3.5) and then inoculated selectively to media. Observing a fungus in a clinical specimen can often be more valuable than merely isolating one without seeing it in the specimen. For example, the isolation of a species of *Rhizopus* may be meaningless, but the observation of hyphae compatible with *Rhizopus* in tissue is diagnostic of zygomycosis.

Once the clinical specimens have been examined macroscopically, suspicious areas are placed in 10% KOH or NaOH and then examined microscopically with either a bright-field or phase-contrast microscope. The KOH preparation is ideal for determining fungal morphology, and whether or not the fungus is dematiaceous. Potassium or sodium hydroxide is used because it readily dissolves the clinical material, but not the fungus. The chitinous cell walls of fungi are somewhat resistant to the hydroxide. Within a few days, the fungus will also be dissolved by the hydroxide unless glycerol has been added to the KOH solution. The clearing effect of the clinical material can be accelerated by gently warming the preparation. Direct examination of clinical specimens provides important information for the physician and the mycologist. The morphology of the fungus, such as the presence of branching, septate hyphae of *Aspergillus fumigatus*, can alert the physician that a particular fungus is probably causing disease. When hyphae compatible with a zygomycete are present, the mycologist can modify the isolation protocols and include sterile bread or malt extract agar with chloramphenicol as an additional isolation medium.

A number of other techniques are available for examining clinical specimens microscopically. For specimens such as spinal fluid, the India ink preparation is excellent. In this technique, ink is used as a dark background to highlight the hyaline yeast cells and any capsular material around them. The India ink technique is not a staining procedure. Many physicians erroneously interpret a positive India ink preparation to be synonymous with *Cryptococcus neoformans*. The India ink preparation is a technique for observation, not identification. Care must be exercised when reporting information gained from this and similar techniques to the physician.

In many instances, fungi are not readily apparent in the clinical specimens. This is especially true with nail and skin (stratum corneum) scrapings. The periodic acid–Schiff stain (PAS) is an excellent staining technique for demonstrating fungi. The staining technique requires additional supplies that are not normally available in the clinical laboratory. However, they are typically present in the pathology laboratory. This technique is not routinely utilized in many laboratories. Burke's modification of the Gram stain is useful for demonstrating the presence of Gram-positive filaments of the actinomycetes, as well as yeasts such as species of *Candida*. There is often substantial distortion of fungi when they are Gram stained. Thus, the Gram stain is of limited mycological value, but it is extremely valuable for determining the degree of bacterial contamination of clinical specimens. Another helpful staining procedure is the Giemsa stain. It is excellent for demonstrating the presence of intracellular yeast cells of *H. capsulatum* in specimens such as bone marrow.

Once the clinical specimens have been examined macroscopically and microscopically, they are ready to be processed and inoculated onto isolation media (Table 3.3). If processing of the specimen must be delayed, antibacterial agents should be added unless an actinomycete infection is suspected. Specimens may be refrigerated (not frozen), but refrigeration should never be used as an excuse for not promptly processing a clinical specimen. Delays in processing will significantly contribute to decreased yields of potential pathogens. Many mycologists prefer to concentrate sputa prior to inoculating the isolation media. This has the advantage of concentrating potential pathogens, but it also concentrates unwanted bacteria and other fungi. Yeast-extract phosphate medium should be used for the recovery of dimorphic fungi from contaminated specimens. The decision to concentrate sputa must be decided by each individual. Without doubt, blood and spinal fluid specimens for mycological study should be processed by the filtration technique. This technique permits the recovery of fungi in 2–3 days, instead of up to 4 weeks in the standard blood bottle

**Table 3.4.** Examination of Clinical Specimens Other Than Hair, Nail, and Stratum Corneum

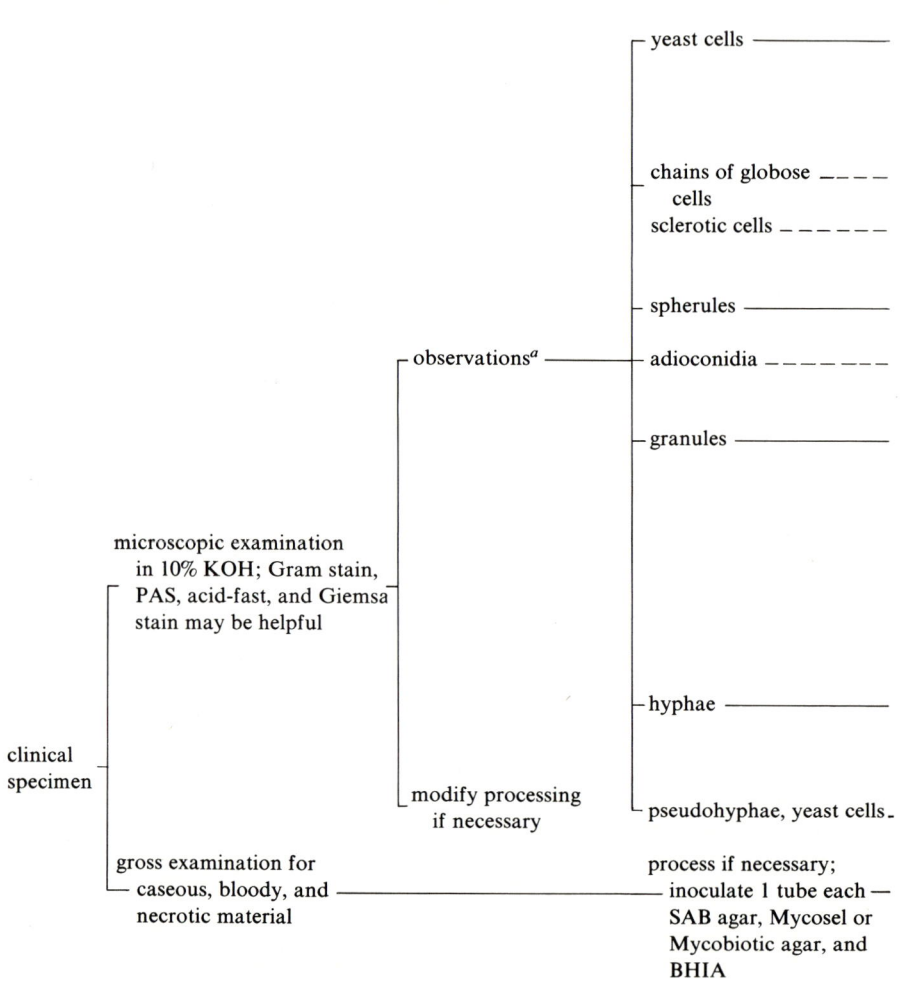

[a] Principal morphology and genera of fungi.
[b] African isolates. Yeast cells are of two sizes: 7–15 μm and 2–3 μm.
[c] Considered by some mycologists to be *Emmonsia*.

# Part 1 General Information

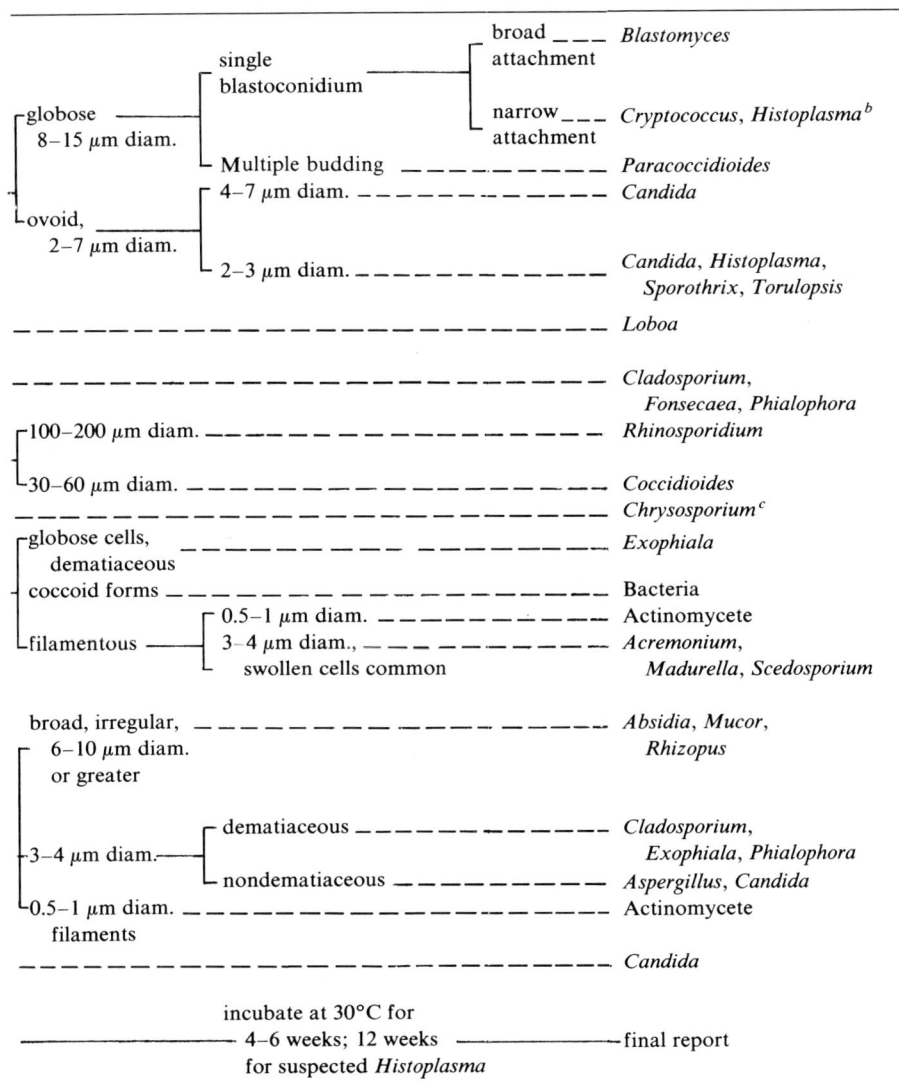

**Table 3.5.** Examination of Hair, Nail, and Stratum Corneum

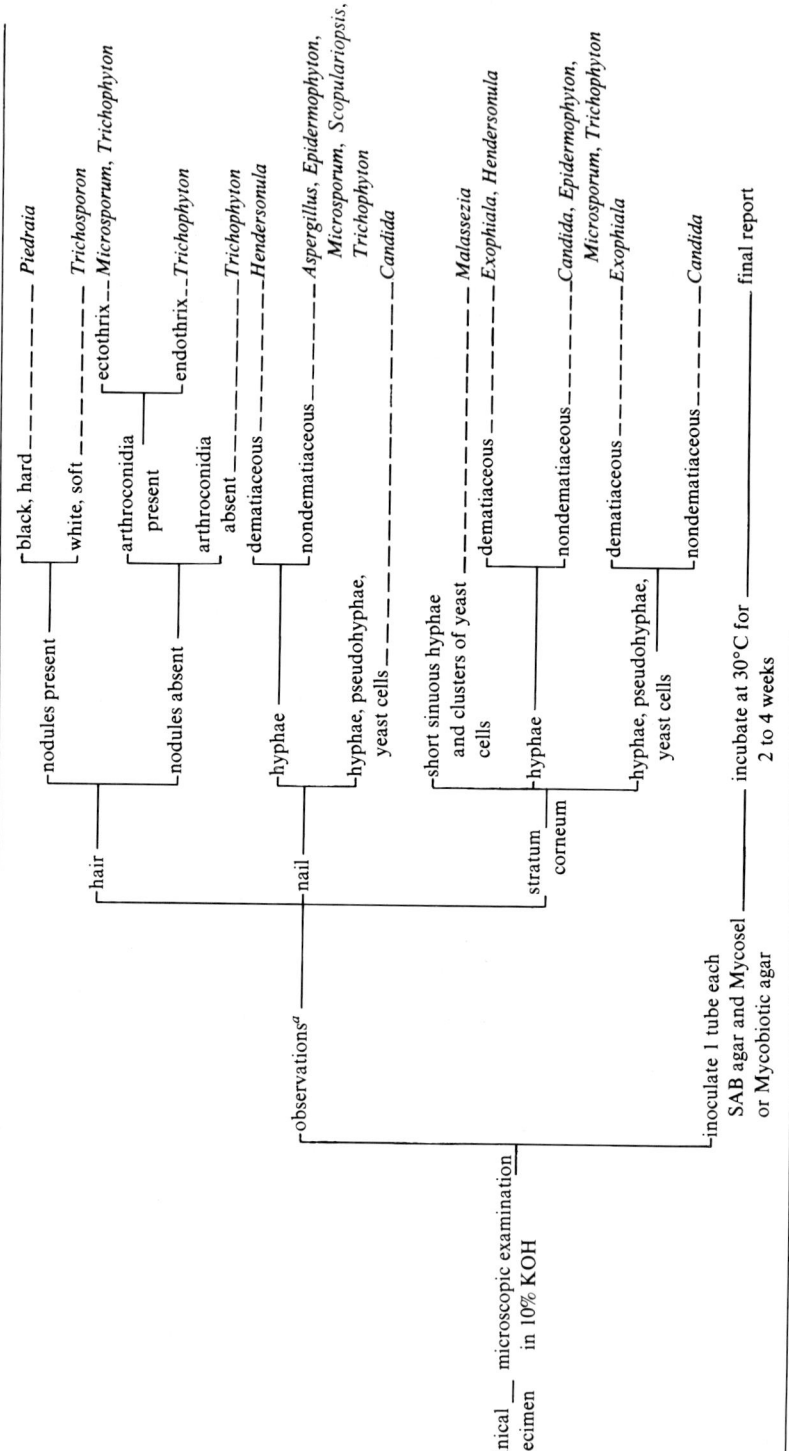

[a] Principal morphology and genera of fungi.

culture techniques. In addition to retaining all the fungal cells present in the specimen on the membrane surface, the fungi can be washed free of antimicrobial, fungistatic, and fungicidal substances that may be present in the clinical specimen. If the filtration technique is not utilized for the recovery of fungi in blood specimens, vented BHIA biphasic blood culture bottles are recommended.

After the fungi are recovered and the cultures have been purified, they should be identified. It is important to identify the fungi recovered to the species level (when appropriate), especially the yeasts. This is important for three reasons. First, unless fungi of medical importance are identified to the species level, we will not know the identity of the pathogens; which ones are predominant in different geographical regions; and which fungi are declining or emerging. Second, the diagnosis of an opportunistic mycosis often requires the demonstration of the same fungus from more than one body site, or the repeated recovery of the same species from repeated specimens. These decisions cannot be made unless the fungus is properly identified. Finally, the identity of the fungus can be a helpful guide to chemotherapy. For example, *C. neoformans* rapidly develops resistance to 5-fluorocytosine during therapy, whereas many other yeasts do not. The probable response to antimycotic agents based upon the identification of the fungus can be important while waiting for susceptibility data.

In small laboratories, clinical specimens and isolates are often mailed to reference laboratories for mycological study and identification assistance. Before a specimen is sent through the mails, the reference laboratory should be contacted for specific instructions pertaining to how specimens are to be prepared for shipment. These instructions will include information on the use of antimicrobial agents, refrigeration requirements, inoculation of media, and other topics. Under no circumstances should Petri dishes be sent through the mails. Dishes are frequently broken and contaminated. Whenever clinical materials or cultures are sent from one laboratory to another, the packaging must conform to federal regulations. These regulations are discussed in Chapter 7.

## Part 1. Selected References

### A. General

1. Ajello, L. (1951). Collecting specimens for the laboratory demonstration and isolation of fungi. *J. Am. Med. Assoc.* **146**:1581–1583.
2. Ajello, L., L. K. Georg, W. Kaplan, and L. Kaufman (1966). "Laboratory Manual for Medical Mycology." U.S. Government Printing Office, Washington, D.C.

3. Brewer, N. S., and L. A. Weed (1976). Diagnostic tissue microbiology methods. *Hum. Pathol.* **7**:141–149.
4. Haley, L. D., and C. S. Callaway (1978). "Laboratory Methods in Medical Mycology," 4th ed., DHEW Publ. No. (CDC) 78-8361. Center for Disease Control, Atlanta, Georgia.
5. Matsen, J. M., and G. M. Ederer (1976). Specimen collection and transport. *Hum. Pathol.* **7**:297–307.
6. Roberts, G. D. (1976). Laboratory diagnosis of fungal infections. *Hum. Pathol.* **7**:161–168.
7. Seabury, J. H., H. A. Buechner, J. F. Busey, L. K. Georg, and C. C. Campbell (1971). The diagnosis of pulmonary mycoses. Report of the committee on fungus diseases and subcommittee on criteria for clinical diagnosis, American College of Chest Physicians. *Chest* **60**:82–86.

## B. Media

1. Bump, C. M. (1973). A survey of procedures used in clinical mycology laboratories. *Am. J. Med. Technol.* **39**:40–51.
2. Caplan, L. M., and W. G. Merz (1978). Evaluation of two commercially prepared biphasic media for recovery of fungi from blood. *J. Clin. Microbiol.* **8**:469–470.
3. Gorman, J. W. (1967). Sabhi, a new culture medium for pathogenic fungi. *Am. J. Med. Technol.* **33**:151–157.
4. Odds, F. C., C. A. Hall, and A. B. Abbott (1978). Peptones and mycological reproductivity. *Sabouraudia* **16**:237–246.
5. Roberts, G. D. (1976). Laboratory diagnosis of fungal infections. *Hum. Pathol.* **7**:161–168.
6. Smith, C. D., and N. L. Goodman (1975). Improved culture method for the isolation of *Histoplasma capsulatum* and *Blastomyces dermatitidis* from contaminated specimens. *Am. J. Clin. Pathol.* **63**:276–280.
7. Smith, R. F., D. Blasi, and S. L. Dayton (1974). Evaluation of media for selective isolation of yeasts from oral, rectal, and burn wound specimens. *Appl. Microbiol.* **28**:112–116.
8. Taplin, D., N. Zaias, G. Rebell, and H. Blank (1969). Isolation and recognition of dermatophytes on a new medium (DTM). *Arch. Dermatol.* **99**:203–209.
9. Thompson, D. W., W. Kaplan, and B. J. Phillips (1977). The effect of freezing and the influence of isolation medium on the recovery of pathogenic fungi from sputum. *Mycopathologia* **61**:105–109.

## Part 2. Techniques

### ABSCESS SPECIMENS

Abscess material is aseptically aspirated from undrained abscesses with a sterile needle and syringe. Pus from miliary abscesses is collected by expressing this material after the abscesses have been opened with a sterile scalpel. The abscess specimens are collected aseptically in sterile tubes and then transported to the laboratory. Swabs are unsatisfactory.

The material is inoculated directly onto the isolation media. If a large amount of this material is available, it can be centrifuged for 15 minutes at 2500 rpm. A small amount of sterile saline or distilled water can be added to it. This makes it easier to find fungal structures and gives a better sediment. If the pus is extremely thick, it can be concentrated by the NALC technique (see sputum). The sediment is then inoculated directly onto isolation media. The media are incubated at 30°C and examined every 2–3 days. The cultures are discarded as negative after 4 weeks. All fungi recovered are identified.

## BLOOD SPECIMENS

Positive blood cultures may result from septicemia or fungemia. Fungemias are usually due to localized colonization at the site of insertion of indwelling intravenous catheters. To distinguish between septicemia and fungemia, take the following steps.

a. Prepare a smear and then culture a portion of the blood that was drawn from the intravenous catheter just prior to its removal from the patient.
b. Prepare a smear and then culture the catheter tip and any exudate that is present at the insertion site. The smears are stained either by the PAS or Giemsa technique.
c. Repeat the blood cultures from the arm that did not have the catheter.
d. Rapidly identify all the fungi isolated.

There are two approaches for the culturing of blood specimens. By far, the membrane filter technique is superior to the vented blood bottle procedure.

1. Membrane filter technique
    a. Collection of blood
        (1) Aseptically collect approximately 8.0 ml of blood in a yellow stoppered Vacutainer containing 0.05% Liquoid (1.7 ml of 0.35% sodium polyanethol sulfonate).
        (2) Mix the blood and anticoagulant thoroughly.
        (3) Place the specimen in a 37°C incubator until processed; do not wait longer than 1 hour.

b. Processing
   (1) A membrane filtration apparatus with a 0.45 μm membrane is used.
   (2) Place 50.0 ml of sterile Triton X-100 solution (0.2%) into the filter apparatus.
   (3) Transfer 4.0 ml of the blood from the Vacutainer to the Triton X-100 solution followed by 2.0 ml of varidase and 50.0 ml of sterile 0.08% sodium carbonate solution.
   (4) Mix by gently rotating the filter apparatus.
   (5) Allow the apparatus to sit for 2–3 minutes, until the erythrocytes are lysed.
   (6) Turn on the vacuum. If the specimen fails to filter, disconnect the vacuum and allow the apparatus to stand for an additional 20–30 minutes. Turn on the vacuum.
   (7) After the contents have passed through the filter, wash the membrane with approximately 50.0 ml of sterile distilled water to remove any residual lysing solution.
   (8) Turn off the vacuum.
   (9) With a sterile scalpel and forceps, remove the membrane from the apparatus and then place it onto SAB agar in a Petri dish, with the inoculated surface of the membrane up. Seal the dish with parafilm or put it in a plastic bag.
   (10) Incubate at 30°C and examine daily for the presence of growth. Growth will be present on the membrane surface in about 18–24 hours.
   (11) Identify all fungi isolated.
2. Routine blood culture
   a. Collection of blood
      (1) Same as for the membrane filter technique.
   b. Processing
      (1) A ratio of 1:10 to 1:20 (blood to broth) is utilized, a minimum of 5.0 ml of blood being required for each culture bottle.
      (2) Inoculate a BHIA biphasic blood bottle and mix the contents well.
      (3) Vent the bottle and incubate at 30°C.
      (4) Prepare smears (PAS, Gram, or Giemsa) and subculture every 2 days onto SAB agar. The agar surface in the blood bottle is examined daily for the presence of colonies. Also wash the broth across the agar surface daily. The bottles are discarded as negative after 4 weeks.
      (5) Identify all fungi isolated.

## BONE MARROW SPECIMENS

Bone marrow specimens are primarily obtained for the isolation of species of *Candida, Cryptococcus neoformans,* and *Histoplasma capsulatum*. Approximately 0.2–0.3 ml of bone marrow are collected aseptically in a heparinized syringe from the sternum or iliac crest. The syringe containing the bone marrow specimen is immediately brought to the clinical laboratory for processing. A smear of this material should be stained by the Giemsa technique.

The specimen is inoculated onto the isolation media. Fragments of marrow from one of the inoculated tubes are removed, mounted in 10% KOH, and then examined microscopically. The syringe should be rinsed with BHI broth, which is then incubated along with the other isolation media. The cultures are incubated at 30°C and examined every 2–3 days. The cultures are discarded after 4 weeks unless *H. capsulatum* is suspected. These are discarded after 12 weeks because many isolates of *H. capsulatum* are not seen until 10–12 weeks of incubation. All fungi recovered are identified.

## CEREBROSPINAL FLUID

Cerebrospinal fluid (CSF) is obtained via lumbar puncture when infections of the central nervous system are suspected. At least 3.0 ml of fluid are necessary for adequate mycological study.

1. Membrane filter technique
    a. Centrifuge the CSF specimen for 15 minutes at 2000 rpm.
    b. Without decanting the supernatant, remove a small amount of the sediment with a sterile capillary pipette.
    c. Place the sediment in either a drop of sterile distilled water or a drop of India ink on a clean microscope slide, and then cover with a cover glass. Examine by phase-contrast or bright-field microscopy.
    d. If the direct preparation is negative for fungi, prepare two additional smears before calling the direct observations negative.
    e. Resuspend the CSF by shaking the tube on a Vortex mixer.
    f. Pass the entire specimen through a sterile membrane filtration apparatus with a 0.45 $\mu$m filter.
    g. Rinse the membrane filter with several milliliters of SAB broth. If the patient is receiving antimycotic therapy, wash the sediment with an additional 50–60 ml of SAB broth.

    h.  With a sterile scalpel and forceps, remove the membrane and place it onto SAB agar in a Petri dish. The inoculated surface of the membrane is placed surface up. Seal the dish with parafilm or put it into a plastic bag. This is necessary to retard the dehydration process.
    i.  Incubate the medium at 30°C and examine every 2–3 days. Growth should be present on the membrane surface in about 24–48 hours. Discard as negative after 2 weeks.
    j.  Identify all fungi isolated.
2. Routine culture technique
    a.  The specimen is handled as in steps a–d in the membrane filter technique.
    b.  Place 0.1 ml of the sediment in tubes containing SAB agar and Sabhi agar.
    c.  Resuspend the remaining sediment and pipette it to a tube containing BHIA.
    d.  Incubate the media at 30°C and examine every 2–3 days. Discard the cultures as negative after 2 weeks.
    e.  Identify all fungi isolated.

## FLUIDS

Bloody specimens should be collected in a heparinized syringe. If the volume is small, fluids are inoculated directly onto the isolation media. If the volume is large, they should be concentrated.

1. Transfer the specimen to sterile 50 ml plastic centrifuge tubes.
2. Centrifuge the specimen for 15 minutes at 2500 rpm.
3. Decant the supernatant and inoculate the sediment with a sterile pipette onto the isolation media. One-tenth milliliter of sediment is inoculated to each tube of medium.
4. Prepare a 10% KOH preparation and examine by bright-field or phase-contrast microscopy.
5. Incubate the media at 30°C and examine every 2–3 days. Discard as negative after 4 weeks.
6. Identify all fungi recovered.

## HAIR

The patient's scalp should be examined with a Wood's lamp for the presence of fluorescing hairs. Not all fungi that invade hair induce fluorescing hairs. When examining patients with a Wood's lamp, allow your eyes to become adjusted to the darkness first, and in the case of older models of lamps, allow the lamp to warm up. With sterile forceps, collect fluorescent hairs or broken hairs for direct examination and culture. Infected hairs are typically loose in the follicles. If epilation of hairs with forceps is difficult (young patients), place a strip of clear tape over the lesion and then remove the tape. Hairs are transported to the laboratory in a Petri dish, between two microscope slides, or in a clean envelope.

1. With sterile forceps, place 1 or 2 hair fragments into a drop of 10% KOH and then cover with a cover glass. Pass the slide several times through a flame.
2. Immediately observe by bright-field or phase-contrast microscopy. Air bubbles racing down the hair shaft are suggestive of *Trichophyton schoenleinii*. The PAS stain may be required if unsatisfactory results are obtained with the 10% KOH preparation.
3. Place 3 or 4 hairs onto a slant of SAB agar and Mycosel or Mycobiotic agar.
4. Incubate the cultures at 30°C and examine every 2–3 days. Discard negative cultures at 3 weeks.
5. Identify dermatophytes to species.

Hair invasion is usually either ectothrix or endothrix. Ectothrix invasion is characterized by the presence of arthroconidia on the outside of the hair shaft and a cuticle that is destroyed. Endothrix hair invasion is characterized by the development of arthroconidia within the hair shaft. The cuticle of the hair shaft is intact.

## NAILS

Nail scrapings are collected by shaving nails that have been cleaned with 70% ethanol. The scrapings are collected from the proximal to the distal end of the nail. The first 4 or 5 scrapings are discarded. The debris under the nail plate should also be collected. Swabs are never used to collect dermatological specimens because fibers can be confused with hyphae in the scrapings. The specimens also typically become trapped in the fibers. The nail scrapings are placed in a sterile Petri dish, between two microscope slides, or in a clean envelope. Large pieces of nail material should be pulverized in a sterile nail pulverizing mill prior to microscopic examination and culture.

1. Place several nail fragments into a drop of 10% KOH and then cover with a cover glass. Pass the slide several times through a flame. Scrapings in KOH may be left overnight in a Petri dish on a piece of moist filter paper or gauze, if the nail has not dissolved.

2. Observe the preparation by bright-field or phase-contrast microscopy. The PAS stain may be required if suspected fungi are not observed in the KOH preparation.
3. Moisten the tip of a sterile long-handled inoculating needle by touching it to the surface of a SAB agar slant and then pick up several scrapings and distribute them across the nutrient agar surface. Repeat the process and inoculate a slant of Mycosel or Mycobiotic agar.
4. Incubate the cultures at 30°C and examine every 2–3 days. Discard negative cultures at 4 weeks.
5. Identify all the fungi recovered. Nail infections are often caused by moulds such as species of *Aspergillus* and *Scopulariopsis*. These should not be discarded simply because they are not dermatophytes.

## SKIN SCRAPINGS (STRATUM CORNEUM)

Dermatophytes typically cause circinate lesions of the glabrous skin with vesicular borders that first heal in the center of the lesion. With an ethanol (70%) gauze square, briskly clean the lesion to include the entire periphery. Sterile distilled water or sterile saline may be substituted for ethanol, especially if a yeast infection is suspected. If the lesion is inflamed or contains fissures, the lesions should be cleaned with a gauze soaked in sterile distilled water. With a sterile scalpel, scrape material from the periphery of the lesion. If dried exudate is present, remove it with sterile forceps. Be sure to collect any moist exudate. Lesions with exudate are usually moist, erythematous, and painful; they are generally caused by species of *Candida*.

Skin scrapings are transported to the clinical laboratory in Petri dishes, between two microscope slides, or in an envelope.

1. Place several scrapings into a drop of 10% KOH and then cover with a cover glass. Pass the slide several times through a flame.
2. Examine the preparation by bright-field or phase-contrast microscopy. The PAS stain may be required if suspected fungi are not observed in the KOH preparation.
3. Moisten the tip of a sterile long-handled inoculating needle by touching it to the surface of a SAB agar slant. Pick up several scrapings and distribute them across the surface of the nutrient agar. Repeat the process and inoculate a slant of Mycosel or Mycobiotic agar.
4. Incubate the cultures at 30°C and examine every 2–3 days. Discard negative cultures at 4 weeks.
5. Identify the fungi recovered. Fungi other than dermatophytes may be present in the stratum corneum.

## SPUTUM

Physicians often exhibit a lack of concern or awareness of the significance of many of the potentially pathogenic fungi recovered from sputum specimens. This is due, in part, to the abundant numbers of "contaminants" that were routinely isolated in the past from poor quality specimens traditionally accepted for mycological study. Sputum is material that comes from deep in the lungs. It is neither saliva nor nasopharyngeal secretions. Since the sputum specimen passes through the oral cavity, it is often contaminated with bacteria and yeasts. Other techniques such as bronchoscopic, transtracheal aspiration, transthoracic needle biopsy, and catheterization procedures give more useful clinical specimens for mycological study, since they are essentially free of "contaminants." Sputum specimens should consist of 10–15 ml of material; be collected first thing in the morning in a sterile wide-mouth container; and be collected after the patient's teeth have been brushed and his mouth washed with mouthwash. Nebulized specimens using mucolytic agents are acceptable, but they must be labeled as such, otherwise, they could be confused with saliva. Twelve- to 72-hour collections are totally unacceptable.

Sputum specimens should be processed within approximately 2 hours. Viscid specimens can be broken up with sterile NALC and mechanical shaking. Digestion of specimens is extremely helpful for the recovery of fungi, but the digestion process must be conducted properly. Gross and microscopic examinations must be done on each specimen. Suspicious areas containing particles, caseous, bloody and necrotic material should be examined microscopically and then inoculated onto isolation media. A discussion in depth of the proper manner to make gross examinations of clinical specimens is included under the next heading: Tissue Specimens.

1. Examination of sputum
   a. Examine the specimen for the presence of suspicious areas. The examination is conducted on the clinical specimen spread out in a Petri dish.
   b. Prepare 10% KOH preparations of all suspicious material and examine them by bright-field or phase-contrast microscopy. The PAS stain may be helpful if the KOH preparation is unsatisfactory.
2. Concentration of sputum
   a. Working in sets of specimens equivalent to one centrifuge load, loosen the caps of the specimen containers.
   b. Transfer the sputum specimens to 50-ml plastic, screw-cap, graduated, sterile centrifuge tubes. Do not put more than 10.0 ml of specimen in each tube. If the specimen exceeds 10.0 ml, use a second centrifuge tube.

c. Add to the specimen an equal volume of freshly prepared digestant (*N*-acetyl-L-cysteine, Dithiothreitol, or Sputalysin) without NaOH. If the specimen is small or very mucoid, the digestant can be added to the specimen while it is in the specimen container. The specimen is then aseptically poured into a sterile centrifuge tube.
   d. Tighten the caps and mix on a Vortex mixer for 5–10 seconds.
   e. Fill each tube to the 50-ml mark with 0.07 $M$ ($M/15$) phosphate buffer with a pH of 6.8–7.1. Tighten the caps and mix the contents by swirling the tubes.
   f. Place the centrifuge tubes into centrifuge safety buckets and then centrifuge for 15 minutes at 2100 rpm.
   g. Decant the supernatant. Chloramphenicol can be added to the sediment to give a final concentration of 0.05–0.1 $\mu g/ml$. Since the yeast form of *Histoplasma capsulatum* is sensitive to chloramphenicol, penicillin (20 units/ml) and streptomycin (40 units/ml) may be substituted for the chloramphenicol. These agents will, of course, kill aerobic actinomycetes.
   h. Mix and inoculate 0.1 ml of the sediment onto the isolation media. A portion of the sediment is examined microscopically in 10% KOH. Two or three smears should be prepared, which can be stained by the PAS technique if necessary.
   i. Incubate the cultures at 30°C and examine every 2–3 days. Negative cultures are discarded after 4 weeks. If *H. capsulatum* is suspected, keep the cultures for 12 weeks before discarding as negative.
   j. Identify the fungi recovered.

## TISSUE SPECIMENS

Tissue specimens must consist of normal tissue and both the center and edge of the lesion. This is especially important when recovering dimorphic fungi. *Histoplasma capsulatum* is usually found in the center of lesions, whereas *Blastomyces dermatitidis* is found at the edge. If the tissue specimen contains only either the edge or center, a pathogenic fungus could be missed. In collecting this material, saline for injection should not be used if it contains antimicrobial agents. Since tissue specimens are theoretically sterile, all fungi recovered are identified to species.

To adequately examine a tissue specimen, it is important that it be spread out. Specimens should therefore be examined in sterile Petri dishes.

It is also important that tissue specimens be protected against dehydration. For this reason, freshly collected tissue specimens are always placed either between two sterile moistened gauze pads or in a sterile tube containing 1.0–2.0 ml of sterile water or sterile saline for transport to the laboratory.

The etiologic agents of actinomycosis, botryomycosis and mycetoma form granules in tissue. The granules may consist of dead or viable organisms. Since the microorganisms could be dead, it is important that the granules be adequately studied.

1. Place the tissue specimen in a 15 × 100 mm plastic Petri dish. The tissue should be teased apart with sterile probes and examined with a dissecting microscope.
2. If granules are absent, inoculate purulent or necrotic material onto the isolation media. If granules are present, mount one or two of them (if enough material is present) in sterile distilled water for microscopic study. Granules can be crushed in a test tube with a glass rod for microscopic examination. Suspected bacterial granules should be Gram stained.
    a. Gram-positive, beaded to branching filaments, 0.5–1.0 $\mu$m in diameter are associated with actinomycetes.
    b. Gram-negative, filamentous, nonbranching bacilli, usually accompanied by Gram-positive cocci are botryomycotic granules (*Escherichia coli, Staphylococcus aureus, Proteus* sp.).
    c. Branching, septate hyphae that are 3.0–7.0 $\mu$m in diameter with swollen cells are characteristic of fungal granules.
3. Tease several granules free from the tissue and place them in a sterile 13 × 100 mm screw cap test tube containing 2.0–3.0 ml of sterile distilled water. Shake the tube gently.
4. With a sterile capillary pipette, transfer the granules to a second 13 × 100 mm tube with sterile distilled water and gently shake again. The washed granules are then transferred with a sterile capillary pipette to a third tube and crushed with a sterile glass rod.
5. The suspension is then inoculated onto the isolation media.
6. Incubate the cultures at 30°C and examine every 2–3 days. Discard the cultures as negative after 4 weeks.
7. Identify the fungi recovered.

When granules are absent, the tissue specimen is processed as follows:

1. Place the tissue in a sterile 15 × 100 mm plastic Petri dish.
2. With sterile dissecting needles, forceps, or scalpels, remove any purulent, necrotic, or caseous material; prepare a KOH preparation and

examine it microscopically. It may be necessary to gently heat the preparation. A PAS-stained smear is often extremely helpful in studying tissue.
3. Inoculate purulent, necrotic, and caseous material directly onto the isolation media. If purulent, necrotic, or caseous material is absent, the specimen is homogenized. Tissue is homogenized to ensure that the greatest amount of surface area of the specimen touches the nutrient agar. This also ensures that intracellular pathogens are released. The fungus must be in contact with the isolation medium before it can be isolated.
   a. Cut the tissue into small fragments with sterile scissors and forceps.
   b. Place the tissue into a sterile 15-ml Ten Broeck tissue homogenizer and thoroughly homogenize; 2–3.0 ml of SAB or BHI broth may be added to the tissue during homogenization.
   c. Pipette 0.05–0.1 ml of the homogenate onto each of the isolation media.
4. Incubate the cultures at 30°C and examine every 2–3 days. Negative cultures are discarded after 4 weeks. If *H. capsulatum* is suspected, discard after 12 weeks.
5. All fungi recovered are identified.

## URINE SPECIMENS

Suprapubic aspirates, catheterized specimens, or clean catch specimens are required. Urines should be processed immediately, but they can be refrigerated for several hours. Approximately 25–50 ml of urine are required for processing.

1. Transfer the urine to a sterile 50-ml plastic centrifuge tube. If more than 50 ml of urine have been collected, use additional centrifuge tubes.
2. Centrifuge the urine for 10–15 minutes at 2000 rpm.
3. Decant the supernatant and pool the sediment if necessary.
4. Inoculate with 0.05–0.1 ml of inoculum. Prepare a direct smear of the sediment in 10% KOH and observe by bright-field or phase-contrast microscopy. An India ink preparation may be helpful.
5. Incubate the cultures at 30°C and examine every 2–3 days. Discard negative cultures after 2 weeks.
6. Identify all fungi isolated.

## Part 2. Selected References

### A. Blood Specimens

1. Caplan, L. M., and W. G. Merz (1978). Evaluation of two commercially prepared biphasic media for recovery of fungi from blood. *J. Clin. Microbiol.* **8**:469–470.
2. Haley, L. D. (1964). "Diagnostic Medical Mycology." Appleton, New York.
3. Komorowski, R. A., and S. G. Farmer (1973). Rapid detection of candidemia. *Am. J. Clin. Pathol.* **59**:56–61.
4. Roberts, G. D., C. Horstmeier, M. Hall, and J. A. Washington (1975). Recovery of yeast from vented blood culture bottles. *J. Clin. Microbiol.* **2**:18–20.
5. Roberts, G. D., and J. A. Washington (1975). Detection of fungi in blood cultures. *J. Clin. Microbiol.* **1**:309–310.

### B. Nails

1. Davies, R. R. (1968). Mycological tests and onychomycosis. *J. Clin. Pathol.* **21**:729–730.
2. Luedemann, G. M., and E. LeBreton (1972). Laboratory mill for pulverizing and homogenizing nail specimens as an aid to microscopy and culture confirmation of onychomycosis. *Appl. Microbiol.* **23**:814–818.
3. Zaias, N. (1967). The longitudinal nail biopsy. *J. Invest. Dermatol.* **49**:406–408.

### C. Skin Scrapings

1. Whiting, D. A., and E. A Bisset (1974). The investigation of superficial fungal infections by skin surface biopsy. *Br. J. Dermatol.* **91**:57–65.

### D. Sputum Specimens

1. Johnston, W. W., and W. J. Frable (1976). The cytopathology of the respiratory tract. A review. *Am. J. Pathol.* **84**:372–414.
2. Kapica, L., C. E. Shaw, and G. W. Bartlett (1968). Inhibition of *Histoplasma capsulatum* by *Candida albicans* and other yeasts on Sabouraud's agar media. *J. Bacteriol.* **95**:2171–2176.
3. Larsh, H. W., and N. L. Goodman (1973). Sputum mycology. *In* "Sputum. Fundamentals and Clinical Pathology" (M. J. Dulfano, ed.), pp. 292–331. Thomas, Springfield, Illinois.
4. Reep, B. R., and W. Kaplan (1972). The use of $N$-acetyl-L-cysteine and dithiothreitol to process sputa for mycological and fluorescent antibody examinations. *Health Lab. Sci.* **9**:118–124.
5. Roberts, G. D., A. G. Karlson, and D. R. DeYoung (1976). Recovery of pathogenic fungi from clinical specimens submitted for mycobacteriological culture. *J. Clin. Microbiol.* **3**:47–48.
6. Thompson, D. W., W. Kaplan, and B. J. Phillips (1977). The effect of freezing and the influence of isolation medium on the recovery of pathogenic fungi from sputum. *Mycopathologia* **61**:105–109.

## Part 3. Direct Examination of Clinical Specimens

### GIEMSA STAIN

The Giemsa stain is used primarily in medical mycology to demonstrate the intracellular nature of the yeast cells of *Histoplasma capsulatum*. The intracellular cells of *H. capsulatum* stain light to dark blue and have a hyaline halo. The halo is not a capsule; it is a staining artifact.

1. Technique for the Giemsa stain

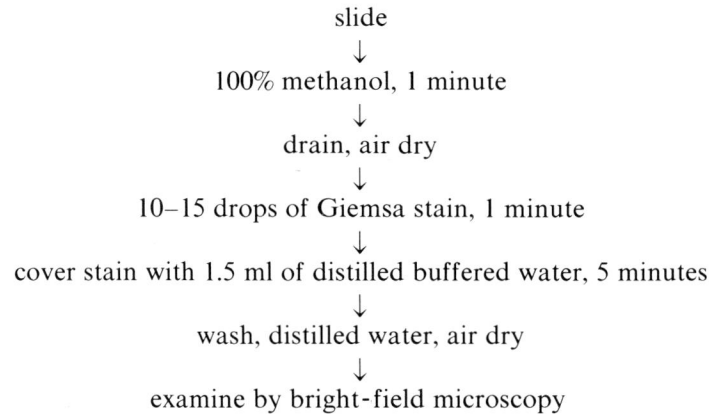

slide
↓
100% methanol, 1 minute
↓
drain, air dry
↓
10–15 drops of Giemsa stain, 1 minute
↓
cover stain with 1.5 ml of distilled buffered water, 5 minutes
↓
wash, distilled water, air dry
↓
examine by bright-field microscopy

### PERIODIC ACID–SCHIFF STAIN

The periodic acid–Schiff stain (PAS) is used when KOH preparations do not demonstrate suspected fungi. In addition to dermatological mycology, the PAS procedure can be used for the demonstration of fungi in many other types of clinical specimens. It is important that the periodic acid and metabisulfite solutions be fresh and protected from the light.

1. For dermatological specimens, using your finger, spread a very light film of albumin fixative slightly off center on a clean glass microscope slide. If the clinical specimen contains protein, the albumin fixative can be omitted. For other types of specimens, prepare a smear and let it air dry.
2. With a clean teasing needle, work several fragments of the dermatological or other clinical specimen into the albumin film. Ensure that the scrapings and hairs are flat.

3. Place the slide on a slide warmer for 2–3 hours. The drying time can be shortened by passing the slide through a flame, but do not overheat.
4. Stain as follows:

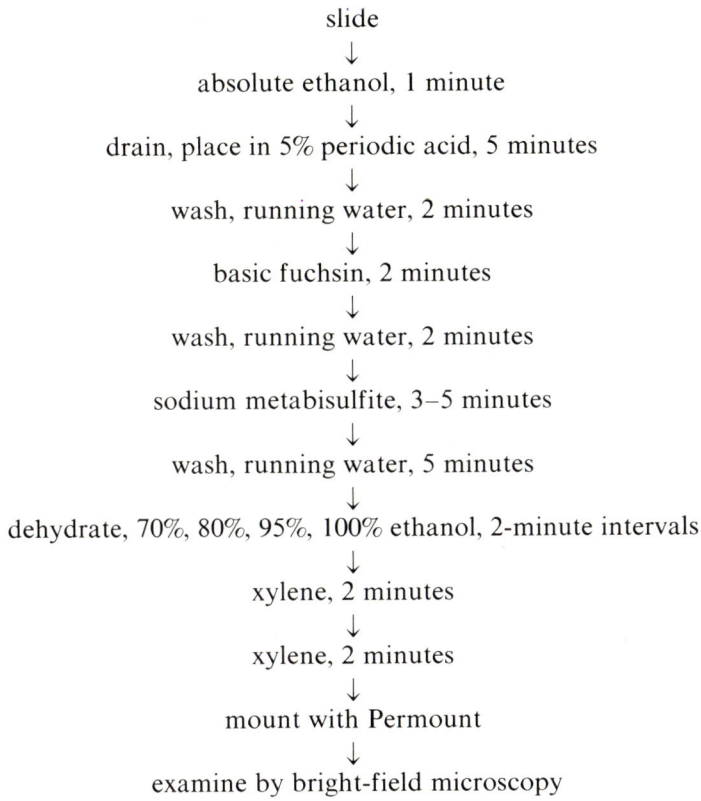

slide
↓
absolute ethanol, 1 minute
↓
drain, place in 5% periodic acid, 5 minutes
↓
wash, running water, 2 minutes
↓
basic fuchsin, 2 minutes
↓
wash, running water, 2 minutes
↓
sodium metabisulfite, 3–5 minutes
↓
wash, running water, 5 minutes
↓
dehydrate, 70%, 80%, 95%, 100% ethanol, 2-minute intervals
↓
xylene, 2 minutes
↓
xylene, 2 minutes
↓
mount with Permount
↓
examine by bright-field microscopy

## POTASSIUM HYDROXIDE PREPARATION

The potassium hydroxide (KOH) preparation is used to clear clinical material so that fungi can be more readily seen. Permanent blue-black ink or Parker 51 can be added to the KOH solution to highlight the fungal cell walls. A potassium hydroxide solution containing dimethyl sulfoxide (DMSO) is excellent for clearing thick pieces of stratum corneum and nail tissue. This results in rapid penetration and clearing of the specimen. It is not recommended for hair and skin scrapings. The KOH technique is excellent for demonstrating the presence or absence of dematiaceous fungal elements.

1. Place a drop of 10% KOH onto a clean glass microscope slide in a slightly off-center position.
2. Place the material to be examined into the KOH and then tease the material apart with two dissecting needles.
3. Place a cover glass over the clinical material. Additional KOH may be required, which can be added at the edge of the cover glass. Excess KOH should be removed with a paper towel.
4. Allow the KOH preparation to sit at room temperature until the material has been cleared. The slide may be passed through a flame to speed the clearing process. Warming will also expel air bubbles.
5. Observe the preparation by bright-field or phase-contrast microscopy. If using bright-field microscopy, reduce the light intensity by slightly closing the iris diaphragm. This is necessary because most fungi are typically hyaline and difficult to see in bright light.
6. The clearing action of KOH will continue until the tissue and fungi are completely destroyed. KOH preparations are not permanent. They can be preserved for several days by adding a small amount of glycerol to the KOH solution or by placing it next to the cover glass; thus permitting the glycerol to flow under the cover glass. If nail material is to be cleared, KOH–DMSO can be substituted for the 10% KOH.

## Part 3. Selected References

### A. Microscopic Examination

1. Forster, R. K., M. G. Wirta, M. Solis, and G. Rebell (1976). Methenamine-silver-stained corneal scrapings in keratomycosis. *Am. J. Ophthalmol.* **82**:261–165.
2. Huppert, M., D. J. Oliver, and S. H. Sun (1978). Combined methenamine-silver nitrate and hematoxylin and eosin stain for fungi in tissues. *J. Clin. Microbiol.* **8**:598–603.
3. Roberts, G. D. (1975. Detection of fungi in clinical specimens by phase-contrast microscopy. *J. Clin. Microbiol.* **2**:261–265.

*Chapter 4*

# Mould Identification

### Part 1. Concepts

The majority of filamentous fungi recovered in the clinical laboratory belong to the class Hyphomycetes, which includes all the filamentous members of the Fungi Imperfecti except for those species that form pycnidia or acervuli. For the most part, the Hyphomycetes can be identified without too much difficulty. Occasionally, isolates are recovered that are difficult, even frustrating, to identify. It soon becomes evident that many of the dichotomous keys for identification, photomicrographs, and illustrations are simply inadequate. Owing to the predominant clinical orientation and training of many medical mycologists, an uncomfortable feeling is not uncommon in deciding which characteristics are most important.

During the late 1800s and early 1900s, Saccardo designed a simple classification system for the Fungi Imperfecti. As new information became available, the system was modified to one degree or another (Table 4.1). Saccardo's classification scheme for the filamentous members of the Fungi Imperfecti currently consists of two classes that are distinguished from each other on the basis of the types of fruiting structures produced. The class Coelomycetes contains two orders, the Melanconiales and Sphaeropsidales. Fungi that produce acervuli are classified in the Melanconiales, whereas pycnidial forms are included in the Sphaeropsidales. The second class of filamentous fungi is the Hyphomycetes, which includes the orders Mycelia Sterilia and Moniliales. The Mycelia Sterilia contains those fungi that produce neither conidia nor spores. All the other members of the class Hyphomycetes are included in the order Moniliales.

The Hyphomycetes were divided by Saccardo into four families. All these families are included in the single order Moniliales. The Mycelia Sterilia does not contain families because the group is so heterogeneous.

**Table 4.1.** Traditional Classification of the Division Fungi Imperfecti

---

A. Class Blastomycetes: Nondematiaceous yeasts; pseudohyphae, hyphae, or both may be present (Chapter 5)
B. Class Coelomycetes: Filamentous fungi that form either acervuli or pycnidia; yeasts absent
   1. Order Melanconiales: Fungi that form acervuli
      a. Family Melanconiaceae
   2. Order Sphaeropsidales: Fungi that form pycnidia
      a. Contains several families
C. Class Hyphomycetes: Filamentous fungi that form neither acervuli nor pycnidia; yeasts typically absent
   1. Order Mycelia Sterilia: Fungi that do not form conidia or spores
      a. There are no families in this order
   2. Order Moniliales: Fungi that form free conidiophores, sporodochia, or synnemata
      a. Family Moniliaceae: Hyaline to light-colored fungi with free conidiophores
      b. Family Dematiaceae: Olive-to-brown-to-black fungi with free conidiophores
      c. Family Tuberculariaceae: Fungi that form sporodochia
      d. Family Stilbellaceae: Fungi that form synnemata

---

The families of the Moniliales were distinguished from each other by the arrangement and color of the conidiophores and conidia. The Moniliaceae (Mucedinaceae of Saccardo) is characterized by the presence of free conidiophores. Free conidiophores are solitary, that is, they are never united into a synnema or formed on an acervulus or sporodochium. The conidiophores and conidia produced by members of the Moniliaceae are always hyaline to light colored, but never olive-to-brown-to-black. The second family, the Dematiaceae, is identical to the Moniliaceae except that the conidiophores, conidia, or both are typically olive-to-brown-to-black. This color range is considered to be dematiaceous. The family Tuberculariaceae was established to accommodate members of the Fungi Imperfecti that produced their conidiophores on sporodochia. The fourth family, the Stilbellaceae (Stilbaceae of Saccardo), contains fungi that produce synnemata.

As a supplement to the families, Saccardo proposed a series of sections that were based upon the shape and septation of the conidia. These sections included (Fig. 4.1) the Amerosporae (1-celled conidia, or ameroconidia), Didymosporae (2-celled conidia, or didymoconidia), Phragmosporae (several-celled conidia having horizontal septa only, or phragmoconidia), Dictyosporae (conidia with vertical and horizontal septa, or dictyoconidia), Scolecosporae (conidia with a width to length ratio of 1:20 or greater, or scolecoconidia), Helicosporae (spiral conidia, or helicoconidia), and Staurosporae (star-shaped conidia, or stauroconidia). Subsections were also established, in which Saccardo used the prefix hyalo- for

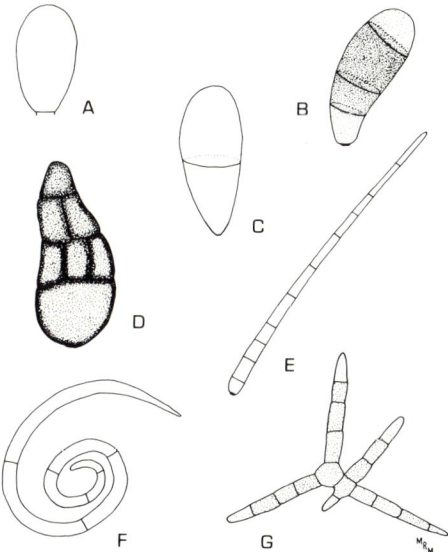

**Fig. 4.1** The Saccardoan classification of the various shapes and septation of conidia and spores. A. Amerosporae, *Chrysosporium* sp., B. Phragmosporae, *Curvularia* sp., C. Didymosporae, *Arthrobotrys* sp., D. Dictyosporae, *Alternaria* sp., E. Scolecosporae, *Cercospora* sp., F. Helicosporae, *Helicosporium* sp., G. Staurosporae, *Tripospermum* sp.

hyaline to lightly colored conidia, and the prefix phaeo- for darkly pigmented conidia (Hyalosporae, Phaeosporae, Hyalodidymae, Phaeodidymae, etc.). The terms amerospore, didymospore, phragmospore, dictyospore, scolecospore, helicospore, and staurospore can be used to describe the shape and septation of spores.

The classification scheme Saccardo proposed was simple and easily understood. The success of his system can be attributed to the simple criteria that he selected as the basis for the system. A number of problems exist in the Saccardoan system; these have stimulated many mycologists to seek a better classification scheme. At first thought, color seems to be an ideal characteristic. However, color is extremely subjective, and no two mycologists interpret colors identically. As a result, some fungi are assigned to the Moniliaceae by one mycologist and to the Dematiaceae by another. There is also an inconsistency in applying this characteristic. For example, no mycologist would transfer *Aspergillus niger,* which produces black conidia, from the genus *Aspergillus* solely upon the basis of color. It has been well established that color is influenced by the age of the isolate, the environmental conditions (especially light) and medium upon which the isolate has been grown. It therefore seems unreasonable to establish genera, as was sometimes done in the Saccardoan system, simply because of color differences.

Septation of conidia presents a similar dilemma. Septation is greatly influenced by substrates and environmental conditions. All conidia are initially one-celled. If immature conidia are being studied, the true septal condition may not be apparent; this could result in misidentifications. Traditionally, there has been too much emphasis placed upon septation.

In many instances, the structures observed on natural substrates are seldom seen on laboratory media. At one stage of fungal taxonomy, the plant from which the fungus was recovered had to be identified before the fungus could be identified. As a result, dichotomous keys will often have a comment to the effect "acervulus present or acervulus absent" or "sporodochium present or sporodochium absent." These structures are very distinct on the host plant, but rarely produced in culture. It is a frustrating experience to try to identify an isolate of *Fusarium* when the dichotomous key states that a sporodochium must be present, especially if a specific host must also be taken into consideration. In fact, if either sporodochia or acervuli were present in culture, it would probably be impossible to tell one from the other.

Similar problems surround the synnematous fungi and their counterparts that produce free conidiophores; development of conidia in balls, chains, or intermediate arrangements; and deciding whether or not the conidiophores are distinctive (Micronemeae and Macronemeae of Saccardo). Those types of problems clearly illustrate that the Saccardoan system crosses many natural boundaries. Even with these problems, Saccardo's artificial classification system is useful and valuable.

In 1953, Hughes proposed an experimental system for the classification of the Hyphomycetes. The proposal was extremely significant because it was based upon the method by which the conidia and their conidiophores developed. The characteristics Saccardo used for his classification system were considered by Hughes to be of secondary importance. Hughes divided the Hyphomycetes into eight sections, one of which was divided into two subsections.

## HUGHES'S EXPERIMENTAL CLASSIFICATION SYSTEM*

### Section IA

Mycelium generally narrow. Conidia usually developing in acropetal succession as blown-out ends at the apex of simple or branched conidiophores, which do not then increase in length. The basal conidia of

---

*Reproduced by permission of S. J. Hughes and the National Research Council of Canada from the *Canadian Journal of Botany* 31:577–659, 1953.

chains aggregated around the apical region of a conidiophore may be morphologically different from the others and in one instance are modified into permanent metulae bearing a terminal conidium and a number of subterminal conidia. Example: *Cladosporium.*

## Section IB

Mycelium generally wide. Conidia developing in acropetal succession as blown-out ends on simple or branched conidiophores; sometimes the lateral branches are modified entirely into a number of conidia or into solitary conidia and in these instances the conidia are borne on conspicuous denticles. The solitary conidia, or short, simple, or branched chains of conidia may be aggregated on well differentiated swollen cells and arise more or less simultaneously on them. In examples with intercalary or lateral swollen and fertile cells bearing simultaneously produced conidia, the main stalk may proliferate to develop further intercalary fertile cells or bear further lateral fertile branches. Example: *Botrytis.*

## Section II

Conidia arising as blown-out ends of apex of simple or branched conidiophores and the ends of successively produced new growing points developing to one side of the previous conidium. The conidiophore, therefore, either increases in length or becomes swollen as a result of conidium production. Acropetal chains of conidia may develop on the primary conidia. Example: *Tritirachium.*

## Section III

Conidia usually thick-walled, arising solitarily as blown-out ends of the apex of simple or branched conidiophores; a plurality of conidia may be produced, each new conidium developing as a blown-out end of successive proliferations *through* the scars of previous conidia so that the conidiophores in such cases become annellate. Example: *Scopulariopsis.*

## Section IV

Conidia (phialospores) developing in rapidly maturing basipetal series from the apex of a conidiophore (phialide) which may or may not possess an evident collarette. Example: *Phialophora.*

## Section V

Conidia developing in gradually maturing basipetal series and originating by the meristematic growth of the apical region of the conidiophore in such a way that the chain of conidia merges imperceptibly with the conidiophore that gives rise to the chain. Example: *Erysiphe*.

## Section VI

Conidia usually thick-walled, developing from pores on conidiophores of determinate or indeterminate length; they are solitary or in whorls, and may occur in acropetal chains. The conidiophore may proliferate through the terminal pore to produce a further terminal conidium or the conidiophore may develop a succession of terminal conidia on successive proliferations developing just below the previous conidium. Example: *Helminthosporium*.

## Section VII

Conidia developing by the basipetal fragmentation of conidiophores of determinate length, and which do not possess a meristematic zone. Example: *Geotrichum*.

## Section VIII

Conidia borne singly at apex, or singly at apex and laterally, often in regular whorls on conidiophores showing basal elongation. Conidia often with longitudinal slit in wall, but this character is by no means restricted to this section. Example: *Arthrinium*.

In sections I through VII, the growth of the conidiophore initial or of the conidiophore itself during conidium formation is restricted to the apical region. In section VIII, the growth of the conidiophore is restricted to the basal region.

The classification system for the Hyphomycetes proposed by Hughes was rapidly accepted. Mycologists, including Subramanian, Tubaki, and Barron, have also proposed similar systems. All these mycologists agreed that the ontogeny of the reproductive structures is as important as the characteristics Saccardo selected for his system—that is, color, shape, and septation of conidia, arrangement of conidiophores, and the presence or absence of synnemata or sporodochia. Unfortunately, many genera could not be readily placed into this new system based upon conidiogenesis, because the genera had been so poorly defined in the past. These mycologists, as well as others, have stimulated a new interest in the Hyphomycetes and fungi in general.

Barron was one of the first mycologists to synthesize the best of each of the proposed systems into an extremely practical classification system for the identification of fungi recovered from soil. In essence, Barron divided Hughes's section III into two parts and adopted Tubaki's concept of naming sections after spore types.

## BARRON'S CLASSIFICATION SYSTEM

### Series Aleuriosporae

Members of this group form solitary (rarely short chains) aleuriospores as blown-out terminal ends of conidiogenous cells. A large number of aleuriospores may develop laterally and below a terminal conidium, resulting in an apical cluster of conidia. These are referred to as botryoaleuriospores. Examples: *Blastomyces, Microsporum,* and *Sepedonium.*

### Series Arthrosporae

Members of this group form arthrospores. The hyphae giving rise to the arthrospores may be morphologically and functionally identical with the vegetative hyphae, or may arise from distinct conidiophores. Examples: *Coccidioides, Geotrichum,* and *Oidiodendron.*

### Series Blastosporae

Members of this series form solitary or catenulate blastospores. The blastospores may form simple or branched chains and usually arise from simple or branching conidiophores. Examples: *Cladosporium* and *Monilia.*

### Series Botryoblastosporae

Members of this series form conidia from a swollen conidiogenous cell called an ampulla. Ampullae are different from similar swellings produced by members of the Sympodulosporae. Ampullae are formed prior to conidium development, whereas the swollen cells found in some members of the Sympodulosporae form as a result of conidium development. The conidia may remain solitary around the ampulla or they may produce secondary blastospores. The conidiophores may be either determinate or indeterminate. Example: *Botrytis*.

### Series Meristem Arthrosporae

Members of this series form a gradually maturing, basipetal series of arthrospores originating by growth at the conidiophore apex. The chain of arthrospores merges imperceptibly with the conidiophore from which it arises. Example: *Trimmatostroma*.

### Series Meristem Blastosporae

Members of this series produce conidia solitarily at the apex, or solitarily and laterally from the conidiophore. They are often in whorls on the conidiophore. The conidiophore elongates by new growth occurring at its base. Example: *Arthrinium*.

### Series Phialosporae

Members of this series produce phialides and phialospores. Examples: *Acremonium*, *Penicillium*, and *Phialophora*.

### Series Porosporae

Members of this series form (usually) thick-walled conidia through channels (pores) in the walls of the conidiophore. The conidia may be solitary or in simple to branching acropetal chains. The channels may be regular, random, solitary, or scattered. The conidiophores may be indeterminate (percurrent or sympodial). Examples: *Stemphylium* and *Ulocladium*.

### Series Sympodulosporae

Members of this series form conidia from sympodial conidiophores. The conidiophores either increase in length or become swollen as a result of conidium production. Examples: *Beauveria*, *Rhinocladiella*, and *Sporothrix*.

In 1969, a group of hyphomycete specialists from around the world gathered at Kananaskis, Alberta, Canada to discuss the terminology that was being applied to the Fungi Imperfecti (see Kendrick, 1971). The purposes of the Kananaskis Conference were to evaluate the terminology and concepts being applied to the Fungi Imperfecti; to develop a scheme for the classification of conidia based upon their individual ontogeny; and to classify the methods by which these fungi produce their conidia. It was not the purpose of the Kananaskis Conference to develop a classification scheme for the Fungi Imperfecti.

On numerous occasions at the conference, it was emphasized that the names applied to conidia should describe their own ontogeny, not the characteristics of the conidiogenous cell from which they developed. For example, the term sympodioconidium was found to be unacceptable because it described a conidium on the basis of how the conidiogenous cell developed. The conidia produced from a sympodial conidiogenous cell (Fig. 4.2) may be either arthroconidia, blastoconidia, or poroconidia, depending upon the fungus.

Conidia were defined as specialized, nonmotile, usually deciduous, asexual propagules that do not develop by progressive cleavage or free-cell formation. All other propagules (ascospores, basidiospores, sporangiospores, and zygospores) were considered to be spores. This is an excellent concept that clearly distinguishes conidia and spores. For this reason, terms such as arthroconidium and blastoconidium are preferred, rather

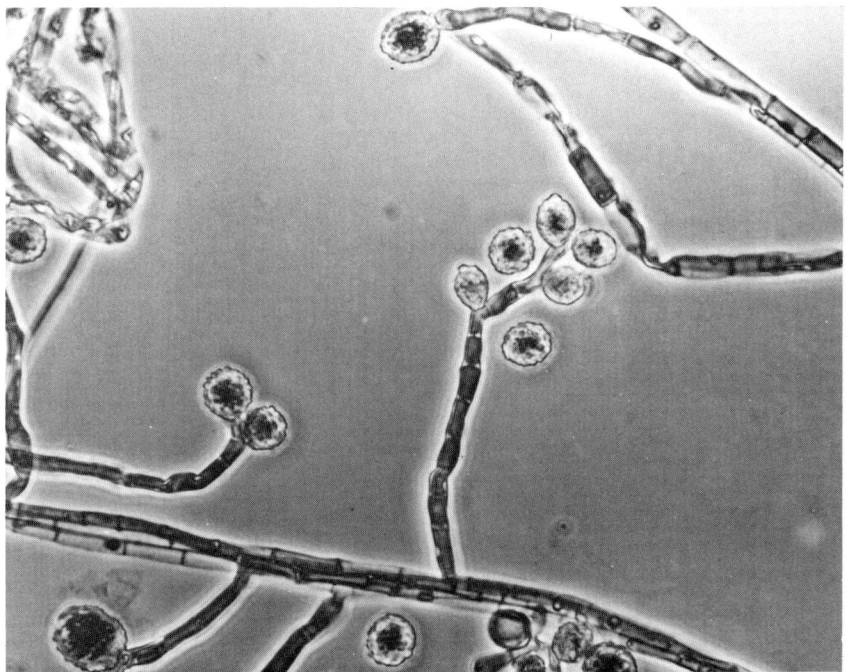

**Fig. 4.2** *Ulocladium atrum.* The muriform conidia develop from sympodial conidiophores. As the conidiophores increase in length, they become geniculate.

than the obsolete expressions arthrospore and blastospore. It was suggested that the term chlamydospore should be discarded because it has been used in a variety of senses in the past. It was felt that the term is of only minimal value. The term chlamydospore is adopted in this handbook because it is felt that it is useful in describing a thallic survival conidium. Chlamydospores are in essence terminal or intercalary holothallic conidia that usually have thick walls and function as survival propagules.

The name tretoconidium was proposed as a replacement for poroconidium (porospore), which is not accepted here. Since the conidium emerges through a pore or channel in the outer cell wall of the conidiogenous cell, the most logical name for such a conidium is poroconidium. The channel is secondary and develops as the holoblastic conidium is released.

Aleuriospore was rejected by the participants of the Kananaskis Conference. This term is of special interest to medical mycologists, since it has been commonly used to describe the holothallic conidia of the dermatophytes and numerous other medically important fungi. The concept in part included a conidium with an annular frill (Fig. 4.3). The term was considered to be unacceptable because it does not characterize the ontogeny of the conidium. It was suggested that these conidia should be referred to simply as terminal thallic conidia. The recommendation to reject the term aleuriospore is accepted in this handbook.

The terminology and concepts that have evolved from the Kananaskis Conference as well as those proposed by Cole and Samson (see Cole and Samson, 1979) are being used for the descriptions and identifications of the Fungi Imperfecti included in this handbook. Many people find it difficult to readjust their thinking from the characteristics Saccardo used to those based upon ontogeny of conidia. Once this transition has been accomplished, the differences between many of the various fungi become obvious, with only minimal gray areas. If the medical mycologist is going to use effectively the mycological literature pertaining to the Fungi Imperfecti, a firm understanding of the terminology and concepts associated with conidiogenesis is imperative. It is important to realize that conidiogenesis cannot be used as the sole basis for classifying fungi. It must be used in conjunction with other types of data.

The division Zygomycota contains two classes, the Zygomycetes and Trichomycetes. The Trichomycetes are associated only with arthropods, upon which they attach themselves to the external cuticle or cuticular lining of the digestive tract by a holdfast. Members of this class are therefore never seen in the clinical laboratory.

The Zygomycetes contain six or seven orders, of which the Entomophthorales and Mucorales are of interest to the medical mycologist.

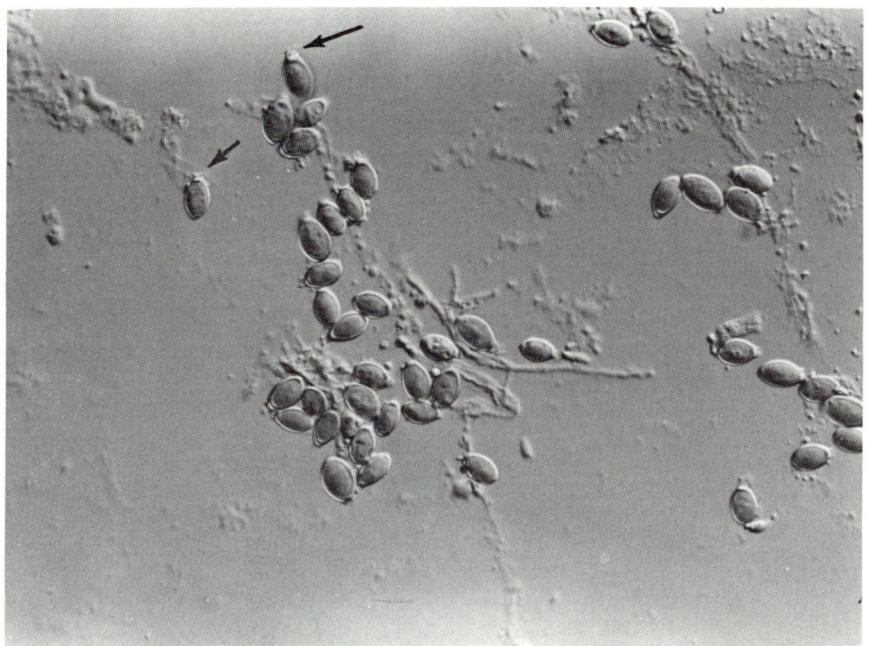

**Fig. 4.3** *Sporotrichum aureum*. When the conidia separate from the conidiophore, an annular frill (arrows) typically remains around their truncate bases.

The Entomophthorales, which contains such genera as *Basidiobolus* and *Conidiobolus*, is characterized by poorly developed mycelium and forcibly discharged sporangiola (conidia). In contrast, members of the Mucorales, such as species of *Absidia, Mucor,* and *Rhizopus*, develop well formed mycelium, but never conidia or spores that are forcibly discharged. *Pilobolus*, which is in the family Pilobolaceae, forcibly discharges its sporangia. All the Zygomycetes have in common, at least theoretically, the formation of zygospores (Fig. 4.4).

The genera within the division Zygomycota are distinguished from each other primarily upon the types of zygospores and sporangia they produce. Speaking from a practical point of view, the various genera are actually distinguished from each other almost entirely on the basis of the types of sporangia formed. For example, the genus *Conidiobolus* is characterized in part by the presence of zygospores that are formed within the larger of two gametangia. *Conidiobolus coronatus*, a major etiologic agent of subcutaneous zygomycosis, does not form zygospores. This species is classified in the genus *Conidiobolus* because it produces forcibly discharged sporangiola and other asexual structures that are included in the generic concept of

**4 Mould Identification**

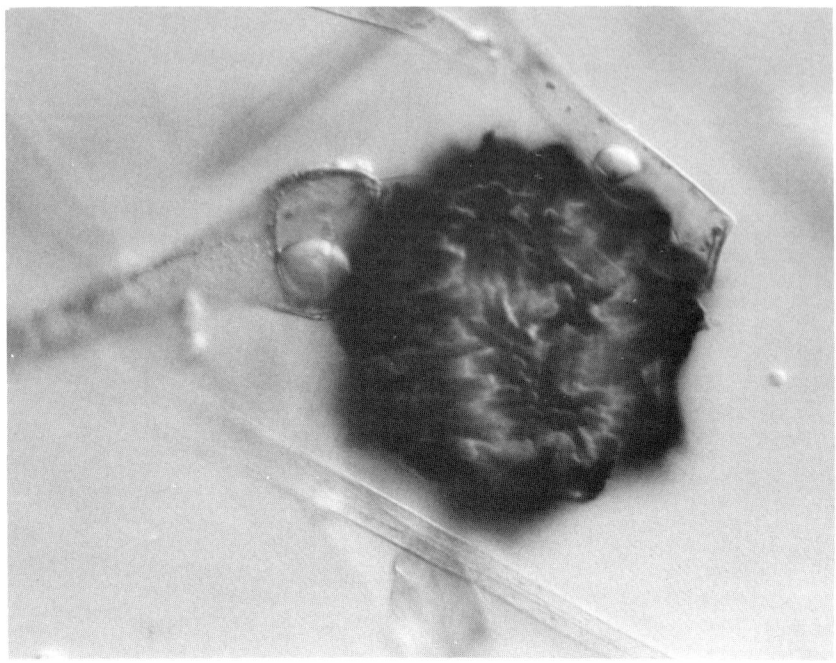

A

**Fig. 4.4** Zygospores are sexual spores that are useful in distinguishing the various genera of Zygomycetes. The suspensor cells are still attached to these zygospores. A. *Mucor bainieri*, B. *Absidia spinosa*.

*Conidiobolus. Conidiobolus coronatus* is an example of a zygomycetous imperfect fungus, classified in a genus based upon sexual characteristics. Similar examples of this approach to the classification of imperfect zygomycetous fungi can be found in genera such as *Absidia, Mucor,* and *Rhizopus*. Since zygospores are usually rare, or absent in the majority of zygomycetous isolates encountered in the clinical laboratory, the distinctive sporangia have assumed the role of the predominant characteristic for the identification of these fungi.

In order for an isolate to be considered an ascomycete, it must produce asci and ascospores. This is an important point because of the tendency of some microbiologists to confuse cleistothecia and perithecia with pycnidia. These misidentifications are primarily a result of basing rapid identifications on the gross morphology of the fruiting body, instead of a careful search for asci and ascospores. Too often, only one or two microscopic fields are examined before it is concluded what the fungus will be called.

The majority of medical mycologists have a good grasp of the various types of ascomycetous fruiting bodies, with the possible exception of the

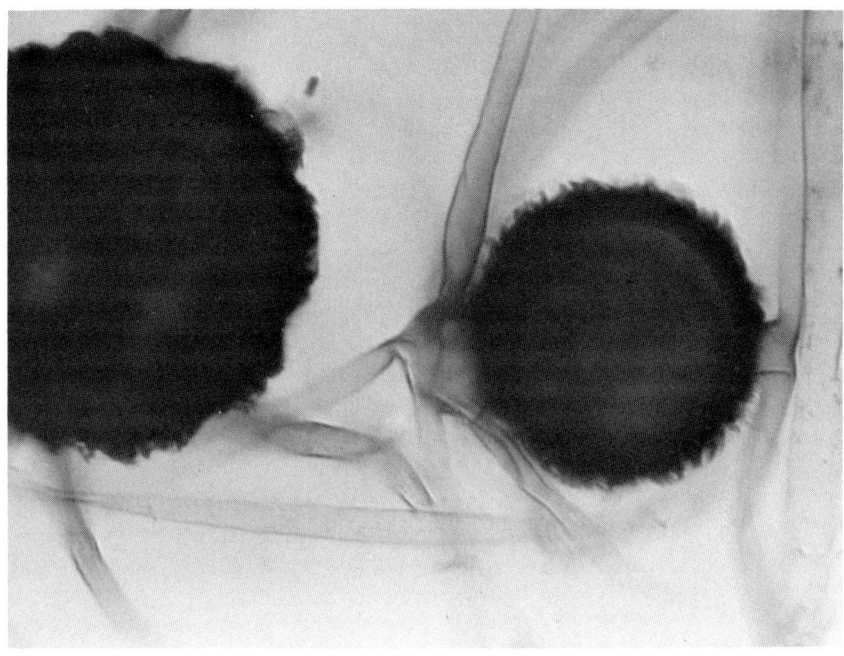

**B**

**Fig. 4.4** Continued

cleistothecium. Occasionally, the medical mycologist will encounter an author who states that a particular fungus forms a cleistothecium, and a second author who refers to the identical structure as a perithecium. The root of the problem involves two different concepts of a cleistothecium. Mycologists more concerned with centrum development, as versus gross morphology of the fruiting body, define cleistothecia as being round and having only randomly dispersed asci. These mycologists would exclude all ascocarps that did not have random asci, regardless of whether they are ostiolate. The second group of mycologists consider all round, nonostiolate ascocarps, regardless of how the centrum develops to be cleistothecia. This concept lumps a number of phylogenetically dissimilar fungi together. The first concept is more ideal because it takes phylogeny into consideration. In recent years, mycologists interested in the Gymnoascaceae, a family classified in the class Plectomycetes, have adopted the term gymnothecium (Fig. 4.5) in lieu of cleistothecium (Fig. 4.6). Gymnothecia are loosely organized ascocarps with randomly dispersed asci. This is an excellent concept for the ascocarps produced by this group of fungi.

For all practical purposes, basidiomycetous fungi are rarely seen in the clinical laboratory. Since most isolates of basidiomycetous fungi are

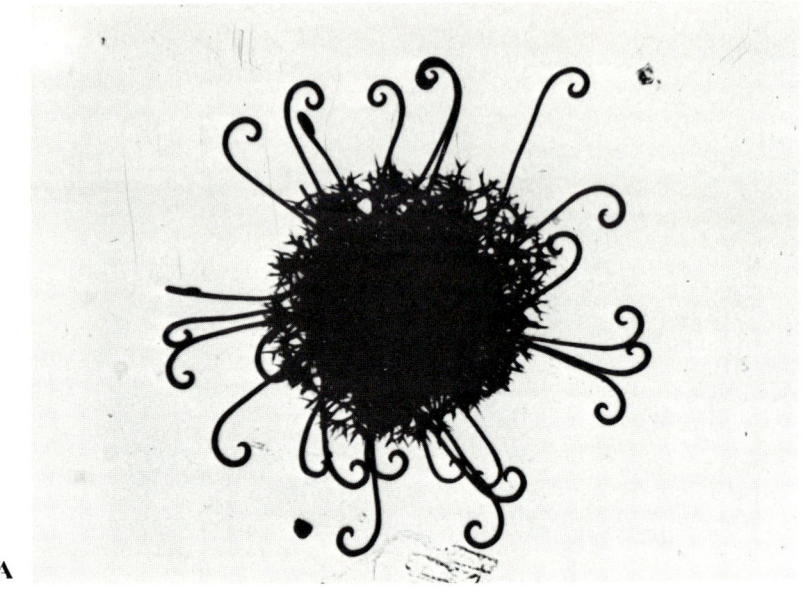

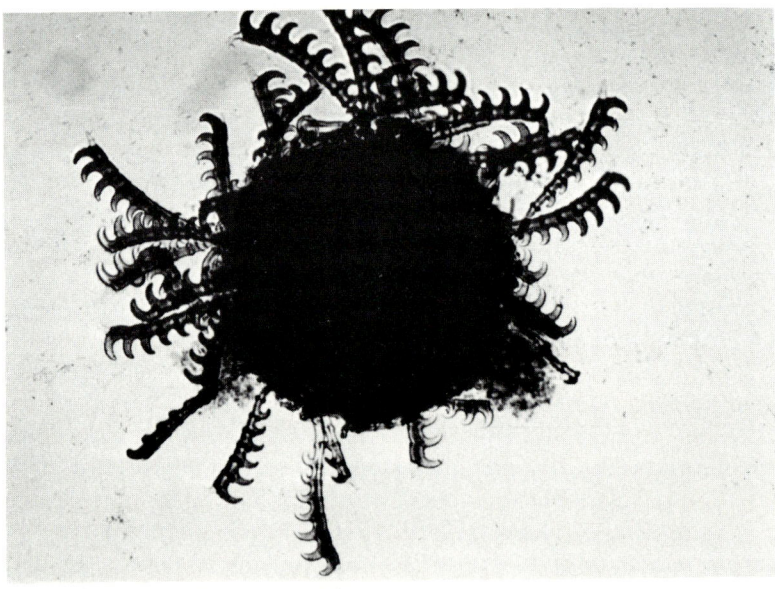

**Fig. 4.5** Mature gymnothecia. A. *Myxotrichum chartarum*, B. *Ctenomyces serratus*, C. *Gymnascella aurantiaca*. Each ascus contains eight ascospores. The loosely woven tuberculate peridial hyphae are visible at the edge of the spore mass. (A reproduced by permission of R. Benjamin and Aliso from *Aliso* 3:301–328, 1956; B courtesy of R. Benjamin.)

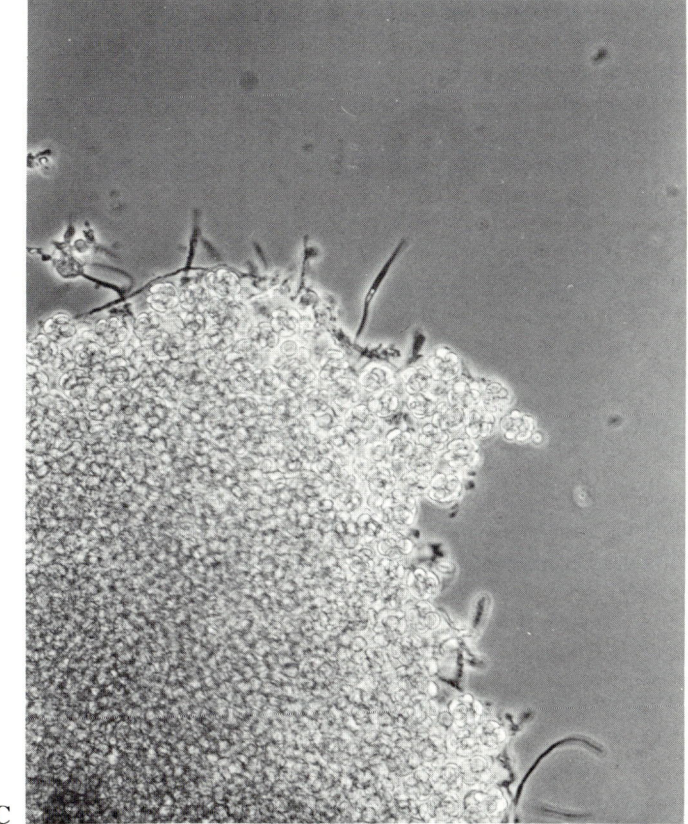

**Fig. 4.5** Continued

heterothallic, fruiting bodies are typically absent. These fungi can be occasionally recognized as such by the presence of clamp connections (Fig. 4.7), or in the case of species of *Rhizoctonia* and *Sclerotium*, by abundant sclerotia (Fig. 4.8) in culture. It is important to mention that some isolates of *Rhizoctonia* are Ascomycetes. Because they are extremely rare in the clinical laboratory, this group of fungi are not included in this handbook.

The last group of filamentous fungi that must be briefly discussed is the Mycelia Sterilia. When sterile isolates are recovered, an attempt should be made to induce the formation of conidia, spores, or other structures that could assist in identifying them. A number of procedures that can be used are included in the techniques portion of this chapter. Sterile isolates represent species of fungi that simply are not producing conidia, spores, pycnidia, ascocarps, or basidiocarps, because of compatibility systems, the lack of appropriate environmental and nutritional needs, or both. Even

**4 Mould Identification**

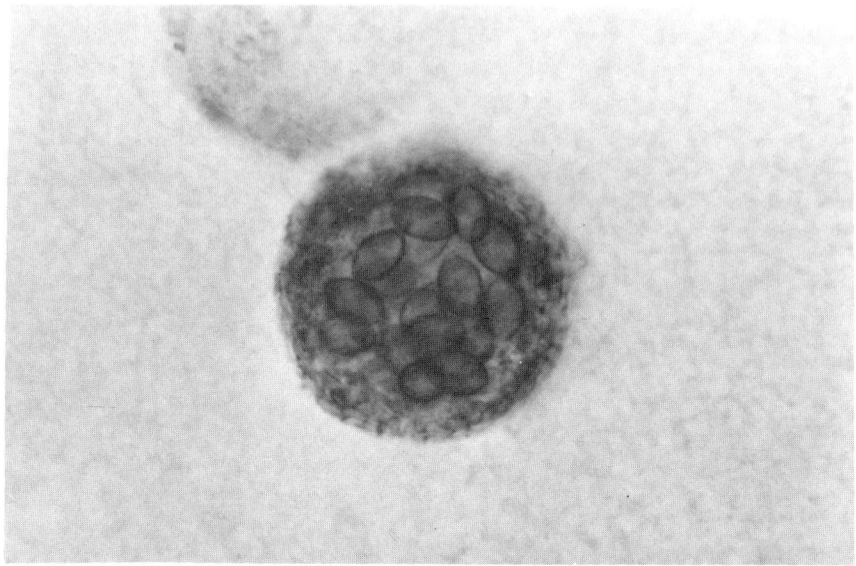

**Fig. 4.6** *Thielavia* sp. A number of free ascospores can be seen within the cleistothecium.

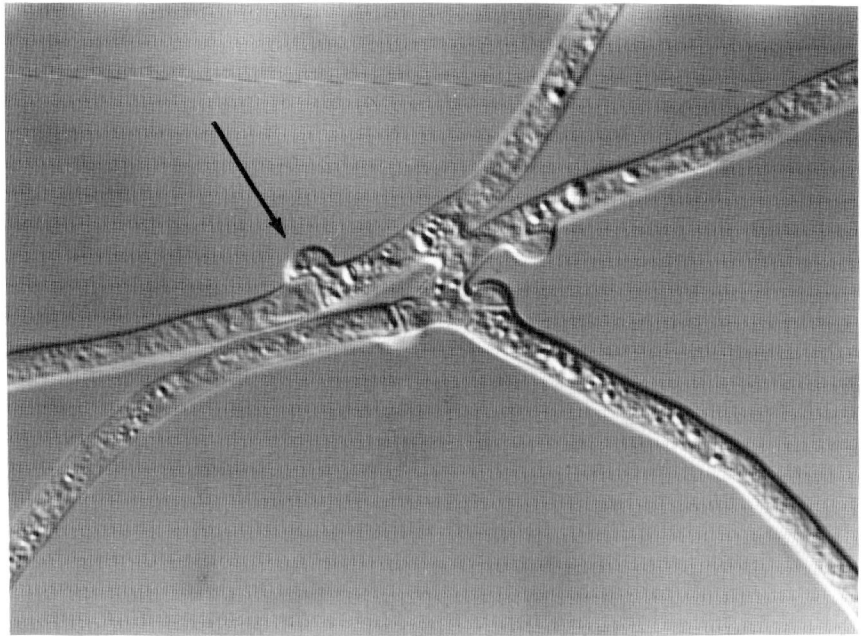

**Fig. 4.7** Clamp connections (arrow) are characteristic of basidiomycete mycelium.

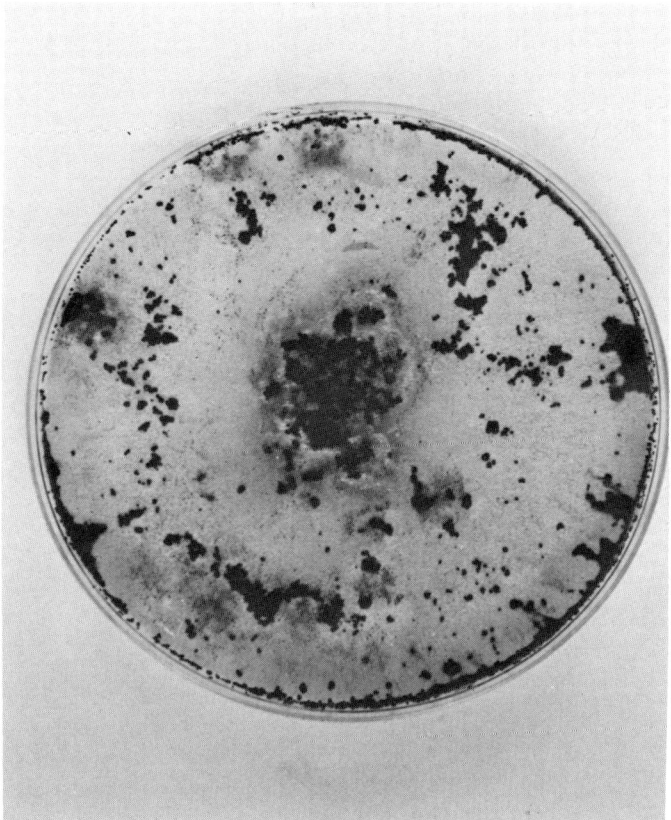

**Fig. 4.8** *Rhizoctonia solani*. The black masses on the surface of the potato dextrose agar are sclerotia.

though these isolates cannot be identified to genus and species in most instances, their vegetative morphology can be compared from one isolate to the next. Observations concerning vesicles, angle of hyphal branching, distance between septa, size of hyphae, frequency of branching, color of hyphae, cell-wall thickness and topography, anastomoses of hyphae, and the presence or absence of fascicles, sclerotia, and other structures can furnish valuable comparative data. In some instances, these fungi are opportunistic pathogens of man. They can no longer be neglected.

In Chapter 1, the terms anamorph, teleomorph, and holomorph were briefly introduced. The term anamorph can be applied to any asexual or somatic reproductive structure, regardless if it is specialized or generalized. The term is not meant to be used for sexual reproductive structures. Sexual reproductive structures are referred to as teleomorphs. When the entire fungus is being considered, it is referred to as the holomorph. For example, under the appropriate conditions, *Histoplasma capsulatum* may form hyphae, macro- and microconidia, and yeast cells. When compatible mating types are crossed, gymnothecia containing asci and ascospores are formed, the sexual stage being called *Ajellomyces capsulatus*. The hyphae, the conidia, and the yeast form are all anamorphs that are used to define the asexual fungus *H. capsulatum*. *Histoplasma capsulatum* can be referred to as the anamorph of *A. capsulatus*. Likewise, *A. capsulatus* is the teleomorph of *H. capsulatum*. When all of the anamorphs and its teleomorph are considered together, the term holomorph is used. For fungi such as *Fonsecaea pedrosoi*, where a teleomorph is unknown, all of its anamorphs together become the holomorph, that is, the whole fungus.

## *General References*

1. Barron, G. L. (1968). "The Genera of Hyphomycetes from Soil." Williams & Wilkins, Baltimore, Maryland.
2. Cole, G., and R. A. Samson (1979). "Patterns of Development in Conidial Fungi." Pitman, London.
3. Goos, R. D. (1956). Classification of the Fungi Imperfecti. *Proc. Iowa Acad. Sci.* **63**:311–320.
4. Hennebert, G. L. (1971). Pleomorphism in Fungi Imperfecti. *In* "Taxonomy of Fungi Imperfecti" (B. Kendrick, ed.), pp. 202–223. Univ. of Toronto Press, Toronto.
5. Hughes, S. J. (1953). Conidiophores, conidia and classification. *Can. J. Bot.* **31**:577–659.
6. Kendrick, B., ed. (1971). "Taxonomy of Fungi Imperfecti." Univ. of Toronto Press, Toronto.
7. Luttrell, E. S. (1963). Taxonomic criteria in *Helminthosporium*. *Mycologia* **55**:643–674.
8. Luttrell, E. S. (1964). Systematics of *Helminthosporium* and related genera. *Mycologia* **56**:119–132.
9. Saccardo, P. A. (1886). "Sylloge fungorum," Vol. 4, pp. 1–807. Published by the author, Pavia, Italy.
10. Saccardo, P. A. (1906). "Sylloge fungorum," Vol. 18, pp. 1–838. Published by the author, Pavia, Italy.
11. Subramanian, C. V. (1962). The classification of the hyphomycetes. *Bull. Bot. Surv. India* **4**:249–259.
12. Talbot, P. H. B. (1971). "Principles of Fungal Taxonomy." Macmillan, New York.
13. Tubaki, K. (1958). Studies on Japanese hyphomycetes. V. Leaf and stem group with a discussion on the classification of hyphomycetes and their perfect stages. *J. Hattori Bot. Lab.* **20**:142–244.
14. Tubaki, K. (1963). Taxonomic study of hyphomycetes. *Annu. Rep. Inst. Ferment., Osaka* **1**:25–54.
15. Vuillemin, P. (1910). Les conidiospores. *Bull. Soc. Sci. Nancy* **11**:129–172.
16. Vuillemin, P. (1911). Les aleuriospores. *Bull. Soc. Sci. Nancy* **12**:151–175.

## Part 2. Techniques

### COLONY CHARACTERISTICS

The identification of filamentous fungi is based upon an evaluation of their colony characteristics and microscopic morphology. Colony characteristics are extremely valuable, but unfortunately they are not often used enough. Most mycologists prefer to study isolates that have been incubated at 25–30°C for approximately 2 weeks on malt agar, potato dextrose agar, or Czapek–Dox-solution agar.

Visual examination of the colony will rapidly reveal important data concerning color, texture, diffusible pigments, exudates, macroscopic structures (such as ascocarps, pycnidia, sclerotia, sporodochia, and synnemata), growth zones, aerial and submerged hyphae, growth rate, and colony topography. In addition to the overall appearance of the colony, a great deal of valuable information can be gained by examining the colony with a dissecting microscope. This tool permits the medical mycologist to bridge the gap between gross colony characteristics and microscopic observations. Unfortunately, the dissecting microscope is often underutilized in the clinical mycology laboratory.

### CONFIRMATION OF DIMORPHIC FUNGI

Dimorphic fungi have the ability to grow vegetatively at 25°C on routine mycological media as moulds. When these fungi are in tissue or on special media incubated at 37°C, they grow vegetatively either as yeasts or as spherules and enlarging endospores (*Coccidioides immitis*). Medical mycologists have taken advantage of this ability to grow in two different vegetative forms, as an aid in distinguishing dimorphic fungi from morphologically similar species. In the past, the conversion of the mould form to its corresponding tissue form was accomplished by infecting laboratory animals and then examining their tissues. Animal studies are no longer necessary except in unusual instances. Special media have been developed that are very reliable for the mould-to-tissue form conversion. Exoantigen techniques are also available at reference centers, but not in the clinical laboratory at this time. These techniques have a great deal of promise.

*Blastomyces dermatitidis*, *Histoplasma capsulatum*, *Paracoccidioides brasiliensis*, and *Sporothrix schenckii* are dimorphic fungi that grow vegetatively as a yeast in tissue and at 37°C. The total conversion of an isolate of one of these species to the yeast form is not necessary for demonstrating that it is dimorphic. The degree of conversion depends upon the isolate. Isolates that are more difficult to convert can usually be completely converted to the yeast form by continuous, rapid subculturing. For the laboratory confirmation of dimorphism, any degree of conversion will suffice. Media containing cycloheximide or chloramphenicol should never be used for the cultivation of the yeast form of *H. capsulatum,* because these antimicrobial agents can inhibit this fungus.

*Sporothrix schenckii* represents a special problem. Several species of *Ceratocystis (C. minor, C. montia, C. multiannulata, C. narcissi, C. nigrocarpa, C. perparvispora, C. pilifera,* and *C. stenoceras)* having a *Sporothrix* anamorph can incite disease in laboratory animals, and produce a yeast form at 37°C that is essentially identical to *S. schenckii.* These observations clearly illustrate that careful morphological study, and the mould-to-yeast conversion, are both necessary in identifying this, as well as other dimorphic fungi.

*Coccidioides immitis,* unlike the other dimorphic fungi of medical interest, produces spherules and endospores at 37°C when it is grown on special media. Sun *et al.* have devised an *in vitro* procedure for inducing the development of spherules on modified Converse medium. Care must be exercised to ensure that the isolate is forming spherules containing endospores and that the endospores are being released. This is necessary because other fungi, such as species of *Malbranchea,* can produce large vesicles under these growth conditions. At 37 and 40°C on routine mycological media, some species of *Chrysosporium* may form large vesicles, thick-walled, spherulelike structures, or both. These enlarged structures do not contain spores. Isolates suspected to be *C. immitis* must at all times be handled in a biological safety cabinet.

Temperature, medium composition, and concentration of $CO_2$ can all affect the mould-to-tissue form conversion. In general, 37°C is necessary for the conversion to occur. Some isolates of *P. brasiliensis* may begin to form yeast cells with blastoconidia at 23–28°C. In this fungus, nutrition appears to be very important. Nutritional requirements are extremely important in the mould-to-yeast conversion of *H. capsulatum,* where cysteine or similar sulfur containing compounds are necessary. The conversion of the mould form to the yeast form in *S. schenckii* and to the spherules of *C. immitis* is enhanced by an increase in atmospheric $CO_2$.

### A. Procedure for Mould-to-Yeast Conversion

1. All procedures are done in a biological safety cabinet.
2. With a long-handled inoculating needle, remove a small portion of the

isolate to be examined and transfer it to two tubes containing the appropriate medium (Table 4.2) for the suspected dimorphic fungus. Incubate one tube at 37°C and one tube at 25°C.
3. Examine the yeastlike areas for the presence of typical yeast cells, conversion of hyphae to yeast growth, or both. If the results are questionable, rapidly subculture the isolate to fresh media. Several weeks may be required for complete conversion. The conversion is considered positive when typical yeast cells are present, regardless of their number. If the suspected conversion does not occur, animal or exoantigen studies will be necessary.

### B. Procedure for Mould-to-Spherule Conversion

1. All procedures are done in a biological safety cabinet.
2. Prepare a standard slide culture preparation using Levine's modification of Converse medium in 1% ionagar No. 2.
3. Add approximately 2.0 ml of Levine's modification of Converse medium to an actively growing isolate suspected to be *C. immitis*.
4. With a sterile loop, transfer a loopful of the floating arthroconidia to the agar block in the slide culture setup.
5. Place a sterile cover glass on the inoculated agar block and then moisten the filter paper with sterile water.
6. Transfer the slide culture to a candle jar, light the candle, and incubate at 40°C for 4–5 days.
7. After 5 days, add 10.0 ml of formalin for each liter of volume to the candle jar and then incubate for an additional 24 hours at 37°C. The formalin will kill the fungus.
8. Examine the preparation microscopically for the presence of spherules and released endospores. Fungi that are similar to *C. immitis* may produce large vesicles, but they do not form spherules with endospores being released.
9. Autoclave the preparation, slide culture, and candle jar.

The mould-to-spherule conversion can also be done on Levine's modification of Converse medium with 1.5% agar in small disposable Petri dishes. The isolate is inoculated on the medium surface in the Petri dish. The conversion occurs in the Petri dish instead of in a slide culture setup. After inoculation of the medium, all the remaining steps are identical. Later, a small amount of growth must be transferred to a microscope slide for examination. These setups can be incubated at 37°C, but this is not recommended because hyphae and arthroconidia are formed too. Arthroconidia are not formed at 40°C.

**Table 4.2.** Mould-to-Tissue Form Conversion of the Dimorphic Fungi

| Fungus | Media and conditions | Morphological form obtained | Some similar fungi at 25°C |
|---|---|---|---|
| *Blastomyces dermatitidis* | Kelley's agar or blood agar, 37°C | Yeast | *Chrysosporium* spp. |
| *Coccidioides immitis* | Modified Converse medium, 40°C, 5–10% $CO_2$ | Spherules and enlarging endospores | *Malbranchea* spp., Gymnoascaceae |
| *Histoplasma capsulatum* | BHI agar[a] plus glutamine or GCB agar,[b] 37°C | Yeast | *Sepedonium* spp., *Chrysosporium* spp. |
| *Paracoccidioides brasiliensis* | BHI agar, 37°C | Yeast | *Chrysosporium* spp., Mycelia Sterilia |
| *Sporothrix schenckii* | BHI agar, 37°C, 5–10% $CO_2$ | Yeast | *Acrodontium* spp. |

[a] Brain heart infusion agar.
[b] Glucose–cysteine–blood agar (1% glucose, 0.1% cysteine, 10% rabbit or sheep blood).

### C. Procedure for Yeast- or Spherule-to-Mould Conversion

1. All procedures are done in a biological safety cabinet.
2. Subculture the yeast or spherule form to media, such as Sabouraud dextrose agar, and incubate at 25°C.
3. Within a few days, typical mould colonies will be present.

## CYCLOHEXIMIDE RESISTANCE

Determining the resistance of isolates to cycloheximide is a useful procedure when screening cultures for *Blastomyces dermatitidis, Coccidioides immitis, Epidermophyton floccosum, Histoplasma capsulatum, Microsporum* spp., *Paracoccidioides brasiliensis, Sporothrix schenckii,* and *Trichophyton* spp. All these fungi will grow in the presence of cycloheximide. Other moulds, such as species *Absidia, Aspergillus, Mucor, Rhizopus, Scedosporium* and many more are inhibited by this agent.

### A. Procedure for Determining Cycloheximide Resistance

1. Remove a small portion of the mould colony with a long-handled inoculating needle from midway between the center and edge of the

colony. Place the inoculum toward the butt in one tube containing Sabouraud dextrose agar (SAB) with cycloheximide and one tube containing SAB without cycloheximide. Mycosel or Mycobiotic agar can be used in lieu of SAB with cycloheximide.
2. Incubate the cultures at 30°C for 7–10 days. Media containing antimicrobial agents must never be incubated at 37°C because many fungi that are not normally sensitive to these agents become so at elevated temperatures.
3. Read and record the results
   a. Growth present on SAB and medium with cycloheximide = resistant.
   b. Growth present on SAB only = susceptible.
   c. No growth on SAB = repeat test.

## FORCIBLY DISCHARGED CONIDIA OR SPORES

Fungi such as members of the genera of *Basidiobolus* and *Conidiobolus* have the ability to produce ballistospores. The technique to demonstrate forcibly discharged spores for these moulds is identical to the one described for the yeasts (Chapter 5).

## *In Vitro* HAIR TEST

A number of dermatophytes have the ability to penetrate hair *in vitro*. This test becomes helpful in distinguishing atypical isolates of dermatophytes, especially *Trichophyton mentagrophytes* from *T. rubrum*. In the test, either the hyphae may penetrate the hair perpendicularly, which results in conical or wedgelike holes called perforations, or the hair may be gradually eroded without the formation of perforations. In the *in vitro* hair test, the presence or the absence of perforations (Fig. 4.9) is the end point for this test. The majority of the perforations are usually present in 10–14 days. The test is not read as negative until 28 days because some isolates produce perforations slowly.

### A. Procedure

1. Place several sterile hairs in a sterile glass Petri dish. Hair from a blond child is preferred because it can be easily seen through. A plastic Petri

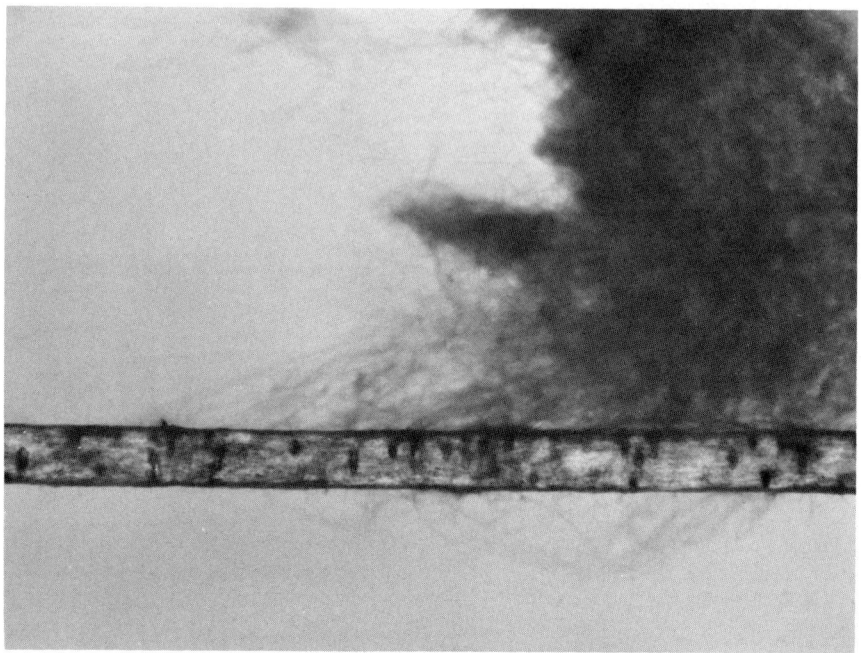

A

**Fig. 4.9** *Trichophyton mentagrophytes*. The conical perforations in the hair were produced in approximately 14 days at 25°C. The hair perforation test is typically used to distinguish *T. mentagrophytes* from *T. rubrum*, the former being able to produce these perforations.

dish is not recommended since they are usually charged with static electricity, which results in the hairs being thrown about.
2. To the Petri dish, add approximately 25 ml of sterile distilled water and 0.1 ml of sterile yeast extract.
3. With a long-handled inoculating needle, transfer a small amount of the fungus from midway between the center and edge of the colony to the hairs in the Petri dish. Known isolates of *T. mentagrophytes* and *T. rubrum* are run concurrently as controls.
4. Incubate the dishes at 25°C and examine weekly for up to 4 weeks. Examination of the hair is accomplished by placing a few hairs in a drop of lactophenol cotton blue or lactophenol mounting medium on a microscope slide, covering the preparation with a cover glass, and then observing it microscopically. The known positive and negative controls must be examined first. If they are unsatisfactory, the test must be repeated.

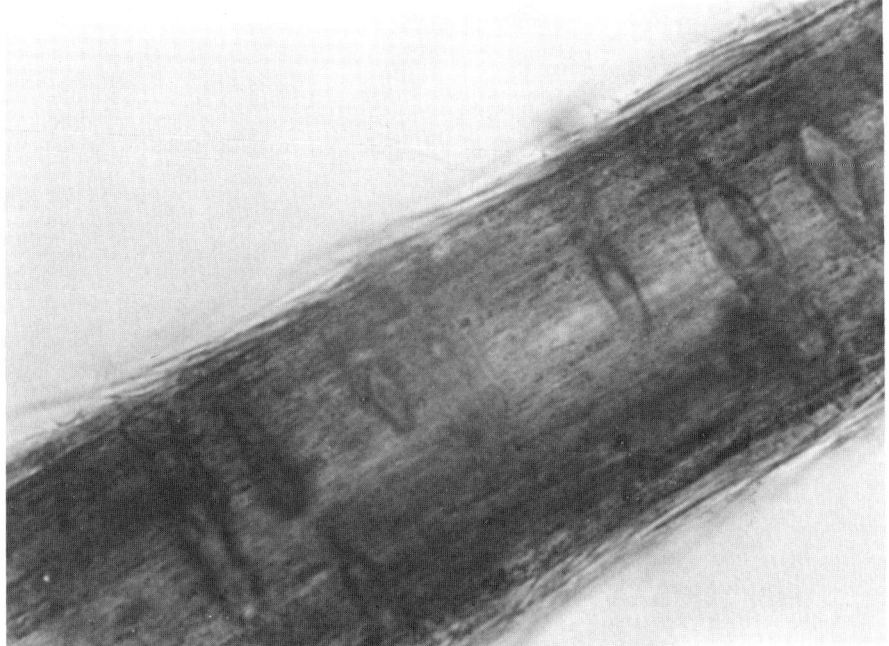

**Fig. 4.9** Continued

## MIXED CULTURES

Pure cultures, regardless of whether they are yeasts or moulds, are always mandatory when identifying fungi. Until demonstrated differently, all isolates should be considered to be contaminated. Since many moulds of medical interest are polymorphic, it is important to know whether or not the various structures present are produced by one fungus or by several fungi. This decision can be made only when pure cultures are being studied. These isolates must also be free of bacterial contamination, because some bacteria may interfere with the development of key morphological structures necessary for the identification of the mould.

### A. *Bacterial contamination*

1. Colony isolation using low temperature
   a. Streak a portion of the isolate to be decontaminated onto the surface of potato dextrose agar (PDA) in a Petri dish.

b. Incubate the culture at 10–15°C for several days. Bacteria do not usually grow at this temperature.
c. Using a dissecting microscope and a sterile needle, transfer hyphal tips to test tubes containing PDA.
d. Incubate the subcultures at 30°C for several days and then Gram stain a portion of the new growth. If the subculture is not pure, further steps are necessary (A2).
2. Colony isolation on 2% water agar
   a. Streak a portion of the isolate to be decontaminated onto the surface of 2% water agar in a Petri dish. The inoculum can also be placed under the agar. This is accomplished by lifting the agar with a sterile spatula, placing the inoculum under the agar, and then setting the agar back down. The agar must be poured in a thin layer and the isolate must be a rapid grower.
   b. Incubate the culture at 30°C for several days. Bacteria do not usually grow on 2% water agar.
   c. Using a dissecting microscope and a sterile needle, transfer hyphal tips to test tubes containing PDA.
   d. Incubate the subcultures at 30°C for several days and then Gram stain a portion of the new growth. If the subcultures are not pure, further steps are necessary (A3).
3. Colony isolation on Sabouraud dextrose agar containing chloramphenicol (SAB + C) or Sabouraud dextrose agar containing penicillin and streptomycin (SAB + P and S)
   a. Streak a portion of the isolate to be decontaminated onto the surface of SAB + C or SAB + P and S in a Petri dish.
   b. Incubate the culture at 30°C for several days and then Gram stain a portion of the new growth. If the subculture is not pure, further steps are necessary (A4).
4. Acidification of Sabouraud dextrose broth
   a. The procedure is identical to that described for the yeasts (Chapter 5).

### B. Mould or Yeast Contamination

1. Colony isolation using hyphal tips
   a. Emulsify a portion of the contaminated culture in sterile distilled water. Streak some of the suspension onto PDA.
   b. Incubate the subculture at 30°C for 2–3 days.
   c. Using either a dissecting microscope and a sterile needle, or a

micromanipulator, transfer several hyphal tips to test tubes containing PDA.
   d. Incubate the subcultures at 30°C for several days. Check the purity of the subcultures.
2. Colony isolation on PDA or 2% water agar
   a. Emulsify a portion of the contaminated isolate in sterile distilled water.
   b. With a sterile inoculating loop, streak a loopful of the suspension onto PDA or 2% water agar.
   c. Incubate the culture at 30°C for 1–2 days.
   d. Using a dissecting microscope and a sterile needle, transfer several individual colonies to test tubes containing PDA.
   e. Incubate the subcultures at 30°C for several days. Check the purity of the subcultures.
3. Isolation of Zygomycetes
   a. Transfer a small portion of the aerial hyphae of the contaminated zygomycete to a Petri dish containing malt extract agar supplemented with 15–20% glucose. Zygomycetes will quickly outgrow other fungi in the presence of this high concentration of glucose.
   b. Incubate the culture at 30°C for 2–3 days.
   c. Using a dissecting microscope and a needle with a moistened tip, or a pair of sterile jeweler's forceps, remove a sporangium and transfer it to a cotton plugged test tube containing PDA.
   d. Incubate the subculture at 30°C for several days. Check the purity of the subculture.
4. Isolation of slow growing fungi contaminated with fast growing fungi
   a. Emulsify a portion of the contaminated culture in sterile distilled water.
   b. Streak a loopful of the suspension on dilute hay infusion agar or soil extract agar. Rapidly growing fungi such as species of *Aspergillus* and *Penicillium* grow slowly on diluted media. Martin's medium, which contains rose bengal, is also effective.
   c. Incubate the cultures at 30°C for 2 or 3 days.
   d. Using a dissecting microscope and a sterile needle, transfer several individual colonies to test tubes containing PDA.
   e. Incubate the subcultures at 30°C for several days. Check the purity of the subcultures.
5. Colony isolation on Sabouraud dextrose agar with cycloheximide (SAB + C)
   a. Emulsify a portion of the contaminated culture in sterile distilled water.
   b. Streak a loopful of the suspension on SAB + C. Dimorphic fungi,

dermatophytes, and a few other fungi are resistant to cycloheximide, whereas many of the common soil fungi are susceptible.
  c. Incubate the culture at 30°C for several days.
  d. Using a dissecting microscope and a sterile needle, transfer several hyphal tips to test tubes containing PDA.
  e. Incubate the subcultures at 30°C for several days. Check the purity of the subcultures.
6. Colony isolation by dilution
  a. Emulsify a portion of the contaminated culture in sterile distilled water.
  b. Prepare a $10^{-2}$ dilution of the suspension in sterile distilled water.
  c. Pipette 1.0 ml of the diluted suspension into a test tube containing 17.0 ml of PDA held at 48–50°C. Mix the contents.
  d. Pour the 18.0-ml volume into a sterile 100-mm plastic Petri dish and allow the medium to harden.
  e. Incubate the culture at 30°C for 2–3 days.
  f. Using a dissecting microscope and a sterile needle, transfer several colonies to test tubes containing PDA.
  g. Incubate the subcultures at 30°C for several days. Check the purity of the subcultures.

The technique can be modified as follows:
  a. Pipette 1.0 ml of the inoculum in step a above to 17.0 ml of PDA held at 48–50°C. Pour the 18.0 ml of PDA into a 100-mm Petri dish.
  b. To the empty test tube, add 17.0 ml of PDA held at 48–50°C. Pour this into a second Petri dish. Repeat the process three additional times.
  c. Continue from step e above.
7. Colony isolation by selective culturing
  a. Using a dissecting microscope and fine-tipped needle that is moistened with water or warm agar, lightly touch the conidia or spores of the desired fungus. Transfer this inoculum to test tubes containing PDA.
  b. Incubate the subcultures at 30°C for several days. Check the purity of the subcultures.

## NUTRITIONAL STUDIES

Nutritional studies can be extremely valuable in identifying some species of moulds, especially dermatophytes. There is probably no experience more frustrating than attempting the identification of a strange isolate of *Microsporum* or *Trichophyton*.

There are two principal types of nutritional or biochemical data that are occasionally used by medical mycologists to assist in the identification of atypical isolates of *Microsporum* and *Trichophyton*. Data of the first type depend upon the isolate's ability, or lack of ability, to assimilate various carbon sources. This biochemical information is based upon the presence or the absence of growth after 21 days of incubation at 25°C on media containing various carbon sources. Data of the second group are based upon the isolate's requirements for selected vitamins. This information is used solely to distinguish a few commonly encountered species within the genus *Trichophyton*.

### A. Procedure for Assimilation Studies (after Philpot, 1977)

1. Inoculum is obtained from isolates that were grown on Hugh and Leifson agar for 7 days at 25°C.
2. With a long-handled inoculating needle, transfer a small portion of the vegetative growth that is approximately 1 mm in diameter to the test tubes or Petri dishes containing the carbon sources to be tested. Avoid transferring nutrient agar along with the vegetative inoculum.
3. Incubate the tests at 25°C for 21 days. The cultures should be examined at weekly intervals.
4. The ability to assimilate a carbon source is read as the presence of growth.

### B. Procedure for Vitamin Studies (after Georg and Camp, 1957)

1. Inoculum is obtained from isolates that were grown on Sabouraud dextrose agar for 7–14 days at 25°C.
2. With a long-handled inoculating needle, transfer a small portion of the vegetative growth that is approximately 1 mm in diameter to the media containing vitamins. Avoid transferring nutrient agar along with the vegetative inoculum.
3. The tests are incubated as indicated in Table 4.3.
4. The effect of the various vitamins is determined by comparing the relative amounts of growth in each independent set of tests. Traces of growth are considered ±, whereas the maximum amount of growth for each series of tubes is assigned a value of 4+. Read the tests and record the results.

**Table 4.3.** Incubation Conditions and Periods for the Vitamin Studies

| Species of *Trichophyton* | Media | Temperature (°C) | Time (days) |
|---|---|---|---|
| *T. concentricum, T. schoenleinii, T. verrucosum* | Casein, casein + inositol, casein + thiamine, casein + inositol and thiamine | 37 | 7 to 14 |
| *T. mentagrophytes, T. rubrum, T. tonsurans* | Casein, casein + thiamine | 25 | 7 to 10 |
| *T. megninii* | Ammonium nitrate, ammonium nitrate + histidine | 25 | 7 to 10 |
| *T. equinum, T. mentagrophytes* | Casein, casein + nicotinic acid | 25 | 7 to 10 |
| *Microsporum ferrugineum, T. violaceum* | Casein, casein + thiamine | 25 | 7 to 10 |

## PROTEOLYTIC ACTIVITY

Many medical mycologists have traditionally relied upon proteolytic activity, or its absence, as a characteristic to distinguish some pathogenic from nonpathogenic isolates. The presence or the absence of proteolytic activity of some medically important fungi when tested on media such as gelatin agar, Löffler's coagulation serum agar, or both, is of questionable value in determining pathogenicity. For example, while studying *Exophiala jeanselmei*, Padhye (1978) showed that isolates obtained from phaeohyphomycosis and natural habitats (such as water cooling towers), lacked proteolytic activity. The absence of proteolytic activity is traditionally associated only with pathogenic isolates. This example clearly casts doubt on the validity of proteolytic activity data in distinguishing pathogenic from nonpathogenic isolates. This obsolete test has been used in the past for determining pathogenicity of isolates of *Cladosporium carrionii, C. bantianum, Exophiala jeanselmei, Fonsecaea pedrosoi,* and *Phialophora verrucosa*.

## RICE GRAIN TEST

The sterile rice grain test is a useful technique as an aid in distinguishing atypical isolates of *Microsporum canis* from *M. audouinii*. *Microsporum audouinii* does not grow on this medium, but some brownish discoloration of the grains usually occurs beneath the inoculum. *Microsporum canis*, as well as most other fungi, will rapidly grow on sterile rice grains. Rice grains also serve as an ideal substrate to stimulate the formation of conidia in many fungi. In this test, it is important that the rice grains are not fortified with vitamins.

### A. Procedure

1. With a long-handled inoculating needle, transfer a small portion of the isolate to be tested to a flask containing sterile rice grains.
2. Incubate the flask at 30°C and examine for growth after 8–10 days.
3. The absence of growth, with or without a brown discoloration of the rice grains at the site of inoculation, is characteristic of *M. audouinii*. Isolates of *M. canis* rapidly grow on the rice grains, typically producing many conidia and a bright yellow pigment.

## SLIDE CULTURE TECHNIQUE

Slide cultures are prepared to aid in the identification of moulds that are difficult to identify with tease mounts. If the slide culture and subsequent slides are prepared properly, a great deal of valuable information can be gained. Slide cultures can be used: to identify rapidly and accurately an unknown mould; to study ontogeny of conidia or spores; for the preparation of photomicrographs and line drawings; as a collection of permanent reference mounts for later identification assistance; and as a record of the isolates maintained in the culture collection.

Media such as cereal agar, cornmeal agar, potato dextrose agar, and V-8 juice agar are excellent for enhancing conidium and spore development. The slide cultures are usually incubated at 25–30°C in the dark for 2 weeks. This can be modified if necessary.

### A. *Preparation of the Slide Culture "Setup"*

1. Place one piece of filter paper in a glass 100 mm-Petri dish. The filter paper should just cover the bottom.

2. On top of the filter paper, place a glass rod that has been bent into the shape of a V. A disposable 1-ml glass pipette works very nicely.
3. Place a clean glass microscope slide on the V-shaped rod. If the microscope slide has a frosted writing edge, be sure it is face up.
4. An 18- to 22-mm glass cover glass should be placed on the microscope slide. The 18-mm cover glass is ideal, but a 22-mm one will work equally well.
5. Sterilize the setup by autoclaving for 15 minutes at 15 psi.
6. Dry the slide culture setups in the autoclave or in a drying oven, and then store them in a metal Petri dish canister.
7. Unused slide culture setups should be resterilized after approximately 4 weeks of storage.
8. Slide culture setups can also be prepared with disposable plastic Petri dishes. Each of the components (filter paper, microscope slides and glass slide covers) are sterilized separately and then added aseptically to the sterile plastic Petri dishes. Sterile, bent, round wooden applicator sticks are an ideal substitute for the glass V-shaped rods. Once the slide culture setup has been used, the entire system can be autoclaved and discarded.

### B. Preparation of the Slide Culture

1. Using a plate of medium that has been poured thick, cut the agar with a sterile scalpel into squares that are approximately 1 cm on each side.
2. Aseptically transfer one agar block with the sterile scalpel to the microscope slide in the slide culture setup. Be sure to place the agar block toward the side opposite the frosted area.
3. With a long-handled inoculating needle, transfer a small amount of the fungus from the edge of the colony to each of the four sides of the agar block.
4. Aseptically place the cover glass on top of the inoculated agar block.
5. Carefully add 1–1.5 ml of sterile water to the bottom of the slide culture. The filter paper must be checked on a regular basis to ensure that it is still moist. The moist filter paper will maintain a humid atmosphere and prevent the agar from drying. Glycerin, 5–20%, can be added to the sterile water to prevent moisture condensation on the microscope slide, cover glass, or both. Generally, this is not necessary.
6. Place the slide culture in a metal Petri dish canister and incubate the fungus for approximately 2 weeks in the dark. The slide can be periodically removed from the Petri dish and examined with the microscope. If the slide culture is not ready, it is simply returned to the

Petri dish and reincubated. If the isolate is sterile, refer to the techniques under the heading Sporulation and Sterile Isolates.

### C. "Taking Down" the Slide Culture

1. Remove the glass slide and wipe off all moisture on the bottom of the slide. Place the slide on the microscope and then determine whether the conidia or spores are mature.
2. Place a small drop of mounting medium (lactophenol is excellent) on a microscope slide that has been cleaned with 70% ethanol. The drop should be placed just off center with a fine-aperture pipette. It is important to ensure that the drop of mounting medium is small. This will ensure that there will not be an excess of mounting medium around the sides of the cover glass.
3. With a pair of forceps, carefully remove the cover glass from the agar block. If the agar block adheres to the cover glass, "flip" it off quickly with a dissecting needle. Care must be exercised that the agar block is not pushed off the cover glass. This will destroy part of the fungal growth on the cover glass.
4. Quickly pass the cover glass once or twice through a flame (blue portion). This will heat-fix the fungus and its conidia or spores in place. If carbon particles are seen on the cover glass after it has been mounted, this means that the cover glass was passed through a cool flame (orange-yellow color). To avoid this problem, the cover glass can be held parallel to the flame for a second or two. The fungus can be heat fixed in this manner without distortion of the diagnostic features. It does not matter which side of the cover glass is exposed to the flame. It is critical, though, to minimize the exposure time in the flame, in order to prevent collapse of the hyphae and conidia or spores.
5. Place the cover glass at the edge of the small drop of mounting medium and then carefully lower the cover glass with a dissecting needle. As the cover glass is lowered, air bubbles and loose conidia or spores will be forced toward the opposite side of the cover glass.
6. Very gently warm the mount. This will expel any air bubbles that may be present; swell and clear the fungus; concentrate the dye in the mounting medium into the hyphae and conidia or spores; and help evaporate excessive mounting medium. If there is excessive mounting medium, be sure to blot it by lightly touching the edge of the cover glass with a paper towel.
7. Ring the outer edge of the cover glass with fingernail polish. The advantage of the 18 mm cover glass is that it allows the nail polish to

flow over a wider area of the microscope slide than do the larger cover glasses. This favors a better sealed mount. Different brands of nail polish behave differently with respect to resistance to cracking and ability to adhere to the glass. A variety of brands should be tried before selecting one for general use. Label the slide on the frosted area.
8. By removing the agar block from the microscope slide in the original slide culture, this slide can be used as a second mount. After the slide has been heat fixed and mounting medium placed on it, a cover glass is placed over the fungus. Since the agar block was originally placed to one side, ample room should be available on the frosted edge for a label.

## SPORULATION AND STERILE ISOLATES

In the past, many medical mycologists incorrectly assumed that sterile isolates were not significant, primarily because they were not known to be pathogenic. Contemporary mycologists realize that these members of the Mycelia Sterilia can cause disease in man under some circumstances. It is therefore important to try to induce these fungi to form conidia, spores, or fruiting bodies so they can be identified. Some of these sterile isolates may represent one of the mating types of heterothallic Ascomycetes or Basidiomycetes, whereas others simply are sterile because the appropriate conditions necessary for the development of reproductive structures have not been met. There is no universal medium or set of environmental conditions that will stimulate conidiogenesis, sporogenesis, or fruiting body development in all fungi. Various media and techniques must be tried until the correct combination of variables is found.

Weak media will often stimulate the development of conidia or spores. Malt extract agar, dilute hay infusion agar, soil extract agar, 2% water agar, filter paper, wooden sticks, leaves, bean pods, carrot wedges, and similar substrates are helpful. All these media and substrates lack high concentrations of sugars, especially monosaccharides. These media are usually manufactured with tap water instead of distilled water because tap water contains trace elements that may be important in stimulating conidiogenesis or sporogenesis. A very simple technique involves inoculating a nonsporulating isolate to a piece of sterile filter paper in the bottom of a plastic Petri dish and moistening it with sterile tap water. Sterile wooden sticks, leaves, carrots, etc. can be placed on the filter paper as additional substrates.

In addition to the substrate upon which the sterile isolate is growing, the photoperiod and quality of light are extremely important. Incandescent lamps should not be used as a source of light because they do not emit the proper radiation needed for the enhancement of conidiogenesis or sporogenesis in many fungi. Near ultraviolet radiation (UV) with a peak of 3650 nm (range 3100 to 4100) is ideal for most fungi. Cool-white daylight fluorescent lamps work well because they emit enough near-UV radiation for most fungi. Plastic Petri dishes permit approximately 70% of the near-UV radiation to pass through them. Near-UV radiation will also penetrate glass Petri dishes. Colonies that are 3–4 days old or older should be exposed to the near-UV light because the light will have little, if any, effect on fungi that are not actively growing. A number of combinations of photoperiods and near UV radiation can be used. The major ones include the following:

1. Expose for 15–20 minutes in full sunlight or cool-white daylight fluorescent lamp, then place in darkness or subdued light.
2. Expose for 2–3 minutes to near-UV radiation, then place in darkness or subdued light.
3. Expose for a few hours to near-UV radiation, then place in darkness or subdued light.
4. Expose to photoperiods of 12 hours of near-UV radiation and then 12 hours of darkness.
5. Expose to near-UV radiation either for 5–10 days or until growth stops.

If a combination of weak media and exposure to UV radiation does not enhance conidiogenesis, sporogenesis, or fruiting body formation, the isolate will probably remain sterile and no further identification will be possible, unless mating studies are conducted. Mating studies are impractical for the clinical laboratory.

## SUBCULTURING ISOLATES

Subculturing is a propagation technique, ensuring that important isolates are maintained in the laboratory. Owing to the potential danger associated with medically important fungi, a long-handled inoculating needle should be used in lieu of short-handled dissecting probes. Inoculum from the colony can also be more easily obtained if the tip of the inoculating needle is bent at a right angle.

Isolates may be subcultured in several ways. The simplest procedure is to transfer a small portion of growth from the edge of the old colony to fresh media in a Petri dish or test tube. The inoculum is taken from the edge of the colony because this is where the fungus is most vegetatively active. When dangerous fungi such as *Coccidioides immitis* or isolates of *Aspergillus*, *Monilia*, etc. which produce abundant numbers of conidia, are being subcultured, the colony should first be flooded with a few milliliters of sterile distilled water. A conidial suspension can then be aspirated with a sterile pipette. A drop or two of this suspension is placed on the fresh media. By using water, aerosols are not created, thereby minimizing the danger of infection, contamination of other cultures, or both.

## TEASE MOUNT

The tease or direct mount is the most common technique used to mount fungi for microscopic examination. Tease mounts are temporary preparations that can be made semipermanent by sealing the edges of the cover glass with nail polish. Since the mould is teased apart with dissecting needles, conidia or spores are seldom found attached to their conidiogenous or sporogenous cells. Identifications are more difficult when using tease mounts instead of slide culture preparations.

### A. Standard Tease Mount

1. Place a very small drop of mounting medium, such as lactophenol (LP), just off center on a clean microscope slide.
2. With a long-handled inoculating needle, gently remove a small portion of growth from midway between the colony center and edge. Gently put this material into the drop of mounting fluid. A jeweler's forceps can be used selectively to obtain special areas, structures, or fruiting bodies.
3. With two dissecting needles or dissecting needle holders fitted with fine insect pins, gently tease the fungus apart so that it is thinly spread out in the mounting medium.
4. Place a cover glass at the edge of the drop of mounting fluid and then lower it with a dissecting needle. By gentle lowering of the cover glass, air bubbles and dislodged conidia or spores are forced toward the opposite edge of the cover glass.
5. Examine the fungus. If the mount is to be kept, the edges of the cover glass can be sealed with nail polish. Excessive LP must be removed with absorbent paper prior to sealing the preparation with nail polish.
6. If only hyphae are seen, prepare a new mount using material taken from the center of the colony. If the mount consists of large numbers of conidia or spores, prepare a new mount using growth at the edge of the colony. Before preparing the mount, it is a good idea to look at the colony first with a dissecting microscope to determine whether or not mature conidia or spores are present.

### B. Mounting Zygomycetes and Fruiting Structures

1. In many instances, sporangia, ascocarps, and other fruiting bodies tend to trap air bubbles, which make preparations unsatisfactory for microscopic study. This problem can be minimized by modifying the standard technique as follows:
    a. Place a drop of 95% ethanol, ethyl acetate, or water with 0.05% Tween 80 on the microscope slide.
    b. Transfer the fungus from the culture to the drop of fluid. These agents are wetting agents, which prevent the formation of air bubbles around the structures to be studied.
    c. Blot the fluid until just enough remains to keep the fungus moist. If 95% ethanol is used, add a drop of 2% KOH to the blotted mount. The KOH is used to reexpand the specimen. The KOH is then blotted.
    d. Add a drop of the usual mounting fluid and proceed as in the standard technique. For Zygomycetes, 1% aqueous phloxine is an excellent mounting medium because it stains the cytoplasm, making it more readily visible.

### C. Tape Technique

1. Place one drop of mounting medium on a clean microscope slide.
2. Remove a short segment of transparent tape approximately 2 cm long from a tape roll.
3. Touch one end of the tape to a round wooden applicator stick and then lightly touch the colony with the sticky loop.
4. Loosen the tape and lay the tape with the surface containing the fungus face down into the mounting medium. Detach the tape from the wooden applicator stick.
5. Examine the mount directly with a microscope. An additional drop of mounting medium can be put on the top of the tape and then covered with a cover glass if desired. This procedure permits the viewing of conidia or spores still attached, as well as other structures in their natural position. Details are often difficult to see owing to the variations in the thickness of the mount.

## TEMPERATURE STUDIES

Thermotolerance is a useful characteristic that can be used as an aid in the identification of several medically important moulds. Since a negative test is based upon the absence of growth at the elevated temperature, two tubes are always necessary. One tube must be incubated at room temperature to ensure that the inoculum was viable, otherwise, the absence of growth at the elevated temperature is meaningless. Media such as potato dextrose agar, cornmeal agar, and Sabouraud dextrose agar are ideal choices for this test. Tubes incubated at the elevated temperature should also be sealed with parafilm or some similar material that will retard the dehydration process, but still permit good aeration.

Thermotolerance (Table 4.4) is a useful test to distinguish isolates of *Trichophyton mentagrophytes* from those of *T. terrestre*. *Trichophyton mentagrophytes* grows at 37°C, whereas *T. terrestre* does not. Isolates of *T. verrucosum* can be readily identified by the property of their growth being enhanced at 37°C. Such growth enhancement at 37°C is not characteristic of any other species of *Trichophyton*. *Wangiella dermatitidis* can be distinguished from similar dematiaceous hyphomycetes by its ability to grow at 40°C. Likewise, *Cladosporium bantianum* can be distinguished from *C. carrionii* and other species of *Cladosporium* by its ability to grow at a temperature range of 42 to 43°C. And finally, *Aspergillus fumigatus* grows well at 48°C, whereas most other species of *Aspergillus* cannot grow at this temperature. Caution must be exercised because other thermotolerant species of *Aspergillus* can also grow at this elevated temperature.

### A. Procedure

1. Remove small portions of the mould colony from midway between the colony center and edge with a long-handled inoculating needle and place it toward the butt in two tubes of media.
2. Incubate one culture at the elevated temperature and one culture at 30°C.

**Table 4.4.** Thermotolerance of Some Medically Important Fungi

| Fungus | Upper growth limits (°C) |
| --- | --- |
| *Aspergillus fumigatus* | 48–50 |
| *Cladosporium bantianum* | 42–43 |
| *C. carrionii* | 35–36 |
| *Fonsecaea pedrosoi* | 38 |
| *Rhizomucor pusillus* | 50–55 |
| *Trichophyton mentagrophytes* | 37 |
| *T. verrucosum* | 37 Enhancement |
| *Wangiella dermatitidis* | 40 |

3. If growth is present at both temperatures, the isolate is thermotolerant. If growth is present at 30°C, but not at the elevated temperature, the test is negative. When growth is absent at 30°C, the test must be repeated.

## UREA HYDROLYSIS

Many medical mycologists use the ability, or inability, to hydrolyze urea as an important characteristic for the identification of some dermatophytes. The test is primarily used to distinguish *Trichophyton mentagrophytes* from *T. rubrum*. These species are usually urease positive and urease negative in 7–8 days, respectively. This test must be used with extreme caution because some isolates of *T. mentagrophytes* are urease negative and others may not hydrolyze urea until after 8 days. Isolates of *T. rubrum* are occasionally encountered that are urease positive within 8 days. In addition, a number of similar species of dermatophytes may be either urease positive or negative, depending upon the species. The principal value of the urea hydrolysis test is to furnish additional data that may be helpful in identifying atypical isolates of *T. mentagrophytes* and *T. rubrum*. Even at this stage of the identification process, the urea hydrolysis test is not definitive.

The ability to produce urease is usually determined with Christensen's urea agar, Philpot's modification of Christensen's urea agar, or Christensen's urea broth. Overall, these three media are basically equivalent. The use of one medium rather than another is based upon personal preference. In each group of urease determinations, an uninoculated tube and two tubes, one each inoculated with *T. mentagrophytes* and *T. rubrum*, are necessary for positive and negative controls.

### A. Procedure

1. With a long-handled inoculating needle, remove a portion of growth from midway between the edge and center of the colony. Inoculate the urea medium.
2. Incubate the test at 25–30°C for 8 days. The tubes should be examined every 2–3 days for the presence of urease, which is detected as a pH indicator color change.
3. The control medium is always read first. The uninoculated medium should be yellow, indicating that there has been no change in the phenol red pH indicator system due to atmospheric gases. The medium

with *T. mentagrophytes* should be pink to red; and that with *T. rubrum* yellow.
a. Medium yellow, urease not produced = negative.
b. Medium pink to red, urease produced = positive.

## Part 2. Selected References

### A. General References

1. Ajello, L., L. K. Georg, W. Kaplan, and L. Kaufman (1966). "Laboratory Manual for Medical Mycology," USPHS Publ. No. 994. Center for Disease Control, Atlanta, Georgia.
2. CMI (1960). "Herb. I.M.I. Handbook. Methods in Use at the Commonwealth Mycological Institute." Commonwealth Mycological Institute, Kew, Surrey, England.
3. CMI (1968). "Plant Pathologist's Pocketbook." Commonwealth Mycological Institute, Kew, Surrey, England.
4. Stevens, R. B., ed. (1974). "Mycology Guidebook." Univ. of Washington Press, Seattle.
5. Tuite, J. (1969). "Plant Pathological Methods. Fungi and Bacteria." Burgess, Minneapolis, Minnesota.

### B. Confirmation of Dimorphic Fungi

1. Campbell, C. C. (1947). Reverting *Histoplasma capsulatum* to the yeast phase. *J. Bacteriol.* **54**:263–264.
2. Carmichael, J. W. (1962). *Chrysosporium* and some other aleuriosporic hyphomycetes. *Can. J. Bot.* **40**:1137–1173.
3. Converse, J. L. (1955). Growth of spherules of *Coccidioides immitis* in a chemically defined liquid medium. *Proc. Soc. Exp. Biol. Med.* **90**:709–711.
4. El-Ani, A. S., J. W. Pickren, and J. E. Fitzpatrick (1978). Coccidioidomycosis in a patient with lymphoma. *Am. J. Clin. Pathol.* **70**:423–428.
5. Emmons, C. W., and W. L. Jellison (1960). *Emmonsia crescens* sp. n. and adiaspiromycosis (haplomycosis) in mammals. *Ann. N. Y. Acad. Sci.* **89**:91–101.
6. Hempel, H., and N. L. Goodman (1975). Rapid conversion of *Histoplasma capsulatum, Blastomyces dermatitidis* and *Sporothrix schenckii* in tissue culture. *J. Clin. Microbiol.* **1**:420–424.
7. Kaufman, L., and P. Standard (1978). Immuno-identification of cultures of fungi pathogenic to man. *Curr. Microbiol.* **1**:135–140.
8. Levine, H. B., J. M. Cobb, and C. E. Smith (1960). Immunity to coccidioidomycosis induced in mice by purified spherule, arthrospore, and mycelial vaccines. *Trans. N. Y. Acad. Sci., Ser. 2*, **22**:436–449.
9. Pine, L., and C. L. Peacock (1958). Studies on the growth of *Histoplasma capsulatum*. IV. Factors influencing conversion of the mycelial phase to the yeast phase. *J. Bacteriol.* **75**:167–174.
10. Sun, S. H., M. Huppert, and K. R. Vukovich (1976). Rapid *in vitro* conversion and identification of *Coccidioides immitis*. *J. Clin. Microbiol.* **3**:186–190.
11. Taylor, J. J. (1970). A comparison of some *Ceratocystis* species with *Sporothrix schenckii*. *Mycopathol. Mycol. Appl.* **42**:233–240.

## C. Cycloheximide Resistance

1. Georg, L. K., L. Ajello, and C. Papageorge (1954). Use of cycloheximide in the selective isolation of fungi pathogenic to man. *J. Lab. Clin. Med.* **44**:422–428.
2. Kuehn, H. H., and G. F. Orr (1962). Tolerance of certain fungi to Actidione and its use in isolation of Gymnoascaceae. *Sabouraudia* **1**:220–229.
3. McDonough, E. S., L. K. Georg, L. Ajello, and S. Brinkman (1960). Growth of dimorphic human pathogenic fungi on media containing cycloheximide and chloramphenicol. *Mycopathol. Mycol. Appl.* **13**:113–120.
4. Salkin, I. F. (1975). Adaptation to cycloheximide: *in vitro* studies with filamentous fungi. *Can. J. Microbiol.* **21**:1413–1419.

## D. In Vitro Hair Test

1. Ajello, L., and L. K. Georg (1957). *In vitro* hair cultures for differentiating between atypical isolates of *Trichophyton mentagrophytes* and *Trichophyton rubrum*. *Mycopathol. Mycol. Appl.* **8**:3–17.

## E. Nutritional Studies

1. Georg, L. K., and L. B. Camp (1957). Routine nutritional tests for the identification of dermatophytes. *J. Bacteriol.* **74**:113–121.
2. Philpot, C. M. (1977). The use of nutritional tests for the differentiation of dermatophytes. *Sabouraudia* **15**:141–150

## F. Proteolytic Activity

1. Berliner, M. D. (1967). Gelatin hydrolysis for identification of the filamentous phase of *Histoplasma, Blastomyces* and *Chrysosporium* species. *Sabouraudia* **5**:274–277.
2. Mackinnon, J. E., L. V. Ferrada, and L. Montemayor (1949). Investigaciones sobre las maduromicosis y sus agentes. *An. Fac. Med. Montevideo* **30**:231–300.
3. Montemayor, L. (1949). Estudio de las propiedades biológicas de varias cepas de hongos patógenos causantes de la cromomicosis, y de especies vecinas saprofitas y patógenas. *Mycopathol. Mycol. Appl.* **4**:379–383.
4. Padhye, A. A. (1978). Comparative study of *Phialophora jeanselmei* and *P. gougerotii* by morphological, biochemical, and immunological methods. *Proc. Int. Conf. Mycosis, 4th,* PAHO Sci. Publ. No. 356, pp. 60–65.
5. Trejos, A. (1954). *Cladosporium carrionii* n. sp. and the problem of Cladosporia isolated from chromoblastomycosis. *Rev. Biol. Trop.* **2**:75–112.

## G. Slide Culture Technique

1. Cole, G. T., T. R. Nag Raj, and W. B. Kendrick (1969). A simple technique for time-lapse photomicrography of microfungi in plate culture. *Mycologia* **61**:726–730.
2. Kohlmeyer, J., and E. Kohlmeyer (1972). Permanent microscopic mounts. *Mycologia* **64**:666–669.
3. McGinnis, M. R. (1974). Preparation of temporary or permanent mounts of microfungi with undisturbed conidia. *Mycologia* **66**:169–170.

4. Riddell, R. (1950). Permanent stained mycological preparations obtained by slide culture. *Mycologia* **42**:265–270.

## H. Sporulation and Sterile Isolates

1. Booth, C. (1971). "The Genus *Fusarium.*" Commonwealth Mycological Institute, Kew, Surrey, England.
2. Stevens, R. B., ed. (1974). "Mycological Guidebook." Univ. of Washington Press, Seattle.

## I. Temperature Studies

1. Borelli, D. (1964). On the importance of temperature in the pathogeny and the clinics of mycoses. *Arch. Dermatol.* **89**:504.
2. Padhye, A. A., M. R. McGinnis, and L. Ajello (1978). Thermotolerance of *Wangiella dermatitidis. J. Clin. Microbiol.* **8**:424–426.
3. Raper, K. B., and D. I. Fennell (1965). "The Genus *Aspergillus.*" Williams & Wilkins Co., Baltimore, Maryland.

## J. Urea Hydrolysis

1. Kane, J., and J. B. Fischer (1971). The differentiation of *Trichophyton rubrum* and *T. mentagrophytes* by use of Christensen's urea broth. *Can. J. Microbiol.* **17**:911–913.
2. Littman, M. L. (1957). An improved method for detection of urea hydrolysis by fungi. *J. Infect. Dis.* **101**:51–61.
3. Philpot, C. (1967). The differentiation of *Trichophyton mentagrophytes* from *T. rubrum* by a simple urease test. *Sabouraudia* **5**:189–193.
4. Philpot, C. M. (1977). The use of nutritional tests for the differentiation of dermatophytes. *Sabouraudia* **15**:141–150.
5. Rosenthal, S. A., and H. Sokolsky (1965). Enzymatic studies with pathogenic fungi. *Dermatol. Int.* **4**:72–79.

## Part 3. Taxonomy

### Key to Some of the Major Groups of Fungi*

1. Ascospores, asci, or both present . . . . . . . . . . . . . . . . . . . . . Ascomycetes
1'. Ascospores and asci absent . . . . . . . . . . . . . . . . . . . . . . . . . . 2
   2. Sporangia, sporangiola, merosporangia, or zygospores present . . . . . Zygomycetes
   2'. Sporangia, sporangiola, merosporangia, and zygospores absent . . . . . . . . . . 3
3. Pycnidia or acervuli present . . . . . . . . . . . . . . . . . . . . . . . Coelomycetes
3'. Pycnidia or acervuli absent . . . . . . . . . . . . . . . . . . . . . . . Hyphomycetes

### Key to Some of the Genera of Ascomycetes

1. Gymnothecia present . . . . . . . . . . . . . . . . . . . . . . . . . . . . . 2
1'. Gymnothecia absent . . . . . . . . . . . . . . . . . . . . . . . . . . . . . 4

---

*Basidiomycetes producing basidiospores and basidia have been excluded. Imperfect Basidiomycetes are treated in the class Hyphomycetes. Yeasts are considered in Chapter 5, except for dematiaceous yeasts, which are considered here.

2. Spirals arising from the center of the gymnothecium, with a network of secondary peridial hyphae arising from the spirals; *Blastomyces* or *Histoplasma* anamorphs usually present . . . . . . . . . . . . . . . . . . . . . . . . . . . . . . *Ajellomyces*

2'. Gymnothecia and anamorphs not as above . . . . . . . . . . . . . . . . . . 3

3. Cells of the peridial hyphae dumbbell-shaped with a deeply constricted central region; *Chrysosporium* or *Trichophyton* anamorphs usually present . . . . . . . . . *Arthroderma*

3'. Cells of the peridial hyphae having a slightly constricted central region; *Microsporum* anamorph usually present . . . . . . . . . . . . . . . . . . . . . . . . . *Nannizzia*

4. Cleistothecia present . . . . . . . . . . . . . . . . . . . . . . . . . . . . 5

4'. Cleistothecia absent . . . . . . . . . . . . . . . . . . . . . . . . . . . . 7

5. Cleistothecia globose, bright yellow; peridium consisting of a 1-cell-thick layer of thin, flattened cells; ascospores purple-red; *Aspergillus* anamorph present . . . . . . *Eurotium*

5'. Cleistothecia globose to subglobose, brown to black; peridium membranaceous; ascospores black, orange to copper . . . . . . . . . . . . . . . . . . . . . . . . . . . 6

6. Ascospores orange to copper with 2 germ pores; peridium 1 to 2 layers thick, nearly transparent, without hairs; *Scedosporium, Graphium,* or both anamorphs usually present . . . . . . . . . . . . . . . . . . . . . . . . . . . . . . . . . *Petriellidium*

6'. Ascospores dark brown with 1 or 2 germ pores; peridium often with hairs; anamorphs *Sepedonium, Botryotrichum,* and other anamorphs usually present . . . . . . *Thielavia*

7. Perithecia globose to flask-shaped, brown to black, ostiolate, with long brown to variously colored hairlike appendages arising from the peridium; ascospores lemon-shaped . . . . . . . . . . . . . . . . . . . . . . . . . . . . . . . . . . . . . *Chaetomium*

7'. Perithecia absent; ascocarps ascostromata; asci bitunicate . . . . . . . . . . . . . 8

8. Asci clavate to cylindrical; ascospores 4- to 9-celled with a constriction at each septum; ascostromata globose to subglobose . . . . . . . . . . . . *Leptosphaeria*

8'. Characteristics not as above . . . . . . . . . . . . . . . . . . . . . . . 9

9. Asci ellipsoidal; ascospores 1-celled, usually curved with a filiform extension; ascostromata irregular to subglobose . . . . . . . . . . . . . . . . . . . . . . . . . . . . *Piedraia*

9'. Asci subglobose to clavate; ascospores 2-celled with a sharply constricted septum; ascostromata globose to ellipsoidal . . . . . . . . . . . . . . . . . . . . *Neotestudina*

### Key to Some of the Genera of Coelomycetes

1. Pycnidia with brown to black setae arising from the upper portion of the fruiting body; pycnidia globose to flask-shaped, black, ostiolate; phialides cylindrical; phialoconidia 1-celled, hyaline . . . . . . . . . . . . . . . . . . . . . . . . . . . . . *Pyrenochaeta*

1'. Pycnidia without setae . . . . . . . . . . . . . . . . . . . . . . . . . . . 2

2. Conidiogenous cells annellides; annelloconidia at first 1-celled and hyaline, becoming 2-celled and dark brown with hyaline longitudinal striations; pycnidia globose, black, ostiolate . . . . . . . . . . . . . . . . . . . . . . . . . . . . . . *Lasiodiplodia*

2'. Conidiogenous cells phialides . . . . . . . . . . . . . . . . . . . . . . . 3

3. Phialoconidia 3-celled, center cell dark brown, end cells lighter, ovoid; phialides short and cylindrical; pycnidia ostiolate, immersed; *Scytalidium* anamorph usually present . . . . . . . . . . . . . . . . . . . . . . . . . . . . . . . . . . . . . . . . . . *Hendersonula*

Key to the Groups of the Hyphomycetes

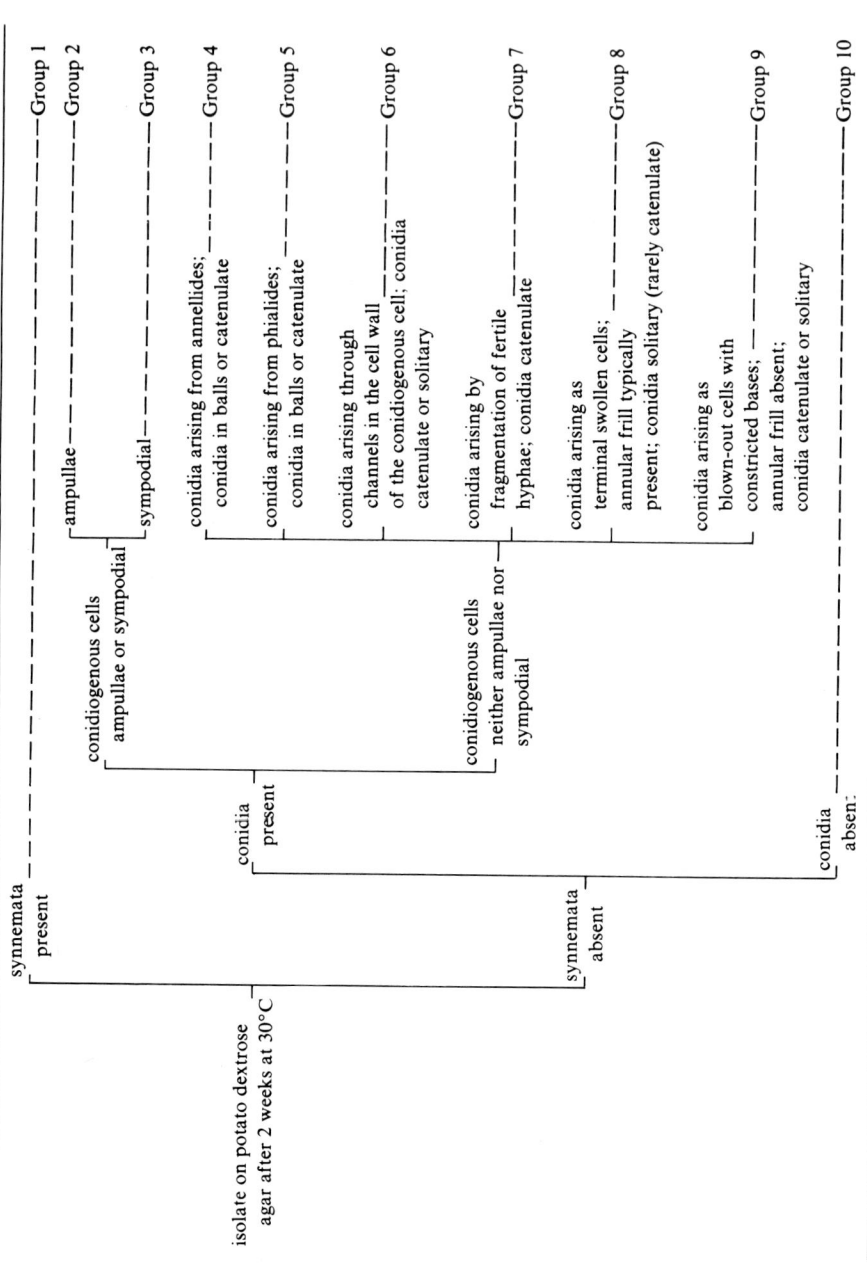

3'. Phialoconidia 1-celled, hyaline; phialides ampulliform; pycnidia ostiolate, superficial
. . . . . . . . . . . . . . . . . . . . . . . . . . . . . . . . . . . . . . . . . *Phoma*

### Key to Some of the Genera of Hyphomycetes

#### Group 1

Group 1 comprises those hyphomycetes that form compact, elongated groups of erect conidiophores that are cemented together, their conidia being produced at the apex, along the sides, or both, from the upper portion of the synnema (Fig. 4.10). Free conidiogenous cells that are identical to those formed by the synnemata may be present. The genera are primarily distinguished from each other on the basis of Saccardoan characteristics. Many of the genera require revision in light of our current concepts of conidiogenesis.

1. Synnemata erect, dark, solitary or in clusters; conidia 1-celled, smooth, hyaline to dark, forming a large slimy ball; conidiogenous cells are annellides; one anamorph being *Scedosporium* . . . . . . . . . . . . . . . . . . . . . . . . . . . . . . . . *Graphium*
1'. Synnemata erect, dark, solitary or in clusters; annelloconidia 1-celled, smooth or rough, hyaline, truncate, forming in chains; *Scopulariopsis* anamorph usually present . . . . . . 2
    2. Setae arising from synnemata . . . . . . . . . . . . . . . . . . . . . . . *Trichurus*
    2'. Setae absent . . . . . . . . . . . . . . . . . . . . . . . . . . . . . *Cephalotrichum*

#### Group 2

Ampullae (Fig. 4.11) are enlarged, usually globose, terminal cells that give rise to several blastic conidia in a synchronized manner. The conidia may be solitary, in simple chains, or in branching chains. The conidiophores are either proliferous or determinate. The conidiophores and their branches terminate in an ampulla.

Isolates of *Arthrobotrys* (Fig. 4.30) produce swollen cells that appear to be ampullae. The blastoconidia of *Arthrobotrys* are formed successively in an asynchronized manner. The conidiophore is proliferous and continues to grow from the apex of the vesicle, which results in several intercalary swellings from which the conidia are produced.

1. Conidiophores erect, branching restricted to apical region; blastoconidia 1-celled, solitary, hyaline to pale brown, forming on denticles . . . . . . . . . . . . . . . . . . . . . *Botrytis*
1'. Conidiophores with nodelike swollen areas that are either terminal, intercalary, or both; blastoconidia developing successively on denticles . . . . . . . . . . . see *Arthrobotrys*

#### Group 3

Sympodial conidiophores are proliferous; that is, they continue to increase in length, even after a terminal conidium is produced (Fig. 4.12). As a conidium is developing at the apex of the conidiophore, a new lateral subterminal growing point forms. From this new apex, a second conidium develops. The process is repeated a number of times and results in either an elongated, or compact, or swollen conidiophore that has a geniculate appearance. The conidia that are formed from a sympodial conidiophore are either arthroconidia, blastoconidia, or poroconidia, and they may occur solitarily or in chains.

1. Conidiogenous cells are swollen at the base, tapering to a long narrow conidium-bearing rachis; blastoconidia 1-celled solitary, hyaline to lightly colored; colonies white to variously colored, but not dematiaceous . . . . . . . . . . . . . . . . . . . . . . . . . . . . . . 2

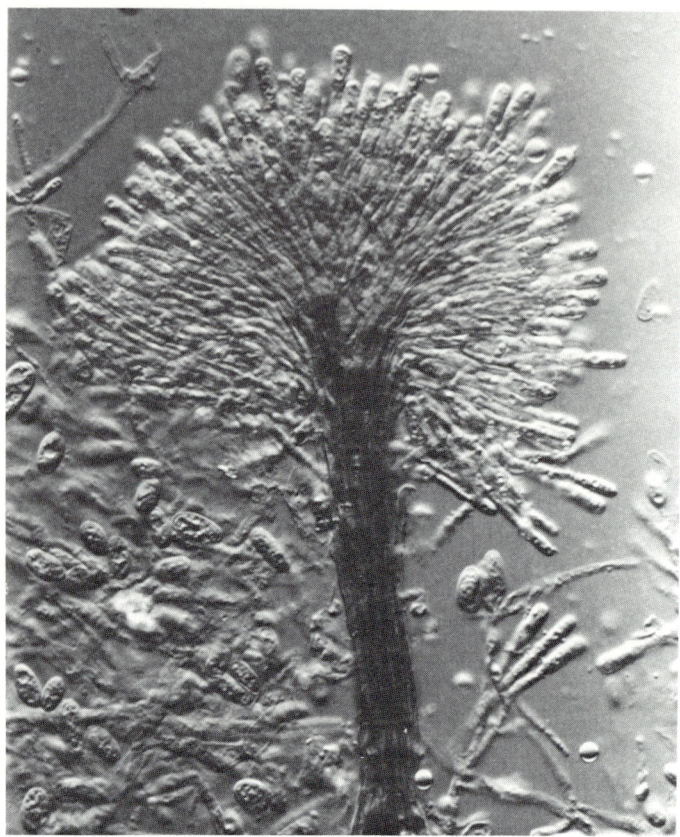

Fig. 4.10 *Graphium* anamorph of *Petriellidium boydii*. The one-celled conidia occur as a mass at the apex of the synnema.

1'. Conidiogenous cells not swollen at base, long narrow conidium-bearing rachis absent . . 3
    2. Sympodial conidiogenous cells arising in dense clusters; conidiophores not verticillate
    . . . . . . . . . . . . . . . . . . . . . . . . . . . . . . . . . . . . . . . *Beauveria*
    2'. Sympodial conidiogenous cells arising in whorls; conidiophores simple or verticillate
    . . . . . . . . . . . . . . . . . . . . . . . . . . . . . . . . . . . . . . *Tritirachium*
3. Conidia muriform, poroconidia solitary or in chains, brown to black . . . . . . . . . . 4
3'. Conidia not muriform . . . . . . . . . . . . . . . . . . . . . . . . . . . . . . . . 5
    4. Conidia in simple or branching chains, ovoid to obclavate; conidiophores erect, simple
    . . . . . . . . . . . . . . . . . . . . . . . . . . . . . . . . . . . . . . . *Alternaria*
    4'. Conidia solitary, obovoid without central constriction; conidiophores simple, occasionally branched, geniculate . . . . . . . . . . . . . . . . . . . . . . . *Ulocladium*
5. Conidia forming in branching chains; blastoconidia 1-celled or 1- to several-celled; pale brown to black . . . . . . . . . . . . . . . . . . . . . . . . . . . . . . . . . . . 6
5'. Conidia not forming branching chains . . . . . . . . . . . . . . . . . . . . . . . . 8

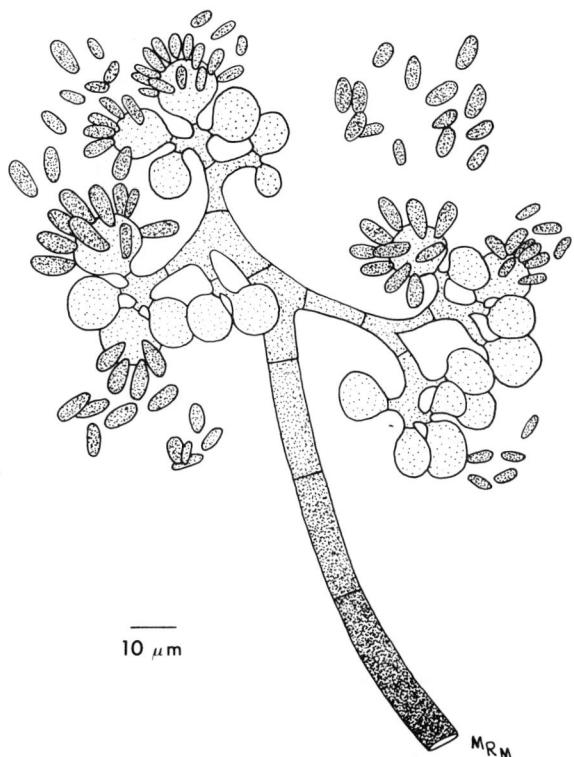

**Fig. 4.11** *Botrytis cinerea*. The blastoconidia are developing in a synchronized manner upon short denticles from the ampullae.

      6. One-celled blastoconidia arising laterally from a parallel-walled sympodial conidiophore; apex may be swollen and irregular; primary blastoconidia producing several 1-celled secondary blastoconidia sympodially; secondary blastoconidia may give rise to tertiary blastoconidia; *Cladosporium, Phialophora,* or both anamorphs may be present . . . . . . . . . . . . . . . . . . . . . . . . . . . . . . . . . . *Fonsecaea*

      6'. Blastoconidia arising from a simple or branched conidiophore in simple or branching acropetal chains; blastoconidia 1- to several-celled . . . . . . . . . . . . . . . 7

7. Blastoconidia 1- to 5-celled, cylindrical, verruculose; forming loosely branching chains; conidiophores simple or sympodial . . . . . . . . . . . . . . . . . . . . . . *Stenella*

7'. Blastoconidia 1- to 4-celled, primarily 1-celled, shield-shaped conidia present, conidia with a distinct dark hilum; branching chains well formed, conidia readily separating from each other; conidiophores erect . . . . . . . . . . . . . . . . . . . . . . . . . . *Cladosporium*

      8. Blastoconidia 1-celled, arising laterally from a parallel-walled conidiophore; conidia pale brown . . . . . . . . . . . . . . . . . . . . . . . . . . . . . . . . . . . . . 9

      8'. Conidia 1-celled or 1- to several-celled; parallel-walled conidiophores present or absent; conidia hyaline or pale brown; combination of characteristics not as in 8 . . 10

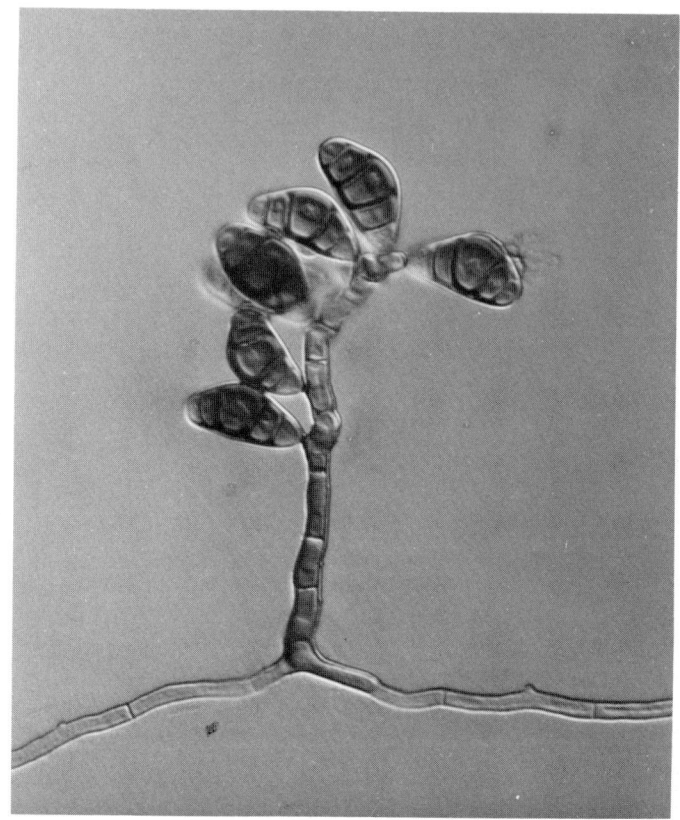

**Fig. 4.12** Sympodial conidiophores are often geniculate in appearance. A. *Curvularia* sp. B. *Alternaria* sp.

9. One-celled blastoconidia arising laterally from a parallel-walled sympodial conidiophore, apex may be swollen and irregular; primary blastoconidia producing several 1-celled secondary blastoconidia sympodially; secondary conidia may form tertiary blastoconidia; *Cladosporium, Phialophora,* or both anamorphs may be present. . . . . . . . . *Fonsecaea*

9′. Blastoconidia not produced from the primary blastoconidia; conidia acropleurogenous . . . . . . . . . . . . . . . . . . . . . . . . . . . . . . . . . . *Rhinocladiella*

    10. Blastoconidia 2- to 4-celled, pale brown, arising from fine tubular denticles; conidia cylindrical to T or Y shaped; conidiophores 1- to several-celled, short clavate to long and hyphalike . . . . . . . . . . . . . . . . . . . . . . . . . . *Scolecobasidium*

    10′. Conidia not arising from tubular denticles, if so, conidia 1-celled only; conidia not T or Y shaped; conidiophores neither short and clavate nor long and hyphalike . . . 11

  11. Blastoconidia 1-celled, arising from denticles; conidia may be either along the hyphae, or from the upper portion of sympodial conidiophores that are swollen or straight, or from both; conidia may be of two types, large and globose (dematiaceous), small and clavate to ovoid (hyaline), or a combination of both kinds . . . . . . . . . . . . . . . *Sporothrix*

  11′. Conidia more than 1-celled; pale brown to black . . . . . . . . . . . . . . . . . . . 12

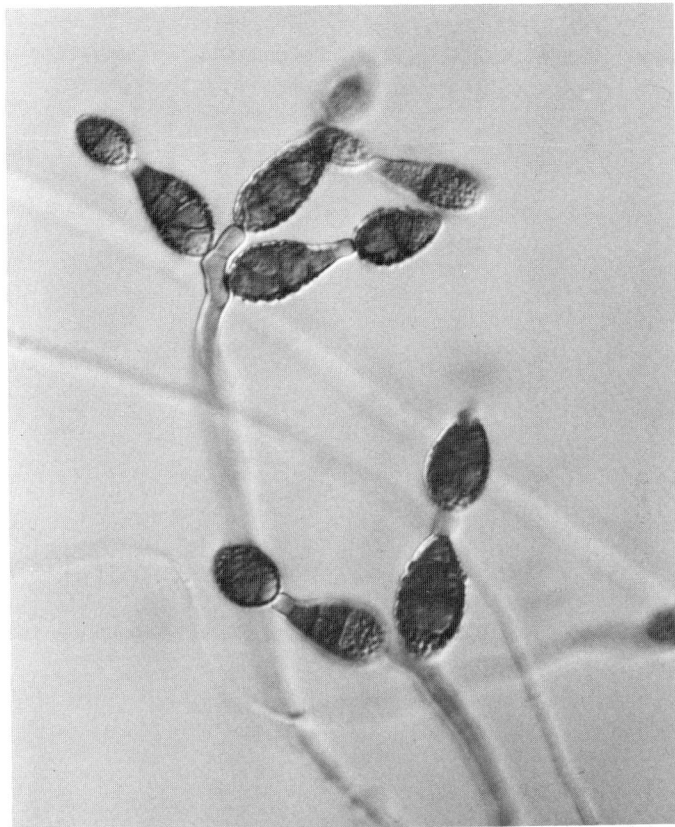

**B**

**Fig. 4.12** Continued

12. Conidia long, narrow, straight, 5- to 26-celled, pale brown, often with a basal appendage, bases convex; conidiophores short with flat to convex conidial scars . . . . . . . . . . . . . . . . . . . . . . . . . . . . . . . . . . . *Mycocentrospora*

12'. Conidia curved-to-cylindrical-to-fusoid; not long and narrow; conidiophores extremely geniculate . . . . . . . . . . . . . . . . . . . . . . . . . . . . . . . . 13

13. Conidia usually curved, several-celled, end cells paler than other cells; brown to black protruding hilum present . . . . . . . . . . . . . . . . . . . . . . . . . *Curvularia*

13'. Conidia cylindrical to fusoid . . . . . . . . . . . . . . . . . . . . . . . *Drechslera*

*Group 4*

Group 4 contains fungi that produce annellides and annelloconidia. Annellides (Fig. 4.13) are proliferous conidiogenous cells that are percurrent in growth. After each blastic conidium is formed and released from the annellide, a ring of outer cell wall material is left behind at the apex of the annellide (annellation). As a result of this type of proliferation, annellides

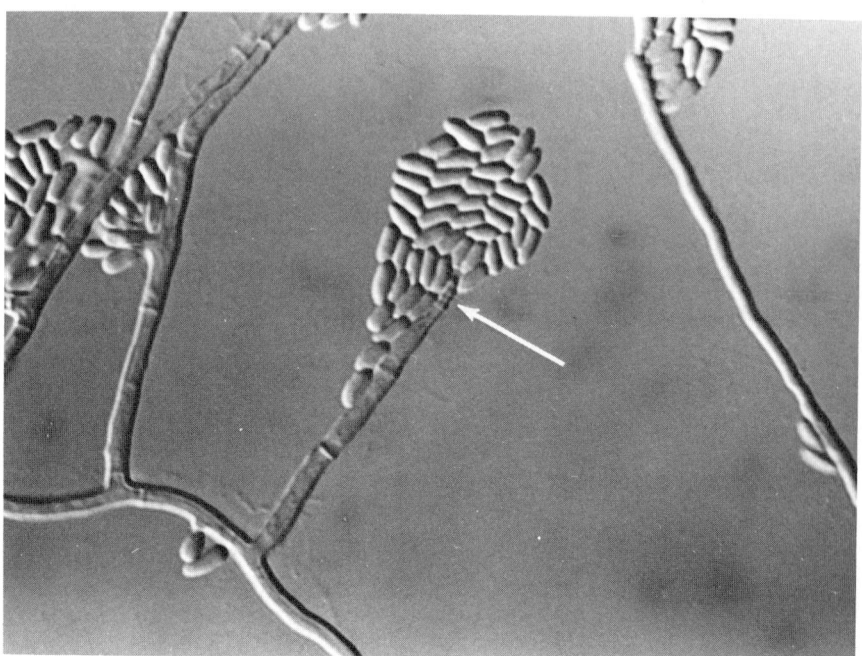

**Fig. 4.13** *Exophiala spinifera*. The annellides in this fungus arise on spinelike conidiophores. Annellations (arrow) can be seen at the apex of the annellide immediately below the ball of annelloconidia. As the ball of conidia increases in size, it slides down the conidiophore.

increase in length and the diameter of the apex becomes smaller. Annelloconidia are usually 1-celled and may occur either in balls or chains. Annellides may be solitary, terminal, intercalary, as yeast cells, or any combination. Simple or branching conidiophores may be present. With the light microscope, they are often recognizable by their narrow, tapering apices.

1. Annelloconidia 1-celled, globose to pyriform, usually with truncate bases, smooth or rough, occurring in simple chains; annellides solitary, in groups, or part of a penicillus; *Cephalotrichum* or *Trichurus* anamorph may be present . . . . . . . . . . *Scopulariopsis*
1'. Annelloconidia occurring in balls . . . . . . . . . . . . . . . . . . . . . . . . . 2
    2. Annellides cylindrical to lageniform, terminal or intercalary; annelloconidia usually 1-celled, may be several-celled in some species (typically not seen in the clinical laboratory), subglobose to cylindrical; toruloid hyphae usually present; *Phaeococcus* anamorph typically present . . . . . . . . . . . . . . . . . . . . . . . *Exophiala*
    2'. Conidium development variable; conidia 1-celled, subglobose to elongate; developing on lateral hyphal outgrowths, or from elongated, cylindrical annellides with a slightly swollen apex; conidia solitary or in balls; *Petriellidium* or similar teleomorph usually present, *Graphium* anamorph may be present . . . . . . . . . . . . *Scedosporium*

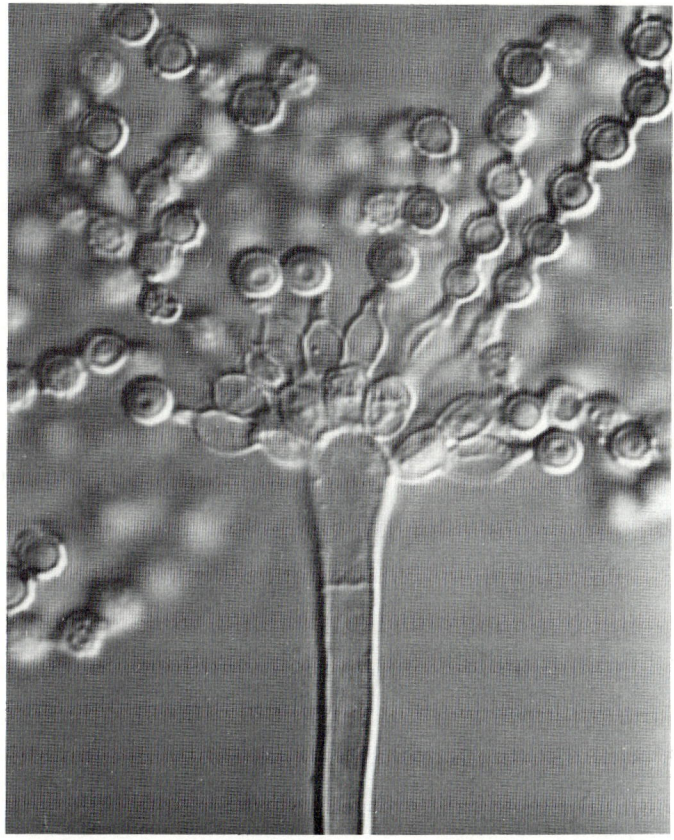

**Fig. 4.14** Phialides are often flask-shaped. A. An *Aspergillus* sp. is forming its phialoconidia in chains. B. *Trichoderma viride* is forming its phialoconidia in balls.

*Group 5*

Phialoconidia produced by phialides is characteristic of group 5. Phialides are determinate conidiogenous cells (Fig. 4.14). The first conidium is holoblastic in origin. Each of the successive conidia arises in a basipetal manner, its cell walls being formed enteroblastically from a fixed locus. The conidia are usually 1-celled and may either develop in simple chains that are solitary or united into a head, or accumulate in balls at the apices of the phialides or as a single large ball at the apices of a group of phialides. In some species, the balls have a tendency to slip (slime) down the phialides. Phialides may be either cylindrical to flask-shaped, solitary, in clusters, in verticils, intercalary, or have a collarette, or any combination of these characteristics. Collarettes may be small, large, cuplike, or cylindrical, depending upon the species. The conidiophores may terminate in a vesicle, be simple, branched, solitary, arranged in verticils, or forming a penicillus. Some phialides without distinct collarettes can be recognized by a thickened apex which appears dark and heavy with the light microscope. Phialides always produce a number of conidia from each conidiogenous locus.

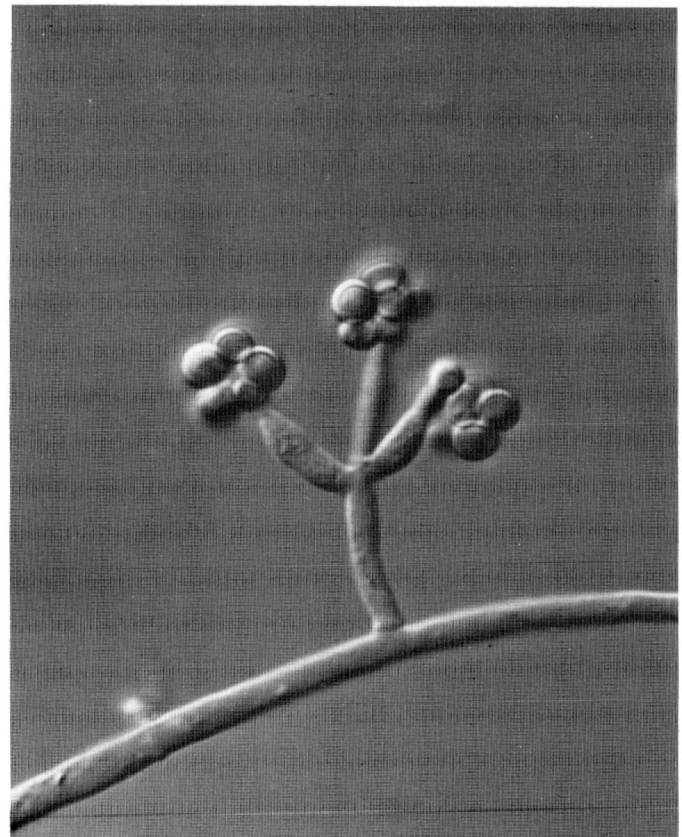

**Fig. 4.14** Continued

1. Conidiogenous cells hyphalike, erect, cylindrical; conidia 2-celled, clavate to ovoid; conidia alternate, forming in a "double row," with their bases becoming wider; conidiophores becoming shorter (retrogressive); colonies pale rose, granular, rapidly growing . . . . . . . . . . . . . . . . . . . . . . . . . . . . . . . . . . . . . . . . . . . . . . . see *Trichothecium*

   1'. Phialoconidia and phialides present . . . . . . . . . . . . . . . . . . . . . . 2

      2. Conidiophores erect, terminating in a vesicle; phialides arising either directly from the vesicle (uniseriate) on metulae (biseriate) or a combination of both; phialoconidia 1-celled, catenulate, forming a head . . . . . . . . . . . . . . . . . . . . . *Aspergillus*

      2'. Conidiophores not terminating in vesicles . . . . . . . . . . . . . . . . . . . 3

3. Hyaline to brown phialides with extremely deep cylindrical collarettes present; phialoconidia 1- to several-celled, cylindrical to ellipsoidal, hyaline to pale brown, solitary, or in chains . . . . . . . . . . . . . . . . . . . . . . . . . . . . . . . . . *Chalara*

   3'. Phialides without extremely deep, cylindrical collarattes . . . . . . . . . . . . . . . . 1

Part 3  Taxonomy                                                              155

    4. Phialoconidia curved to cylindrical, 2 or more celled; microconidia usually present . 5
    4'. Phialoconidia 1-celled; microconidia absent . . . . . . . . . . . . . . . . . . 6
5. Macroconidia cylindrical to curved, usually boat-shaped, with a distinct foot cell and tapering ends, 2- to several-celled, forming in balls that tend to slide down the phialides; phialides tapering, solitary, or as a component of a complex branching system; microconidia 1- or 2-celled, ovoid to cylindrical, in chains or more commonly balls; sporodochia may be present . . . . . . . . . . . . . . . . . . . . . . . . *Fusarium*
5'. Macroconidia cylindrical to curved, without a distinct foot cell, with rounded ends, 2- to 11-celled, solitary, occasionally in chains; phialides solitary or from branched conidiophores that resemble a penicillus; microconidia 1- or 2-celled, ovoid to cylindrical, in chains or balls; sporodochia may be present . . . . . . . . . . . . . . . *Cylindrocarpon*
    6. Conidiophores erect, simple or branched, branching verticillate; phialides in verticillate clusters; conidia 1-celled, hyaline, ovoid to allantoid, in balls . . . . . *Verticillium*
    6'. Verticillately arranged conidiophores absent . . . . . . . . . . . . . . . . . . 7
7. Conidiophores erect, repeatedly branching toward their apices, forming a penicillus; conidia in chains or as a large ball . . . . . . . . . . . . . . . . . . . . . . . 8
7'. Repeatedly branching, erect conidiophores forming a penicillus are absent . . . . . . 10
    8. Phialoconidia 1-celled, ovoid, hyaline to green, forming a large green ball at the apex of the penicillus, occasionally forming a loose column . . . . . . . . . . *Gliocladium*
    8'. Phialoconidia in chains, not forming a large green ball at the apex of the penicillus . 9
9. Phialides swollen at the base and gradually tapering towards the apex; phialoconidia are 1-celled, ovoid to fusoid, forming long simple chains that commonly become entangled; conidia tend to slip down upon each other. The phialides may also occur solitarily, in pairs, or in verticils . . . . . . . . . . . . . . . . . . . . . . . . . . . . . . *Paecilomyces*
9'. Phialides flask-shaped, in groups; phialoconidia 1-celled, globose to ovoid; in simple chains or chains forming a brushlike structure . . . . . . . . . . . . . . . *Penicillium*
    10. Phialides swollen at base and gradually tapering toward the apex, solitary, in pairs, in verticils; simple or branched conidiophores present; conidia 1-celled, ovoid to fusoid, forming long, simple chains that commonly become entangled; conidia tend to slip down upon each other . . . . . . . . . . . . . . . . . . . . . . . . *Paecilomyces*
    10'. Characteristics not as above . . . . . . . . . . . . . . . . . . . . . . . . 11
11. Phialides, conidia, or both dematiaceous . . . . . . . . . . . . . . . . . . . . 12
11'. Phialides and conidia not dematiaceous . . . . . . . . . . . . . . . . . . . . 15
    12. Phialides cylindrical with slightly swollen basal regions, typically hyaline, solitary or in groups; conidia 1-celled, green to black, globose to fusoid, smooth or rough, in balls or chains . . . . . . . . . . . . . . . . . . . . . . . . . . . . . . *Gliomastix*
    12'. Cylindrical phialides with slightly swollen basal regions absent; phialides typically pigmented . . . . . . . . . . . . . . . . . . . . . . . . . . . . . . . . 13
13. Phialides flask-shaped to cylindrical, terminal, integrated, rarely percurrent, solitary, with a distinct flared collarette; phialoconidia 1-celled in balls . *Phialophora* (also see *Madurella*)
13'. Collarettes absent . . . . . . . . . . . . . . . . . . . . . . . . . . . . . 14
    14. Phialides cylindrical with swollen upper portions, in clusters of 3 to 10 at apex of erect conidiophores; conidia 1-celled, smooth or rough, sliming down the phialides or forming chains . . . . . . . . . . . . . . . . . . . . . . . . . . . *Stachybotrys*

14'. Phialides lageniform to flask-shaped, solitary, terminal or integrated; conidia 1-celled, smooth, accumulating in balls; *Phaeococcus* anamorph typically present . . . . . . . . . . . . . . . . . . . . . . . . . . . . . . . . . . . . . . . . . . . . . . . . *Wangiella*

15. Colonies rapid growing, white, flat, developing green tufts; phialides ovoid to flask-shaped, swollen in center, tapering toward the apex, solitary, in pairs, clusters, or verticils, forming at wide angles to each other; phialoconidia 1-celled, hyaline to green, in balls . . . . . . . . . . . . . . . . . . . . . . . . . . . . . . . . . . . . . . . . *Trichoderma*

15'. Colonies not white with green tufts . . . . . . . . . . . . . . . . . . . . . . . 16

    16. Phialides swollen in the central or upper portion; phialoconidia 1-celled, in chains . 17

    16'. Phialides not swollen in the central or upper portion; phialoconidia 1-celled, in chains, balls, or both . . . . . . . . . . . . . . . . . . . . . . . . . . . . 18

17. Phialides cylindrical, swollen in upper portion, tapering toward the apex, arising directly from the hyphae; phialoconidia ellipsoidal to obovoid, truncate at both ends . *Monocillium*

17'. Phialides cylindrical, swollen in the central portion, tapering toward the apex, arising from cylindrical conidiophores; phialoconidia globose . . . . . . . . . . . *Torulomyces*

    18. Phialides long, narrow, flexuous, slightly swollen at base, gently tapering toward apex, arising from hyphae; phialoconidia ovoid, cylindrical to elliptical, truncate at both ends, in chains . . . . . . . . . . . . . . . . . . . . . . . . . *Sagrahamala*

    18'. Phialides cylindrical, arising from hyphae and fascicles; phialoconidia globose to cylindrical, typically in balls, occasionally in chains . . . . . . . . . . *Acremonium*

*Group 6*

Poroconidia form through a channel in the outer wall layer(s) of the conidiogenous cell (Fig. 4.46). The conidiogenous cell may be either a distinct conidiophore as in *Helminthosporium* (Fig. 4.64), or another conidium as in *Alternaria* (Fig. 4.29). Poroconidia are recognized by the presence of a minute pore at their bases. The conidia are typically thick-walled, septate, and dematiaceous. The conidiogenous cells giving rise to the conidia may be either determinate or proliferous. Proliferous conidiogenous cells are either percurrent or sympodial. With the oil objective, the pores in the wall of the conidiogenous cell appear as a small hyaline or lightly pigmented circle.

1. Conidia brown to black, in simple or branching acropetal chains . . . . . . . . . . . 2

1'. Conidia brown to black, solitary, not forming in chains . . . . . . . . . . . . . . . 3

    2. Conidia muriform, ovoid to obclavate; conidiophores septate, sympodial . . *Alternaria*

    2'. Conidia not muriform; conidia cylindrical, 3- to 15-celled, with a constriction at each septum, apical cell darkly pigmented and functions as conidiogenous cell, verrucose; chains acropetal; conidiophores hyphalike with a swollen apical cell . . . . . *Torula*

3. Conidiophores proliferating percurrently through the scar left by the previous terminal conidium, apex of conidiophore swollen; conidia solitary, muriform, usually with a central constriction; conidiophores simple or branched . . . . . . . . . . . . . *Stemphylium*

3'. Conidiophores not proliferating percurrently . . . . . . . . . . . . . . . . . . . . 4

    4. Conidiophores proliferous, growing sympodially, geniculate . . . . . . . . . . . 5

    4'. Conidiophores determinate, paralled-walled, erect; conidia several-celled, obclavate, forming laterally from the conidiophore, basipetal, youngest conidia toward base of the conidiophore; brown to black protruding hilum present . . . . *Helminthosporium*

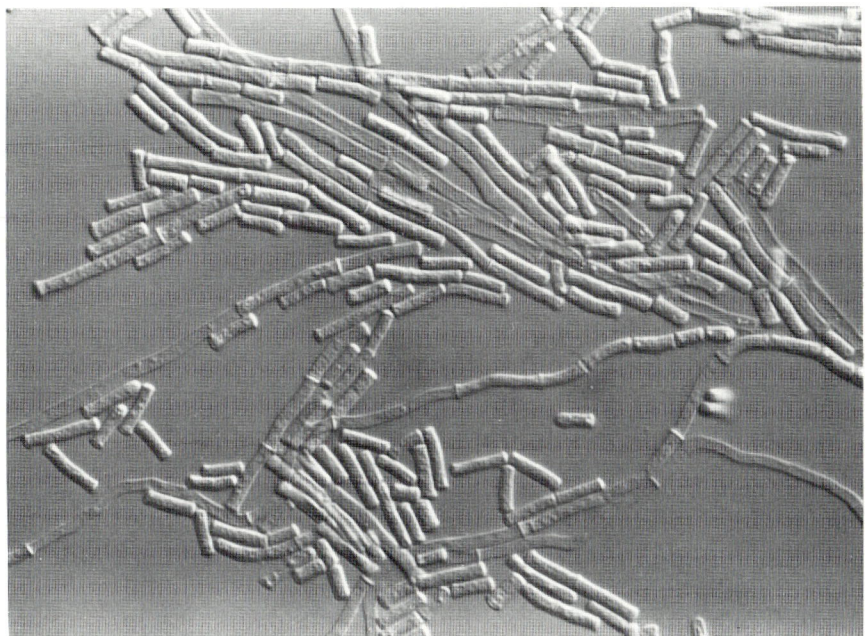

**Fig. 4.15** *Geotrichum candidum*. The fertile hyphae are forming arthroconidia, which are then released by fission through double septa.

5. Conidia muriform, obovoid, solitary, without central constriction; conidiophores simple, occasionally branched . . . . . . . . . . . . . . . . . . . . . . . . . . . . . *Ulocladium*
5'. Conidia not muriform . . . . . . . . . . . . . . . . . . . . . . . . . . . . . . . . 6
    6. Conidia usually curved, several-celled, end cells paler than other cells; brown to black protruding hilum typically present . . . . . . . . . . . . . . . . . . . . . *Curvularia*
    6'. Conidia cylindrical to fusoid . . . . . . . . . . . . . . . . . . . . . . . . *Drechslera*

*Group 7*

Arthroconidia are thallic conidia that occur in simple or branching chains (Fig. 4.15). The conidia are released by either splitting through a double septum or by the lysis or fracture of a disjunctor cell. The fertile hyphae may be identical to the vegetative hyphae, or they may be either larger or smaller. Distinct conidiophores may be present or absent. Arthroconidia may be quite variable, 1-celled or several-celled, globose, ovoid, rectangular, square, swollen, hyaline or dematiaceous, terminal or intercalary, and with rounded or truncate ends. If an isolate is forming blastoconidia in addition to arthroconidia, genera such as *Trichosporon, Moniliella,* and others should be considered. These are discussed in Chapter 5.

1. Blastoconidia developing from the conidiophores, conidiophores becoming shorter (retrogressive); conidia 2-celled, clavate to ovoid, forming in a "double row," bases becoming wider; colonies pale rose, rapidly growing, granular . . . . . . . . . . see *Trichothecium*

1'. Arthroconidia present . . . . . . . . . . . . . . . . . . . . . . . . . . . . . 2
    2. Conidiophores erect, narrow, simple, dematiaceous, repeatedly branching at their apices, giving rise to delicate heads of fertile hyphae; arthroconidia 1-celled, globose to cylindrical; chains of conidia held together by gelatinouslike strands (actually conidial wall) . . . . . . . . . . . . . . . . . . . . . . . . . . . . . . . . . *Oidiodendron*
    2'. Erect conidiophores absent . . . . . . . . . . . . . . . . . . . . . . . . . 3
3. Disjunctor cells present between the arthroconidia . . . . . . . . . . . . . . . . . 4
3'. Disjunctor cells absent . . . . . . . . . . . . . . . . . . . . . . . . . . . . 5
    4. Spherules containing endospores formed at 37°C on special media or in tissue . . . . . . . . . . . . . . . . . . . . . . . . . . . . . . . . . . . . *Coccidioides*
    4'. Spherules and endospores absent; some isolates may form enlarged cells at 37°C on special media . . . . . . . . . . . . . . . . . . . . . . . . . *Malbranchea*
5. Arthroconidia pale brown to black, 1-celled, occasionally 2-celled, and often with a constriction at the septum, smooth or verrucose, often thick-walled, oblong . . *Scytalidium*
5'. Arthroconidia hyaline, slimy, 1-celled, smooth, thin-walled, subglobose to cylindrical . . . . . . . . . . . . . . . . . . . . . . . . . . . . . . . . . . . *Geotrichum*

*Group 8*

The fungi in group 8 form swollen terminal conidia that are typically solitary. They are released either by lysis or fracture of the supporting cell. With careful observation, an annular frill is usually seen at the base of each conidium, which is a remnant of the supporting cell's cell wall. The conidia are 1- to several-celled, globose to cylindrical, thin- or thick-walled, solitary (rarely in short chains), hyaline to black, and smooth to verrucose. The conidia may form along the hyphae or upon distinct conidiophores.

1. Conidia muriform, brown to black, rough with a warty crust, subglobose; sporodochia usually present; colonies dirty yellow to orange . . . . . . . . . . . . . . . *Epicoccum*
1'. Muriform conidia and sporodochia absent . . . . . . . . . . . . . . . . . . . . 2
    2. Conidia 2- or more celled . . . . . . . . . . . . . . . . . . . . . . . . . . 3
    2'. Conidia 1-celled . . . . . . . . . . . . . . . . . . . . . . . . . . . . . . 5
3. Conidia clavate, often poorly differentiated from hyphae, thick-walled, smooth, 3- to 5-celled, solitary or in clusters of 3 to 5; microconidia absent; chlamydosphores common, especially upon subculturing . . . . . . . . . . . . . . . . . . . . . *Epidermophyton*
3' Conidia spindle-shaped to clavate, thick- or thin-walled, smooth or echinulate, solitary; microconidia typically present . . . . . . . . . . . . . . . . . . . . . . . . . 4
    4. Macroconidia spindle-shaped, thin- to thick-walled, echinulate, 2- to several-celled; arising from micronematous conidiophores; microconidia usually present, 1-celled, clavate, smooth with thin walls . . . . . . . . . . . . . . . . . . . . *Microsporum*
    4'. Macroconidia cylindrical to clavate, thin- to thick-walled, smooth 2- to several-celled, arising from micronematous conidiophores; microconidia 1- to several-celled, smooth with thin walls . . . . . . . . . . . . . . . . . . . . . . . . . *Trichophyton*
5. Conidia 1-celled, dark brown to black, globose to ovoid, solitary, or in short chains . . . 6
5'. Conidia not dark brown to black . . . . . . . . . . . . . . . . . . . . . . . . . 7

6. Conidia black, solitary, smooth, subglobose to ovoid, horizontally flattened; conidiophores hyaline, swollen basally and tapering toward the conidium; colonies becoming dematiaceous . . . . . . . . . . . . . . . . . . . . . . . . . . . . . . . . . *Nigrospora*

6'. Conidia dark brown to black, solitary or in short chains, smooth, globose to ovoid; conidiophores absent or short, cylindrical to slightly inflated; *Sagrahamala* anamorph may be present . . . . . . . . . . . . . . . . . . . . . . . . . . . . . . . . . . *Humicola*

7. Conidia globose to ovoid, large, 1-celled, thick-walled, solitary or in clusters; cylindrical, erect conidiophores present; second condial form usually present . . . . . . . . . . . 8

7'. Conidia not as above . . . . . . . . . . . . . . . . . . . . . . . . . . . . . . . . . . 9

8. Yeast form produced at 37°C; macroconidia 8–14 μm in diameter, hyaline, smooth to tuberculate, with fingerlike projections; microconidia 2–4 μm in diameter, smooth to echinulate; both types of conidia forming on short conidiophores . . . . *Histoplasma*

8'. Yeast form absent at 37°C; macroconidia 1-celled, 15–25 μm, solitary or in clusters, globose to ovoid, hyaline to amber, smooth or verrucose, usually with a thick wall; conidiophores short to long; *Verticillium* anamorph may be present . . . . *Sepedonium*

9. Conidia 1-celled, ovoid, truncate with a broad base, thick-walled, golden-brown with annular frill; clamp connections present; conidiophores short with broad denticles . . . . . . . . . . . . . . . . . . . . . . . . . . . . . . . . . . . . . . . . . . . . *Sporotrichum*

9'. Conidia not ovoid, thick-walled, golden-brown; clamp connections absent; conidiophores without broad denticles . . . . . . . . . . . . . . . . . . . . . . . . . . . . . . . . . 10

10. Macroconidia typically present . . . . . . . . . . . . . . . . . . . . . . . . . 11

10'. Macroconidia absent . . . . . . . . . . . . . . . . . . . . . . . . . . . . . . . . 12

11. Microconidia 1-celled, globose to pyriform, produced along the hyphae, in clusters, or both; cylindrical to clavate macroconidia may be present . . . . . . . . . . . *Trichophyton*

11'. Microconidia 1-celled, clavate, produced along the hyphae; spindle-shaped macroconidia usually present . . . . . . . . . . . . . . . . . . . . . . . . . . . . . . . . . *Microsporum*

12. Yeast form present at 37°C; conidia 1-celled, solitary, hyaline, globose to subglobose, usually truncate; conidiophores arise at right angles to hyphae . . . . . . . *Blastomyces*

12'. Yeast form absent at 37°C; conidia 1-celled, solitary or rarely in chains of 2–3 conidia, hyaline, globose to clavate, usually truncate; pedicels and conidiophores arise at right angles to hyphae; thick-walled, large globose vesicles may be formed by some species at 37 and 40°C . . . . . . . . . . . . . . . . . . . . . . . . . . *Chrysosporium*

*Group 9*

The conidia found in group 9 appear to be "blown-out" and constricted at their bases. The conidia are released by a double-septum mechanism. The conidia may occur solitarily, accumulate in balls, or develop in acropetal chains that may be simple or branched (Fig. 4.16). The conidia may form from yeast cells, hyphae, or distinct conidiophores. They are extremely variable in shape, size, septation, and color.

1. Ampullae present, blastoconidia 1-celled, hyaline to pale brown, solitary; arising in a synchronized manner on denticles from ampullae; conidiophores erect, branching restricted to apical region . . . . . . . . . . . . . . . . . . . . . . . . . . . . . . . . . . . *Botrytis*

1'. Ampullae absent . . . . . . . . . . . . . . . . . . . . . . . . . . . . . . . . . . . . . 2

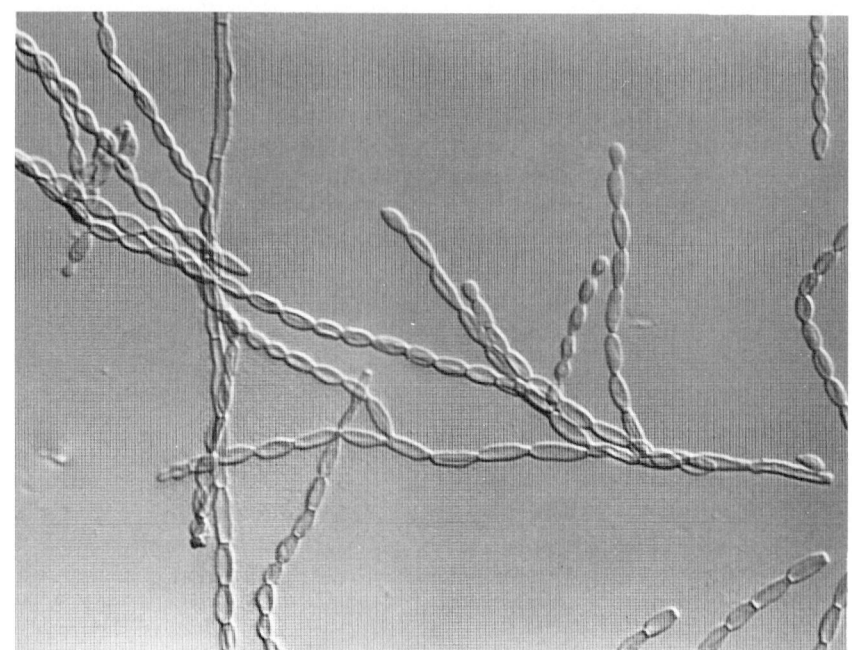

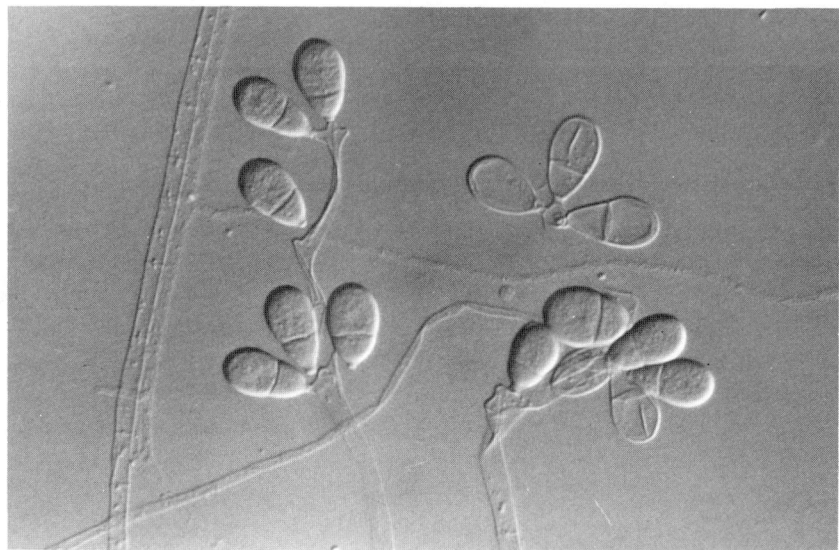

**Fig. 4.16** Blastoconidia are formed by a blowing-out process. A. *Cladosporium bantianum* typically forms long, sparsely branching chains of one-celled blastoconidia. B. *Arthrobotrys* sp. is forming two-celled blastoconidia at nodelike swellings along its conidiophores.

2. Conidiophores retrogressive; conidia usually 2-celled, bases becoming wider, alternate, forming in a "double row"; conidiophores hyphalike . . . . . . . . . *Trichothecium*
   2'. Conidiophores not retrogressive . . . . . . . . . . . . . . . . . . . . . . . 3
3. Conidia cylindrical, 3- to 15-celled, with a constriction at each septum; apical cell darkly pigmented and functions as a conidiogenous cell, verrucose; chains acropetal; conidiophores with a swollen apical cell . . . . . . . . . . . . . . . . . . . . *Torula*
3'. Not as above . . . . . . . . . . . . . . . . . . . . . . . . . . . . . . . . . 4
   4. Conidia forming in acropetal chains . . . . . . . . . . . . . . . . . . . . . 5
   4'. Conidia solitary or in balls . . . . . . . . . . . . . . . . . . . . . . . . . 8
5. Conidia and hyphae approximately 1–2 μm in diameter; conidia 1-celled, fusoid to cylindrical, with either truncate or rounded ends; chains simple or branched . . . *Fusidium*
5'. Conidia and hyphae 3–4 μm or greater in diameter . . . . . . . . . . . . . . . 6
   6. Conidia 1-celled, globose to ovoid, hyaline to subhyaline; chains branching and beadlike; conidiophores hyphalike, simple or branched . . . . . . . . . . . *Monilia*
   6'. Conidia 1- to several-celled; pale brown to black; chains not beadlike; conidiophores usually distinctive . . . . . . . . . . . . . . . . . . . . . . . . . . . . . . 7
7. Conidia 1- to 5-celled, cylindrical, verrucose; forming loosely branching chains; conidiophores simple or sympodial . . . . . . . . . . . . . . . . . . . . . . . *Stenella*
7'. Conidia 1- to 4-celled, primarily 1-celled, shield-shaped conidia present, conidia with a distinct dark hilum; branching chains well formed, conidiophores erect . . . *Cladosporium*
   8. Conidia 1-celled, arising solitarily, in clusters, or synchronously from denticles along a hypha; secondary blastoconida common; *Scytalidium* anamorph commonly present . . . . . . . . . . . . . . . . . . . . . . . . . . . . . . . . . . *Aureobasidium*
   8'. Dematiaceous yeast cells producing 1-celled conidia; hyphae and pseudohyphae typically absent or sparse . . . . . . . . . . . . . . . . . . . . . . *Phaeococcus*

## Group 10

The Mycelia Sterilia consists of those fungi that produce neither conidia nor spores. This order is in essence a "garbage can" that contains a large number of nondistinctive filamentous fungi. The fungi are Zygomycetes, Ascomycetes, and Basidiomycetes that either lack an anamorph or teleomorph, or simply are not producing conidia or spores under the laboratory procedures being employed. The presence of clamp connections, bulbils, or sclerotia are helpful in recognizing some genera, such as *Papulaspora*, *Sclerotium*, and *Rhizoctonia*. The identification of isolates of *Madurella* and *Paracoccidioides* requires clinical data.

1. Black granules from a mycetoma; hyphae in culture nondistinctive; colonies dematiaceous . . . . . . . . . . . . . . . . . . . . . . . . . . . . . . . . . . . . . . *Madurella*
1'. Isolate dimorphic, hyphae in culture at 25°C nondistinctive; multiple budding yeast form at 37°C; colonies white . . . . . . . . . . . . . . . . . . . . . . . *Paracoccidioides*

### Key to Some of the Genera of Zygomycetes

1. Merosporangia or 1-celled sporangiola arising from terminal vesicles at the apices of the sporangiophores and their branches . . . . . . . . . . . . . . . . . . . . . . . 2
1'. Merosporangia absent; if sporangiola present, not arising from terminal vesicles . . . . 3

2. Merosporangia present, sporangiospores 1-celled, globose; sporangiophores branching sympodially with curved lateral branches . . . . . . . . . . . . . *Syncephalastrum*

2'. Merosporangia absent; 1-celled sporangiola developing on swollen denticles from a terminal vesicle; sporangiophores erect, straight with branching below the apex . . . . . . . . . . . . . . . . . . . . . . . . . . . . . . . . . . . . . . . . . . *Cunninghamella*

3. One-celled spores forcibly discharged; sporangia containing many sporangiospores typically absent; hyphae sparse in most isolates . . . . . . . . . . . . . . . . 4

3'. Spores not forcibly discharged; sporangia containing many sporangiospores; hyphae abundant . . . . . . . . . . . . . . . . . . . . . . . . . . . . . . . . . . . . . . 5

    4. Zygospores with 2 closely appressed beaklike appendages; primary spores 1-celled, solitary, arising from sporophores with swollen region below spore; secondary spores 1-celled, solitary, passively released, with a knoblike adhesive tip . . . . . *Basidiobolus*

    4'. Zygospores, when present, formed in the larger of two gametangia, without 2 closely appressed beaks; primary spores 1-celled, solitary, arising from simple sporophores . . . . . . . . . . . . . . . . . . . . . . . . . . . . . . . . . . . . . . *Conidiobolus*

5. Sporangia formed at the apices of circinate sporangiophores that branch sympodially; sporangial walls encrusted with calcium oxalate crystals, breaking into pieces; irregular collarettes present . . . . . . . . . . . . . . . . . . . . . . . . . . . . . . *Circinella*

5'. Circinate sporangiophores absent . . . . . . . . . . . . . . . . . . . . . . . . . . 6

    6. Sporangiophores erect, delicate, simple or branched and tapering toward their apices; sporangia globose without columellae; collarettes present . . . . . . . . *Mortierella*

    6'. Sporangiophores not tapering toward their apices; columellae present . . . . . . . 7

7. Sporangiophores solitary, in clusters of 2 or more, or both, arising opposite rhizoids at nodes; sporangia globose with flattened base; columellae hemispherical; collarettes absent . . . . . . . . . . . . . . . . . . . . . . . . . . . . . . . . . . . . . . . *Rhizopus*

7'. Sporangiophores not arising opposite rhizoids at nodes . . . . . . . . . . . . . . 8

    8. Stolons and rhizoids absent; sporangiophores solitary, simple or branched; sporangia globose; columellae variable in shape; collarette may be present . . . . . . . *Mucor*

    8'. Stolons and rhizoids present . . . . . . . . . . . . . . . . . . . . . . . . . . 9

9. Apophyses absent; sporangia globose; thermophilic . . . . . . . . . . . . *Rhizomucor*

9'. Apophyses present, sporangia pyriform . . . . . . . . . . . . . . . . . . . . *Absidia*

## ASCOMYCETES

*Ajellomyces* McDonough et Lewis emend. McGinnis et Katz, 1979

Diagnostic features: Members of the genus *Ajellomyces* produce globose to stellate, tan gymnothecia (Fig. 4.17) that have several radiating broad spirals originating from the center of the ascocarps. From the spirals, a

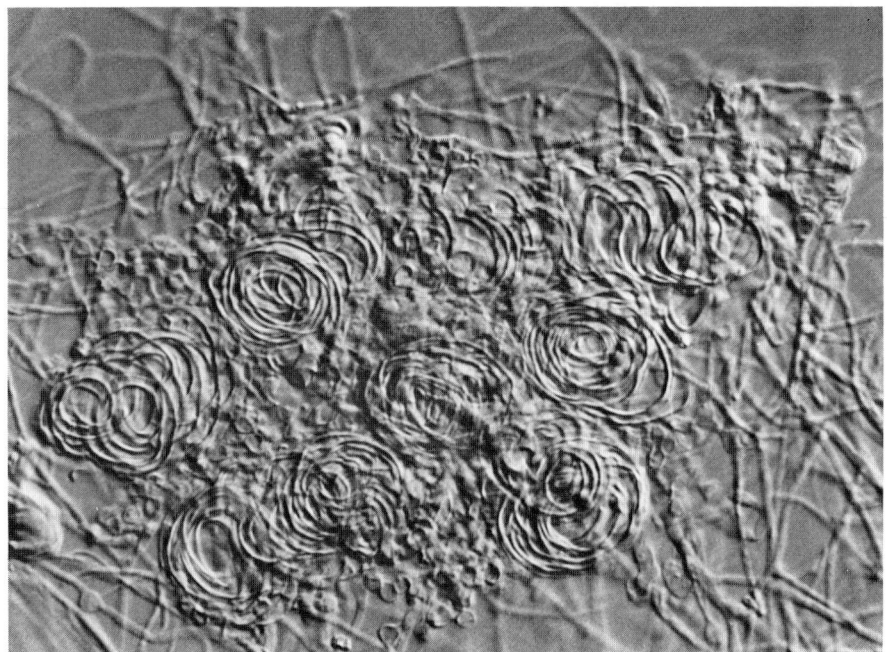

A

Fig. 4.17 *Ajellomyces dermatitidis*. A and B. The mature gymnothecium has several spirals that radiate from a common point in the center of the ascocarp. The peridial hyphae consists of swollen cells in this species.

network of secondary peridial hyphae forms. These are thin-walled, hyaline, with either parallel walls or regularly swollen cells. The asci are subglobose to pyriform, evanescent, with 8 ascospores. The ascospores are hyaline, 1-celled and globose. The species are heterothallic.

Comments: The genus *Ajellomyces* was established by McDonough and Lewis in 1968 (135) for the teleomorph of *Blastomyces dermatitidis*. Four years later, Kwon-Chung (121) discovered the teleomorph of *Histoplasma capsulatum* and established the genus *Emmonsiella*. The two genera were distinguished from each other by Kwon-Chung primarily upon differences in the ascocarp initials, secondary peridial hyphae, and shape of the asci. McGinnis and Katz (143) studied the type material for both genera and concluded that the ascocarp initials and shape of the asci were essentially the same. They emended the genus *Ajellomyces,* placed *Emmonsiella* into synonymy with *Ajellomyces,* and made the new combination *A. capsulatus*. *Ajellomyces dermatitidis* and *A. capsulatus* are readily distinguished from each other by their regularly swollen and parallel-walled secondary peridial hyphae, respectively. In addition, *A. dermatitidis* produces a *B. dermatitidis* anamorph, whereas *A. capsulatus* has a *H. capsulatum* anamorph.

164                                                4  Mould Identification

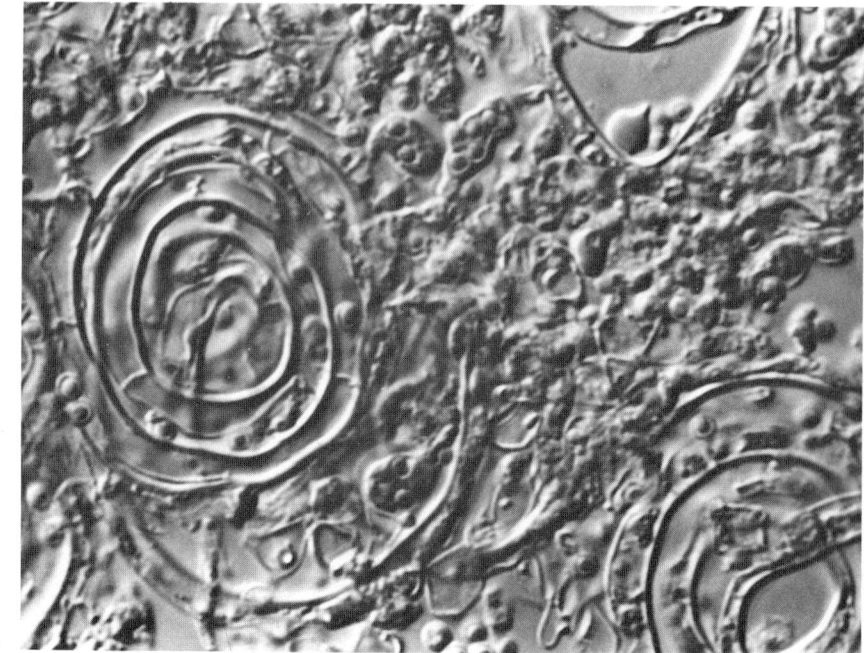

B

Fig. 4.17  Continued

Gymnothecia of *Ajellomyces* are not seen in the clinical laboratory unless the appropriate mating types are crossed.

*Arthroderma* Currey ex Berkeley, 1860

Diagnostic features: The genus *Arthroderma* is characterized by small, globose gymnothecia with dumbbell-shaped cells (Fig. 4.18) in the peridial hyphae. Each cell of the outer portion of the peridial hyphae is swollen at both ends, with a deeply constricted central region. The swollen portion is echinulate and thick-walled, whereas the central portion is smooth with a thin wall. The peridial hyphae are straight to curved, branched and often recurved. Long, slender, septate, thin-walled, smooth appendages arise from the peridial hyphae. The asci are globose to subglobose, evanescent, with 8 ascospores. The ascospores are small, hyaline (yellow in mass), 1-celled, smooth, and oblate. There are heterothallic and homothallic species in this genus.

Comments: The genus *Arthroderma* (164) is the teleomorph for some species of *Trichophyton* and *Chrysosporium* (Table 4.5). *Arthroderma* is extremely similar to the genus *Nannizzia*, which was established by Stock-

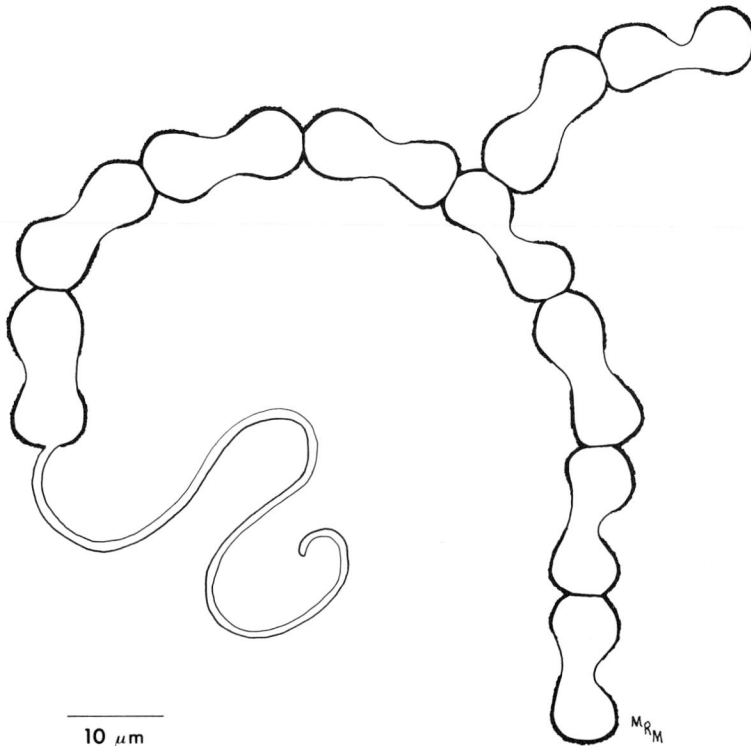

**Fig. 4.18** *Arthroderma* sp. The cells of the peridial hyphae have a constricted central portion that is smooth. The ends of the cells are swollen and echinulate. Sterile appendages may be present.

dale (206) as the teleomorph for some members of *Microsporum*. The principal difference in the two genera involves the peridial hyphae. *Arthroderma* forms pronounced dumbbell-shaped cells, whereas *Nannizzia* does not.

Isolates of *Arthroderma* may be occasionally recovered in the clinical laboratory if they are homothallic. Otherwise, gymnothecia of *Arthroderma* are not seen in the clinical laboratory unless mating studies are conducted.

### *Chaetomium* Kunze ex Fries, 1829

Diagnostic features: Members of the genus *Chaetomium* form globose, ovoid, barrel to flask-shaped, dark brown to black, ostiolate (rarely nonostiolate) perithecia. Long, hairlike, brown to black or variously colored appendages arise from the peridium (Fig. 4.19). The peridium is brittle, fragile, and membranaceous. The asci are clavate to cylindrical, evanes-

Table 4.5. The Genus *Arthroderma*

| Teleomorph | Anamorph |
|---|---|
| *A. benhamiae* | *Trichophyton mentagrophytes* |
| *A. ciferrii* | *T. georgiae* |
| *A. cuniculi* | *Chrysosporium* anamorph |
| *A. curreyi* | *Chrysosporium* anamorph |
| *A. flavescens* | *T. flavescens* |
| *A. gertleri* | *T. vanbreuseghemii* |
| *A. gloriae* | *T. gloriae* |
| *A. insingulare* | *T. terrestre* |
| *A. lenticularum* | *T. terrestre* |
| *A. multifidum* | *Chrysosporium* anamorph |
| *A. quadrifidum* | *T. terrestre* |
| *A. simii* | *T. simii* |
| *A. tuberculatum* | *Chrysosporium* anamorph |
| *A. uncinatum* | *T. ajelloi* |
| *A. vanbreuseghemii* | *T. mentagrophytes* |

cent, with 8 (rarely 4) ascospores. The ascospores are 1-celled, light to dark (usually olive brown) in color and lemon-shaped. Chlamydospores and solitary conidia may be formed.

Comments: Members of the genus *Chaetomium* (8, 197) are infrequently isolated in the clinical laboratory. *Chaetomium* species are associated with the soil.

## *Eurotium* Link ex Fries, 1829

Diagnostic features: Species of *Eurotium* produce yellow, globose, nonostiolate cleistothecia (Fig. 4.20) and a conspicuous *Aspergillus* anamorph. The asci are globose to subglobose, evanescent, with 8 ascospores. The ascospores are typically lenticular, smooth-walled, with equatorial crests and a purple-red color. Hülle cells may be present.

Comments: The genus *Eurotium* (27) is one of several perfect genera associated with the anamorph *Aspergillus*. Occasionally, cleistothecia of *Eurotium* are seen in isolates of *Aspergillus* that are recovered in the clinical laboratory.

## *Leptosphaeria* Cesati et de Notaris, 1861

Diagnostic features: *Leptosphaeria* is a loculoascomycete that forms nonostiolate, globose to subglobose, black ascostromata. The peridium consists of several layers of cells. The asci are clavate to cylindrical,

Part 3  Taxonomy

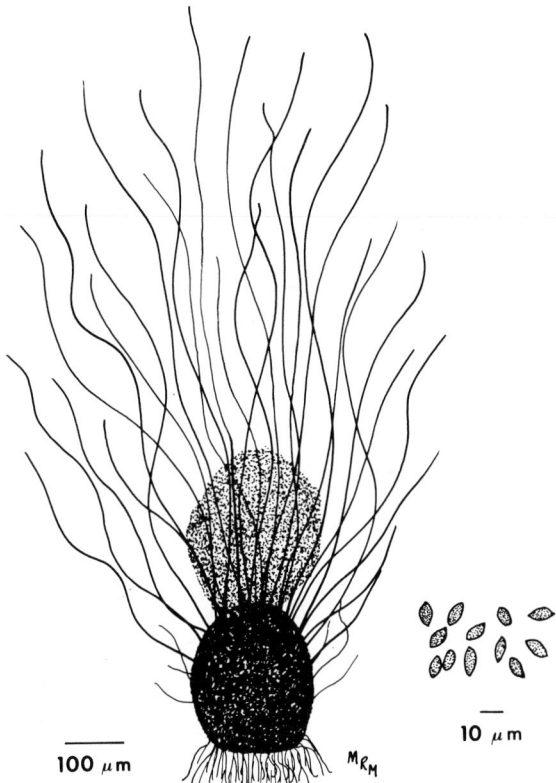

**Fig. 4.19** *Chaetomium globosum*. The perithecia of this fungus have long dark setae. The ascospores are pale brown and lemon-shaped.

bitunicate, with 8 ascospores. The ascospores are 4- to 9-celled, fusoid to curved, hyaline to pigmented, and with a constriction at each septum. *Leptosphaeria senegalensis* and *L. tompkinsii* are homothallic. An anamorph is absent.

Comments: The description of *Leptosphaeria* is based upon *L. tompkinsii*. Both *L. senegalensis* and *L. tompkinsii* are etiologic agents of mycetoma (Fig. 4.21). They are not usually recovered in the clinical laboratory unless they are isolated from a case of mycetoma. Members of the genus *Leptosphaeria* (81, 92, 93, 151) are associated with dead plant material.

*Nannizzia* Stockdale, 1961

Diagnostic features: Members of the genus *Nannizzia* are characterized by the development of globose gymnothecia (Fig. 4.22) that usually have

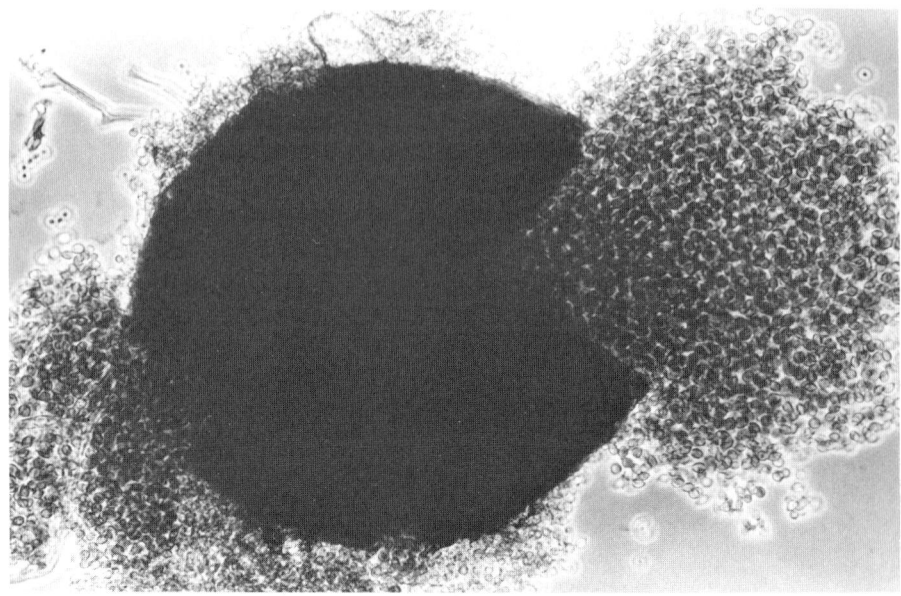

**Fig. 4.20** *Eurotium* sp. The cleistothecium has ruptured. A mass of asci and ascospores can be seen escaping from the ascocarp into the mounting medium.

appendages arising from the peridial hyphae. The peridial hyphae consist of hyaline, septate, verticillately branching hyphae. The outer cells of the peridium are long, symmetrical, slightly constricted in the middle portion, and uniformly rough. Appendages may be of three basic types: long, slender, smooth-walled, septate, straight or curved hyphae; long, slender, smooth-walled, septate, tightly spiraled hyphae; and macroconidia. The asci are globose to ovoid, hyaline, smooth, evanescent, with 8 ascospores. The ascospores are hyaline (yellow in mass) and lenticular in shape. Members of this genus are heterothallic.

Comments: The genus *Nannizzia* (206) was established to accommodate the sexual form of some species of *Microsporum* (Table 4.6). *Nannizzia* is distinguished from *Arthroderma* by its uniformly roughened, slightly constricted cells in the outer portion of the peridial hyphae, and the development of a *Microsporum* anamorph.

*Nannizzia* is not seen in the clinical laboratory unless the appropriate mating types are crossed.

*Neotestudina* Segretain et Destombes, 1961

Diagnostic features: The description presented here is based primarily upon *Neotestudina rosatii*. *Neotestudina* is a loculoascomycete that forms

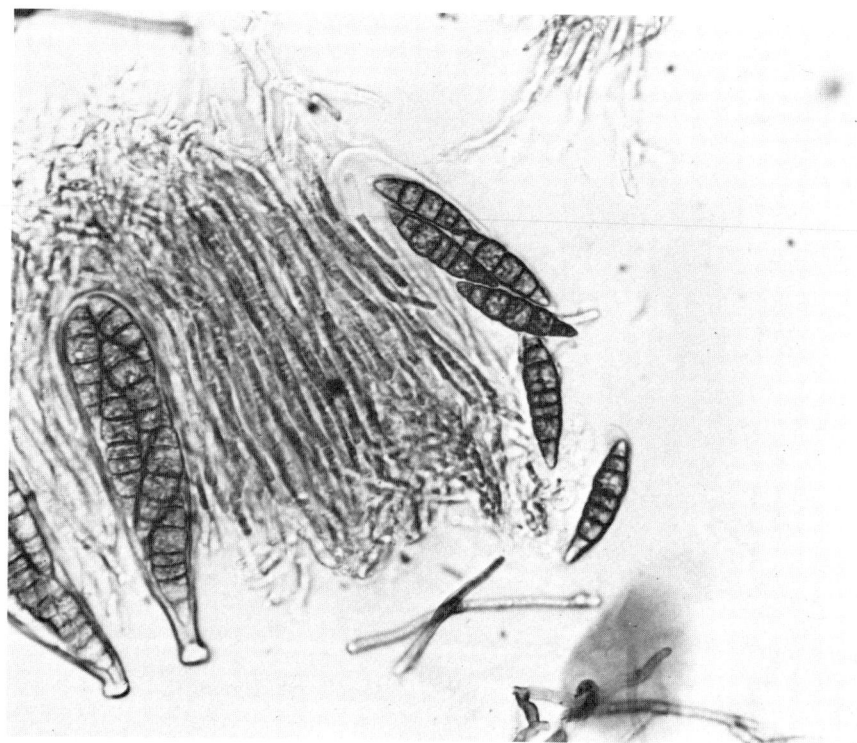

Fig. 4.21 The asci and ascospores of *Leptosphaeria* are formed in an ascostroma. A. *L. tompkinsii* produces ascospores that are predominantly seven-celled. B. *L. senegalensis* produces ascospores that are predominantly five-celled. (Reproduced by permission of A. El-Ani and Mycologia from *Mycologia* **58**:406–311, 1966 and *Mycologia* **57**:275–278, respectively.)

nonostiolate, globose to ellipsoidal, carbonaceous, black ascostromata. The peridium consists of pseudoparenchymatous cells organized into *textura angularis*. The pseudoparaphyses are sparse, hyaline, and hyphalike. They begin to develop at the same time the asci are forming. The asci occur in the center of the ascostroma and are globose, subglobose to clavate, thick-walled, bitunicate, evanescent, with 8 ascospores. The ascospores are ellipsoidal to variable in shape, dark brown (black in some species), smooth (rough in some species), random within the ascus, and with a single transverse septum that is sharply constricted. An anamorph is absent.

Comments: Segretain and Destombes (196) described the genus *Neotestudina* for an etiologic agent of mycetoma that formed white granules. Hawksworth and Booth studied *N. rosatii*, concluded that it was a loculoascomycete, and transferred it to the genus *Zopfia*. Later, Hawks-

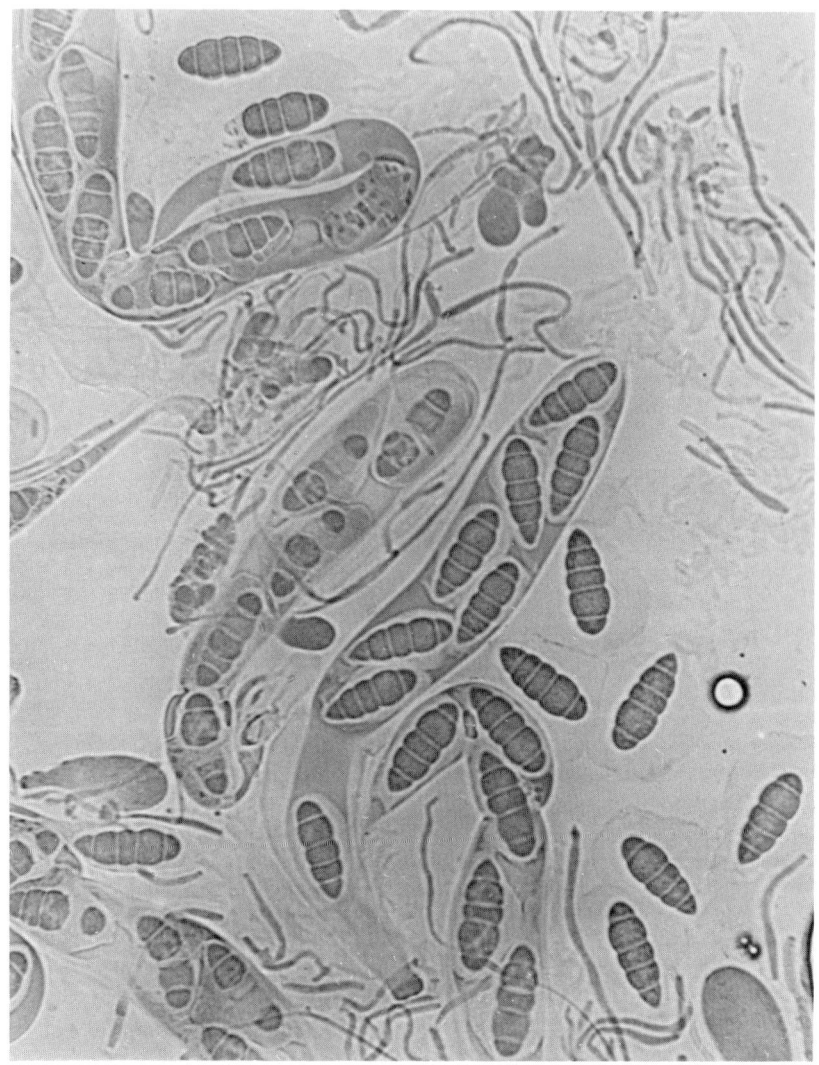

**Fig. 4.21** Continued

worth (84) felt that their original concept of *Zopfia* was too broad. He now considers *Neotestudina* to be the most appropriate genus for *N. rosatii*. Thus, *N. rosatii* is the best name for this agent of mycetoma.

Isolates of *Neotestudina* are rarely, if ever, seen in the clinical laboratory unless they are recovered from a case of mycetoma. Members of the genus *Neotestudina* are associated with plant roots and soil.

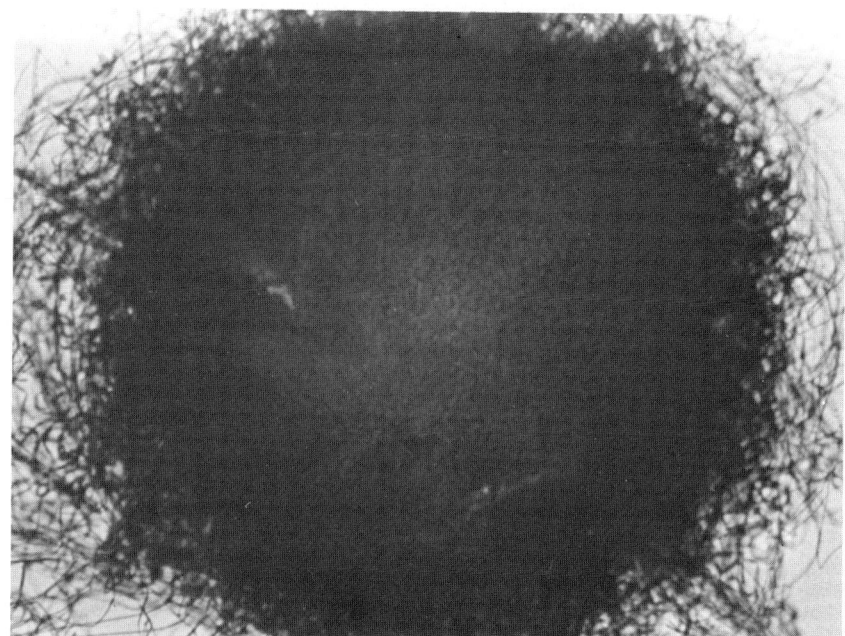

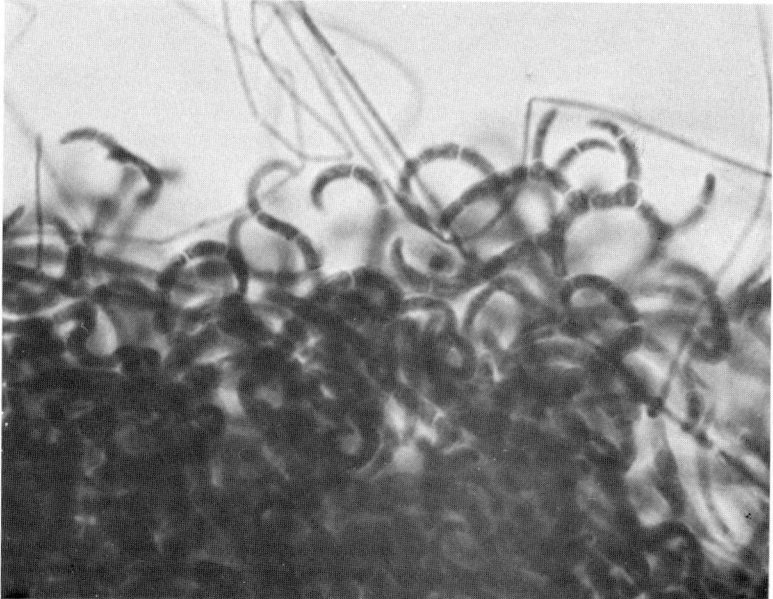

**Fig. 4.22** *Nannizzia grubyia*. The gymnothecium is a large, loosely organized, globose body. The cells of the peridial hyphae are smooth and they are not constricted in the middle.

**Table 4.6.** The Genus *Nannizzia*

| Teleomorph | Anamorph |
|---|---|
| *N. borellii* | *Microsporum amazonicum* |
| *N. cajetani* | *M. cookei* |
| *N. fulva* | *M. fulvum* |
| *N. grubyia* | *M. vanbreuseghemii* |
| *N. gypsea* | *M. gypseum* |
| *N. incurvata* | *M. gypseum* |
| *N. obtusa* | *M. nanum* |
| *N. otae* | *M. canis* |
| *N. persicolor* | *M. persicolor* |
| *N. racemosa* | *M. racemosum* |

*Petriellidium* Malloch, 1970

Diagnostic features: Species of *Petriellidium* form globose, nonostiolate, light brown to black, membranaceous cleistothecia (Fig. 4.23) that are frequently produced beneath the agar surface. The peridium consists of pseudoparenchymatous tissue that is 1 or 2 cells deep. The asci are subglobose to globose, evanescent, with 8 ascospores. The ascospores are ovoid to ellipsoidal, pale yellow-brown to copper, smooth-walled and with 2 germ pores.

Comments: The genus *Allescheria* was established in 1899 by Saccardo and Sydow for a fungus known as *Eurotiopsis gayoni*. In 1922, Shear (198) described the second species in the genus *Allescheria* as *A. boydii*, a fungus that was isolated from a case of mycetoma (37). While reevaluating members of the Microascaceae, Malloch (130) concluded that the description of *E. gayoni* fits the genus *Monascus*. Since the genus *Allescheria* was based upon *E. gayoni*, *Allescheria* becomes a synonym of *Monascus*. The fungus described as *A. boydii* by Shear is completely different from the genus *Monascus*. Thus, Malloch established the new genus *Petriellidium* for *A. boydii*. This was necessary because there was no genus available that could adequately accommodate *P. boydii*. Presently, there are seven species in the genus *Petriellidium* (12, 130, 131).

Shear (198) illustrated and discussed two anamorphs for *P. boydii*. Judging from his illustrations and descriptions and from study of his original slide preparations, the synnemata he found can be assigned to the genus *Graphium* (Fig. 4.10), even though he considered them to be *Dendrostilbella boydii*. The second anamorph was described by Shear as *Cephalosporium boydii*. This state is *Scedosporium apiospermum*, which Emmons (66) also demonstrated was an anamorph of *P. boydii*.

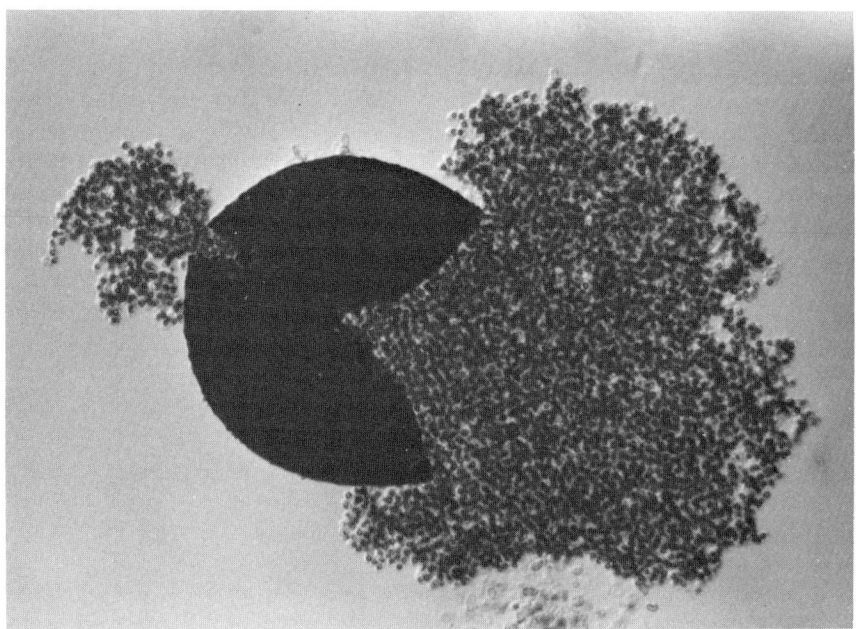

**Fig. 4.23** *Petriellidium boydii*. The cleistotheium has ruptured and a mass of ascospores is escaping.

Based upon the *S. apiospermum* anamorph (Fig. 4.88), many medical mycologists tend to identify an isolate as *P. boydii*, regardless of whether cleistothecia are present or absent. This is unwarranted because other members of the Microascaceae, such as species of *Petriella*, may also form a *Scedosporium* anamorph that is identical to the one formed by *P. boydii*. In addition, the seven species of *Petriellidium* are distinguished from each other on the basis of sexual structures, not of their conidial forms. Many isolates have probably been misidentified as *P. boydii* in the past.

Species of *Petriellidium* are frequently recovered in the clinical laboratory. Most of them are first recognized as *S. apiospermum*. The frequency of isolation of the other six species is difficult to determine because of the tendency of medical mycologists to lump all isolates of *Petriellidium* into the single species *P. boydii*. Members of this genus are usually associated with soil.

### *Piedraia* Fonseca et Arêa Leão, 1928

Diagnostic features: *Piedraia* is a loculoascomycete that forms dark brown to black, slow growing, small, velvety, folded colonies. The ascostromata are dark and irregular to subglobose in shape. The asci are ellipsoidal, solitary or in small groups, evanescent, with 8 ascospores. The ascospores are hyaline to darkly pigmented, 1-celled, fusoid, usually curved, tapering toward each end with a filiform extension. An anamorph is absent.

Comments: *Piedraia hortae* is the etiologic agent of black piedra, an infection of the hair shaft. The identification of this fungus is based upon examining the hard, black, firm nodules around the hair shaft (Fig. 4.24). The production of ascostromata with ascospores in the laboratory is unusual (211). Von Arx's study of the Myriangiales should be consulted for additional information on *Piedraia* (9).

## *Thielavia* Zopf, 1876

Diagnostic features: The genus *Thielavia* is characterized by the development of globose, nonostiolate, smooth, dark colored cleistothecia (Fig. 4.6). The cells of the peridium are flattened (*textura epidermoidea*). The asci are

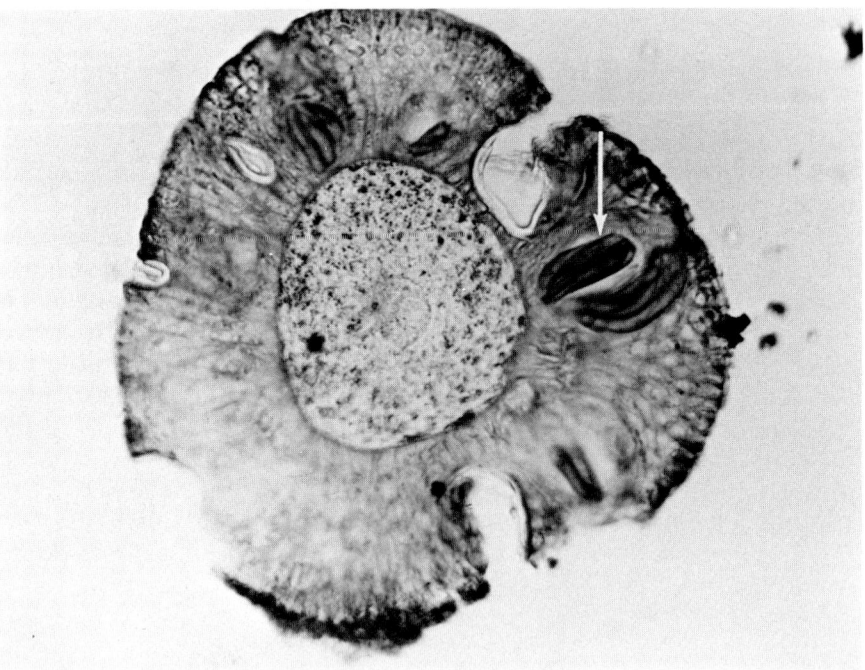

**Fig. 4.24** *Piedraia hortae*. An ascostroma containing several locules has formed around the hair. Each ascus (arrow) contains eight ascospores. (Reproduced by permission from *Mycopathologia Mycologia et Applicata* **45**:269–283, 1971.)

either irregularly distributed or in fascicles. They are globose to clavate, evanescent, with 4–8 ascospores. The ascospores are ellipsoidal, clavate to fusiform, 1-celled, brown, smooth, with 1 or 2 conspicuous germ pores.

Comments: Isolates of *Thielavia* (13, 132) are occasionally recovered in the clinical laboratory. In most instances, an anamorph is absent. When conidia are present, they are either phialoconidia, arthroconidia, or solitary conidia and represent genera such as *Sepedonium, Chrysosporium*, and *Acremonium*. Species of *Thielavia* are readily recognized by their off-white colonies and numerous black cleistothecia in the thallus.

## COELOMYCETES

*Hendersonula* Spegazzini, 1880

Diagnostic features: The genus *Hendersonula* is characterized by black, ostiolate pycnidia. Hyaline, simple, lageniform to flask-shaped phialides

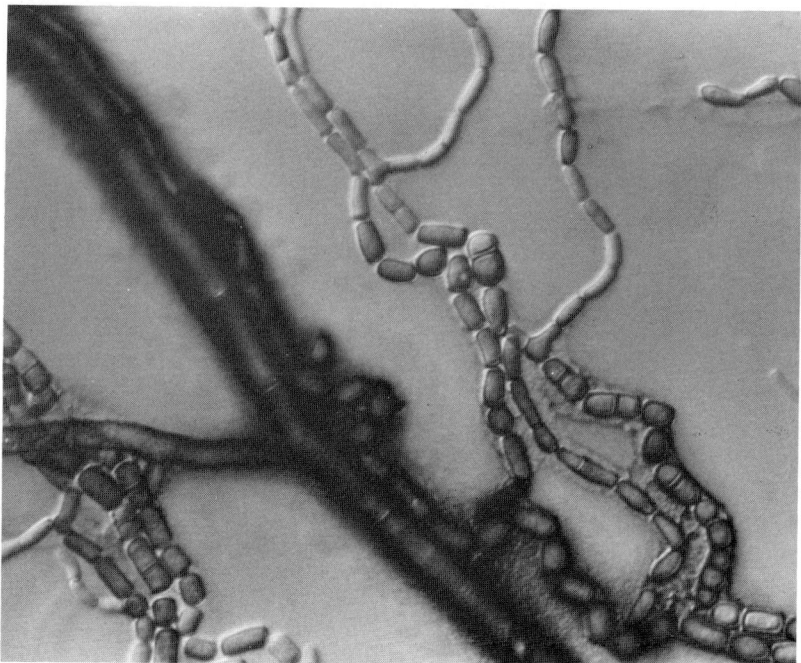

**Fig. 4.25** *Scytalidium* anamorph of *Hendersonula toruloidea*. The dark arthroconidia may either be one- or two-celled.

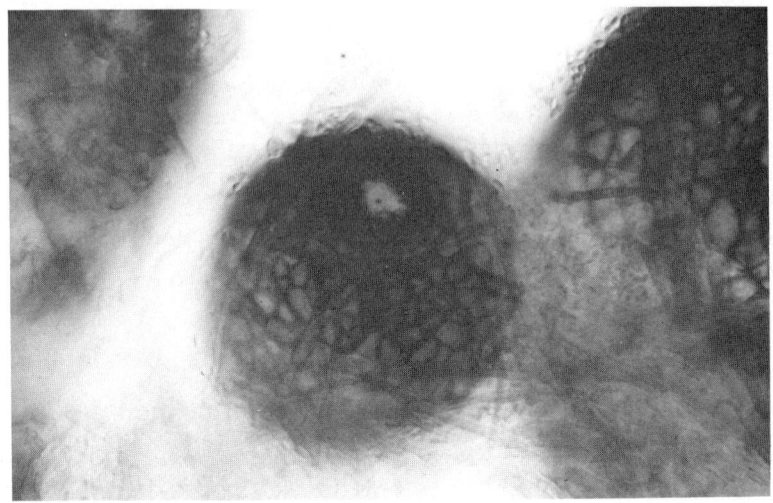

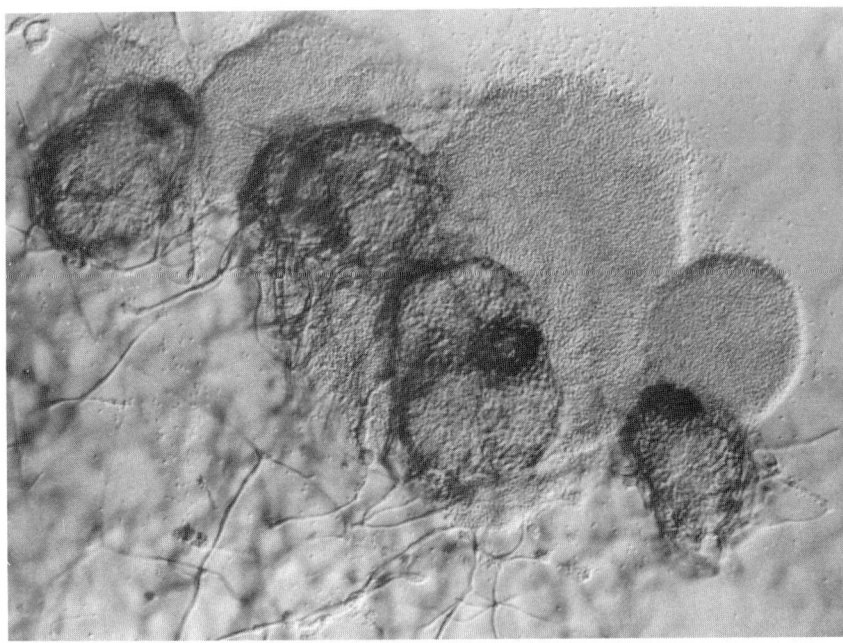

**Fig. 4.26** *Phoma* sp. A. The ostiole is very evident in this pycnidium. B. Masses of phialoconidia are accumulating around four ostiolate pycnidia.

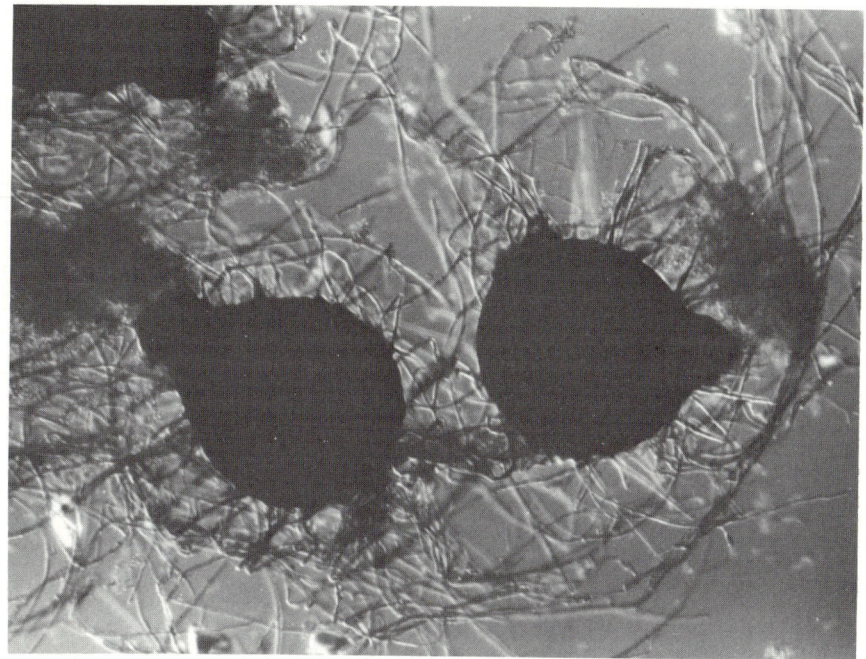

**Fig. 4.27** *Pyrenochaeta unguis-hominis.* A and B. The characteristic setae of this genus can be seen arising from the pycnidia. The phialoconidia develop in the pycnidium, after which they escape through the ostiole.

with collarettes arise from the inner walls of the pycnidia. The conidia are at first 1-celled and hyaline, later becoming 3-celled, brown, with the center cell darker than the end cells. The phialoconidia are ovoid to ellipsoidal. A *Scytalidium* anamorph is typically present. This description is based upon *H. toruloidea*.

Comments: *Hendersonula toruloidea* is a plant pathogen (168) as well as an etiologic agent of onychomycosis and superficial skin infections. In culture, a *Scytalidium* anamorph (Fig. 4.25) consisting of chains of 1- to 2-celled, brown, smooth-walled, subglobose to cylindrical (with truncate ends) arthroconidia is present. Most of the human infections have apparently originated in the tropics. The fungus is rarely, if ever, seen in the clinical laboratory.

*Lasiodiplodia* Ellis et Everhart apud Clendenin, 1896

Diagnostic features: The pycnidia of *Lasiodiplodia* are globose, black, ostiolate, and carbonaceous. The conidiophores are simple, short, hyaline,

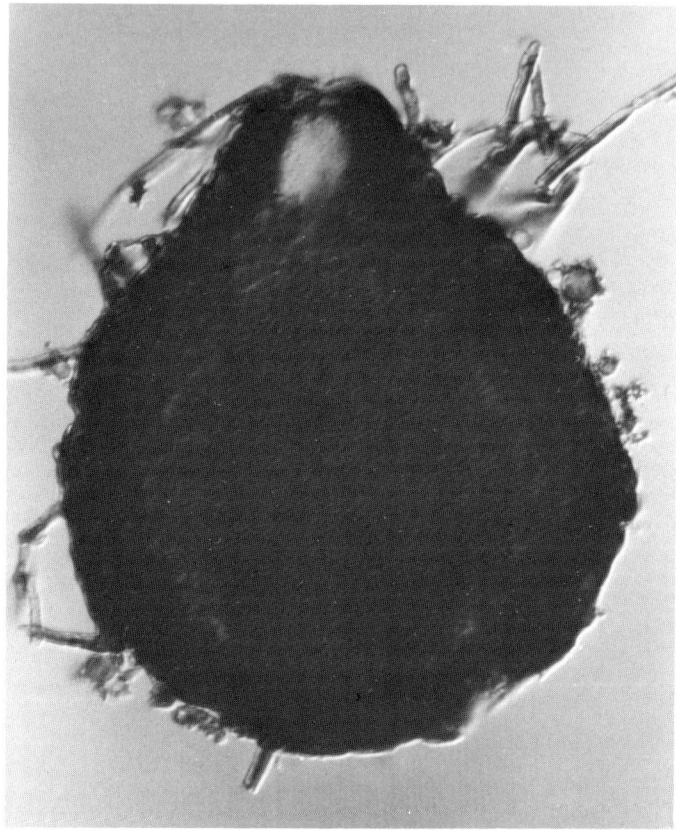

**Fig. 4.27** Continued

and arise within the pycnidia from the peridium. The conidia are at first 1-celled, hyaline, and at maturity, they are 2-celled, brown, ovoid to elongate with narrow hyaline longitudinal striations. The conidia appear to be annelloconidia. The description is based upon *L. theobromae*.

Comments: *Lasiodiplodia theobromae* has been referred to as *Botryodiplodia theobromae* by some medical mycologists (6) in the past. This coelomycete is an etiologic agent of nail and eye infections. It is also a plant pathogen in the tropics.

*Phoma* Saccardo, 1880 *nom. cons.*

Diagnostic features: *Phoma* produces globose to lens-shaped, membranous to leathery, black, ostiolate pycnidia (Fig. 4.26) that may have a short apical neck. The conidiogenous cells are ampulliform phialides. The phialoconidia are globose to cylindrical, 1-celled, hyaline, and usually with 2 oil droplets.

Comments: Isolates of *Phoma* (29, 30, 109) are occasionally recovered in the clinical laboratory. This genus consists primarily of soil organisms and phytopathogens.

### *Pyrenochaeta* de Notaris, 1849

Diagnostic features: Members of the genus *Pyrenochaeta* form globose to flask-shaped, membranous to carbonaceous, black, ostiolate pycnidia with sterile, brown to black setae arising from the upper portion of the fruiting body (Fig. 4.27). The conidiogenous cells are phialides that arise from branching conidiophores. The phialoconidia are ovoid to cylindrical (may be slightly curved), 1-celled, hyaline and with two oil droplets per conidium.

Comments: Members of the genus *Pyrenochaeta* (167, 192) are rarely isolated in the clinical laboratory.

## HYPHOMYCETES

### *Acremonium* Link ex Fries, 1821

Diagnostic features: Isolates of *Acremonium* are readily recognized by the presence of solitary, erect, hyaline, tapering phialides that arise from (Fig. 4.28) hyphae or fascicles. At the apex of each phialide, a ball (rarely a chain) of 1-celled, globose to cylindrical, hyaline conidia forms. When viewed microscopically, the fungus appears to be very delicate. The common species of *Acremonium* form white, low spreading colonies that are moist to dry in appearance.

Comments: Gams (72) studied the genera *Acremonium* and *Cephalosporium* and concluded that they were congeneric (one and the same). Based upon priority, *Acremonium* was considered to be the correct name for this group of fungi. Gams proposed that the monophialidic species of *Paecilomyces* as well as the members of the genus *Gliomastix* should be included in his revised concept of *Acremonium*. This concept of *Acremonium* appears to be a little too broad; therefore, *Gliomastix* is being maintained as a separate genus, and the monophialide species of *Paecilomyces* (162) are considered in this handbook to be members of the genus *Sagrahamala* (208). Gams (73a) has recently treated the genus

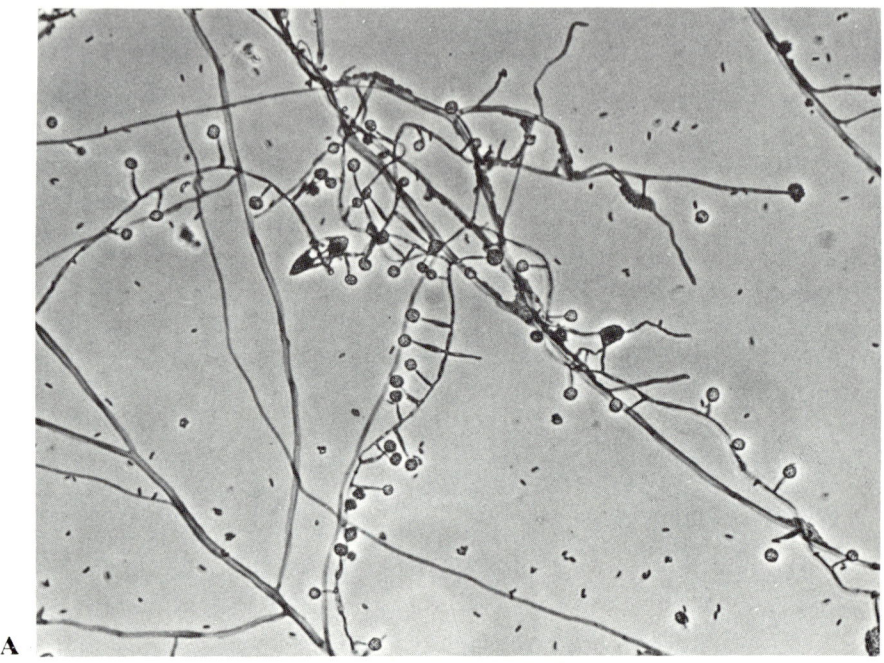

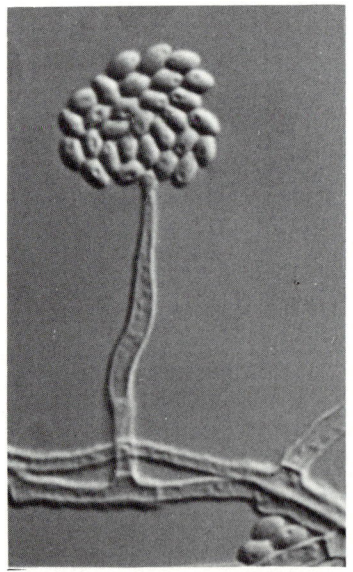

**Fig. 4.28** *Acremonium* sp. A and B. The tapering phialides are rising from the vegetative hyphae. The one-celled phialoconidia typically occur in balls at the apices of the phialides.

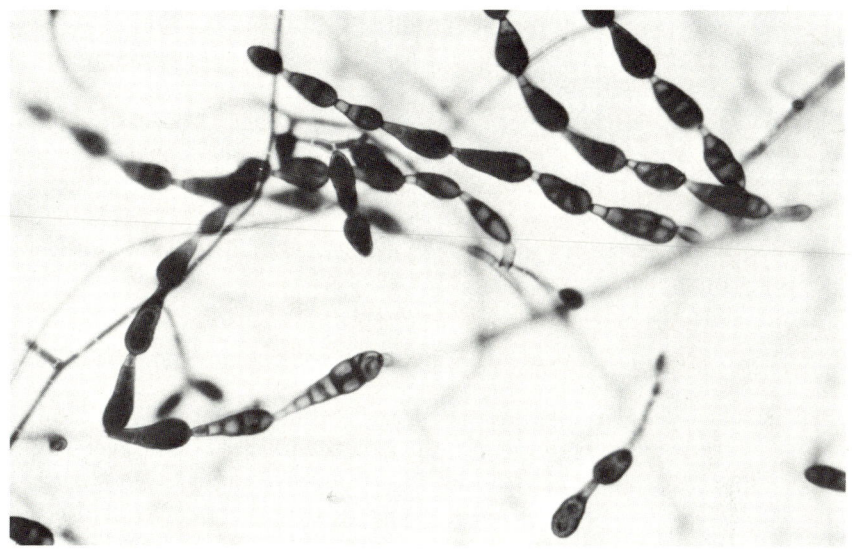

**Fig. 4.29** *Alternaria* sp. Members of this genus are characterized by chains of dark, muriform conidia that arise from sympodial conidiophores. The conidia are usually swollen at their bases and taper toward their apices.

*Sagrahamala* as a synonym of *Acremonium* and established the new genus *Sagenomella* for the monophialidic species of *Paecilomyces*.

*Acremonium* is similar to *Cylindrocarpon, Fusarium, Monocillium, Phialophora hoffmannii, Torulomyces*, and *Verticillium*. The gently tapering solitary phialides distinguish *Acremonium* from these other genera of fungi. Both *Cylindrocarpon* and *Fusarium* typically have an *Acremonium* anamorph.

Species of *Acremonium* are frequently recovered in the clinical laboratory. A number of *Acremonium* spp. are recognized as opportunistic pathogens of man and animals. The Ascomycetes *Emericellopsis, Nectria, Neocosmospora*, and others may form an *Acremonium* anamorph.

*Alternaria* Nees ex Wallroth, 1833 *nom. cons.*

Diagnostic features: Members of the genus *Alternaria* form dematiaceous, muriform, ovoid to obclavate conidia in simple or branching acropetal chains (Fig. 4.29). The chains arise from dark, septate conidiophores that may be sympodial.

Comments: The conidia of *Alternaria* arise through channels in the conidiophore wall, which can be readily seen with oil immersion. The conidia of *Alternaria* are poroconidia. The conidia are variable in shape, size, and septation, which makes the identification (108, 201) of members of this genus difficult. The black to gray colonies are not distinctive.

Isolates of *Alternaria* are occasionally encountered in the clinical laboratory. Several species have been reported as pathogens of man. In most instances, the isolate of *Alternaria* recovered was probably a skin contaminant and did not contribute to the disease process. A commonly encountered species of *Alternaria* is *A. alternata* (syn. *A. tenuis*). The ascomycetous fungi *Clathrospora, Leptosphaeria, Pleospora*, and others may form an *Alternaria* anamorph.

### *Arthrobotrys* Corda emend. Schenck, Kendrick et Pramer, 1977

Diagnostic features: *Arthrobotrys* forms hyaline, septate, solitary, simple or rarely branched conidiophores. The conidia are 1- to several-celled (usually 2-celled) and are ovoid-to-obovate-to-cylindrical. They form on denticles that arise from nodelike swellings (Fig. 4.30). Chlamydospores may be present.

Comments: The first conidium is formed on a denticle at the apex of the conidiophore. A second conidium forms just below the first conidium. The process is repeated, which results in a cluster of basipetal blastic conidia on denticles arising from a swollen area (description based upon *A. amerospora*). The conidiophore may then increase in length from the top of the vesicle, the entire process being repeated. This results in a conidiophore with intercalary nodelike areas and clusters of conidia. *Arthrobotrys* is similar to *Dactylaria* and *Sporothrix*. The latter two genera form sympodial conidiogenous cells.

Members of the genus *Arthrobotrys* (18, 50, 79, 176, 190) are rarely seen in the clinical laboratory. Species of *Arthrobotrys* are often pathogens of nematodes.

### *Aspergillus* Micheli ex Link, 1821

Diagnostic features: Members of the genus *Aspergillus* produce distinct, hyaline to brown, erect, simple conidiophores that arise from a foot cell. The apex of the conidiophore expands into a vesicle from which flask-shaped phialides may arise either directly from the vesicle (uniseriate)(Fig. 4.31), from metulae on the vesicle (biseriate)(Fig. 4.32), or a combination of both. The phialoconidia are 1-celled, usually globose, and in simple, long, dry, basipetal chains.

Comments: The aspergilli (70, 170, 185) are classified upon the basis of colony characteristics (Table 4.7) and microscopic morphology (Table 4.8). Czapek–Dox-solution agar containing 3% sucrose is the standard medium

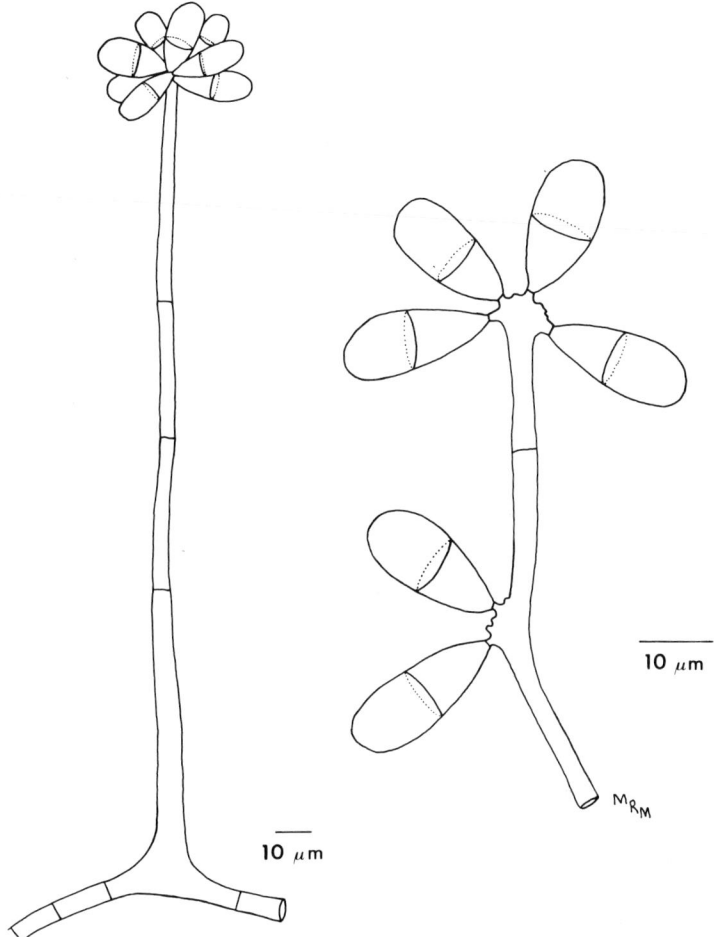

**Fig. 4.30** *Arthrobotrys* sp. The blastoconidia are typically two-celled and arise in clusters at nodelike swellings.

used for determining colony color and morphology. Colony development is studied by placing three drops of an aqueous suspension of conidia an equal distance apart on the medium surface in a Petri dish containing 25 ml of medium. Other media, such as malt extract agar, are also useful. Sabouraud dextrose agar should not be used for studying the aspergilli because a defined medium is necessary if the results are to be meaningful. A special medium (36, 182) has been developed for the identification of the members of the *A. flavus* group. Colony age, exposure to light, incubation temperature and medium composition must be held constant when identi-

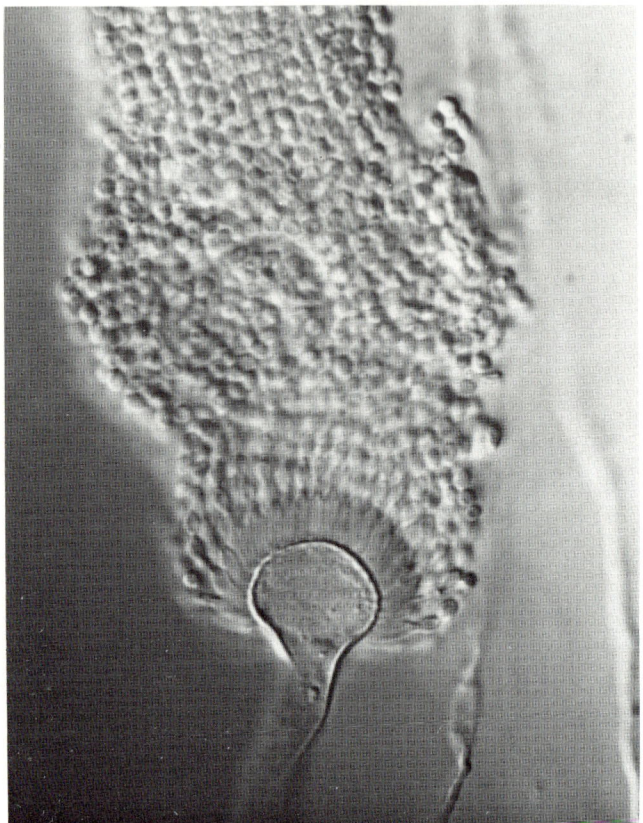

**Fig. 4.31** *Aspergillus fumigatus*. The phialides are arising directly from the vesicle in an uniseriate arrangement. The chains of phialoconidia are forming a columnar head.

fying species of *Aspergillus*. As with *Fusarium* and *Penicillium*, only isolates derived from single conidia or hyphal tips should be used.

The uniseriate, uniseriate and biseriate, or biseriate arrangement of phialides (sterigmata of Raper and Thom) is a major characteristic used to distinguish the various *Aspergillus* groups. The arrangement of phialides is best seen either by focusing on the edge of the row of phialides or by smashing the heads and then looking to see whether or not the phialides are attached to metulae. The arrangement of conidial chains (radiate, columnar, etc.) should be determined with a dissecting microscope.

It is often difficult, if not impossible, in many instances to determine which species of *Aspergillus* have actually caused disease in man and animals. Many medical mycologists have used species epithets and *Asper-*

Part 3  Taxonomy

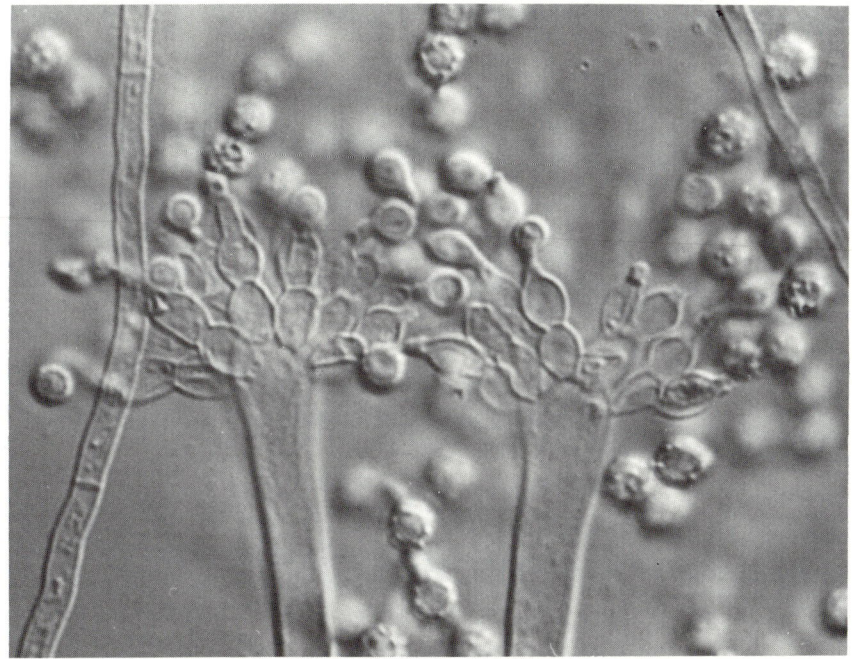

**Fig. 4.32** *Aspergillus* sp. The phialides formed on metulae, which resulted in a biseriate arrangement.

*gillus* group names interchangeably. For example, *A. glaucus* is occasionally reported in the literature as an etiologic agent of aspergillosis. *Aspergillus glaucus* was originally described in vague terms and was subsequently used for a number of different *Aspergillus* species. The name *A. glaucus* has no real value since it does not represent any particular species of *Aspergillus*. Owing to historical reasons, the name is maintained for a group of the aspergilli.

Species of *Aspergillus* are frequently recovered in the clinical laboratory. *Aspergillus fumigatus*, *A. flavus*, and *A. niger* are the most commonly encountered species. In addition to its uniseriate arrangement of phialides, echinulate, globose, 2.5–3.0 μm conidia forming compact columnar heads, isolates of *A. fumigatus* are thermotolerant and can grow at 48°C. A yellow-green colony and conidial heads with both uniseriate and biseriate arrangement of phialides typify most members of the *A. flavus* group. *Aspergillus niger*, which is one member of the *A. niger* group, forms distinctive black conidial heads with large metulae and small phialides. The ascomycetous genera *Emericella*, *Eurotium*, *Sartorya*, and others may form an *Aspergillus* anamorph.

## *Aureobasidium* Viala et Boyer, 1891

Diagnostic features: The conidiophores of *Aureobasidium* species are undifferentiated (micronematous) from the vegetative hyphae, and are hyaline to light brown in color. The hyaline, 1-celled, ovoid conidia arise on short denticles in a cluster or solitarily (Fig. 4.33). Secondary blastoconidia may form from the primary conidia. The colonies are usually pasty and black. Arthroconidia are typically present.

Comments: To most medical mycologists, *Aureobasidium* is characterized in part by the presence of 1- to 2-celled, thick-walled arthroconidia commonly called chlamydospores. These arthroconidia actually represent the *Scytalidium* anamorph of *Aureobasidium* and are only of secondary importance in recognizing members of this genus. If an isolate is producing only dematiaceous arthroconidia, it would probably be identified as a species of *Scytalidium* (200), not of *Aureobasidium*.

Hermanides-Nijhof (88) has recently studied the genera *Aureobasidium* and *Hormonema*. She concluded that *Hormonema* is different from *Aureobasidium* because it produces conidia in a basipetal manner instead of synchronously. Judging by her illustrations and study of several of her isolates, there is some question whether or not *Hormonema* should be considered a separate genus. Until additional information is available, *Hormonema* is being considered as a synonym of *Aureobasidium* in this handbook.

Most "black yeasts" (51, 52) are typically identified by laboratorians without careful study as *A. pullulans*. This is misleading since there are a number of species of *Aureobasidium* besides *A. pullulans*. In fact, many of these black yeasts may actually be species of *Exophiala, Phaeococcus*, or *Wangiella*. Isolates believed to be *Aureobasidium* should be carefully studied by the slide culture technique.

Isolates of *Aureobasidium* are occasionally encountered in the clinical laboratory. By far the most common black yeasts are species of *Phaeococcus* and the yeast form of *E. jeanselmei*. The pycnidial fungi *Dothichiza* and *Sarcophoma*, and ascomycetous fungi such as *Dothidea, Guignardia, Muellerites, Potebniamyces, Pringsheimia*, and *Sydowia*, may form an *Aureobasidium* anamorph.

## *Beauveria* Vuillemin, 1912

Diagnostic features: The genus *Beauveria* is characterized by dense clusters of hyaline, flask-shaped, conidiogenous cells that form along the hyphae. From each flask-shaped cell, a zigzag-appearing rachis develops in a sympodial manner. Along the rachis, 1-celled, hyaline, globose to ovoid, blastic conidia are produced (Fig. 4.34).

## Part 3 Taxonomy

**Table 4.7.** Classification of the Aspergilli Based Primarily on Color[a]

| | | |
|---|---|---|
| 1. | Conidial heads showing some shade of green during development | 2 |
| 1.′ | Conidial heads in some other color | 12 |
| | 2. Vesicles clavate or subclavate; phialides uniseriate | 3 |
| | 2.′ Vesicles not clavate; phialides uniseriate or biseriate | 4 |
| 3. | Vesicles strongly clavate; conidial heads blue-green, becoming gray in age | *A. clavatus* group |
| 3.′ | Vesicles subclavate; phialides uniseriate; conidial heads yellow-green, gray-green, or blue-green when young, darkening in most species | *A. ornatus* group |
| | 4. Conidial heads bright yellow-green when young, sometimes becoming brown in age, loosely radiate; phialides biseriate in most species | *A. flavus* group |
| | 4.′ Conidial heads in other green shades; phialides uniseriate or biseriate | 5 |
| 5. | Colonies mostly showing naked yellow cleistothecia and yellow or red encrusted hyphae | *A. glaucus* group |
| 5.′ | Colonies lacking naked yellow cleistothecia and yellow and red encrusted hyphae | 6 |
| | 6. Conidial heads definitely columnar | 7 |
| | 6.′ Conidial heads globose, radiate, or loosely columnar | 9 |
| 7. | Phialides uniseriate | 8 |
| 7.′ | Phialides biseriate; globose to subglobose hülle cells common; cleistothecia in some species; ascospores orange-red to violet | *A. nidulans* group |
| | 8. Conidial heads columnar, long, narrow (often twisted) to irregular; conidia usually formed as cylindrical segments from the phialides; cleistothecia lacking; typically osmophilic | *A. restrictus* group |
| | 8.′ Conidial heads columnar, compact and typically uniform in diameter throughout; conidia not formed as cylindrical segments; cleistothecia in some species; not typically osmophilic | *A. fumigatus* group |

*continued*

Comments: *Acrodontium*, *Isaria*, *Lomentospora*, and *Tritirachium* are similar to *Beauveria* (87, 95). *Beauveria* can be distinguished from these genera by its distinctive conidiogenous cells with a zigzag-appearing rachis (114).

*Beauveria* species are occasionally recovered in the clinical laboratory. The most common species is *B. bassiana*, which was the first fungus discovered to be a pathogen of animals (3).

### *Blastomyces* Gilchrist et Stokes, 1898

Diagnostic features: *Blastomyces dermatitidis*, the single species within the genus, forms solitary, hyaline, globose to subglobose, 1-celled, terminal conidia upon conidiophores that arise at right angles to the hyphae.

**Table 4.7.** *Continued*

---

9. Vesicles small, variable in shape . . . . . . . . . . . . . . . . . . . . . . . . . . 10
9.′ Vesicles large, strictly globose; conidiophores constricted below the vesicle . . . . 11

    10. Conidial heads blue-green, dull yellow-green, or gray blue-green, radiate to loosely columnar; hülle cells globose to subglobose . . . . . . *A. versicolor* group
    10.′ Conidial heads olive, olive-gray, drab, to light brown; radiate to broadly columnar; hülle cells elongate to twisted . . . . . . . . . . . . . . . *A. ustus* group

11. Conidial heads graying in age from blue-green or olive-buff shades . . *A. sparsus* group
11.′ Conidial heads pale yellow-green, blue-green, or buff-brown . . . . *A. cremeus* group
                                         (see also *A. wentii* group)

    12. Growth very sparse and sporulation poor on Czapek's agar . . *A. cervinus* group
    12.′ Growth and sporulation usually abundant on Czapek's agar . . . . . . . . 13

13. Heads loosely to compactly columnar . . . . . . . . . . . . . . . . . . . . . 14
13.′ Heads globose to radiate . . . . . . . . . . . . . . . . . . . . . . . . . . . . 15

    14. Heads loosely columnar, white, flesh colored, or cream-buff . . *A. flavipes* group
    14.′ Heads compactly columnar, avellaneous to cinnamon . . . . . *A. terreus* group

15. Heads persistently white; larger heads definitely globose or radiate . *A. candidus* group
15.′ Heads not white . . . . . . . . . . . . . . . . . . . . . . . . . . . . . . . . 16

    16. Heads in yellow, ochraceous or light brownish shades . . . . . . . . . . 17
    16.′ Heads in black or dark brown shades . . . . . . . . . . . . *A. niger* group

17. Heads in sulphur yellow to ochraceous shades . . . . . . . . . . *A. ochraceus* group
17.′ Heads in yellow-brown to dull buff shades . . . . . . . . . . . . *A. wentii* group
                                        (also *A. cremeus* group in part)

---

[a] Reproduced and modified by permission of K. Raper and Williams & Wilkins Co. from "The Genus *Aspergillus*," 1965.

*Blastomyces* grows as a globose, large (10–15 µm), thick-walled yeast with unipolar blastoconidia that are attached by a broad base in animal tissue and at 37°C (Fig. 4.35).

Comments: There is considerable confusion surrounding the generic name *Blastomyces*. Costantin and Rolland (53) established the genus *Blastomyces* in 1888. Their mould, which was isolated from bear dung, is identical to *Chrysosporium merdarium*. In 1896, Gilchrist and Stokes (76) isolated a white mould from a case of blastomycosis that they tentatively identified as a species of *Oidium*. In a later study during 1898 (77), they proposed the genus *Blastomyces* for their fungus because it developed a yeast form in tissue. Gilchrist and Stokes were unaware that the generic name *Blastomyces* had already been proposed for a different fungus. Thus,

Table 4.8. Classification of the Aspergilli Based Primarily on Morphology[a]

I. Phialides strictly uniseriate
   A. Conidial heads clavate with conidial masses splitting at maturity, in blue-green shades; vesicles strongly clavate . . . . . . . . . . . . . . . *A. clavatus* group
   B. Conidial heads radiate to columnar, variable in color; vesicles variable, from globose or nearly so to subclavate or turbinate
      1. Conidial heads radiate, variable in size, in bluish green or olive green shades (brown in one species); osmophilic; bright yellow cleistothecia abundant in most species . . . . . . . . . . . . . . . . . . . . . . . *A. glaucus* group
      2. Conidial heads radiate to very loosely columnar, comparatively large, in grayish or yellowish green to olive-brown shades; white to purplish or olive cleistothecia produced in some species . . . . . . . . . . *A. ornatus* group
      3. Conidial heads radiate (short columnar in one species), small, in pinkish fawn shades; cleistothecia lacking . . . . . . . . . . . . . . . *A. cervinus* group
      4. Conidial heads loosely to definitely columnar, often long, thin and twisted, in green shades; conidia cylindrical when young; osmophilic; cleistothecia lacking . . . . . . . . . . . . . . . . . . . . . . . . . . . . . *A. restrictus* group
      5. Conidial heads compactly columnar, in pale gray-green to dark blue-green shades; conidia not cylindrical when young; not osmophilic . . . . . . . . . . . . . . . . . . . . . . . . . . . . . . . . . . . . . . . . . . . . *A. fumigatus* group
         a. Cleistothecia lacking . . . . . . . . . . . . . . *A. fumigatus* series
         b. Cleistothecia present, white to yellowish . . . . . . . . *A. fischeri* series

II. Phialides biseriate or uniseriate (the former predominant), or with both conditions in the same head
   A. Conidial heads usually globose when young, radiate or splitting in age, rarely loosely columnar; vesicles globose to subglobose or somewhat elongate; conidiophores not constricted below the vesicle; sclerotia produced in many species
      1. Conidial heads globose when young, sometimes remaining so but usually splitting into more or less well defined columns at maturity
         a. Conidial heads in yellow, buff, or ochraceous shades; conidiophores commonly roughened and often pigmented; cleistothecia in one species . . . . . . . . . . . . . . . . . . . . . . . . . . . . . . . . *A. ochraceus* group
         b. Conidial heads in shades of black; conidiophores usually smooth and colorless or becoming pigmented below the vesicle . . . . *A. niger* group
         c. Conidial heads white or cream colored; conidiophores smooth and colorless . . . . . . . . . . . . . . . . . . . . . . . . . . . *A. candidus* group
      2. Conidial heads typically radiate with conidial chains usually separate, sometimes forming poorly defined columns
         a. Conidial heads in yellow-green to deep olive-brown shades; conidiophores usually roughened, colorless . . . . . . . . . . . . . . *A. flavus* group
         b. Conidial heads in yellow-brown to dull buff shades; conidiophores smooth or delicately roughened, colorless or lightly pigmented . . *A. wentii* group

*continued*

**Table 4.8.** *Continued*

- B. Conidial heads large, radiate; vesicles strictly globose; conidiophores definitely constricted below the vesicles; sclerotia lacking
  1. Conidial heads of one type, buff-brown, pale yellow-green, or blue-green; conidiophores usually colorless, smooth; osmophilic; cleistothecia produced in some species . . . . . . . . . . . . . . . . . . . . . . *A. cremeus* group
  2. Conidial structures of two types: large heads light gray, green, or olive-buff with conidiophores usually in brown shades and encrusted; fragmentary structures borne near or beneath the agar surface . . . . . . . .*A. sparsus* group

III. Phialides strictly biseriate
- A. Conidial heads typically in definite green shades; hülle cells usually globose but sometimes irregularly ovate to pyriform
  1. Conidial heads typically radiate, becoming loosely columnar in some species; conidiophores colorless or light brown, commonly exceeding 300 µm in length; vesicles variable, elongate, subglobose, hemispherical, or only slightly expanded; hülle cells sometimes abundant, more often limited or lacking . . . . . . . . . . . . . . . . . . . . . . . . . . . . . . . . . *A. versicolor* group
     a. Conidial heads uniformly pigmented, small or fragmentary structures sometimes present; hyphal masses or sclerotia occasionally produced . . . . . . . . . . . . . . . . . . . . . . . . . . . . . . *A. versicolor* series
     b. Conidial heads not uniformly pigmented, both white and green heads present (at least on some substrates) . . . . . . . . . . . *A. janus* series
  2. Conidial heads typically columnar, usually dark yellow-green but occasionally gray blue-green or brownish; conidiophores brown walled, commonly less than 300 µm long; vesicles subglobose, hemispherical, or terminally flattened; hülle cells typically produced, usually abundant, clustered, forming crusts, or enveloping ascocarps; cleistothecia common, purplish at maturity; ascospores in orange-red to blue-violet shades . . . . . . . . . . . . . *A. nidulans* group
- B. Conidial heads in shades other than true green; hülle cells, when present, elongate to strongly curved and twisted
  1. Conidial heads radiate to broadly columnar, in drab, olive, or dull brown shades; conidiophores typically brown-walled; vesicles variable from globose to elongate or hemispherical; hülle cells elongate, often strongly curved or twisted . . . . . . . . . . . . . . . . . . . . . . . . . . . . *A. ustus* group
  2. Conidial heads broadly to irregularly columnar, white to avellaneous or vinaceous; conidiophores with walls brown or uncolored; vesicles subglobose to elongate; elongate hülle cells or heavy-walled hyphal elements present . . . . . . . . . . . . . . . . . . . . . . . . . . . . . . . . . . *A. flavipes* group
  3. Conidial heads compactly columnar, typically in cinnamon to orange-brown or pale buff shades; conidiophores colorless; vesicles hemispherical . . . . . . . . . . . . . . . . . . . . . . . . . . . . . . . . . . . . . *A. terreus* group

[a] Reproduced and modified by permission of K. Raper and Williams & Wilkins Co. from "The Genus *Asperigillus*," 1965.

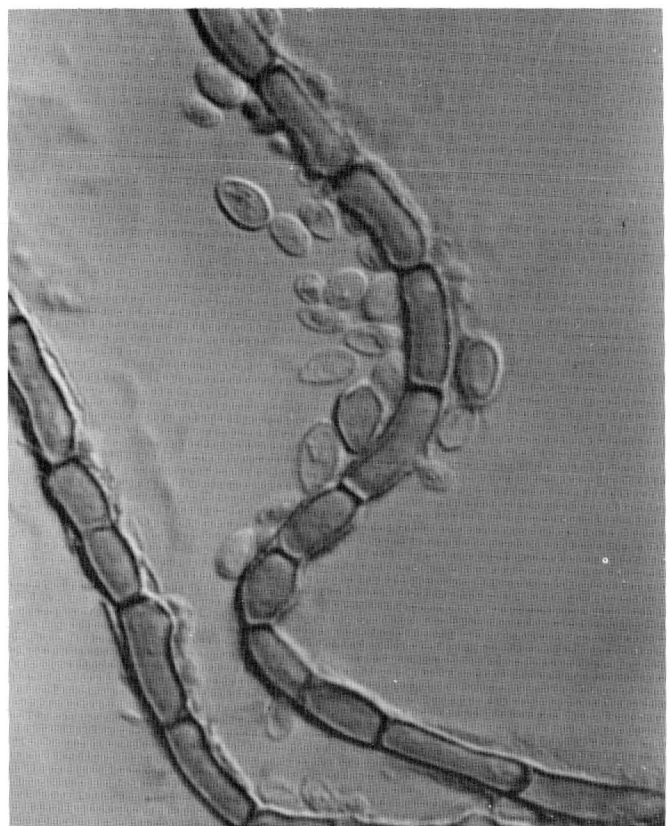

**Fig. 4.33** *Aureobasidium pullulans.* The hyaline one-celled conidia of this fungus arise on short denticles from the hyphae.

*Blastomyces* Gilchrist et Stokes is a later homonym, and according to the International Code of Botanical Nomenclature, is illegitimate and must be rejected, even though *Blastomyces* Costantin et Rolland is a synonym of *Chrysosporium.* Owing to its ability to grow as a mould or a yeast, and its historical value and common usage, steps are being initiated to have the name *Blastomyces* Gilchrist et Stokes conserved.

Carmichael (43) considers *Blastomyces* in the senses of Costantin and Rolland, and Gilchrist and Stokes to be synonyms of *Chrysosporium.* He proposed the new combination *C. dermatitidis* for *B. dermatitidis.* This proposal has not been accepted by most medical mycologists. The distinctive terminal conidia that arise solitarily on micronematous conidiophores developing at right angles to the hyphae, and its ability to grow at 37°C in a yeast form, clearly distinguish *B. dermatitidis* from species of *Chrysosporium* and similar hyphomycetes. In tissue, *B. dermatitidis* rarely forms both hyphae and yeast cells (82).

Because of its similarity to *Chrysosporium*, isolates of *B. dermatitidis* must be confirmed as such by converting the mould form to the yeast form, or vice versa. The fungus has been reported from soil (57) and pigeon manure (188), but these reports are questionable. It is generally agreed by medical mycologists that the natural habitat is unknown. *Blastomyces dermatitidis* is the anamorph of *Ajellomyces dermatitidis*.

### *Botrytis* Micheli ex Saint-Amans, 1821

Diagnostic features: *Botrytis* forms dematiaceous, erect, septate conidiophores that branch (often dichotomously), the branches being restricted to the apical region. The terminal cell of each branch becomes swollen, forming an ampulla. From the ampullae, 1-celled, hyaline to

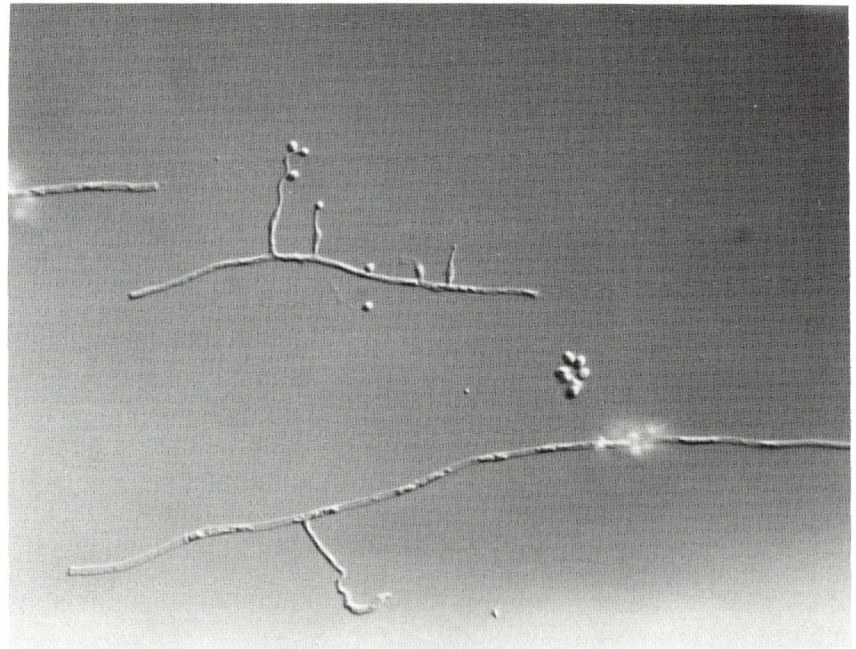

**Fig. 4.34** *Beauveria bassiana.* Each sympodial conidiogenous cell is slightly swollen at its base, gradually tapering toward its apex to form a long rachis. Along the rachis, one-celled conidia can be seen. The conidiogenous cells occur in dense clusters along the hyphae.

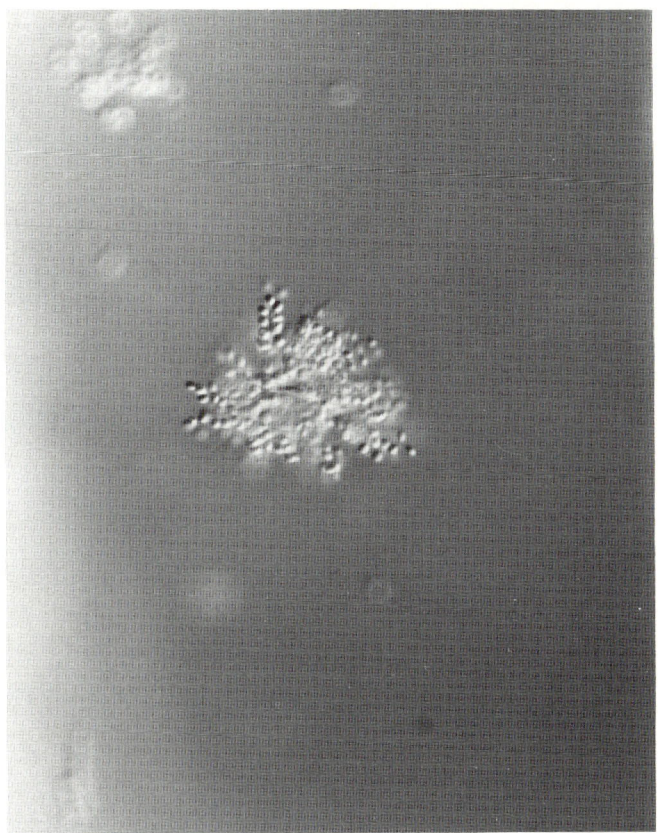

**B**

**Fig. 4.34** Continued

pale-brown, spherical to ellipsoidal, blastic conidia develop on denticles (Fig. 4.36). The conidia are produced in a synchronized manner.

Comments: *Botrytis cinerea* is one of the more common species of *Botrytis* (17, 86, 106). It commonly occurs as a "gray mould" on plants. Species of *Botrytis* are rarely encountered in the clinical laboratory. The ascomycetous fungi *Botryotinia* and *Sclerotinia* may form a *Botrytis* anamorph.

*Cephalotrichum* Link ex Gray, 1821

Diagnostic features: Members of the genus *Cephalotrichum* form a synnema (Fig. 4.37) having a sterile stalk with the region of conidiogenesis restricted to the upper portion of the fruiting structure. The conidiogenous

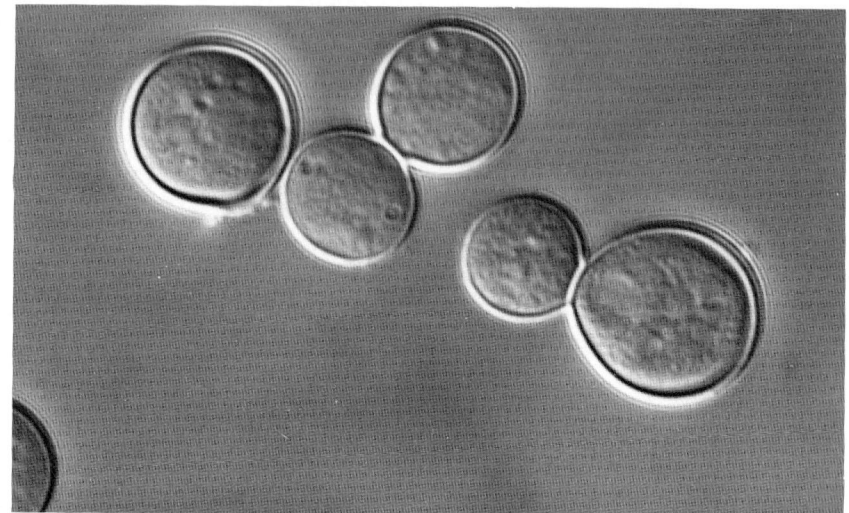

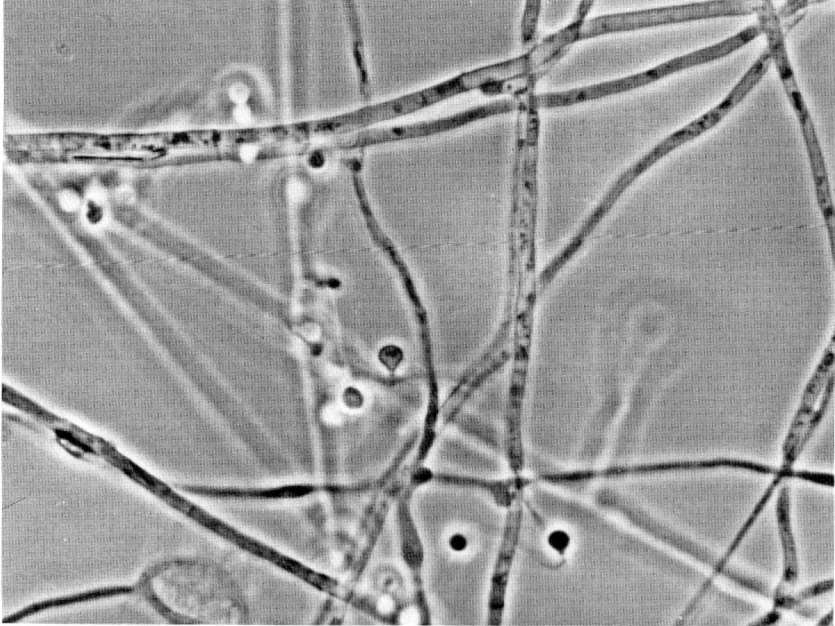

**Fig. 4.35** *Blastomyces dermatitidis*. A. The yeast form of this dimorphic fungus develops at 37°C on media such as Kelley's agar. B and C. At 25°C, the typical one-celled conidia are produced on short conidiophores. (C reproduced by permission from *Clinical Microbiology Newsletter* **1**(5):1–3, 1979.)

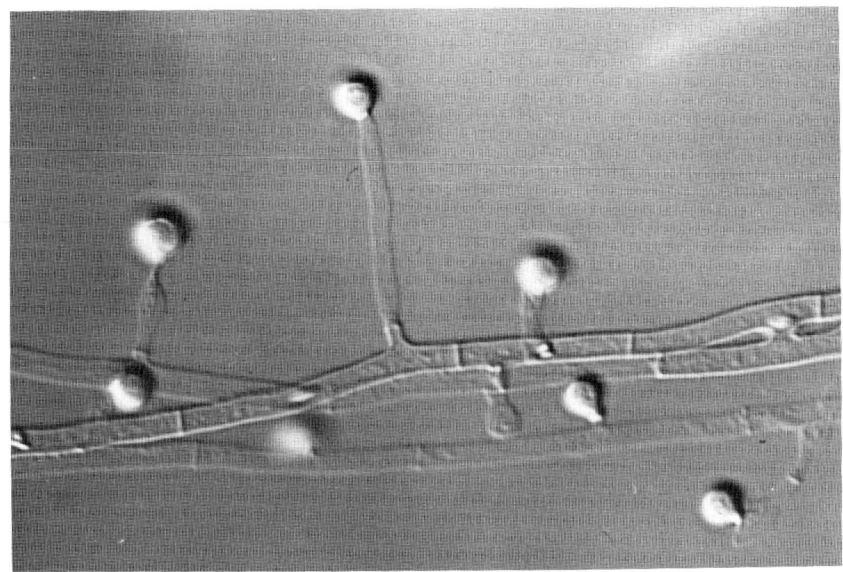

C

Fig. 4.35 Continued

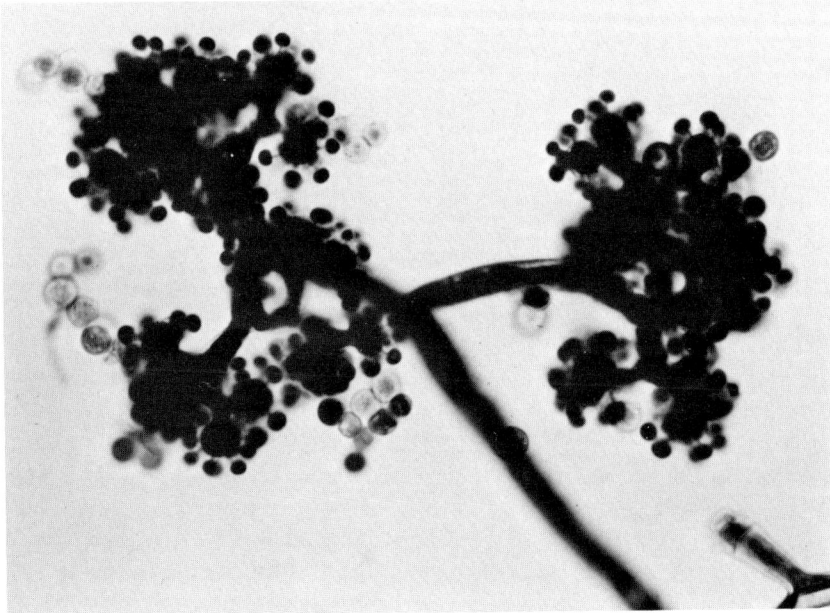

Fig. 4.36  *Botrytis cinerea*. The blastoconidia develop on short denticles from the ampullae in a synchronized manner. The conidiophore is branching dichotomously at its apex.

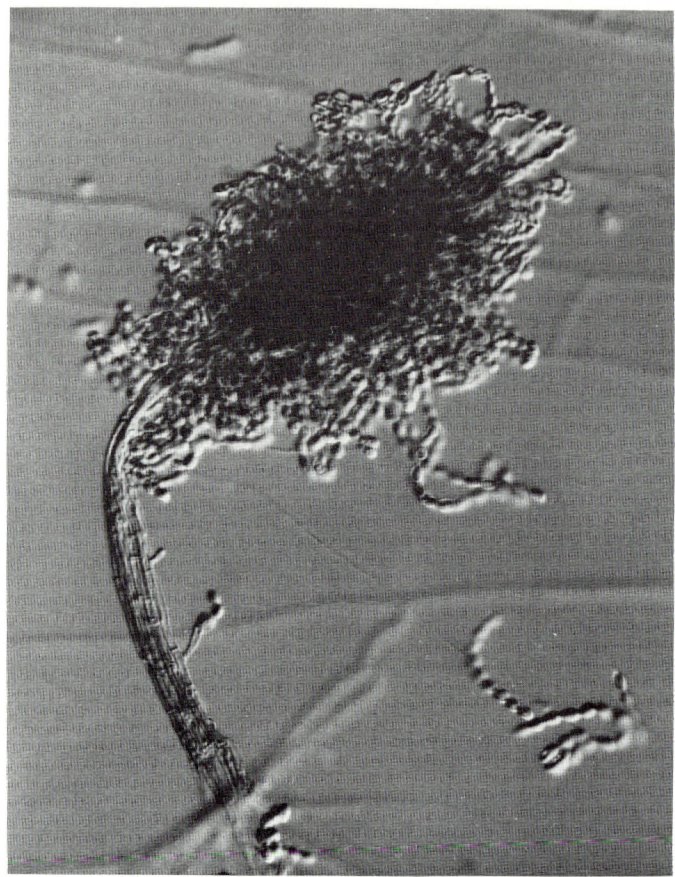

**Fig. 4.37** *Cephalotrichum* sp. The conidia occur in chains along the sides of the synnema.

cells are annellides. The annelloconidia are 1-celled, smooth or rough, catenulate, globose to ovoid and usually truncate at the base.

Comments: The generic names *Doratomyces* and *Stysanus* were both proposed well after the name *Cephalotrichum*. *Cephalotrichum* (149) is essentially a *Trichurus* that does not have setae, or vice versa. Isolates of *Cephalotrichum* are rarely encountered in the clinical laboratory. When they are isolated, a *Scopulariopsis* anamorph is also usually present. For all practical purposes, *Cephalotrichum* is the synnematous form of *Scopulariopsis* (150), even though an *Echinobotryum* anamorph may be produced too. *Cephalotrichum* is a soil organism that may be associated with the ascomycete *Microascus*.

### *Chalara* (Corda) Rabenh. emend. Nag Raj et Kendrick, 1975

Diagnostic features: *Chalara* species produce hyaline to brown phialides with extremely deep, cylindrical collarettes (Fig. 4.38). The conidiophores may be simple (rarely branched) or absent. The phialoconidia are 1- to several-celled, cylindrical to ellipsoidal, hyaline to pale brown, and either solitary or in chains. Chlamydospores may be present.

Comments: Species of *Chalara* are rarely recovered in the clinical laboratory. Members of this genus are usually pathogens of higher plants. They are occasionally isolated from the soil and forest litter. The monograph by Nag Raj and Kendrick (155) should be consulted for additional information. *Chalara* is the anamorph of several species of *Ceratocystis*.

### *Chrysosporium* Corda, 1833

Diagnostic features: Species of *Chrysosporium* are characterized by hyaline, 1-celled conidia that are terminal, on pedicels or long branches, along the sides of the hyphae, or both (Fig. 4.39). Arthroconidia are usually present in a random arrangement. Both the solitary conidia and arthroconidia are swollen, that is, they are broader than the parent hyphae.

Comments: Carmichael's (43) concept of *Chrysosporium* is broad. As a result, not all mycologists have completely accepted it. The revised concept of *Chrysosporium* and its relationship to similar genera by Sigler and Carmichael (200) offers a practical approach to this group of difficult fungi. *Chrysosporium* is similar to *Geomyces, Malbranchea*, and *Myceliophthora. Geomyces* forms acutely branched fertile hyphae on erect conidiophores; *Malbranchea* forms nonswollen, regular, narrow alternate arthroconidia; and *Myceliophthora* produces conidia directly from the hyphae on pedicels or from swollen conidiogenous cells. *Myceliophthora* does not form arthroconidia (163).

The hyphomycetous genus *Emmonsia* (47) was established to accommodate *Haplosporangium parvum*. This was necessary because the genus *Haplosporangium* was originally established for a zygomycete (221). In culture at 25°C, the two species *E. crescens* and *E. parva* are identical (68). On enriched media at 37°C, the conidia of *E. crescens* enlarge to approximately 250–400 µm and have a cell wall that is up to 70 µm thick, whereas *E. parva* remains the same size. At 40°C, the conidia of some isolates of *E. parva* enlarge to 10–25 µm in diameter and have a cell wall up to 2 µm in thickness. The enlarged cells of *E. crescens* are multinucleate and those of *E. parva* are uninucleate. Subsequently, Carmichael (43) considered *Emmonsia* to be a synonym of *Chrysosporium* and *E. crescens* as a variety of *C. parvum*. This treatment appears to be the most ideal.

198                                                                    4  Mould Identification

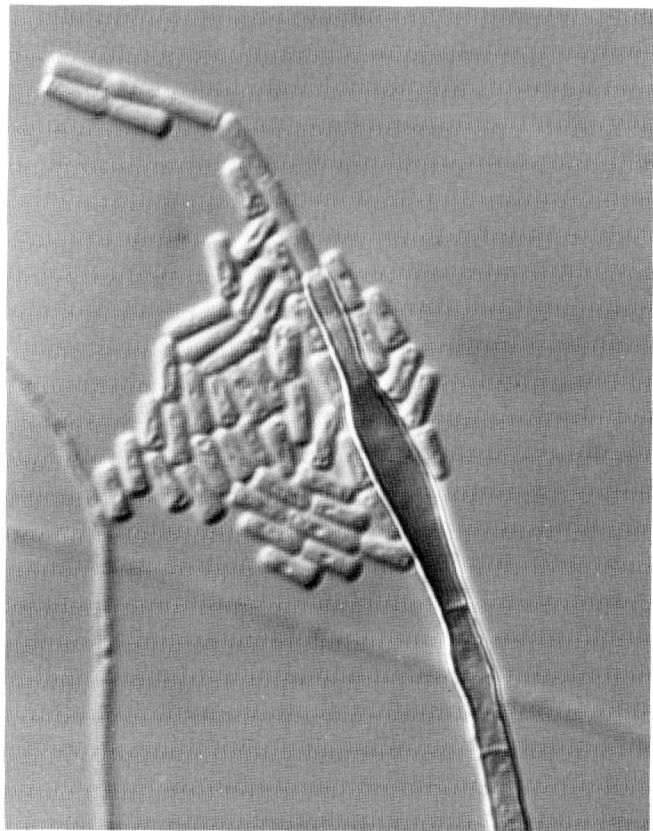

**Fig. 4.38** *Chalara* sp. The phialoconidia are formed by a phialide that has an extremely deep, cylindrical collarette.

Species of *Chrysosporium* are occasionally isolated in the clinical laboratory, especially from skin and nail specimens. *Chrysosporium* is a fairly common soil organism. Members of this genus have been reported as pathogens, but most likely only represented contaminants. *Chrysosporium* is the anamorph of some species of *Arthroderma* and other members of the Gymnoascaceae.

*Cladosporium* Link ex Gray, 1821

Diagnostic features: The genus *Cladosporium* is characterized by branching chains of blastoconidia that are formed in an acropetal manner from a distinct, erect, pigmented conidiophore, which is sympodial. The conidia are smooth to echinulate (occasionally), pale brown to dark brown, 1- to

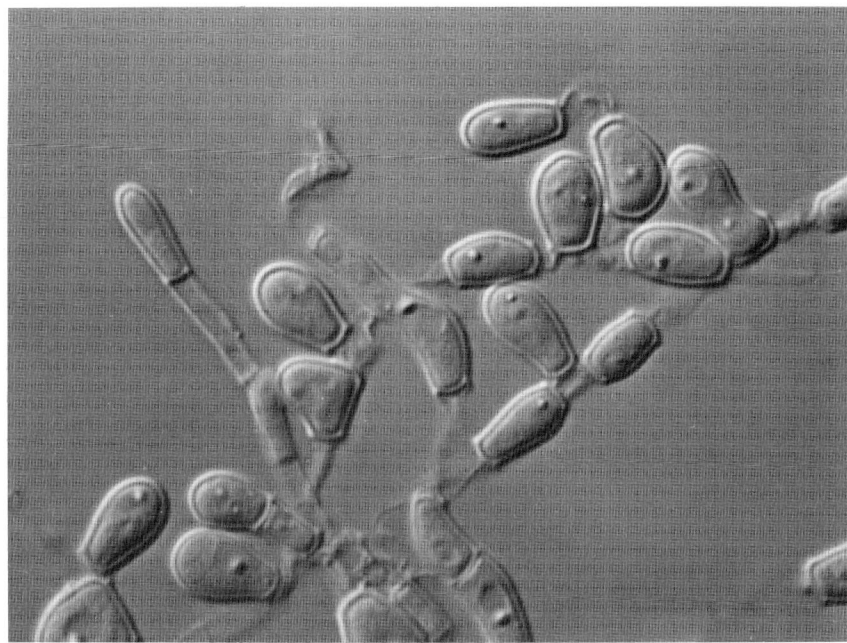

**Fig. 4.39** *Chrysosporium pruinosum.* The abundant one-celled lateral conidia and arthroconidia are typical of this genus.

4-celled, with a distinct dark hilum. The conidia closest to the conidiophore, and where the chains branch, are usually "shield-shaped." The presence of shield-shaped conidia, a distinct dark hilum, and chains of conidia that readily disarticulate, are diagnostic for the common species of *Cladosporium.*

Comments: In the older mycological literature, species of *Cladosporium* were commonly referred to as *Heterosporium* and *Hormodendrum* spp. Species of *Heterosporium* originally included plant pathogens that produced 1- to several-celled conidia and conidia that were solitary or in short to long chains. One-celled conidia were segregated into the genus *Hormodendrum* (occasionally spelled incorrectly *Hormodendron*). Both these genera are now considered to be synonyms of *Cladosporium*, at least in part. Some species of *Heterosporium* have been transferred to the genus *Scolecobasidium.*

There is considerable confusion surrounding the status of *C. bantianum* (180) and *C. trichoides* (26). Borelli (34) believes that these species are one and the same, whereas Emmons *et al.* (67) consider them to be different. The disagreement involves the size ranges for the conidia and the number of conidia composing the chains. Even though the conidia of *C. bantianum* were reported to be larger than those of *C. trichoides*, these two species can be considered conspecific (one and the same species). Emmons *et al.* point out that the conidia of some isolates of *C. trichoides* are initially larger than the accepted size range, but upon subculture, they become smaller. This was probably the case in *C. bantianum*. Unfortunately, only dried material was preserved for this species. I have had the opportunity to examine this type material as well as Saccardo's original photomicrographs, and believe that *C. trichoides* should be considered a synonym of *C. bantianum* (Fig. 4.40).

*Cladosporium carrionii* (Fig. 4.41), an etiologic agent of chromoblastomycosis, can be distinguished from *C. bantianum*, which causes

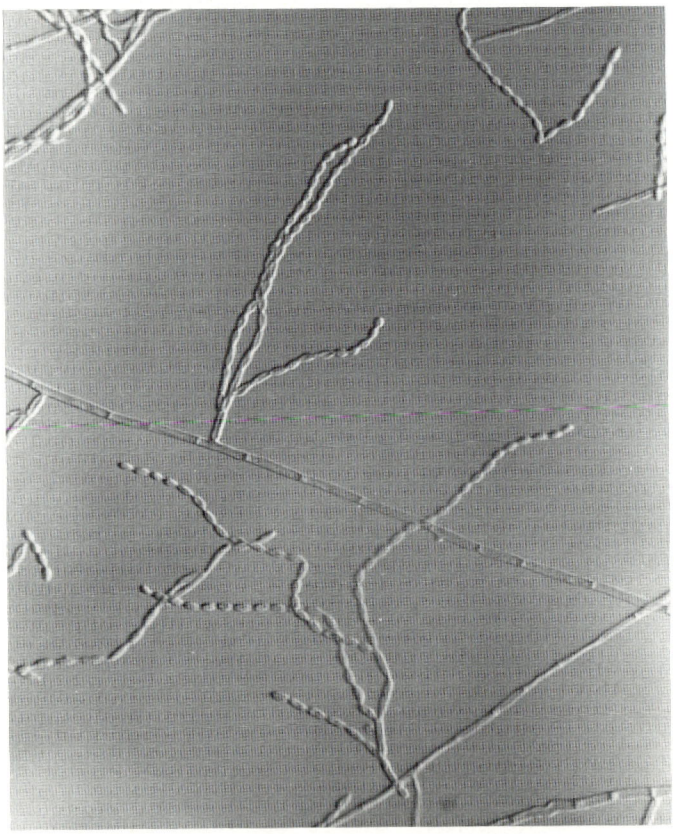

**Fig. 4.40** *Cladosporium bantianum*. The one-celled blastoconidia occur in long, sparsely branching chains.

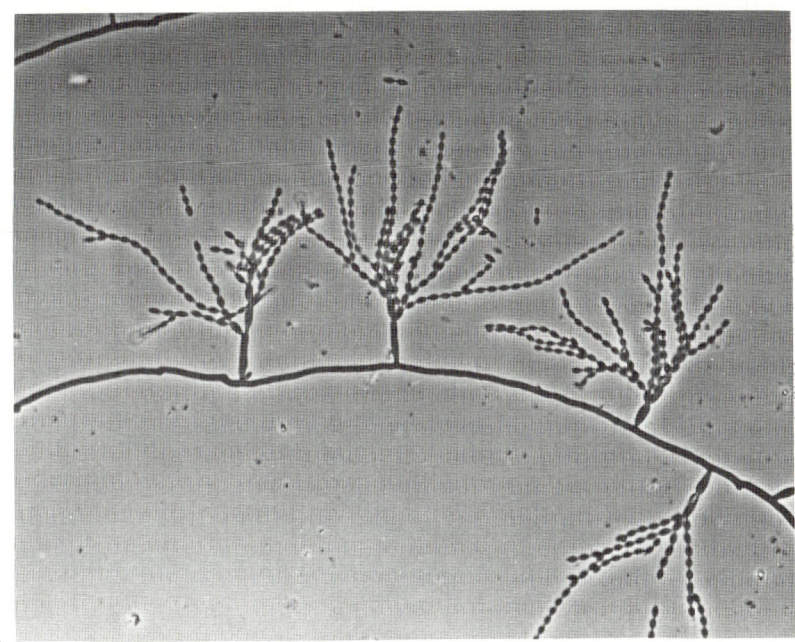
**Fig. 4.41** *Cladosporium carrionii.* A and B. The one-celled blastoconidia occur in branching chains.

phaeohyphomycosis, by its inability to grow beyond 35–36°C (42–43°C for *C. bantianum*) (35), slower growth rate on artificial media, shorter blastoconidia (4.8–5.2 μm for *C. carrionii* and 7.3–7.6 μm for *C. bantianum*), and an absence of neurotropism in man and experimental animals. *Cladosporium carrionii* and *C. bantianum* have been separated from nonpathogenic species of *Cladosporium* by their inability to digest Löffler's coagulated serum medium (214). This test is questionable and should not be used as the sole basis of determining pathogenicity.

Isolates of *Cladosporium* (Fig. 4.42) are commonly recovered in the clinical laboratory. Most of the more common species of *Cladosporium* are soil fungi. The works by de Vries (217) and Ellis (64, 65) should be consulted for additional information. Some Ascomycetes such as *Mycosphaerella* and *Venturia*, may produce a *Cladosporium* anamorph. The genus *Hyalodendron* is essentially a fragile *Cladosporium* that is hyaline instead of dematiaceous.

### *Coccidioides* Rixford et Gilchrist, 1896

Diagnostic features: *Coccidioides immitis* forms 1-celled, hyaline, rectangular to barrel-shaped, alternate arthroconidia, terminally and intercalary

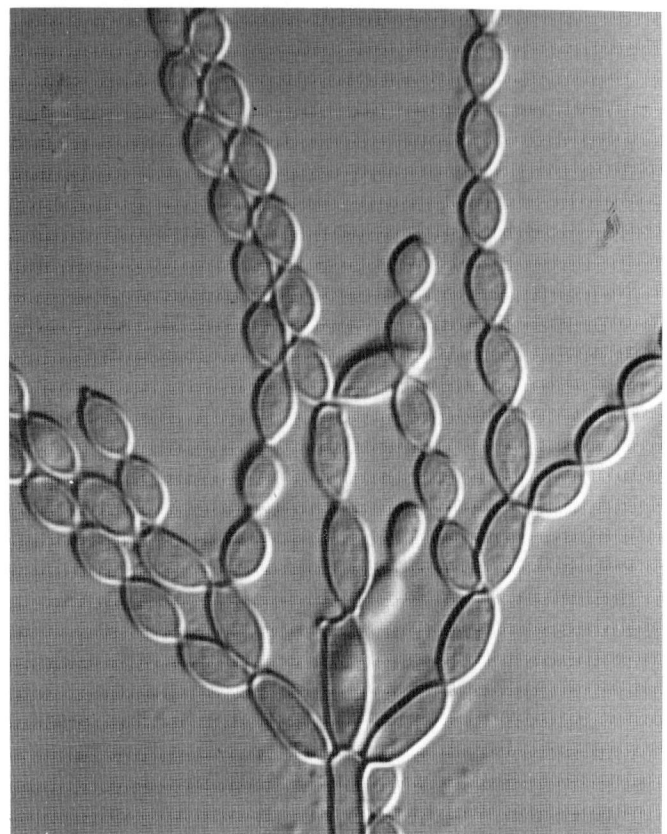

Fig. 4.41 Continued

on short to long lateral fertile hyphae that arise at a right angle to the vegetative hyphae (Fig. 4.43). Spherules with endospores are formed in animal tissue and at 37°C on special media.

Comments: Rixford and Gilchrist proposed the genus *Coccidioides* with the single species *C. immitis* for a "protozoan" in tissue that they (177) could not isolate. The taxonomy for their new genus and species was handled by Stiles. The fungus may have been recovered, but its dimorphic nature went unrecognized. Since the spherule is actually a sporangium with sporangiospores, some mycologists in the past have considered *C. immitis* to be a zygomycete. At present, the consensus is that *C. immitis* is most likely the anamorph of an ascomycete, probably a member of the Gymnoascaceae.

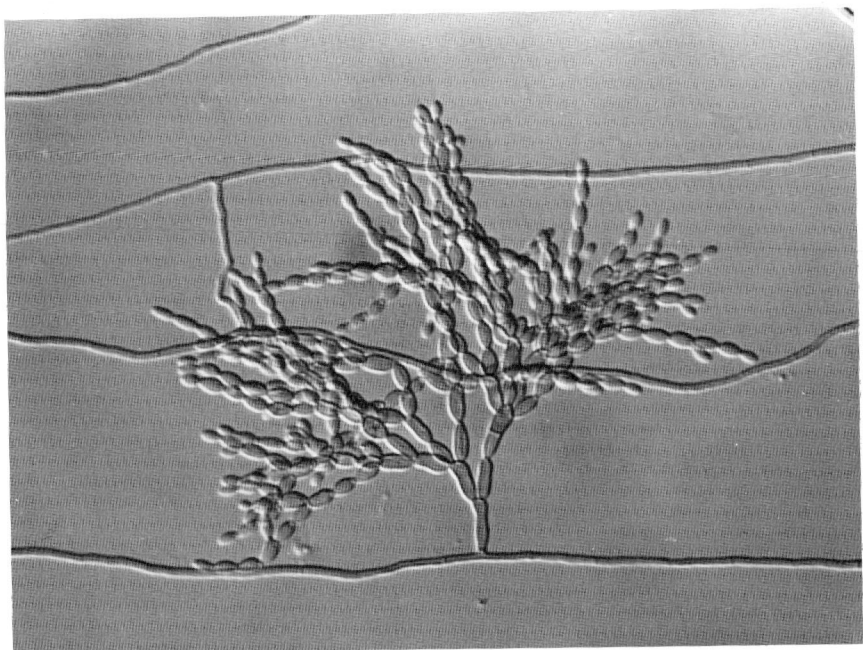

**Fig. 4.42** *Cladosporium* sp. Branching chains of dematiaceous blastoconidia, arising from an erect conidiophore, are characteristic of the common species of *Cladosporium*.

In their study of the genus *Malbranchea*, Sigler and Carmichael (200) pointed out that the mould form of *C. immitis* could be accommodated in the genus *Malbranchea*, and they used the name *Malbranchea* state of *C. immitis*. *Coccidioides immitis* is similar to species of *Sporendonema*, but can be easily distinguished from them as well as other species of *Malbranchea* by the development of spherules. The development of spherules in tissue or at 37°C on special media (209) is necessary before an isolate can be identified as *C. immitis*. An exoantigen technique (103, 113) is also available for identifying colonies of *C. immitis*.

*Coccidioides immitis* is a soil organism associated with the Lower Sonoran Life Zone of North, South, and Central America. The fungus is extremely dangerous and should be worked with only in a Class II or Class III biological safety cabinet. The isolation of *C. immitis* is never considered to be insignificant.

### *Curvularia* Boedijn, 1933

Diagnostic features: The conidiophores of *Curvularia* are brown, simple or branched, solitary or in groups, borne laterally or terminally from the

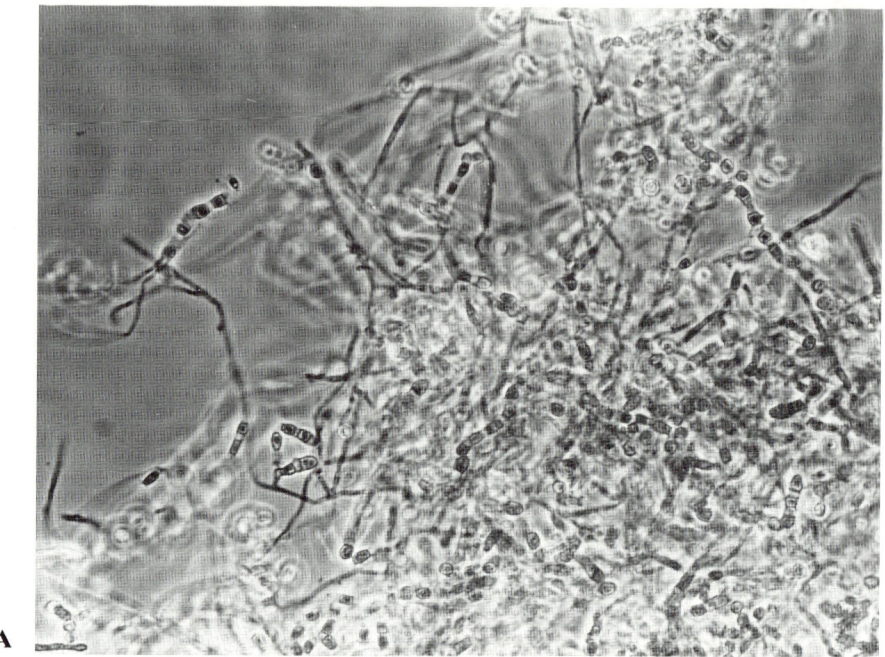

**Fig. 4.43** *Coccidioides immitis.* The one-celled arthroconidia are separated from each other by disjunctor cells. The fertile hyphae are larger in diameter than the vegetative hyphae.

hyphae, septate, and sympodial in development. The poroconidia are usually curved, occasionally straight to pyriform, several-celled, smooth to verrucose, pale brown to dark brown, and usually with a protuberant hilum. The end cells of the conidia are frequently paler than the rest of the conidium. The conidia are acropleurogenous or in whorls about the conidiophore (Fig. 4.44).

Comments: Isolates of *Curvularia* are periodically recovered in the clinical laboratory. Species of *Curvularia* (63, 111, 203) are usually pathogens and saprophytes of plants. They are occasionally found in the soil. As etiologic agents of disease, they are most frequently associated with mycotic keratitis. *Curvularia* is the anamorph of some species of *Cochliobolus.*

*Cylindrocarpon* Wollenweber, 1913 *nom. cons.*

Diagnostic features: The conidiogenous cells of *Cylindrocarpon* are phialides that arise from the hyphae, lateral branches, or from branched conidiophores that resemble a penicillus. The phialides may be either solitary or in groups. The macrophialoconidia are hyaline, straight to

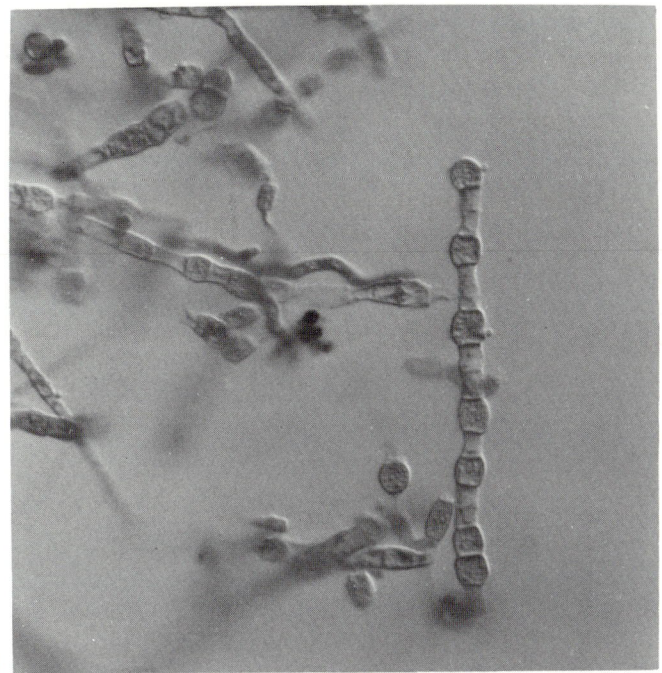

**Fig. 4.43** Continued

curved, cylindrical to fusiform, with rounded ends, 2- to 11-celled, and usually not in chains (Fig. 4.45). A *Fusarium* type foot cell is absent. Microphialoconidia may be present, which are hyaline, 1- to 2-celled, and forming either chains or balls. Chlamydospores and sporodochia may be either present or absent. The colonies are usually floccose and white to purple.

Comments: *Cylindrocarpon* (31) is similar to *Fusarium* and *Cylindrocladium* (28, 102). It can be distinguished from *Fusarium* by the absence of a foot cell at the base of the macrophialoconidia and by having rounded ends. It differs from *Cylindrocladium* by lacking a sterile appendage arising from the top of the conidiophore. The microphialoconidia of *Cylindrocarpon* are very similar to the conidia of *Acremonium*.

Species of *Cylindrocarpon* are mainly soil organisms and are infrequently recovered in the clinical laboratory. Because of their similarity to *Fusarium* and *Acremonium*, medical mycologists should always consider this genus when identifying isolates of *Fusarium* and *Acremonium*. The Ascomycetes *Nectria* and *Calonectria* may produce a *Cylindrocarpon* anamorph.

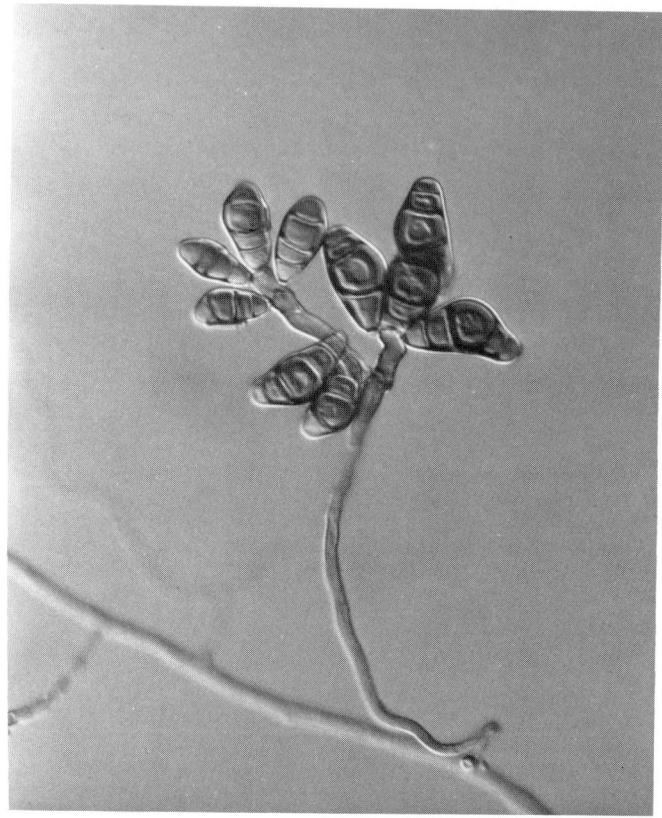

**Fig. 4.44** *Curvularia* sp. The conidia are curved, swollen in the central portion, multicelled, and with end cells that are paler in color than the central cells. The geniculate conidiophores are sympodial.

## *Drechslera* Ito, 1930

Diagnostic features: Species of *Drechslera* produce brown, simple or branched, geniculate, sympodial conidiophores. Through small channels in the conidiophore wall, darkly pigmented, cylindrical, multicelled poroconidia arise (Fig. 4.46).

Comments: The genus *Angiopoma* is an earlier name for *Drechslera*. Sutton (210) has proposed that *Drechslera* be conserved against *Angiopoma*. In anticipation that the generic name *Drechslera* will be conserved against *Angiopoma*, *Drechslera* is being used in this handbook. Shoemaker (199) has suggested that *Drechslera* should be divided into two genera, *Drechslera* and *Bipolaris*. *Bipolaris* in part may be a synonym of

Part 3  Taxonomy

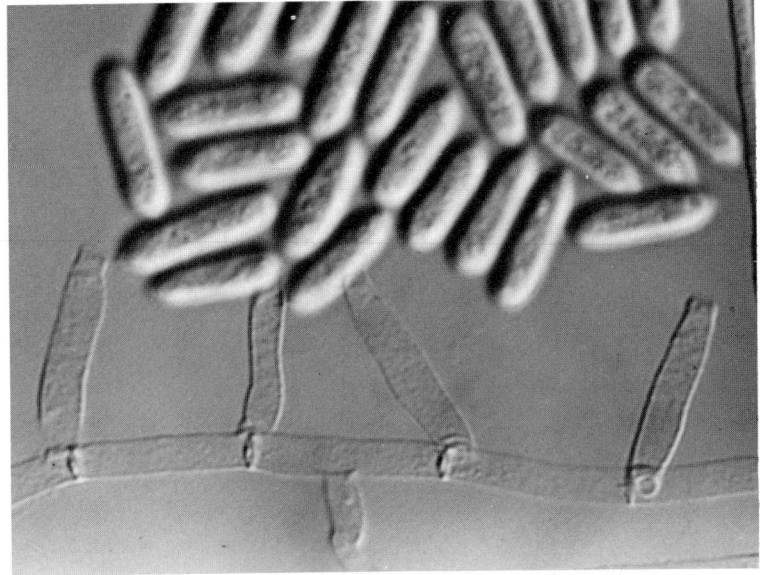

A

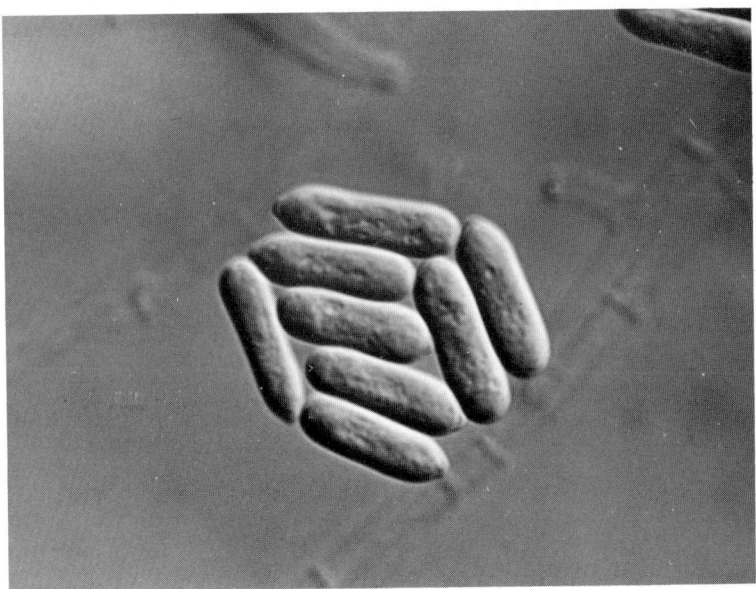

B

**Fig. 4.45** *Cylindrocarpon* sp. A and B. The phialides produce balls of phialoconidia. Unlike species of *Fusarium*, the conidia are rounded at their bases and do not have a foot cell.

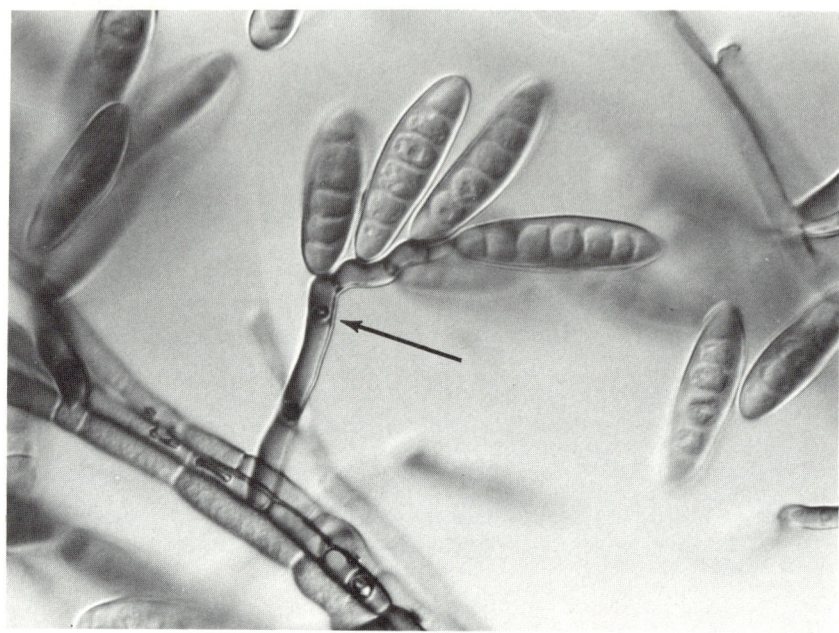

**Fig. 4.46** *Drechslera* sp. Each poroconidium arises through a channel (arrow) in the cell wall of the sympodial conidiophore.

*Curvularia*. *Drechslera* as defined by Shoemaker would contain those species that formed cylindrical poroconidia that could germinate from any cell, whereas isolates with fusoid conidia and only bipolar germination would be classified in *Bipolaris*. Until additional information is available, *Drechslera* will be used in this handbook to encompass all isolates with cylindrical to fusoid conidia, regardless of their method of germination. The confusion surrounding this concept is compounded because Luttrell (126) has suggested that *Cuspidosporium* and *Podosporiella* may be prior names for *Bipolaris*.

*Drechslera* is quite distinct from *Helminthosporium*, which forms determinate, nongeniculate conidiophores. These two genera are commonly confused in medical mycology, with isolates of *Drechslera* commonly misidentified as *Helminthosporium*.

*Drechslera* is frequently recovered in the clinical laboratory. Members of this genus are common soil organisms, and some species are plant pathogens. Isolates of *Drechslera* are most frequently associated with mycotic keratitis, and rarely phaeohyphomycosis. *Cochliobolus* and *Pyrenophora* species may form a *Drechslera* anamorph.

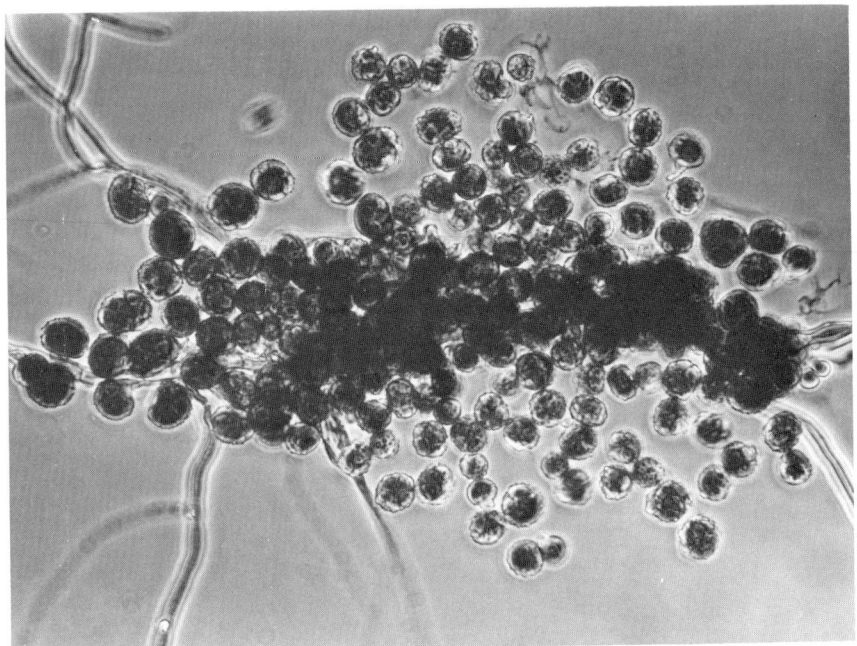

**Fig. 4.47** *Epicoccum nigrum.* The muriform, rough-walled conidia are forming on a sporodochium.

## *Epicoccum* Link ex Steudel, 1824

Diagnostic features: The genus *Epicoccum* is characterized by sporodochia, upon which short conidiophores produce dark brown, terminal, sometimes lateral, muriform, large (15–30 µm), rough, warty crusted, subglobose, holoblastic conidia (Fig. 4.47). The colonies are usually yellow to orange. The conidia may be released by rhexolytic or schizolytic processes.

Comments: Isolates of *Epicoccum* are occasionally recovered in the clinical laboratory. They are rapidly recognized by their yellow to orange colonies. This is a fairly common soil fungus. There appear to be two species within the genus (193).

## *Epidermophyton* Sabouraud, 1907

Diagnostic features: Members of the genus *Epidermophyton* form large, thick-walled, 3- to 5-celled, smooth, holothallic, club-shaped conidia that may be solitary or in clusters (Fig. 4.48). Older colonies typically contain numerous chlamydospores. Microconidia are absent.

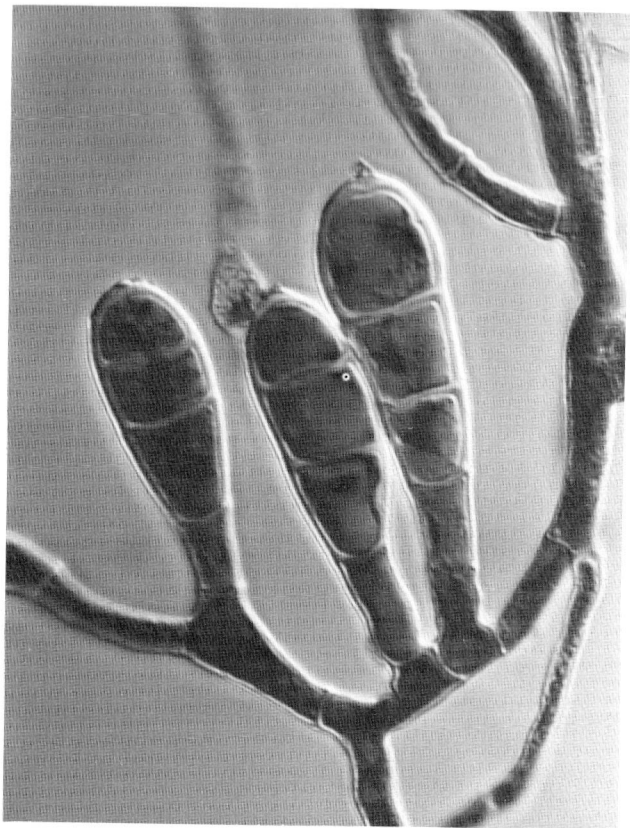

**Fig. 4.48** *Epidermophyton floccosum*. The large, thick-walled, smooth, clavate, several-celled conidia produced by this fungus may occur solitarily or in clusters.

Comments: *Epidermophyton* Sabouraud, 1907 is a homonym of *Epidermidophyton* Lang, 1879 and *Epidermophyton* Mégnin, 1881. Loeffler's (123a) proposal to conserve *Epidermophyton* Sabouraud against *Epidermidophyton* Lang and *Epidermophyton* Mégnin has been rejected by the Special Committee for Fungi and Lichens of the International Botanical Congress. A new conservation proposal is being submitted for consideration.

The genus *Epidermophyton* contains two species, *E. floccosum* and *E. stockdaleae*, which form large thallic conidia. During repeated subculture, most isolates begin to form large numbers of chlamydospores in lieu of the other conidia. *Epidermophyton floccosum* is a common cause of tinea cruris, tinea pedis and onychomycosis (172), whereas *E. stockdaleae* is known only from the soil.

## *Exophiala* Carmichael, 1966

Diagnostic features: The genus *Exophiala* is characterized by the development of cylindrical to lageniform, pale brown, terminal and integrated annellides. One- to several-celled, hyaline to brown annelloconidia form in a ball at the tip of each annellide. Most isolates produce yeast cells and toruloid hyphae.

Comments: Owing to their polymorphic nature, and the use of fungal morphology in tissue for classification purposes, a substantial amount of confusion and misunderstanding has surrounded many species of *Exophiala*. In the past, *Exophiala jeanselmei* (Fig. 4.49) has been considered a species of *Phialophora*, even though the fungus does not produce phialides. The fungus known as *Sporotrichum gougerotii*, in the sense of Borelli and many contemporary medical mycologists, represents a misidentification of *E. jeanselmei*. *Sporotrichum gougerotii*, in the original sense of Matruchot, was simply a morphological variant of *Sporothrix schenckii* that was more yeastlike than usual (144).

The fungus that Nielson and Conant described as *P. spinifera* is actually a species of *Exophiala*. De Hoog (97) considers *E. spinifera* to be a member of the genus *Rhinocladiella*. *Exophiala spinifera* (Fig. 4.50) forms annellides on distinct spinelike conidiophores (136); it cannot be classified in the genus *Rhinocladiella*, which is characterized by sympodial conidiogenous cells. In his monograph of *Exophiala*, de Hoog (97) considered *Wangiella dermatitidis* and *Cladosporium mansonii* to be species of *Exophiala*. These treatments are not accepted because *W. dermatitidis* forms distinctive phialides (137), and *C. mansonii* in the original sense of Castellani was proposed for the tissue form of *Malassezia furfur* (140). The fungus Castellani sent to the major culture collections as *C. mansonii* is actually a fungus he recovered from a different patient several years after the original name was proposed. The living culture of "*C. mansonii*" (Fig. 4.51) is a species of *Wangiella*.

The last species of medical interest is *E. werneckii* (Fig. 4.52), which was originally described as *C. werneckii*, an agent of tinea nigra. In her study of *Sarcinomyces crustaceus*, Hermanides-Nijhof (88) placed *E. werneckii* in synonymy with *S. crustaceus*. After studying the appropriate cultures and herbarium specimens, McGinnis showed that *S. crustaceus* (Fig. 4.53) and *E. werneckii* are entirely different fungi (140). *Exophiala werneckii* is considered to be the best name for this hyphomycete.

*Exophiala jeanselmei* is frequently recovered in the clinical laboratory. In many instances, it is recovered as a black yeast that could be identified as a species of *Phaeococcus*. Upon subculture to potato dextrose agar or cornmeal agar, its typical mycelial nature becomes evident. Other species

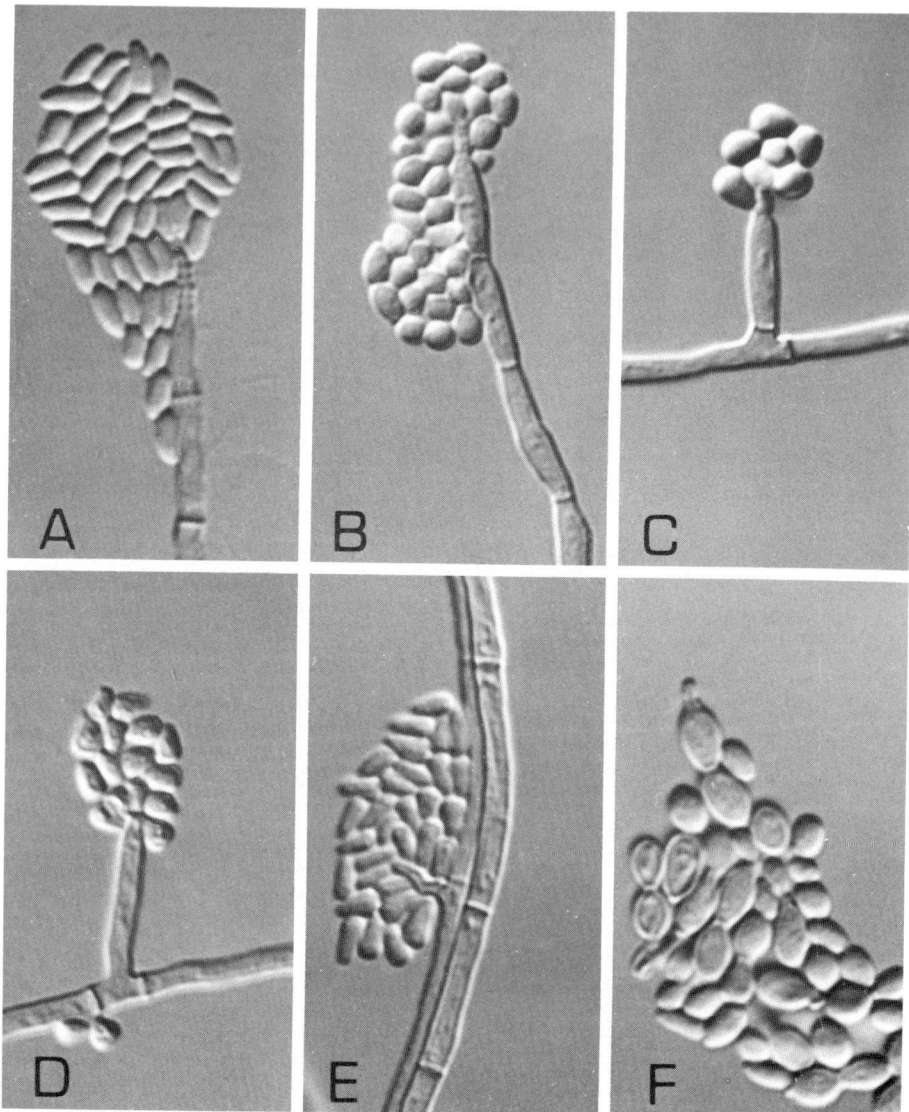

**Fig. 4.49** *Exophiala jeanselmei*. A-E. The one-celled annelloconidia accumulate in balls at the apices of erect and intercalary annellides. F. A yeast form is often present. (Reproduced by permission from *Mycopathologia* **65**:79–87, 1979.)

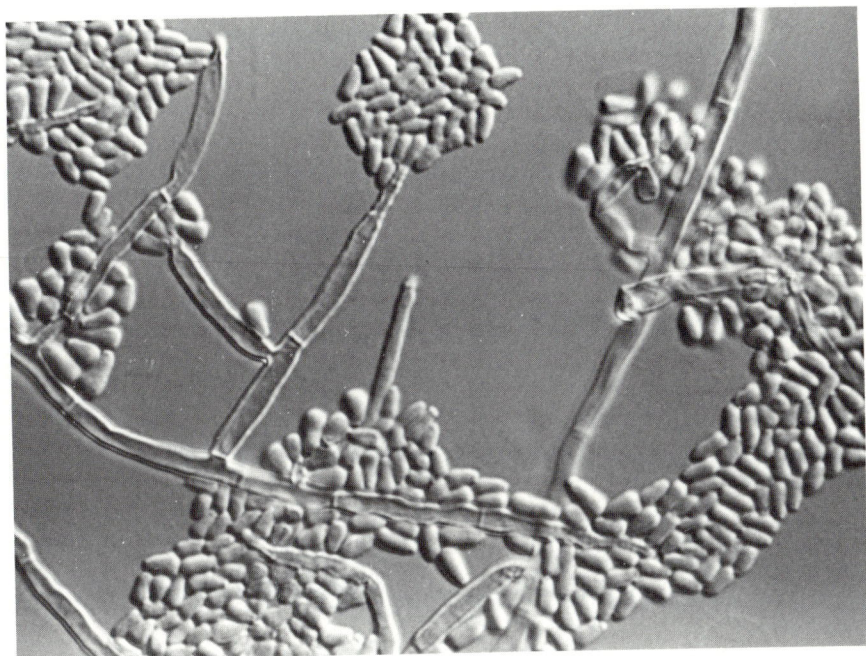

**Fig. 4.50** *Exophiala spinifera*. The annellides develop on spinelike conidiophores and produce annelloconidia that accumulate in balls.

of *Exophiala* are rarely encountered. Recently, *E. moniliae* was demonstrated to be the etiologic agent of phaeohyphomycosis in a patient in Australia. Thus, all species in the genus *Exophiala* have caused disease either in fish (44, 142), animals, or man at one time or another.

### Key to the Medically Important Species of Exophiala

1. Spinelike conidiophores present. . . . . . . . . . . . . . . . . . . . . . *E. spinifera*
1'. Spinelike conidiophores absent . . . . . . . . . . . . . . . . . . . . . . . . . . 2
    2. Annellides swollen (toruloid) with an elongate neck; annelloconidia are abundantly produced . . . . . . . . . . . . . . . . . . . . . . . . . . . . . *E. moniliae*
    2'. Not as above. . . . . . . . . . . . . . . . . . . . . . . . . . . . . . . . 3
3. Annellides reduced to yeast cells (usually 2-celled); hyphae and hyphae with intercalary annellides usually sparse . . . . . . . . . . . . . . . . . . . . . . . . *E. werneckii*
3'. Annellides cylindrical to lageniform; abundant hyphae; yeast cells 1-celled. . *E. jeanselmei*

### *Fonsecaea* Negroni, 1936

Diagnostic features: Members of the genus *Fonsecaea* may exhibit four basic forms of conidium development. *Fonsecaea* (157, 158) was originally

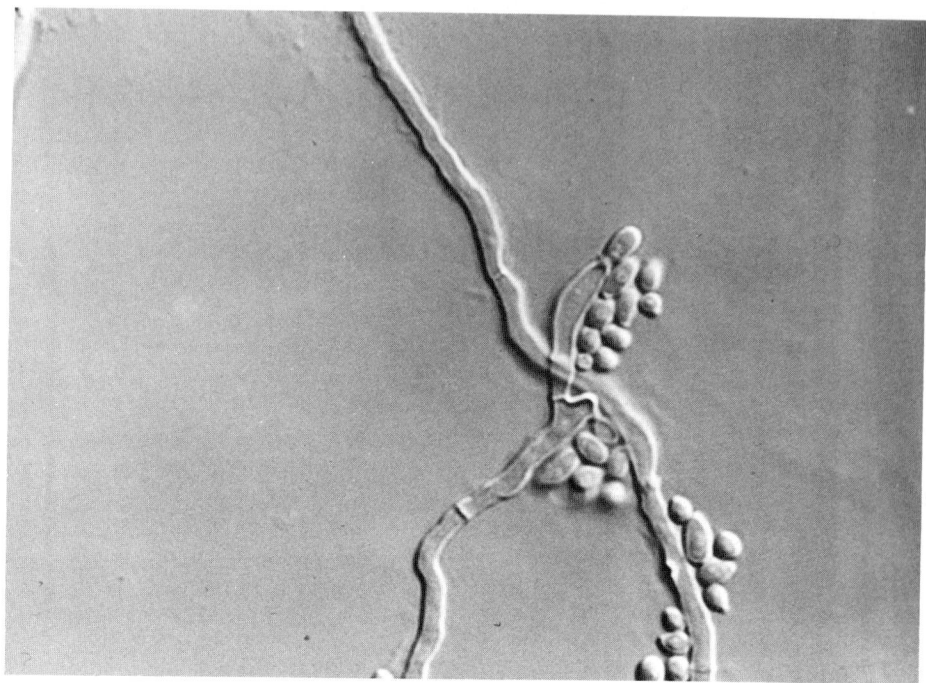

**Fig. 4.51** *Wangiella* sp. The phialide does not have a collarette. A ball of one-celled phialoconidia are at the apex of the phialide.

based upon dark, sympodial conidiophores with the conidiogenous zone confined to the upper portion of the conidiogenous cell as well as its morphology in tissue. From this region, 1-celled, pale brown, holoblastic conidia were formed on denticles. From these conidia, secondary 1-celled, pale brown, conidia may form in a sympodial manner on denticles that are confined to the upper portion of the primary conidium (Fig. 4.54). Some isolates produce dematiaceous, flask-shaped phialides with a distinct collarette. The 1-celled, pale brown phialoconidia produced by these phialides remain in a ball at the apex of the phialide (Fig. 4.54). A *Cladosporium* anamorph (Fig. 4.55) may also be present.

Comments: *Fonsecaea* presently contains two species, *F. pedrosoi* and *F. compacta*. Since the generic name *Fonsecaea* is feminine, *compacta* and not *compactum* is the correct spelling for this species epithet. At one time or another, these fungi have been placed in seven other genera. The two more common ones are *Rhinocladiella* (194) and *Phialophora* (67). The confusion surrounding *F. pedrosoi* and *F. compacta* has resulted from their polymorphic nature and disagreement among medical mycologists as to which characteristics should be used to identify them.

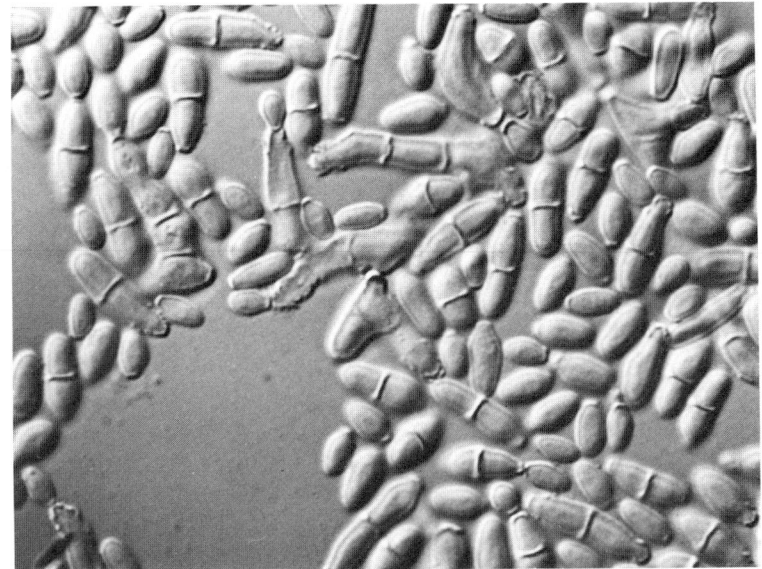

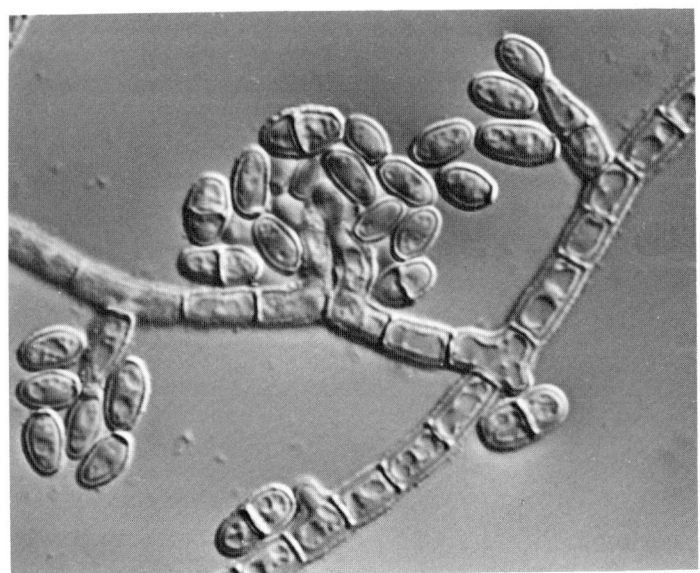

**Fig. 4.52** *Exophiala werneckii*. A and B. The annellides may either be yeast cells that are typically two-celled or they may arise from the hyphae. The annelloconidia are either one- or two-celled. (B reproduced by permission from *PAHO Scientific Publ. No.* 356, pp. 37–59, 1978.)

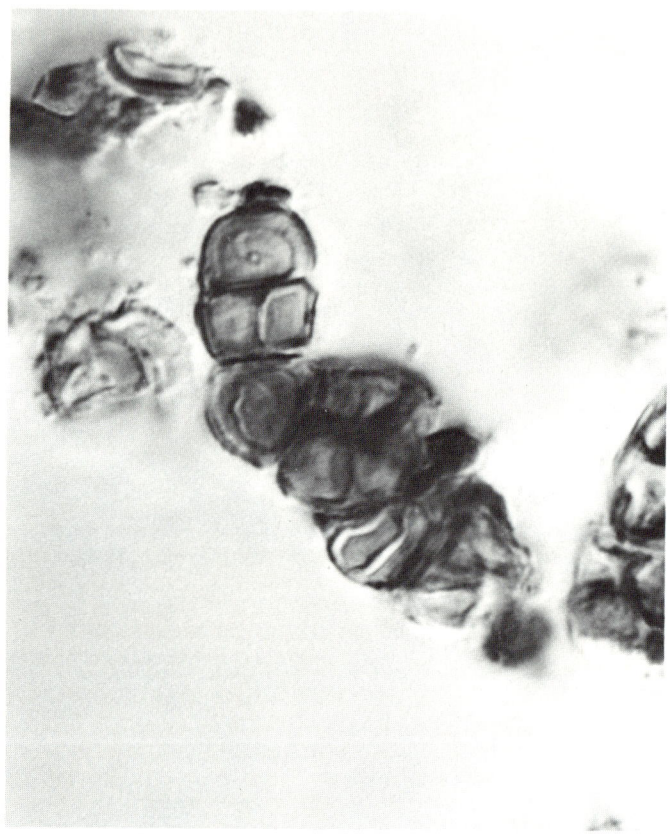

**Fig. 4.53** *Sarcinomyces crustaceus.* The vegetative form of this fungus consists mainly of muriform, dark cells.

The initial sympodial development of *Fonsecaea* is similar to that seen in *Rhinocladiella*. *Fonsecaea* differs in that the conidiogenous zone is confined to the upper portion of the conidiogenous cell and typically becomes slightly swollen, in an irregular manner, and the conidia in turn typically function as conidiogenous cells themselves, producing additional blastic conidia in a sympodial manner (48). When these additional conidia are present, the conidial head begins to resemble the genus *Cladosporium*. Some isolates of *Fonsecaea* may form phialides with collarettes that are typical of the genus *Phialophora*. The amount and proportion of these different modes of conidiogenesis varies from one isolate to the next. Since the sympodial development of the erect conidiphores, as well as the primary conidia functioning as sympodial conidiogenous cells is both

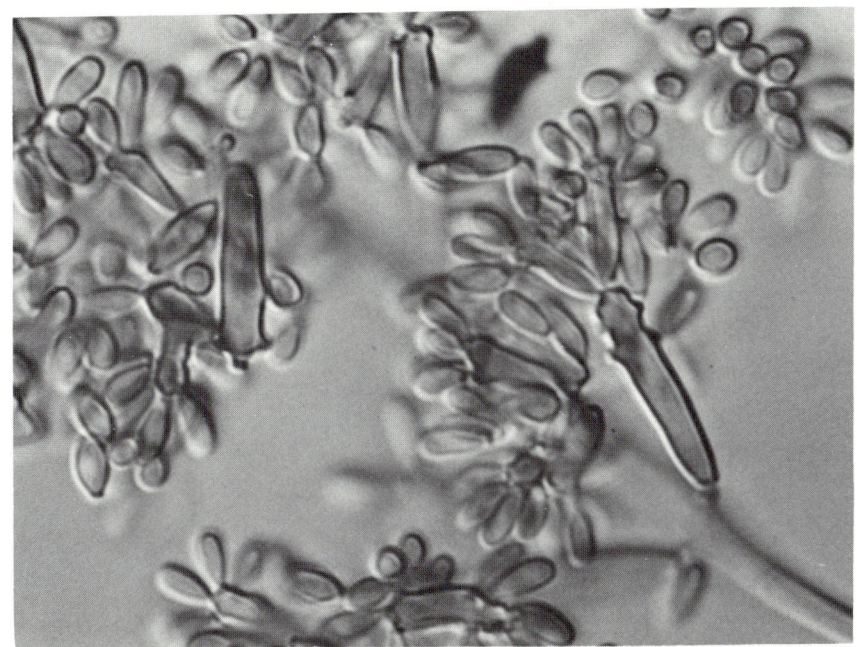

**Fig. 4.54** *Fonsecaea pedrosoi*. A. The primary conidia typically function as sympodial conidiogenous cells to produce secondary conidia. B. Phialides with collarettes and one-celled phialoconidia accumulating in balls are found in some isolates.

distinctive and stable, this mode of development should be used as the basis for defining the genus *Fonsecaea*. The *Cladosporium*-like and *Phialophora*-like types of development are best referred to as additional anamorphs of *Fonsecaea*. The expression *Acrotheca*-like has been applied in the past to the sympodial or *Rhinocladiella*-like form found in *Fonsecaea*. This is incorrect because *Acrotheca* is a synonym of *Ramularia*, a hyphomycete that is entirely different from *Fonsecaea*.

There is some debate whether or not *F. compacta* is a distinct species of *Fonsecaea*. This species is very rare and known only from a few collections (45). De Hoog has suggested (97) that its morphology is similar to that of species of *Xylohypha* (101), probably *X. curta*. *Xylohypha* and *F. compacta* are entirely different fungi. Without doubt, *F. compacta* should be classified in the genus *Fonsecaea*. *Fonsecaea pedrosoi* (Figs. 4.54 and 4.55) and *F. compacta* (Fig. 4.56) are readily distinguishable from each other by their loose conidial heads, prominent scars, elongated conidia, and by compact conidial heads, blunt scars, and subglobose to ovoid conidia,

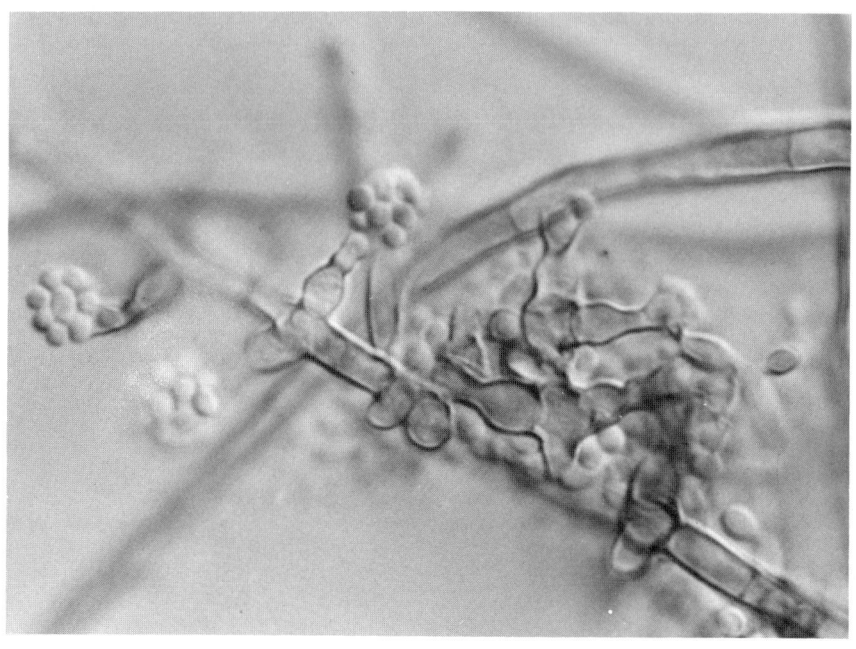

**Fig. 4.54** Continued

respectively. Isolates of *F. pedrosoi* are occasionally encountered in the clinical laboratory. Both species are soil fungi and *F. pedrosoi* is also associated with forest litter decomposition.

## *Fusarium* Link ex Gray, 1821

Diagnostic features: Species of *Fusarium* typically produce both macro- and microphialoconidia. The macrophialoconidia are hyaline, 2- to several-celled, cylindrical to curved (usually boat-shaped), and with a distinctive foot cell (Fig. 4.57). The conidia tend to form in balls and then slime down the tapering phialides, which are borne solitarily or as a component of a complex branching hyphal system. The microphialoconidia are 1- or 2-celled, small, hyaline, ovoid to cylindrical, catenulate or more commonly in balls. In some isolates, secondary blastoconidia may be formed from the phialoconidia. Chlamydospores may be present or absent. In culture, sporodochia are usually absent.

Comments: Many mycologists find isolates of *Fusarium* (32, 33, 107) difficult to identify. This is primarily owing to the variability of such characteristics as conidium size and shape, colony color, and the absence

## Part 3 Taxonomy

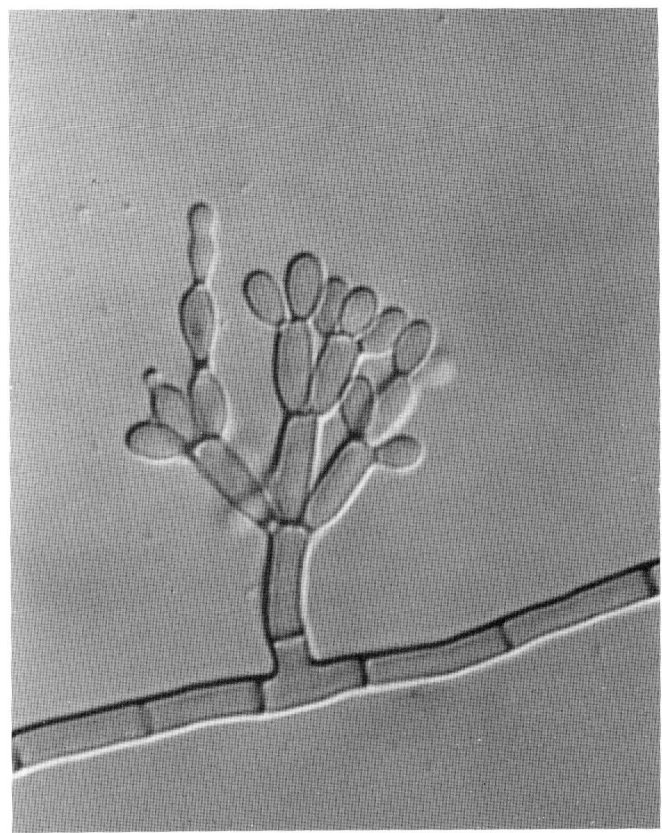

A

**Fig. 4.55** *Fonsecaea pedrosoi.* A and B. The chains of blastoconidia produced by most isolates are typical of those seen in the genus *Cladosporium.*

of macrophialoconidia in some isolates after several subcultures. The two key considerations in identifying a *Fusarium* are the need to start with a pure culture (single conidium or hyphal tip isolate) and to make all observations on a standard medium. Factors such as pH, carbon:nitrogen ratio in the medium, glucose concentration, $CO_2$ concentration, phosphates, and exposure to light affect the microscopic and macroscopic morphology. The various formulations of media used by Booth (32, 33) are recommended whenever one is identifying isolates of *Fusarium.*

Occasionally, infections are attributed to *F. roseum* and *F. episphaeria. Fusarium roseum* consists of several species of *Fusarium*, and therefore has no real meaning. Most mycologists feel that *F. episphaeria* represents two distinct species, one of which is *F. dimerum.* Occasionally, *Gibberella fujikuroi* is reported as a pathogen, which is the ascomycetous teleomorph

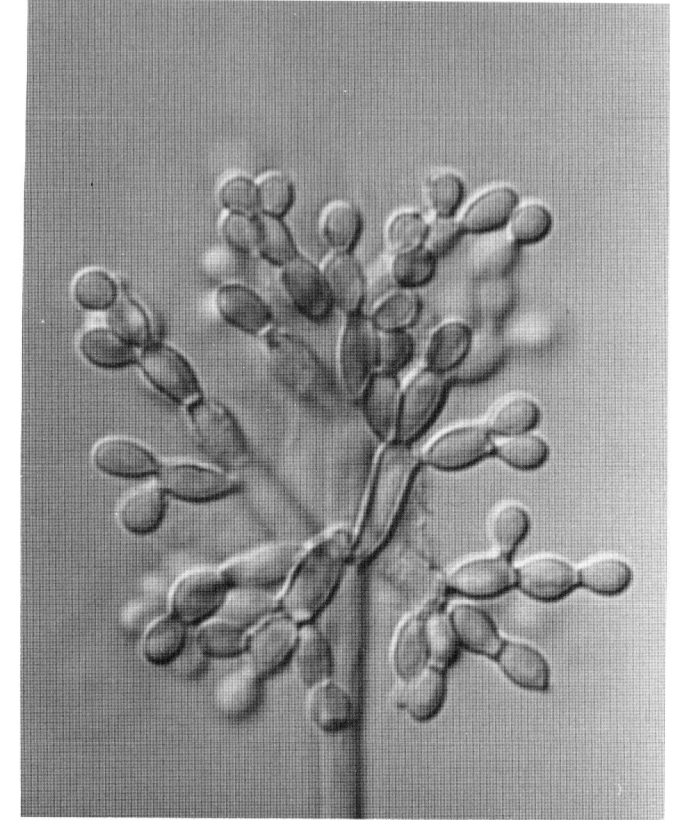

**Fig. 4.55** Continued

of *F. moniliforme*. Since the microconidia of *Fusarium* are essentially the same as *Acremonium*, isolates of *Fusarium* not producing macroconidia would probably be identified as species of *Acremonium*.

Isolates of *Fusarium* are often recovered in the clinical laboratory. The majority of these are *F. oxysporum*. Species of *Fusarium* may cause disease in man and animals, produce mycotoxins, and cause serious plant diseases. The Ascomycetes *Calonectria*, *Gibberella*, *Micronectriella*, and *Nectria* may form a *Fusarium* anamorph.

*Fusidium* Link ex Gray, 1821

Diagnostic features: *Fusidium* species form hyaline to pale brown, simple or branching chains of blastoconidia (Fig. 4.58). The conidia are 1-celled, fusoid to cylindric, with either truncate or rounded ends, and

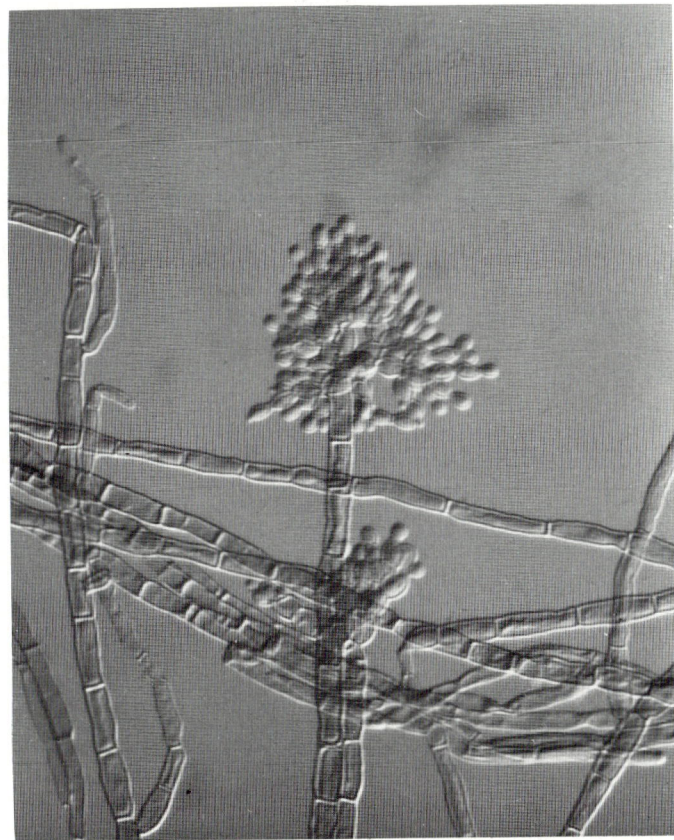

**Fig. 4.56** *Fonsecaea compacta*. A and B. The one-celled blastoconidia occur in compact heads.

develop from undifferentiated vegetative hyphae. Its mycelium is approximately the size of that produced by an aerobic actinomycete.

Comments: *Fusidium* (123) has been included in this handbook because of its resemblance to the aerobic actinomycetes. The occurrence of members of this genus in the clinical laboratory is unknown.

### *Geotrichum* Link ex Persoon, 1822

Diagnostic features: Species of *Geotrichum* produce chains of hyaline, smooth, 1-celled, subglobose to cylindrical, slimy arthroconidia from undifferentiated hyphae. The arthroconidia are released by separation at a double septum. Thus, they are fission arthroconidia (Fig. 4.59). Blas-

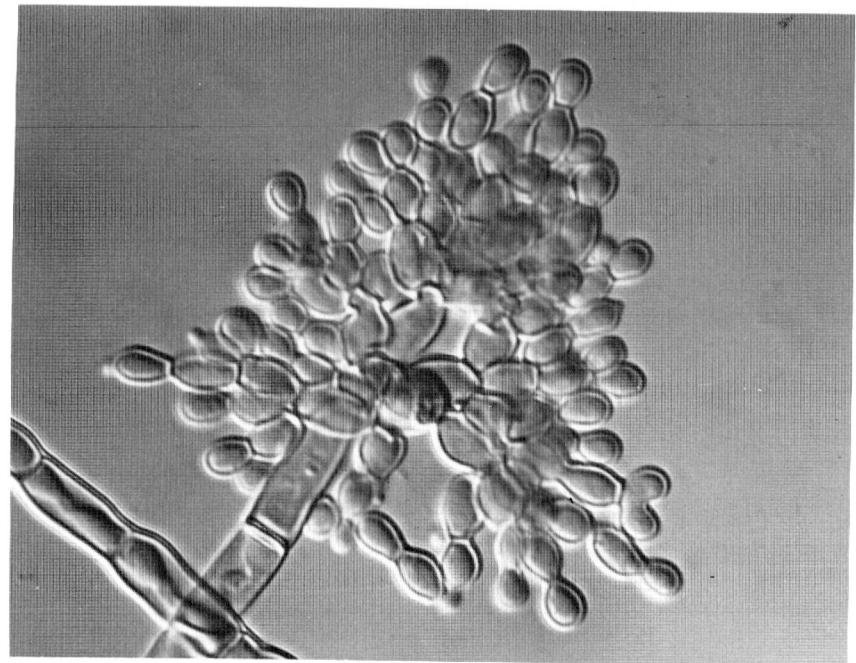

**Fig. 4.56** Continued

toconidia are absent. The various species of *Geotrichum* are differentiated from each other with biochemical data (78).

Comments: The genus *Geotrichum* (14, 78, 148), and more specifically *G. candidum*, has become a collecting point for almost any hyaline fungus producing arthroconidia (42). Sigler and Carmichael (200) have recently redefined *Geotrichum* and a number of similar genera. Their excellent monograph of *Malbranchea* should be consulted for additional details. Von Arx *et al.* (15) have modified the concept of *Geotrichum* by accepting species in the genus that occasionally produce a few blastoconidia. Weijman (218) believes *Geotrichum* must be restricted to fungi with ascomycetous affinities and *Dipodascus* teleomorphs.

In the past, species of *Geotrichum* were commonly referred to as *Oidium*, *Oospora* and a number of other generic names. *Oidium* (94) is restricted for the anamorph of *Erysiphe* and similar genera. *Oospora* was used for species in several different genera besides *Geotrichum*. *Oospora* is a *nomen illegitimum* because one of those previous genera should have been retained for this fungus (100).

*Geotrichum* is frequently recovered in the clinical laboratory. Care must be exercised in deciding whether it has a role in the disease process. The

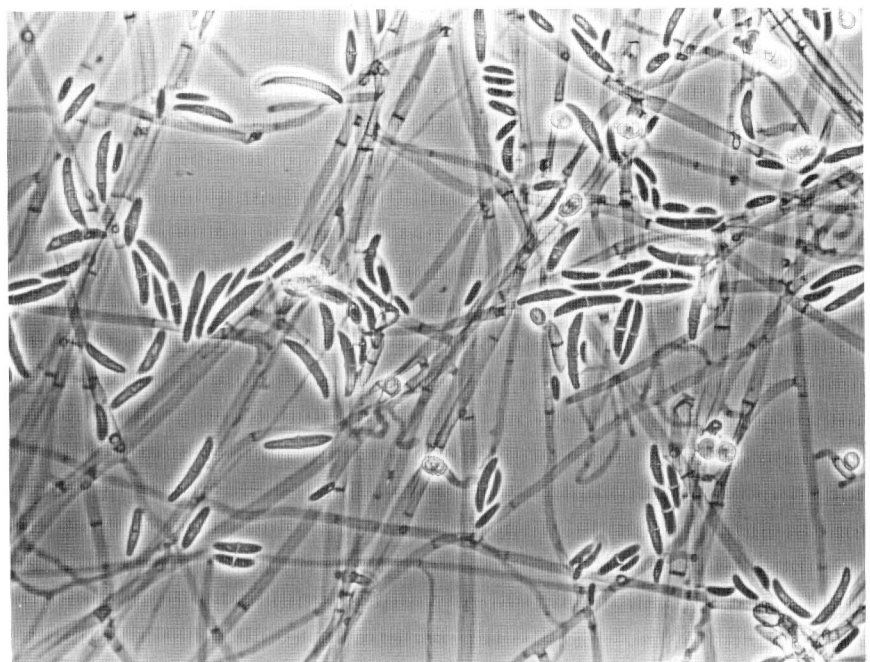

**Fig. 4.57** *Fusarium solani*. The macrophialoconidia are curved, multicelled, and have a distinctive foot cell. The microphialoconidia are one-celled and are typical of those seen in the genus *Acremonium*. Chlamydospores are usually produced, too.

presence of *Geotrichum* in large quantities, especially in sputum, may simply reflect a diet rich in dairy products, not pulmonary disease as occasionally reported in the literature. Members of this genus are also common soil organisms.

Great care must be exercised when identifying members of this genus. Many isolates being identified as *Geotrichum*, especially *G. candidum*, in clinical laboratories may actually be fungi such as *Arthrographis*, *Oidiodendron*, and others (200, 207). The Ascomycetes *Dipodascus* and *Endomyces* may form a *Geotrichum* anamorph (173).

### Key to *Geotrichum* and Some Similar Genera Producing Arthroconidia

1. Conidiophores, hyphae, or arthroconidia dematiaceous . . . . . . . . . . . . . . .
. . . . . . . . . . . . . . . . . . . . . . . . *Coremiella, Oidiodendron, Scytalidium*
1'. Arthroconidia hyaline . . . . . . . . . . . . . . . . . . . . . . . . . . . . . 2
    2. Arthroconidia and blastoconidia present . . . *Aciculoconidium, Moniliella, Trichosporon*
    2'. Arthroconidia only; blastoconidia absent . . . . . . . . . . . . . . . . . . 3

224                                                                                  **4  Mould Identification**

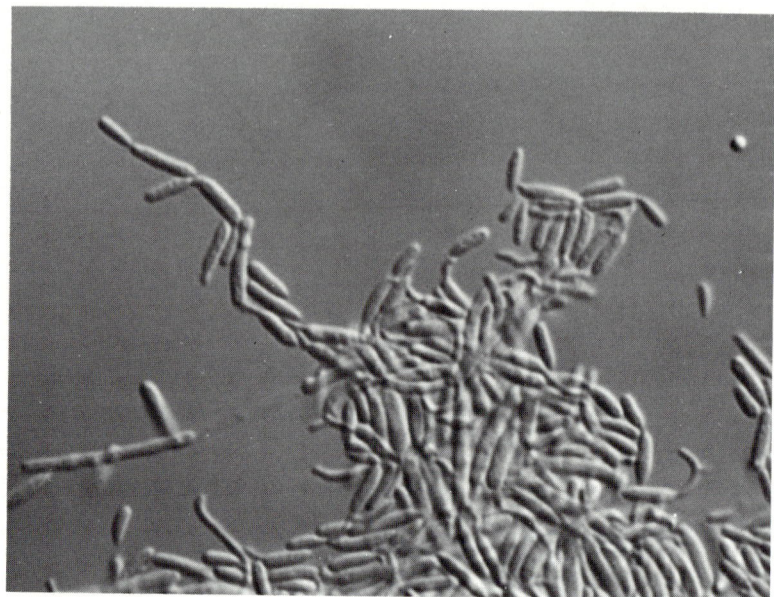

**Fig. 4.58** *Fusidium*. sp. Isolates of this genus form hyaline to pale brown chains of blastoconidia. The hyphae are approximately the same size as the filaments produced by the aerobic actinomycetes.

3. Distinct, differentiated conidiophores present. . . . *Arthrographis, Geomyces, Oidiodendron*
3'. Distinct, differentiated conidiophores absent . . . . . . . . . . . . . . . . . . . . 4
    4. Arthroconidia released by fission through double septa; annular frill absent
    . . . . . . . . . . . . . . . . . . . . . . . . . . . . . . . . . . . . *Geotrichum*
    4'. Arthroconidia released by disjunctor cells; annular frill usually present. . . . . . .
    . . . . . . . . . . . . . . . . *Coccidioides, Sporendonema, Malbranchea, Ovadendron*

## *Gliocladium* Corda, 1840

Diagnostic features: Members of the genus *Gliocladium* produce a very distinctive erect conidiophore that repeatedly branches toward its apex, forming a penicillus, with phialides arising at the apex of the branches. The hyaline to green, 1-celled, ovoid phialoconidia typically form as a large gloeoid ball at the top of the penicillus (Fig. 4.60). The conidia may also form as a loose column.

Comments: *Gliocladium* (17) is occasionally recovered in the clinical laboratory. Members of this genus are common soil fungi and are associated with the Ascomycetes such as *Hypocrea* and *Nectria*.

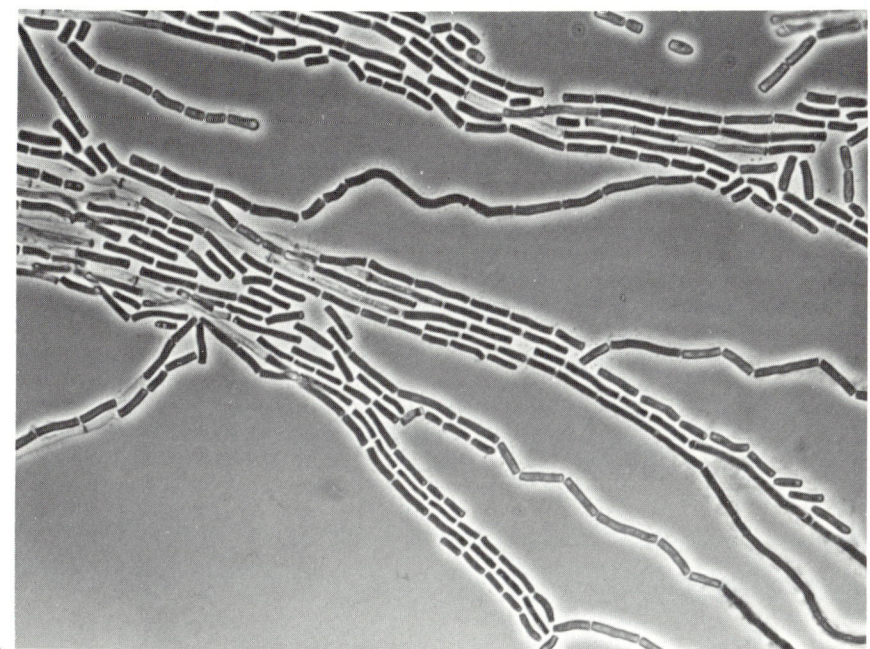

A

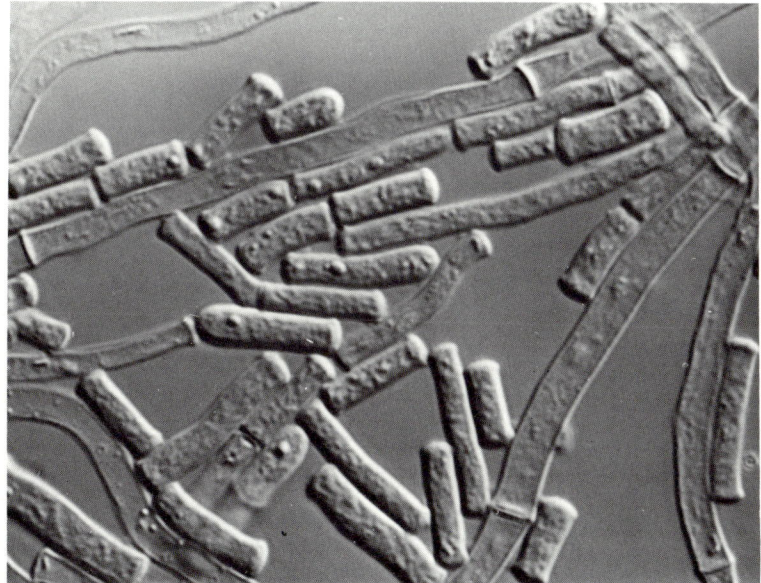

B

**Fig. 4.59** *Geotrichum candidum*. The fertile and vegetative hyphae are the same size. As the arthroconidia mature, they are separated from each other by fission through double septa.

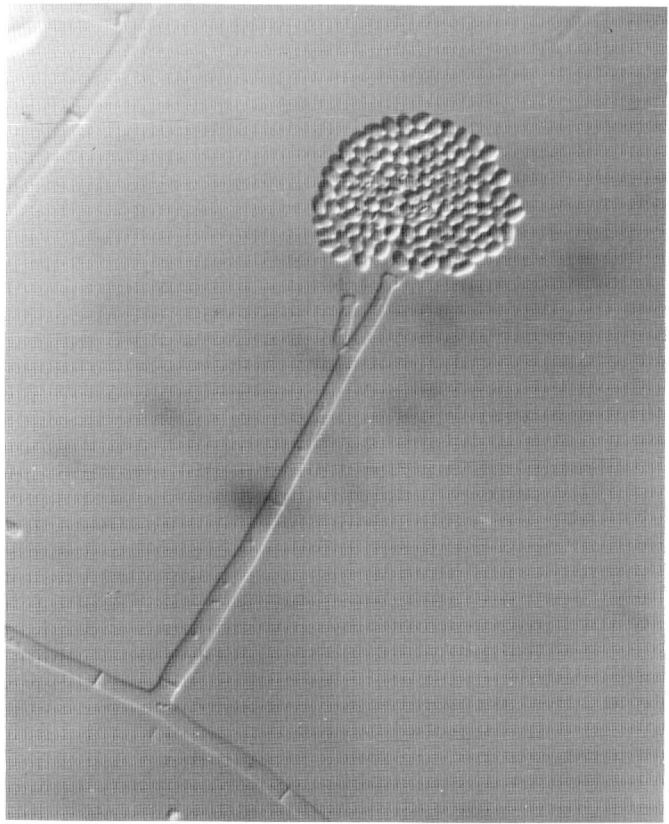

**Fig. 4.60** *Gliocladium* sp. The phialoconidia accumulate in a large, single, green ball at the apices of a cluster of phialides. The phialides are on a branched, erect conidiophore.

## *Gliomastix* Guéguen, 1905

Diagnostic features: Members of the genus *Gliomastix* form phialides that are cylindrical with a slightly swollen basal region that gradually tapers toward the apex. They are straight to slightly bent toward the apex, hyaline to slightly pigmented, and arise directly from the hyphae or on short conidiophores. The phialides are usually solitary, but may occur in groups. The phialoconidia are 1-celled, green to black, smooth to rough walled, globose to fusoid, forming as a ball or chain at the apex of the phialide (Fig. 4.61).

Comments: *Gliomastix* (58) is similar to *Acremonium*. Gams (72) considered the genus *Gliomastix* to be a synonym of *Acremonium*. This has not been accepted by most mycologists. *Gliomastix* is similar to several species included in *Acremonium* and *Sagrahamala*.

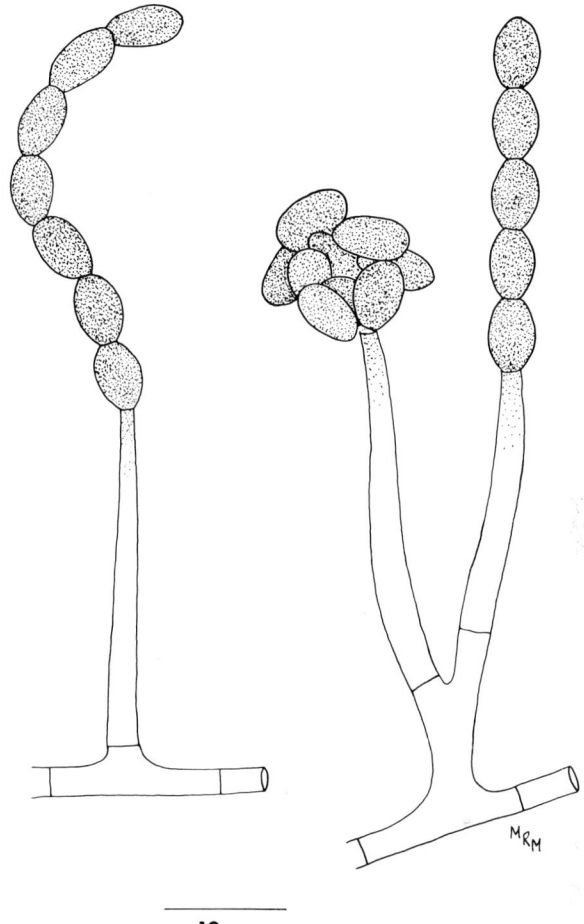

**Fig. 4.61** *Gliomastix murorum*. Dark colored phialoconidia, either in balls or chains arising from gradually tapering phialides, are characteristic of this genus and species.

Isolates of *Gliomastix* are occasionally recovered in the clinical laboratory even though they are mainly soil fungi.

*Graphium* Corda, 1837

Diagnostic features: The genus *Graphium* is characterized by synnemata (Fig. 4.62) that are dark, erect, solitary or in clusters, that become divergent at the apex. Hyaline, 1-celled, smooth, subglobose to ovoid conidia form a large, slimy ball at the apex of the synnema. The conidiogenous cells are annellides.

Comments: *Graphium* (149) is of interest to medical mycologists because it is one of the anamorphs of *Petriellidium* (Fig. 4.23) and *Petriella.* (Fig. 4.63). It is also associated with other Ascomycetes, such as *Ceratocystis. Graphium* is rarely encountered in the clinical laboratory. Species of *Graphium* are commonly found on wood plant material.

*Helminthosporium* Link ex Fries, 1821 *nom. cons.*

Diagnostic features: *Helminthosporium* species form determinate, parallel-walled, erect, brown to dark brown conidiophores. As the conidiophore increases in length, several-celled, obclavate, pale to dark brown poroconidia form laterally (often in verticils) in a basipetal manner (Fig. 4.64). Once the terminal conidium is formed, the conidiophore does not continue to increase in length. The poroconidia usually have a distinct brown to black protruding hilum.

Comments: The generic name *Helminthosporium* is commonly misapplied to isolates of *Drechslera* by some medical mycologists. *Helminthosporium* (62, 127) is relatively uncommon and probably is not isolated in clinical laboratories. *Helminthosporium* can be readily distinguished from

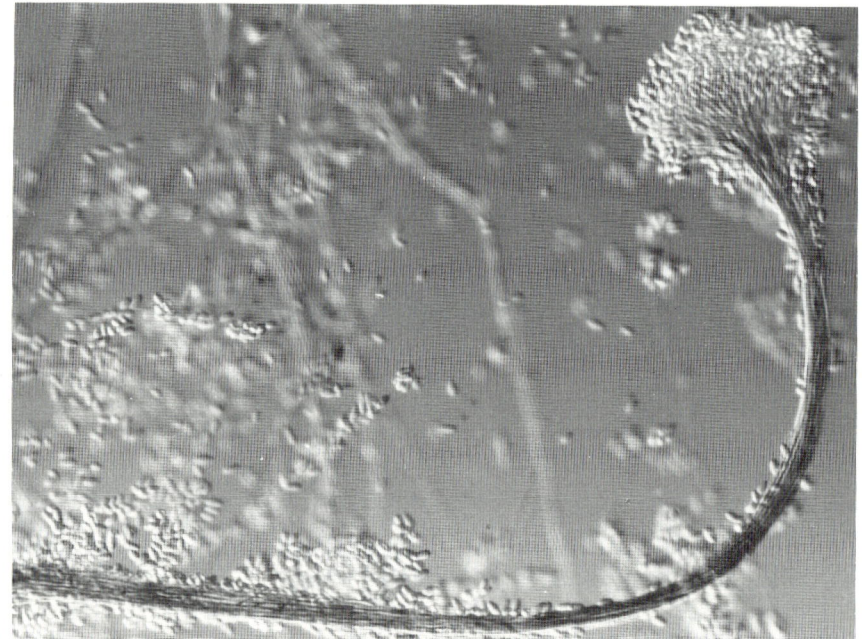

**Fig. 4.62** *Graphium* sp. A ball of conidia is formed at the apex of the synnema.

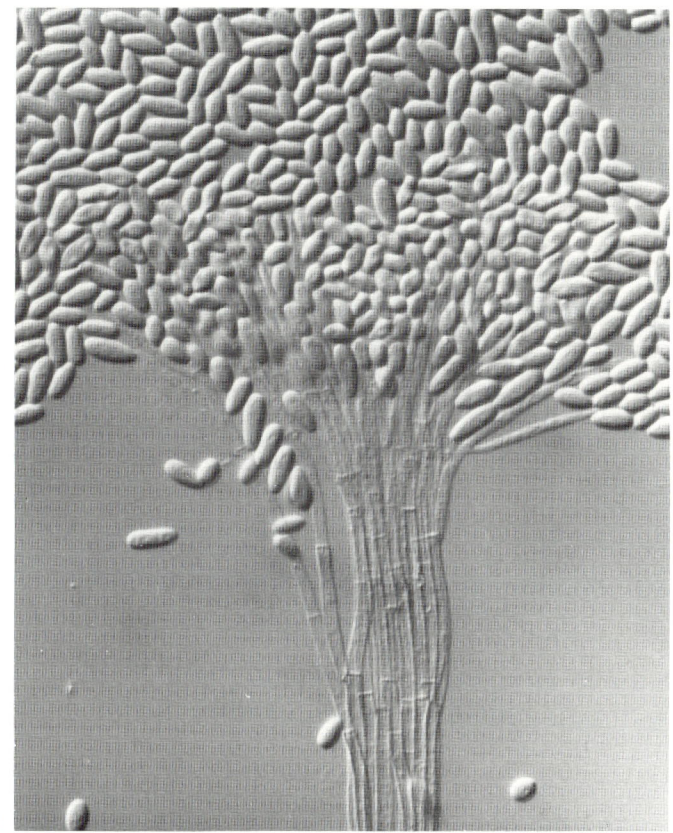

Fig. 4.62  Continued

*Drechslera* by its parallel-walled, determinate conidiophore that ceases growth when a terminal conidium is formed.

*Histoplasma* Darling, 1906

Diagnostic features: The genus *Histoplasma* is characterized by macro- and microconidia that develop from hyaline, short, narrow conidiophores arising at a 90° angle to the parent hyphae. The conidiophores rarely branch. The macroconidia are large, 8–14 μm, 1-celled, smooth to tuberculate, with fingerlike projections. The microconidia are hyaline, small, 2–4 μm, and smooth to echinulate. At 37°C on enriched media, *Histoplasma* will grow as a yeast (Fig. 4.65).

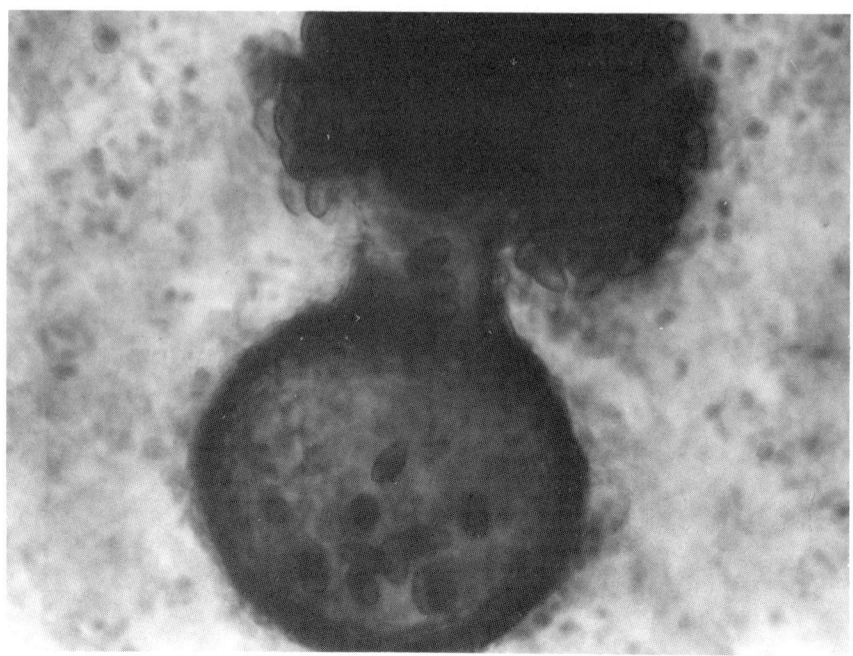

**Fig. 4.63** *Petriella* sp. The ascospores escape through an ostiole that is at the apex of the perithecium. Setae are near the ostiole.

Comments: The genus *Histoplasma* was proposed by Darling (55) for an intracellular parasite he considered to be a protozoan. The genus contains two species, *H. capsulatum* var. *capsulatum*, *H. capsulatum* var. *duboisii*, and *H. farciminosum*. *Histoplasma duboisii* is considered to be a variety of *H. capsulatum* because in culture they are identical, even though their yeast forms in tissue are of different sizes. *Histoplasma farciminosum* is maintained in the genus *Histoplasma* solely because it forms an intracellular yeast in tissue (horses and mules). In culture, it produces arthroconidia, blastoconidia, and chlamydospores. Thus, the generic concept of *Histoplasma* is based, in part, upon tissue morphology and pathogenicity.

In culture, *Histoplasma* most closely resembles species of *Sepedonium* and the *Chyrsosporium* anamorph of *Renispora flavissima*. The three genera are differentiated from each other on the basis that *Histoplasma* will convert from a mould form to a yeast form at 37°C on enriched media. The microconidia of *H. capsulatum* are morphologically similar to the conidia of *Blastomyces dermatitidis* and *Chrysosporium parvum*.

Mycoses caused by *H. capsulatum* var. *capsulatum* and *H. capsulatum* var. *duboisii* can be referred to as histoplasmosis capsulati and histoplas-

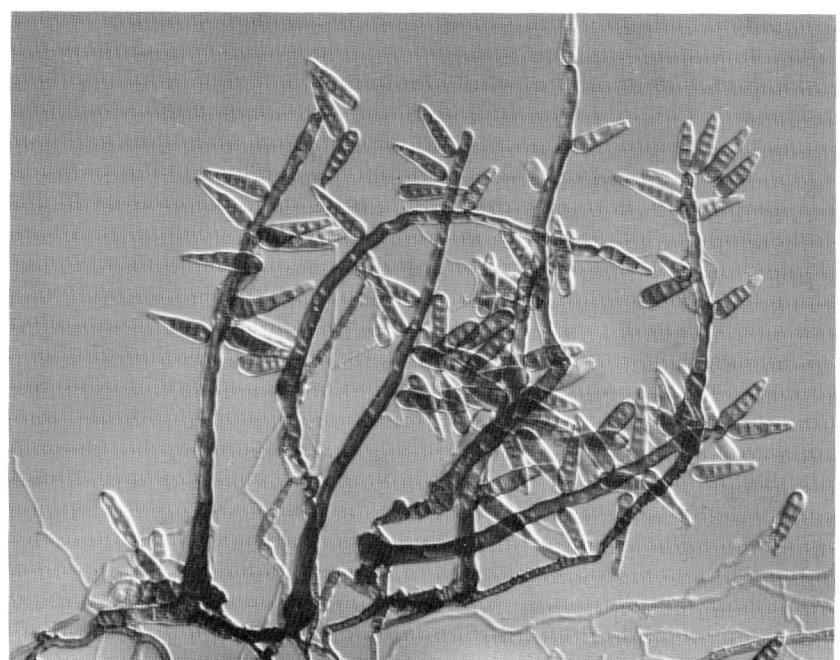

**Fig. 4.64** *Helminthosporium solani*. The erect conidiophores are determinate and have poroconidia along their sides.

mosis duboisii, respectively. These terms are comprehensive and clearly denote which etiologic agent is causing the disease. To be grammatically correct, capsulati and not capsulatum (neuter) should be attached to histoplasmosis (probably feminine).

The isolation of *H. capsulatum*, and its subsequent mould-to-yeast conversion is confirmation that the fungus is *H. capsulatum*. *Histoplasma capsulatum* normally occurs in soil or compost that is enriched with bird dung, especially dung from starlings and chickens. McGinnis and Katz (143) have transferred the ascomycetous teleomorph of *H. capsulatum* to the genus *Ajellomyces* as *A. capsulatus*. An exoantigen is available.

### *Humicola* Traaen, 1914

Diagnostic features: *Humicola* forms hyaline to dark hyphae with globose to ovoid, dark brown to black, solitary, 1-celled, smooth conidia (Fig. 4.66). The holoblastic conidia may occur in short chains arising from either the hyphae or short cylindrical to slightly inflated conidiophores. Chlamydospores, phialides, or both may be present.

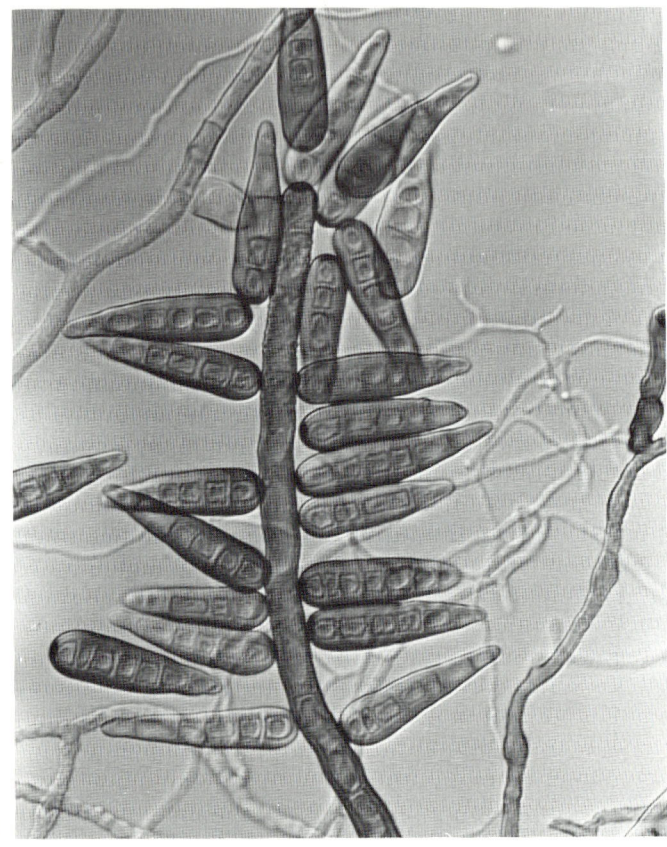

**Fig. 4.64** Continued

Comments: *Humicola* (23, 216, 220) is similar to the genera *Gilmaniella* and *Thermomyces*. *Gilmaniella* forms conidia in a cluster at the apex of the conidiogenous cell, whereas *Thermomyces* produces rough-walled conidia. *Thermomyces* and *Humicola* could be considered congeneric.

*Humicola* isolates are occasionally recovered in the clinical laboratory. This genus and *Gilmaniella*, are extremely common soil fungi. The phialides produced by some species of *Humicola* are similar to those formed by *Sagrahamala*.

*Madurella* Brumpt, 1905

Diagnostic features: The genus *Madurella* was based upon hard, black granules observed in several cases of mycetoma. An isolate is considered to

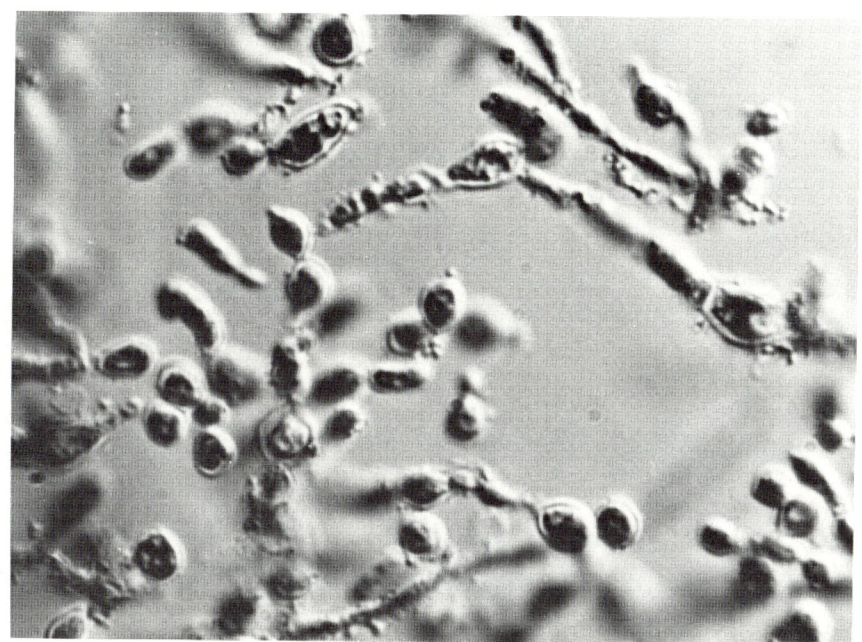

**Fig. 4.65** *Histoplasma capsulatum.* A. The yeast form develops at 37°C on special media such as cysteine–blood agar. B. At 25°C, the characteristic tuberculate macroconidia are formed on hyphalike conidiophores.

be a species of *Madurella* when it is isolated from a case of mycetoma with black granules and forms sterile colonies on mycological media.

Comments: Brumpt *et al.* (41) in 1901 described a case of black grain mycetoma. A year later, Laveran (122) studied their material and named the etiologic agent *Streptothrix mycetomatis* (as "*mycetomi*") without having cultures. Using material from a different case, Brumpt (40) proposed the genus *Madurella* in 1905 for this fungus. Like Laveran, Brumpt based his name upon the fungus in tissue. *Madurella mycetomatis* was first studied in culture in 1912 by Brault (38).

Two species are accepted by most medical mycologists, *M. mycetomatis* and *M. grisea*. The term mycetoma is a Greek word and its genitive in Latin becomes *mycetomatis*, not *mycetomi*. *Madurella mycetomatis* is distinguished from *M. grisea* (129) by its ability to grow at 37°C (30°C for *M. grisea*) and inability to assimilate sucrose as a sole carbon source.

The genus *Madurella* and especially *M. mycetomatis*, is in need of revision. The genus *Madurella* is a member of the Mycelia Sterilia, yet some isolates of *M. mycetomatis* are recovered that form phialides with

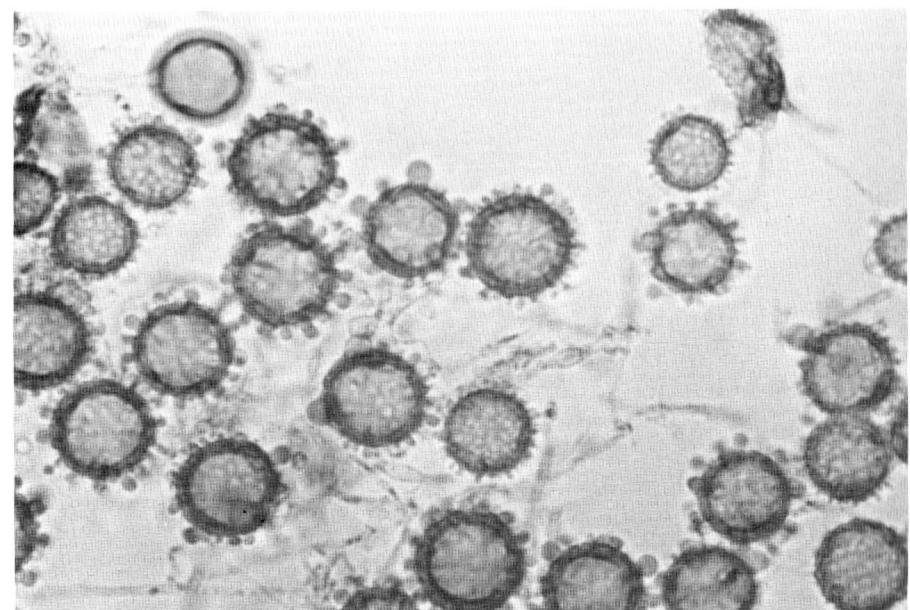

B

Fig. 4.65 Continued

collarettes (Fig. 4.67). The problem involves the use of tissue morphology for the identification of fungi in lieu of fungal morphology in culture. With our current definition of *Madurella*, this fungus is seen in the clinical laboratory only when it has been recovered from a case of mycetoma with black granules. *Madurella* may consist of a complex of soil organisms.

*Malbranchea* Saccardo, 1882

Diagnostic features: Members of the genus *Malbranchea* are characterized by the presence of hyaline, 1-celled, cylindrical, truncate, alternate arthroconidia (Fig. 4.68). Distinct conidiophores are absent. The fertile hyphae arise from the vegetative hyphae either as curved or straight branches that are 1.5–3.0 $\mu$m (no more than 4$\mu$m) wide. The arthroconidia are released by the lysis of the disjunctor cells. Arthroconidia may become yellow to greenish yellow at maturity.

Comments: The genus *Malbranchea* (200) has been overlooked by most mycologists. In the past, many isolates of *Malbranchea* were probably misidentified as species of *Chrysosporium*, or simply referred to as the arthroconidial form of various members of the Gymnoascaceae. Species of

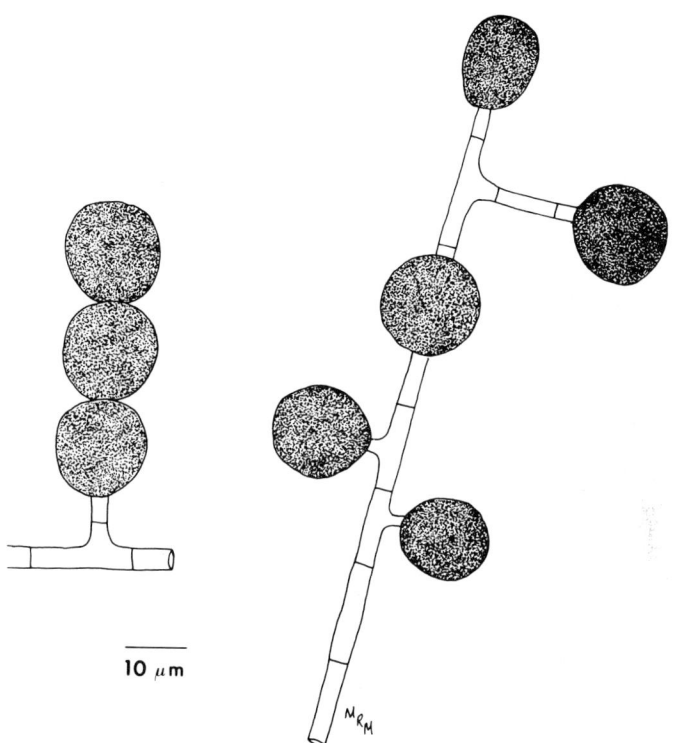

**Fig. 4.66** *Humicola grisea*. Dark colored, one-celled, globose, large conidia that may occur in short chains, solitarily, or intercalary are typical of the genus *Humicola*.

*Malbranchea* are similar to members of the genera *Coremiella*, *Sporendonema*, and *Ovadendron*. *Coremiella* is dematiaceous; *Ovadendron* forms swollen arthroconidia; and *Sporendonema* has wide hyphae and arthroconidia. *Scytalidium* forms dematiaceous fission arthroconidia in contrast to the alternate hyaline arthroconidia of *Malbranchea*.

Isolates of *Malbranchea* are occasionally recovered in the clinical laboratory. This group of fungi are soil organisms having a worldwide distribution. *Coccidioides immitis* is in essence a *Malbranchea*. The production of spherules on special mycological media at 37°C or in tissue, is diagnostic for *C. immitis*. Some species of *Auxarthron*, *Myxotrichum*, *Uncinocarpus* and related genera may form a *Malbranchea* anamorph.

### *Microsporum* Gruby, 1843

Diagnostic features: *Microsporum* species form macro- and microconidia on short conidiophores. The macroconidia are 2- to several-celled, spindle-shaped, hyaline, echinulate, with a thickened cell wall. An annular frill is usually present at the base of the conidia. Microconidia are 1-celled, hyaline, smooth, and clavate. The microconidia are not distinctive for any one particular species.

Comments: *Microsporum canis* (Fig. 4.69) and *M. gypseum* (Fig. 4.70) are two commonly isolated species. At one time in the United States, *M. audouinii* (Fig. 4.71) was frequently isolated as the etiologic agent of tinea capitis, but it has now been replaced by *Trichophyton tonsurans*. Table 4.9 summarizes the major features of the more commonly encountered species of *Microsporum*. The data in Table 4.10 are modified from an approach Philpot (166) has taken in identifying some isolates with nutritional data. Even though a large number of isolates representing each species were not tested, the data are useful.

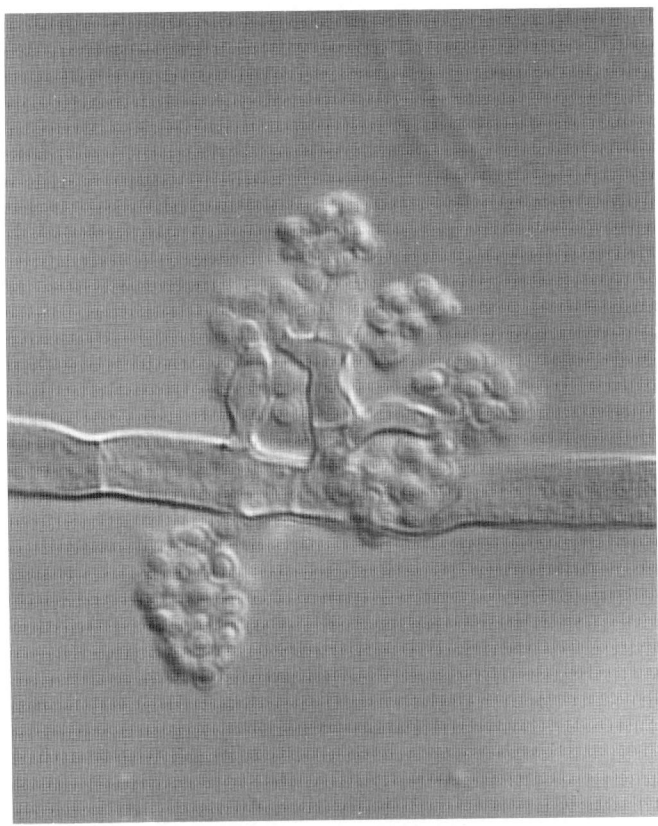

**Fig. 4.67** *Madurella mycetomatis*. On cornmeal agar, some isolates of *M. mycetomatis* produce phialides with collarettes (arrow) and one-celled phialoconidia that accumulate in balls.

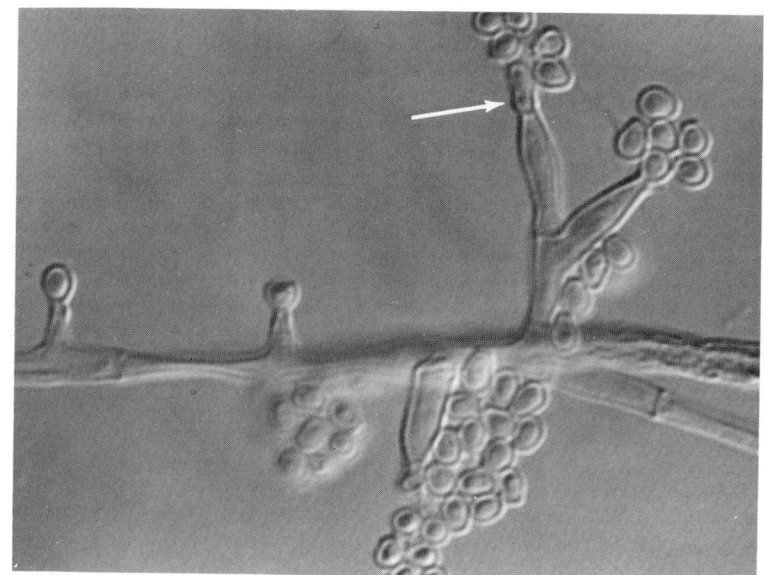

**Fig. 4.67** Continued

For those isolates of *M. canis* and *M. audouinii* that are not producing macroconidia, they should be transferred to sterile rice grains, and media for the enhancement of conidium production for the dermatophytes. On sterile rice grains *M. canis* rapidly grows and forms a bright yellow pigment. In the case of *M. audouinii*, a slight brown discoloration beneath the inoculum is usually observed with only a little growth, if any. In some instances, development of macroconidia may be stimulated in both species.

The macroconidia of *M. audouinii*, when formed, are extremely distinctive. They are similar to the distorted, twisted, multicelled echinulate macroconidia of *M. distortum*. In contrast, the macroconidia of *M. canis* and *M. gypseum* are spindle-shaped, but never distorted. Most isolates of *M. canis* produce macroconidia having 6 or more cells that have a thick cell wall, thin cross-walls, and a knoblike terminal beak. *Microsporum gypseum* forms macroconidia that are more spindle-shaped, with the cell and septal walls of approximately the same thickness. An apical beak is absent. The macroconidia of most isolates of *M. gypseum* have a very distinct taillike annular frill at their bases.

When conidia are absent, most isolates of *M. audouinii* on Sabouraud dextrose agar (4% glucose, with neopeptone) form a spreading, dense, off-white colony with a salmon to peach color under the central portion of the colony. Isolates of *M. audouinii* tend to form vesicles, some of which

## 4 Mould Identification

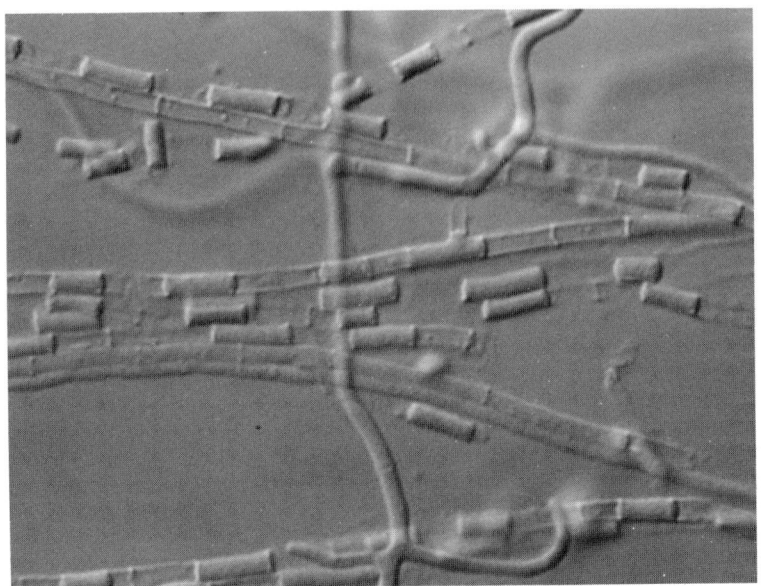

**Fig. 4.68** *Malbranchea albolutea.* The arthroconidia are separated from each other by disjunctor cells.

are terminal with a spinelike projection. These forms are helpful in making an identification, but they are not diagnostic. For more specific information concerning this species as well as other members of the genus *Microsporum* (2, 71), Rebell and Taplin's monograph (172) should be consulted.

Few dermatophytes are seen in most clinical laboratories because dermatologists traditionally do their own mycology. However, isolates of *Microsporum* are occasionally encountered. The ascomycetous genus *Nannizzia* is the teleomorph for members of the genus *Microsporum* that have been shown to reproduce by sexual means (Table 4.11).

*Monilia* Bonorden, 1851 nom. cons.

Diagnostic features: Isolates of *Monilia* are rapid growing. The conidiophores are hyphalike, variable, hyaline, erect to flat, and simple or branched. The blastoconidia are hyaline to subhyaline, catenulate, in branching chains, globose to ovoid, with a beadlike appearance (17) (Fig. 4.72)

Comments: The mould *Monilia* and the yeast *Candida* were originally confused by the early medical mycologists (see discussion of *Candida* in

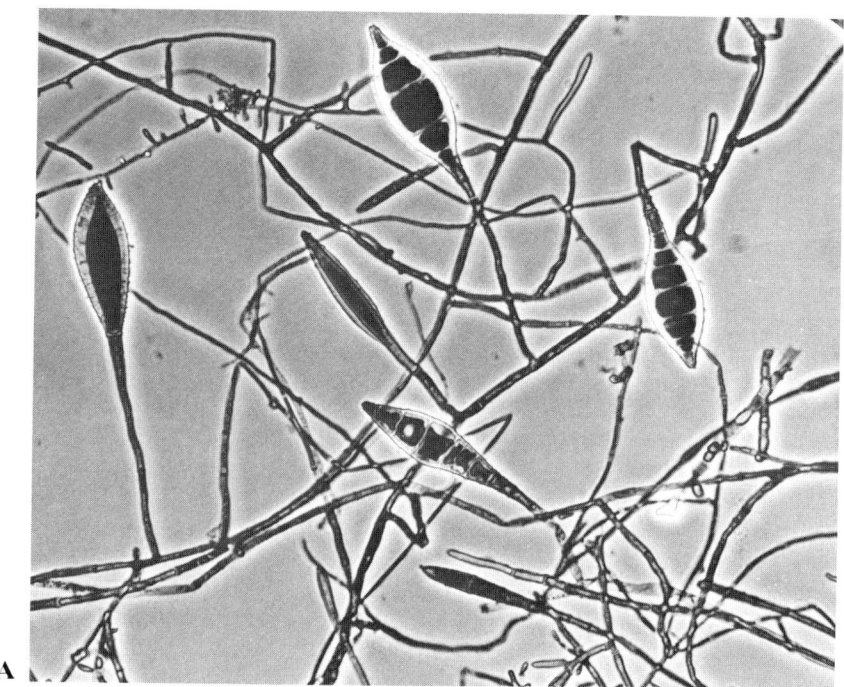

**Fig. 4.69** *Microsporum canis*. A and B. The macroconidia are spindle-shaped with rough walls. In this species, the cross walls of the macroconidia are thinner than the outer wall. The microconidia are not distinctive enough to be used for identification purposes.

Chapter 5). As a result of this confusion, many yeasts were incorrectly classified as species of *Monilia*.

*Monilia* is occasionally recovered in the clinical laboratory. It should be handled with care, since it has a tendency to become a laboratory contaminant. *Monilia* is the anamorph of *Monilinia* and *Neurospora*.

## *Monocillium* Saksena, 1955

Diagnostic features: In the genus *Monocillium*, phialides arise directly from the hyphae. They have a cylindrical basal stalk, a swollen middle region, and a tapering apex. The phialoconidia are hyaline, 1-celled, ellipsoidal to obovoid, truncate, and occur in fragile nonbranching chains (Fig. 4.73). The conidia may slime down to form balls.

Comments: The genera *Monocillium, Acremonium, Torulomyces,* and *Sagrahamala* are very similar. In fact, there is a natural transition from one genus to the next. Phialides arising directly from the vegetative hyphae with a swollen central to apical portion with a tapering apex that gives rise

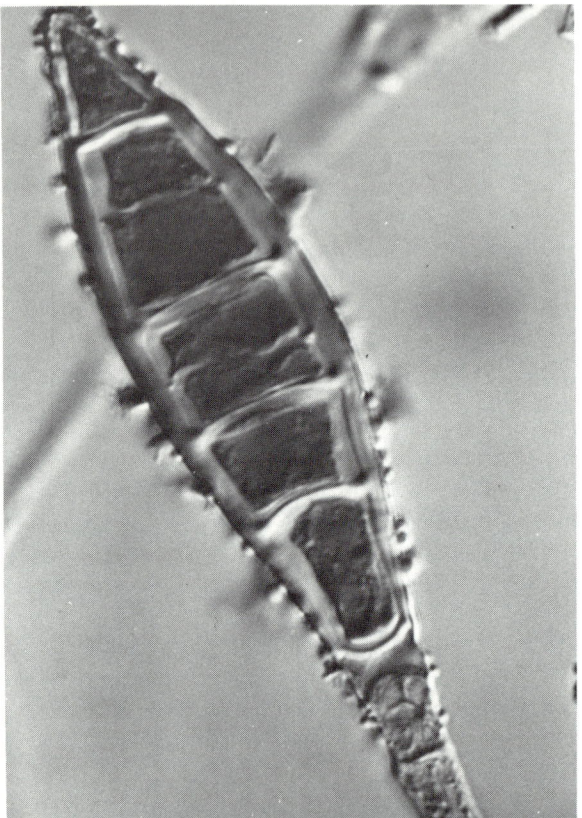

Fig. 4.69 Continued

to chains of phialoconidia distinguish *Monocillium* (181) from the other listed genera.

Isolates of *Monocillium* are occasionally recovered in the clinical laboratory. Members of this genus are soil fungi. *Monocillium* has been associated with the ascomycete *Niesslia*.

## *Mycocentrospora* Deighton, 1972

Diagnostic features: The genus *Mycocentrospora* is characterized by short, lateral, sympodial, simple, pale brown, septate, smooth conidiophores that have convex to flat conidial scars. The conidia are pale brown, straight, narrow, obclavate, smooth, and long with 5–26 cells (Fig. 4.74). There are no constrictions at the septa and a basal appendage may be present from the conidium.

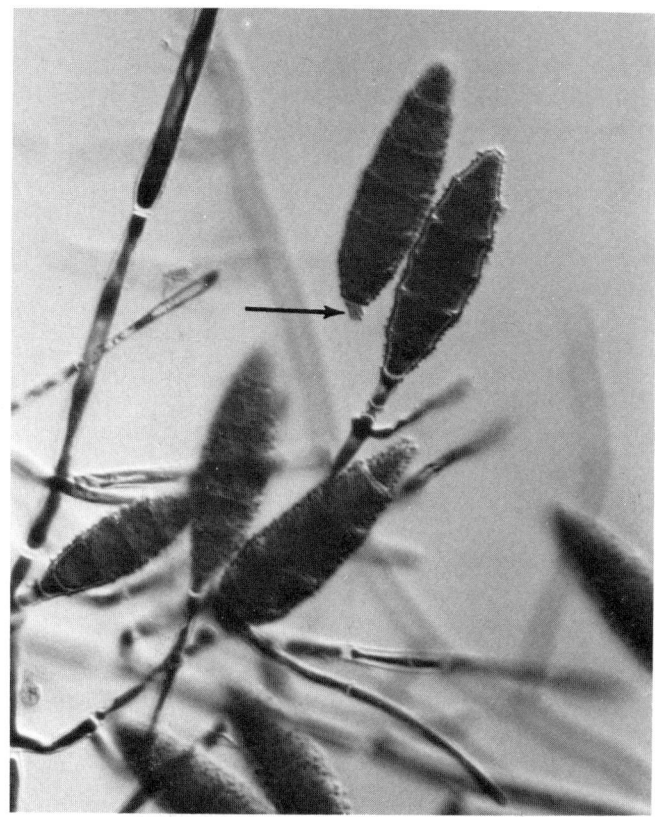

**Fig. 4.70** *Microsporum gypseum*. The cross walls and echinulated outer cell wall of the macroconidia are of the same thickness. The outer cell wall tends to collapse slightly between each of the septa. An annular frill (arrow) can be seen at the base of one conidium.

Comments: The genus *Mycocentrospora* is included in this handbook because of its close resemblance to *Cercospora* and the misidentification of *M. acerina* (56) by Emmons *et al.* as *C. apii* (69). *Mycocentrospora acerina* was shown to be the etiologic agent of a case of phaeohyphomycosis.

Isolates of *Mycocentrospora* are probably not encountered in the clinical laboratory. Members of this genus are associated with plants and soil.

### *Nigrospora* Zimmerman, 1902

Diagnostic features: *Nigrospora* species produce distinctive black, 1-celled, solitary, smooth, subglobose to ovoid, horizontally flattened holoblastic conidia that develop upon hyaline conidiophores. The co-

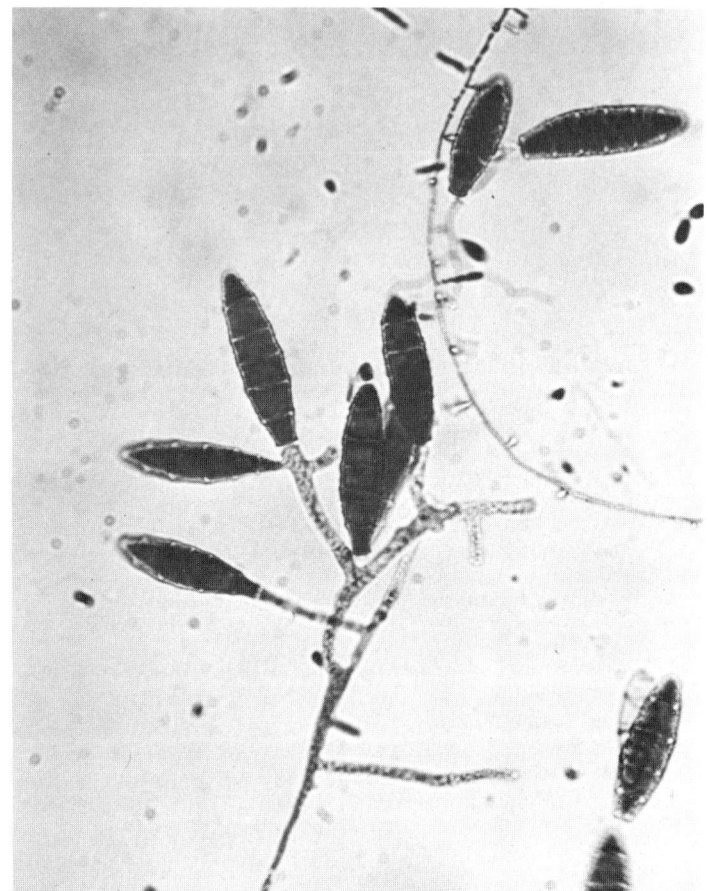

**Fig. 4.70** Continued

nidiophores arise at a 90° angle to the vegetative hyphae, may be determinate or percurrent, are swollen at the basal region, and taper to the point where the conidia are attached (Fig. 4.75). The vegetative hyphae are initially hyaline, but usually become darkly pigmented with age.

Comments: Isolates of *Nigrospora* are occasionally encountered in the clinical laboratory. Species of *Nigrospora* (64) are usually plant pathogens. The ascomycete *Khuskia* may form a *Nigrospora* anamorph.

*Oidiodendron* Robak, 1932

Diagnostic features: Members of the genus *Oidiodendron* typically produce narrow, erect, simple (occasionally branched), usually pigmented

Part 3  Taxonomy                                                                                           243

Table 4.9. Cultural Characteristics of Selected Species of *Microsporum* on Sabouraud Dextrose Agar[a]

| Species | Macroscopic | Microscopic |
|---|---|---|
| *M. audouinii* | Colonies slow growing, flat, velvety, slightly raised in center, white-tan to off brown. Reverse color absent or salmon to orange-tan | Mycelium usually sterile with numerous vesicles. Microconidia rare, clavate, smooth. Macroconidia when present large, irregularly spindle-shaped, thick-walled, smooth to echinulate. Abortive to bizarre macroconidia most common |
| *M. canis* | Colonies rapid growing, at first silky, white with bright yellow color in peripheral growth, later cottony, tan, occasionally with irregular tufts or concentric rings. Reverse color bright yellow, becoming dull orange-brown | Microconidia scarce, 1-celled, clavate, smooth. Macroconidia abundant, 8- to 15-celled, spindle-shaped, often with distinct terminal knob, walls thick and echinulate. Walls of septa thin |
| *M. distortum* | Colonies rapid growing, flat with a tendency to form radial grooves, velvety to cottony, white to tan. Some isolates appear waxy. Reverse color colorless to dull yellow-tan | Microconidia pyriform, 1-celled, smooth. Macroconidia numerous, thick-walled, echinulate, several celled, distorted |
| *M. ferrugineum* | Colonies slow growing, glabrous with numerous small folds, yellow to | Micro- and macroconidia absent or extremely rare. Macroconidia when present, similar to *M. canis* |

*continued*

conidiophores that repeatedly branch at their apices to form a delicate head of fertile hyphae. Erect conidiophores may be absent or reduced in length. The fertile hyphae become 1-celled, smooth to rough, globose to cylindrical, hyaline to pigmented arthroconidia. As the arthroconidia separate via a double septum, a gelatinous appearing connection remains between each arthroconidium. The connection is actually conidial cell wall that resulted from polar growth of the cells in the chain. The overall appearance of *Oidiodendron* is a repeatedly branching, erect conidiophore that is forming delicate chains of arthroconidia, each arthroconidium being separated by a connection (Fig. 4.76).

Comments: The connectives between the arthroconidia of *Oidiodendron*

**Table 4.9.** *Continued*

| Species | Macroscopic | Microscopic |
|---|---|---|
|  | deep rust color. Reverse color yellow or orange |  |
| *M. gypseum* | Colonies rapid growing, flat, granular, buff to deep cinnamon brown. Sterile white tufts rapidly developing. Reverse color yellow to tan, rarely pink to red | Microconidia usually rare, 1-celled, smooth. Macroconidia abundant, 3- to 9-celled, ellipsoidal, thin walls, echinulate. Septal and conidial walls approximately same thickness. Distinct annular frill present at base of macroconidia |
| *M. nanum* | Colonies rapid growing, flat, granular to cottony, white to cinnamon-tan. Reverse color orange, becoming brown-red to dark red | Microconidia pyriform, 1-celled, smooth. Macroconidia numerous, 1- to 3-celled, ovoid to elliptical, thin walls, echinulate |
| *M. vanbreuseghemii* | Colonies rapid growing, flat, granular to cottony, white, yellow to tan, or pink to deep rose. Reverse color absent to light yellow | Microconidia common, pyriform to obovate, 1-celled, smooth. Macroconidia numerous, 5- to 12-celled, cylindrical, thick, and echinulate |

[a] Reproduced and modified by permission of L. Ajello from "Laboratory Manual for Medical Mycology," USPHS, 1966.

distinguishes it from *Arthrographis*. *Geotrichum* forms fission arthroconidia, and *Malbranchea* and *Ovadendron* alternate arthroconidia. *Oidiodendron* is occasionally encountered in the clinical laboratory, but it is primarily a wood or soil organism (16). The anamorph *Oidiodendron* has been associated with some members of the Gymnoascaceae such as *Byssoascus* and *Myxotrichum*.

### *Paecilomyces* Bainier, 1907

Diagnostic features: Species of *Paecilomyces* typically form simple or branched, hyaline to pigmented conidiophores. The phialides, which are

**Table 4.10.** Nutritional Tests for the Identification of the More Common Species of *Microsporum*[a]

A. Assilimation of carbon compounds[b]

| Species | No. of isolates tested | L-Arabinose | Dextrin | Erythritol | D-Galactose | D-Glucitol | Glycerol | Maltose | Ribitol | Ribose | Sucrose | Trehalose |
|---|---|---|---|---|---|---|---|---|---|---|---|---|
| *M. audouinii* | 6 | 0 | 0 | 100 | 0 | 50 | 0 | 100 | 0 | 0 | 100 | 0 |
| *M. canis* | 9 | 0 | 0 | 100 | 0 | 67 | 0 | 100 | 0 | 0 | 100 | 89 |
| *M. cookei* | 4 | 0 | 25 | 100 | 0 | 50 | 0 | 0 | 25 | 0 | 0 | 100 |
| *M. equinum* | 4 | 0 | 100 | 100 | 0 | 0 | 0 | 0 | 0 | 0 | 100 | 100 |
| *M. ferrugineum* | 4 | 0 | 25 | 0 | 0 | 75 | 0 | 0 | 0 | 0 | 0 | 75 |
| *M. gypseum* | 6 | 0 | 0 | 50 | 100 | 100 | 0 | 100 | 0 | 0 | 100 | 50 |
| *M. persicolor* | 3 | 0 | 0 | 100 | 0 | 100 | 0 | 0 | 0 | 33 | 0 | 66 |

[a] Reproduced and modified by permission of C. Philpot from *Sabouraudia* 15:141-150, 1977.
[b] Values equal percentage positive of isolates tested.

B. Hydrolysis of urea[c]

| Species | No. of isolates tested | Days to become positive | | | | Negative |
|---|---|---|---|---|---|---|
| | | 0–7 | 8–10 | 11–14 | 14–21 | |
| *M. audouinii* | 11 | 0 | 27 | 27 | 18 | 27 |
| *M. canis* | 12 | 25 | 67 | 8 | 0 | 0 |
| *M. cookei* | 6 | 0 | 83 | 17 | 0 | 0 |
| *M. distortum* | 4 | 50 | 25 | 25 | 0 | 0 |
| *M. equinum* | 7 | 0 | 29 | 71 | 0 | 0 |
| *M. fulvum* | 7 | 57 | 29 | 14 | 0 | 0 |
| *M. gypseum* | 17 | 53 | 24 | 24 | 0 | 0 |
| *M. nanum* | 4 | 100 | 0 | 0 | 0 | 0 |
| *M. persicolor* | 24 | 13 | 29 | 54 | 4 | 0 |

[c] Values equal percentage positive of isolates tested.

**Table 4.11.** The Genus *Microsporum*

| Anamorph | Teleomorph |
|---|---|
| *M. amazonicum* | *Nannizzia borellii* |
| *M. audouinii* | Unknown |
| *M. boullardii* | Unknown |
| *M. canis* | *N. otae* |
| *M. cookei* | *N. cajetani* |
| *M. distortum* | Unknown |
| *M. equinum* | Unknown |
| *M. ferrugineum* | Unknown |
| *M. fulvum* | *N. fulva* |
| *M. gallinae* | Unknown |
| *M. gypseum* | *N. gypsea, N. incurvata* |
| *M. magellanicum* | Unknown |
| *M. nanum* | *N. obtusa* |
| *M. persicolor* | *N. persicolor* |
| *M. praecox* | Unknown |
| *M. racemosum* | *N. racemosa* |
| *M. ripariae* | Unknown |
| *M. vanbreuseghemii* | *N. grubyia* |

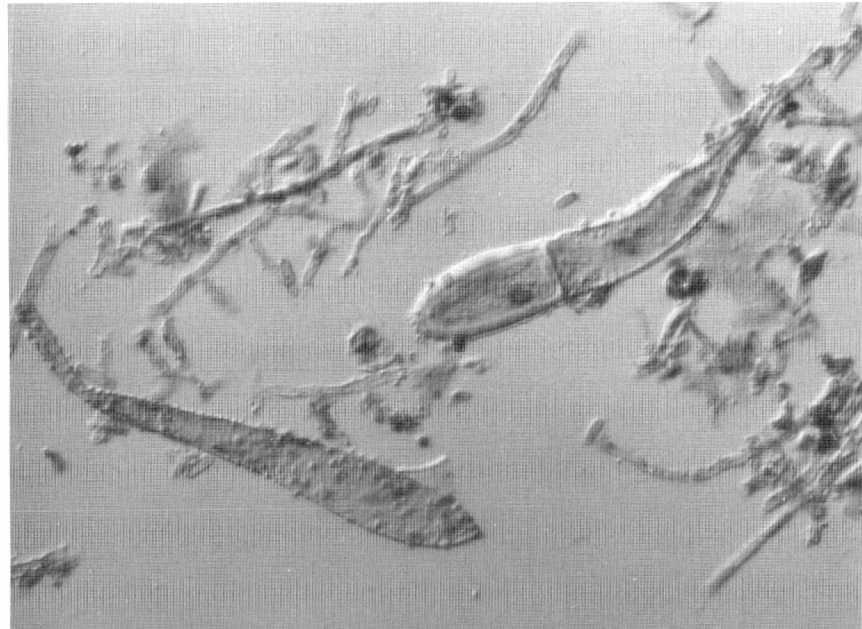

**Fig. 4.71** *Microsporum audouinii*. The echinulate macroconidia are irregular in shape and size. Macroconidia are infrequently seen in clinical isolates.

Part 3 Taxonomy 247

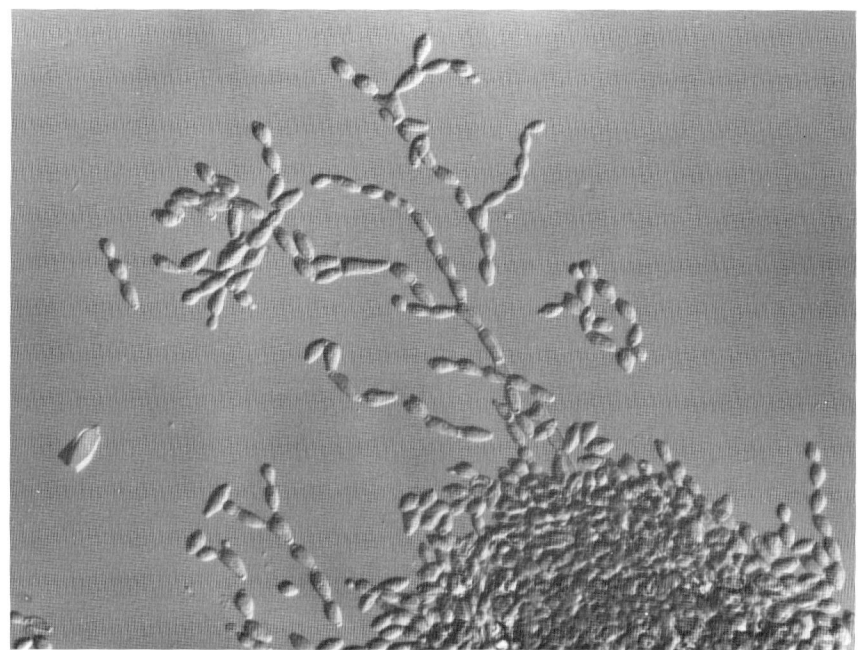

**Fig. 4.72** *Monilia sitophila.* A and B. Hyaline blastoconidia occurring in branching chains that readily break apart are characteristic of this fungus.

generally swollen at the basal region and gradually taper toward the apex, occur solitarily, in pairs, as verticils, and in penicillate heads. The phialoconidia are 1-celled, hyaline to dark, smooth or rough, ovoid to fusoid, and occur in long dry chains that do not branch, but tend to become entangled with each other (Fig. 4.77). The phialoconidia tend to slip slightly down upon each other in the chains.

Comments: The genus *Paecilomyces* (39, 184) is similar to the genera *Penicillium* and *Verticillium.* Basally swollen phialides that taper toward their apex, forming long chains of conidia that tend to slip slightly downward, readily distinguish *Paecilomyces* from *Penicillium* and *Verticillium.*

There is considerable controversy concerning the proper genus for the "monophialide species of *Paecilomyces.*" Onions and Barron (162) expanded the concept of *Paecilomyces* to include fungi that produced phialides and phialoconidia typical of the genus *Paecilomyces* directly from the vegetative hyphae or individually on short conidiophores. During his revision of the genus *Acremonium,* Gams (72) did not accept this concept, and transferred the monophialide species of *Paecilomyces* to the genus *Acremonium.* In his monograph on *Paecilomyces,* Samson (184) agreed with

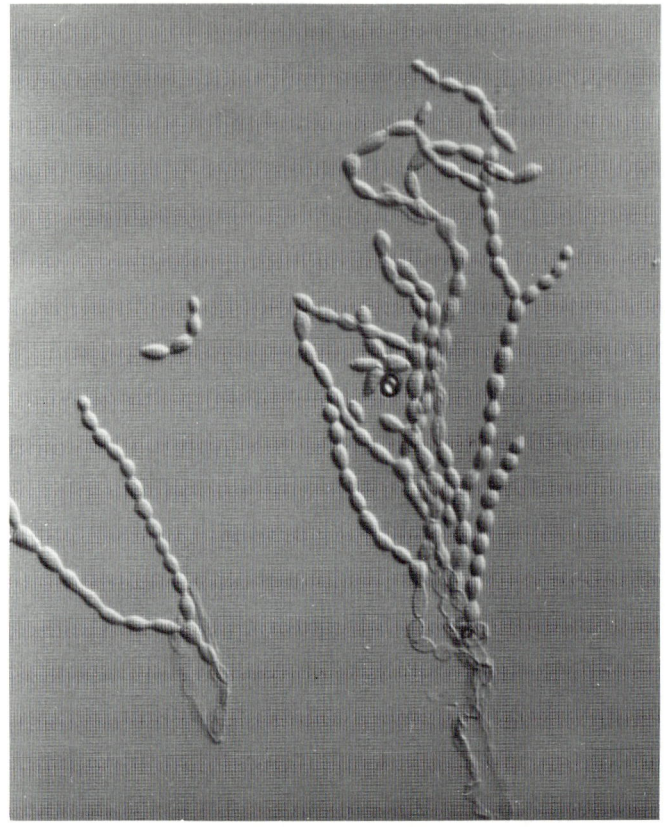

B

Fig. 4.72 Continued

Gams. While studying monophialidic hyphomycetes, Subramanian established a new genus, *Sagrahamala*, that included the monophialide species of *Paecilomyces*. Gams (73a) has recently rejected the genus *Sagrahamala* and established the new genus *Sagenomella* for these fungi. *Sagrahamala* (208) appears to be the best place for these fungi for the present.

Isolates of *Paecilomyces* are frequently isolated in the clinical laboratory. Species of *Paecilomyces* are common soil fungi and pathogens of insects. The Ascomycetes *Byssochlamys*, *Cephalotheca*, and *Thermoascus* may develop a *Paecilomyces* anamorph.

*Paracoccidioides* de Almeida, 1930

Diagnostic features: Isolates of *Paracoccidioides brasiliensis*, the only species in the genus, grow slowly and are typically sterile. Some isolates

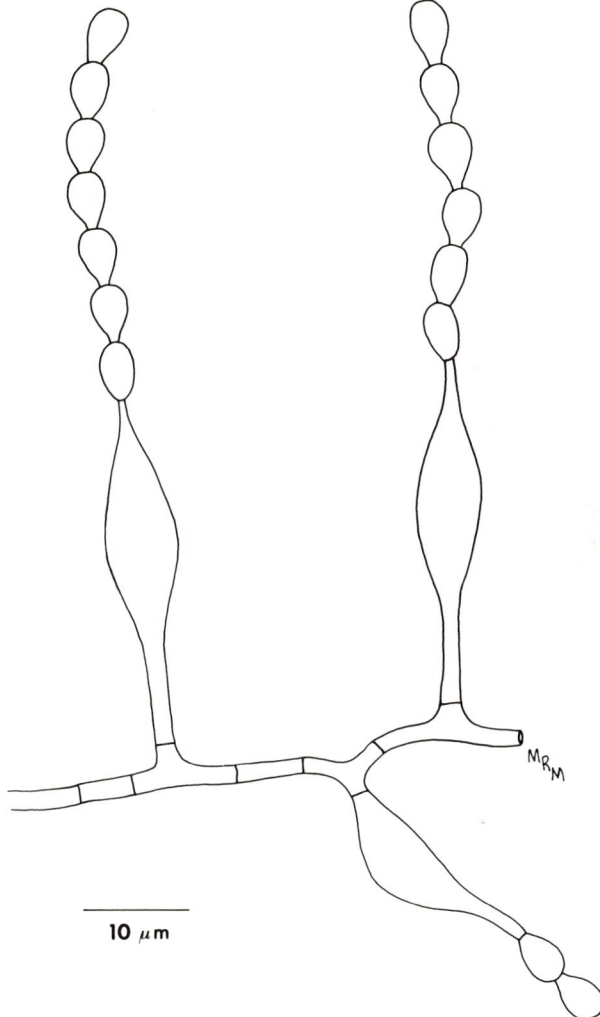

**Fig. 4.73** *Monocillium indicum*. The one-celled phialoconidia arise in chains from phialides that are swollen near their apices.

produce solitary conidia and arthroconidia that are similar to those found in *Chrysosporium*. The identification of *P. brasiliensis* is based upon the conversion of the mould form to the yeast form at 37°C on special media. The yeast form consists of globose cells with blastoconidia attached to the parent cell by a tubular denticle. The blastoconidia remain attached and in turn form secondary blastoconidia, which remain attached to their parent

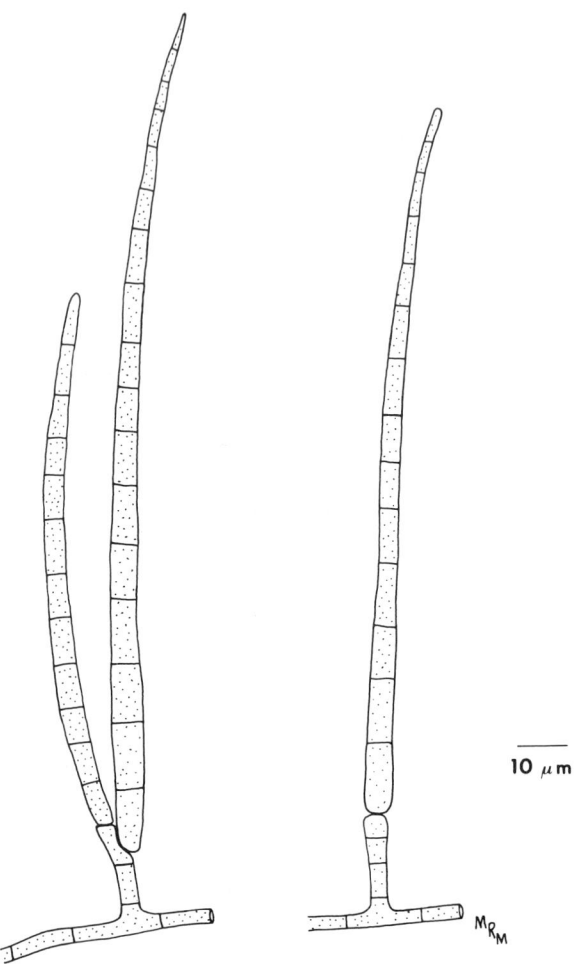

**Fig. 4.74** *Mycocentrospora acerina.* The conidia are long, several-celled, and arise from conidiophores that are sympodial in development.

cells. The process is repeated, resulting in "multiple" budding from each cell (Fig. 4.78).

Comments: *Paracoccidioides brasiliensis* was first isolated and studied in tissue by Lutz in 1908 (128), but he did not propose a name for the fungus. In 1912, Splendore (204) proposed the name *Zymonema brasiliense* and later de Almeida (7) established the genus *Paracoccidioides* for *P. brasiliensis*.

Occasional isolates of *P. brasiliensis* are found that produce conidia that are typical of *Chrysosporium*. The majority of isolates of *P. brasiliensis*

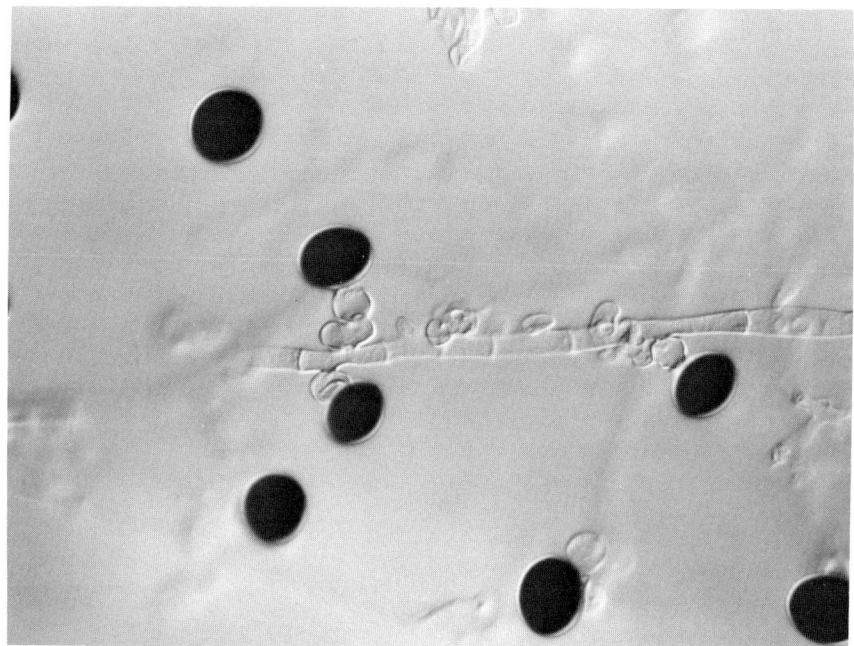

**Fig. 4.75** *Nigrospora oryzae*. The conidia are one-celled, horizontally flattened, and black in color. The conidia develop upon hyaline conidiophores that are swollen at their bases and taper toward the conidia.

remain sterile regardless of the media and growth conditions employed. Isolates of *P. brasiliensis* have been recovered from soil as well as woody plant material, suggesting that these are its natural habitats.

## *Penicillium* Link ex Gray, 1821

Diagnostic features: The genus *Penicillium* is characterized by the development of distinct, erect, usually branched, smooth to rough, hyaline to colored conidiophores. If the conidiophore branches, the metulae, branches, or both may be either adpressed to the main axis or divergent (separating from it). Flask-shaped, hyaline phialides form in groups at the apices of the metulae. From the phialides, 1-celled, hyaline to darkly pigmented, smooth or rough walled, globose to ovoid phialoconidia arise in chains. Each phialoconidium is separated from its neighbor by a connection. The overall impression of the fruiting head is a penicillus (Fig. 4.79). Sclerotia and sexual fruiting bodies may be present.

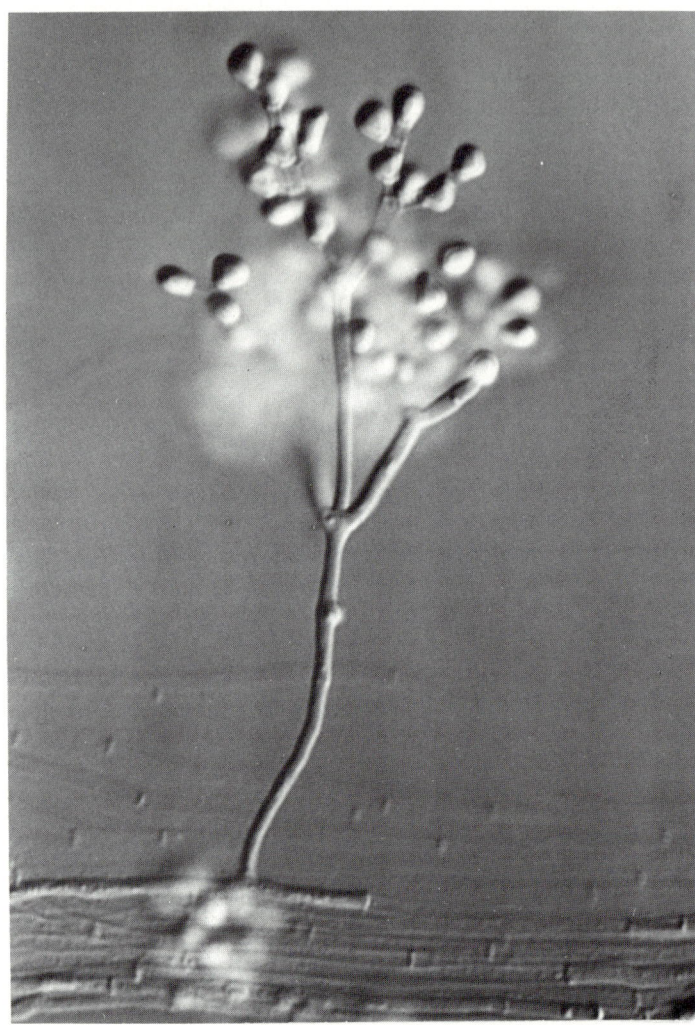

**Fig. 4.76** *Oidiodendron* sp. The conidiophores are erect and form an apical branching network of fertile hyphae. The fertile hyphae give rise to arthroconidia that are held together by connections.

Comments: The Latin term *penicillus*, which means brush or broom, is commonly used to describe the brushlike structure formed by members of the genus *Penicillium*. The penicillus is measured from the base of the lowest branch to the tip of the phialides, excluding all the phialoconidia that might be present. The term sterigmata has been used in the past for

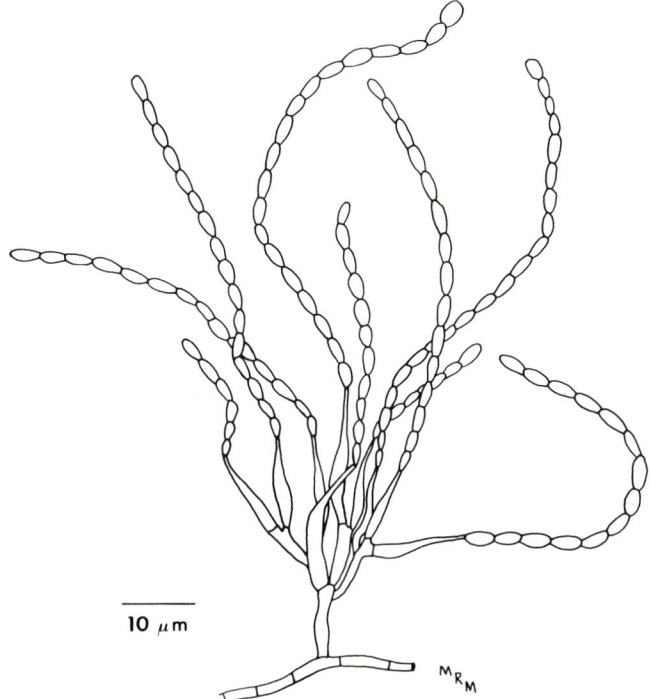

**Fig. 4.77** *Paecilomyces variotii*. The phialoconidia develop in long entangled chains from phialides that are swollen at their bases, gradually tapering toward their apices. The phialides and phialoconidia may form a penicillus.

the conidiogenous cells of *Penicillium*. Sterigmata should be restricted to the denticle-like structures upon which basidiospores develop, and not used for the phialides of *Penicillium*.

The sterile cells found directly beneath the phialides are referred to as metulae. In many species of *Penicillium*, additional levels of sterile cells may occur directly below the metulae. These cells are called branches. If branches are present, they arise directly from the conidiophore. The major sections of the genus *Penicillium* (Table 4.12) are based upon the presence or absence of metulae and branches, as well as their arrangement about the central axis of the conidiophore.

When the phialides arise directly from the apex of the conidiophore (metulae and branches are absent), the isolate is considered to be monoverticillate. The phialides and chains of phialoconidia stand out as being separate and distinct. Monoverticillate isolates are classified in the section Monoverticillata. More commonly, isolates of *Penicillium* with two, or rarely three, levels of branching are encountered. The levels of branching include both metulae and branches. Penicilli with two or three levels of branching are biverticillate (Fig. 4.80). A biverticillate penicillus is considered symmetrical when the metulae and branches are regular and evenly spaced about the central axis of the conidiophore. Penicillia with a biverticillate symmetrical arrangement of their penicillus are classified in the section Biverticillata-Symmetrica. Other isolates of *Penicillium* may form a biverticillate penicillus that is one-sided or lopsided. Such penicillia are classified in the section Asymmetrica. On rare occasions, isolates of *Penicillium* having several levels of branching are found. These complex heads are polyverticillate and such isolates are classified in the section Polyverticillata. There is question as to whether or not the Polyverticillata are actually species of *Penicillium*. The penicillia are variable, and most isolates will probably contain more than one type of penicillus. In this event, the overall predominant type of penicillus should be used to identify the isolate. Each section contains several series, which represent groups of similar species.

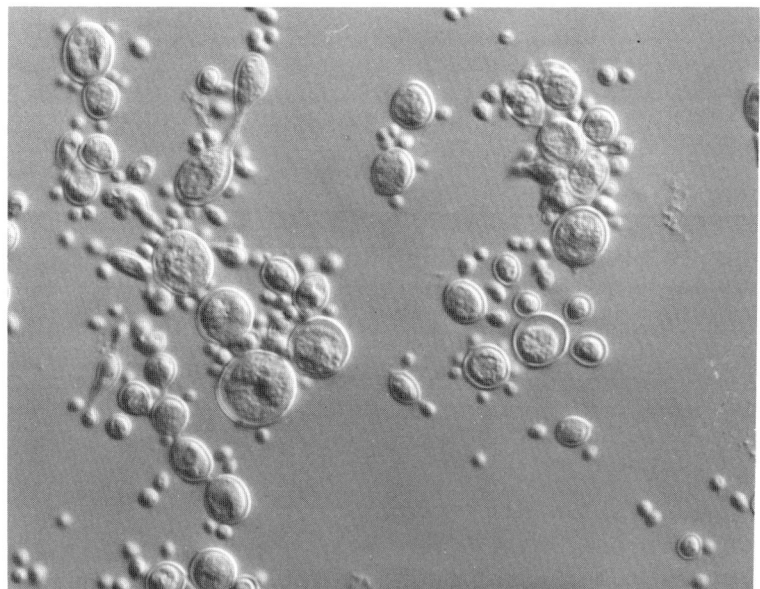

**Fig. 4.78** *Paracoccidioides brasiliensis*. The development of many blastoconidia around each of the parent cells is commonly referred to as multiple budding. At 37°C, the yeast form develops on special media such as cysteine–blood agar. At 25°C, conidia that are similar to those formed by members of the genus *Chrysosporium* are occasionally seen in fresh isolates.

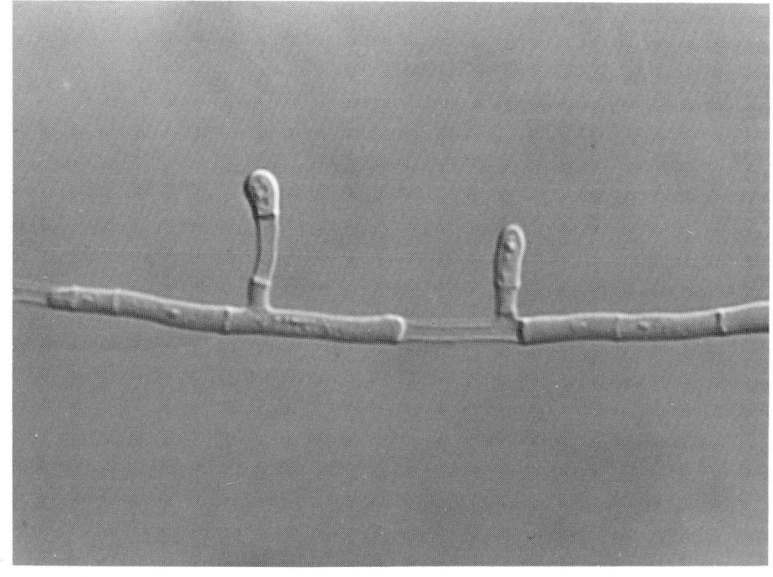

**Fig. 4.78** Continued

The penicillia are extremely variable in culture. It is therefore important to work with cultures that originated from a single conidium or hyphal tip. Czapek–Dox-solution agar is used as the standard medium for identifying isolates of *Penicillium*. Malt extract agar is used more or less as a backup medium. In addition to penicillus morphology, culture characteristics on Czapek–Dox-solution agar are extremely important in differentiating the penicillia. Culture characteristics of importance include color, texture, margins, growth rate, zonation, exudates, and odors. Other characteristics, such as the presence of sclerotia and ascocarps, are important in identifying *Penicillium* species.

Isolates of *Penicillium* are commonly recovered in the clinical laboratory. Occasionally, species of *Penicillium* are reported to cause disease in man. Two of the more commonly cited pathogenic species are *P. glaucum* and *P. crustaceum*. *Penicillium glaucum* has been frequently used for any green, yellow-green, or blue-green penicillia that was not otherwise identified. Likewise, *P. crustaceum* has been used in a similar manner. As a result, *P. glaucum* and *P. crustaceum* are meaningless. Two other species that are commonly cited as pathogens in review papers are *P. bertai* and *P. mycetomagenum*. *Penicillium bertai* appears to be monoverticillate and resembles *P. citreo-viride*, whereas *P. mycetomagenum* cannot be identified from its original description, but could be a member of the Biverticillata-

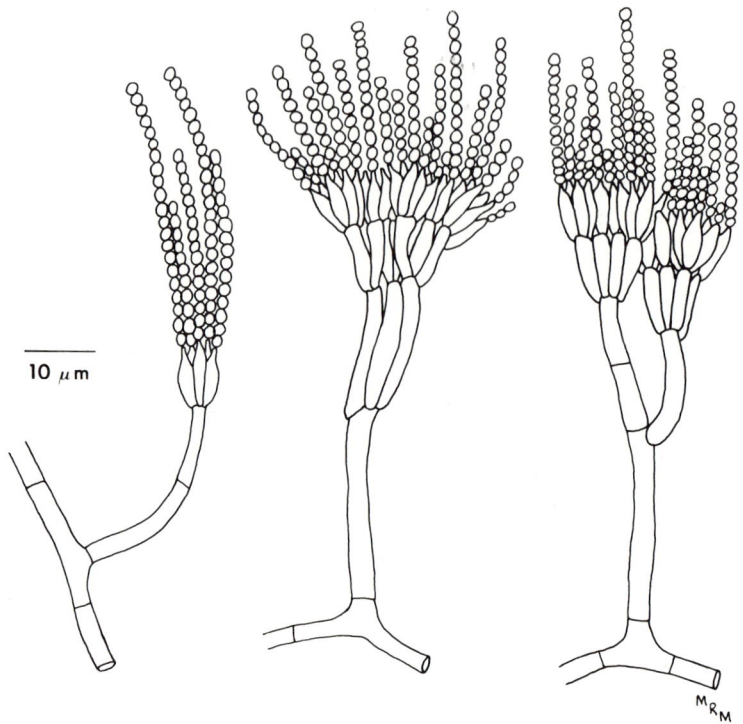

**Fig. 4.79** *Penicillium* sp. The most frequently encountered sections of the genus *Penicillium* are from left to right, Monoverticillata, Biverticillata-Symmetrica, and Asymmetrica.

Symmetrica group. In most instances, the penicillia are most likely contaminants, not pathogens. Species of *Penicillium* (120, 171, 186, 187) are probably the most ubiquitous group of fungi. *Penicillium* is an anamorph for a number of the Ascomycetes. The more common genera include *Eupenicillium, Penicilliopsis,* and *Talaromyces.*

*Phaeococcus* de Hoog, 1977

Diagnostic features: The genus *Phaeococcus* was established for fungi that produce black, glistening, colonies composed of dark brown to black, thick-walled, globose to ellipsoidal yeast cells producing secondary conidia (Fig. 4.81). Hyphae are absent, but pseudohyphae, chains of globose cells, or both may be present.

Comments: De Hoog (97) established the genus *Phaeococcus* for black yeasts that form neither hyphae nor other diagnostic structures. These

Part 3  Taxonomy

**Table 4.12.** General Key to the Series of the Penicillia[a]

I. Penicilli consisting of single clusters, or verticils of phialides at the tips of fertile hyphae, or conidiophores; conidiophores usually unbranched, in some forms irregularly branched but with each branch terminating in a distinct and separate monoverticillate penicillus · · · · · · · · · · · · · · · · · · · · · · · MONOVERTICILLATA Section
   A. Colonies producing either cleistothecia or sclerotia.
      1. Colonies producing fertile cleistothecia which are commonly sclerotioid and often ripen late · · · · · · · · · · · · · · · · · · · · *P. javanicum* series
      2. Colonies producing sclerotia, often suggestive of young cleistothecia but never developing an ascogenous stage · · · · · · · · · · · · · · · *P. thomii* series
   B. Colonies producing neither cleistothecia nor sclerotia.
      1. Conidiophores generally unbranched and bearing single, strictly monoverticillate penicilli.
         a. Colonies velvety or nearly so; conidiophores arising mostly from the substratum.
            1'. Colonies generally spreading broadly.
               aa. Conidia globose or subglobose · · · · · · *P. frequentans* series
               bb. Conidia elliptical · · · · · · · · · · · · · *P. lividum* series
            2'. Colonies growing rather restrictedly, especially on Czapek's solution agar · · · · · · · · · · · · · · · · · · · · · · · *P. implicatum* series
         b. Colonies appearing velvety or lightly floccose, but with conidiophores borne as short branches from interwoven aerial hyphae · · · · · · · · · · · · · · · · · · · · · · · · · · · · · · · · · · · · · · · · · · · *P. decumbens* series
         c. Colonies floccose or floccose-funiculose with conidiophores arising primarily from aerial hyphae.
            1'. Colonies predominantly floccose with funiculose habit lacking or limited · · · · · · · · · · · · · · · · · · · · · · *P. restrictum* series
            2'. Colonies with funiculose habit predominant or well-developed · · · · · · · · · · · · · · · · · · · · · · · · · · · · · · · · · *P. adametzi* series
      2. Conidiophores mostly irregularly branched but with each branch bearing a terminal, well-marked monoverticillate penicillus · · · The Ramigena series

II. Penicilli characteristically once- or twice-branched below the level of the phialides; typically asymmetrical, irregular, or one-sided; phialides not lanceolate · · · · · · · · · · · · · · · · · · · · · · · · · · · · · · · · · · · · · · · · · · · · · · ASYMMETRICA Section
   A. Penicilli characteristically strongly divaricate, with individual elements strongly divergent, often appearing monoverticillate but so arranged as to produce the appearance of a single branched penicillus · · · · · · · Divaricata Sub-section
      1. Colonies producing cleistothecia, sclerotia, or masses of thick-walled cells.
         a. Colonies producing true cleistothecia, parenchymatous or sclerotioid throughout; ripening from the center outward and often late · · · · · · · · · · · · · · · · · · · · · · · · · · · · · · · · · · · · · · · · · *Carpenteles* series
         b. Colonies producing sclerotia or masses of thick-walled cells; never developing asci or ascospores · · · · · · · · · · · · · · · · *P. raistrickii* series
      2. Colonies not producing cleistothecia, sclerotia, or masses of thick-walled cells.
         a. Conidial areas not showing green, gray-green, or blue-green shades—lilac, vinaceous or avellaneous shades usually produced · · · *P. lilacinum* series
         b. Conidial areas showing green, gray, gray-green, or blue-green shades.
            1'. Conidial areas in pale blue-green or gray-green shades; colony reverse often brightly colored.

*continued*

**Table 4.12.** *Continued*

    aa. Conidial chains strongly divergent; phialides abruptly tapered to narrow conidium bearing tubes . . . . . . *P. janthinellum* series
    bb. Conidial chains tending to form columns, at least when young; phialides not abruptly tapered. . . . . . . . . *P. canescens* series
  2′. Conidial areas in dull gray to olive-gray shades; colony reverse usually in dull yellow to orange-brown shades . . . *P. nigricans* series
B. Penicilli seldom strongly divaricate, usually compact, with branches and metulae tending to be parallel rather than divergent.
 1. Colonies typically velvety, with conidiophores arising characteristically from the substratum in a dense even stand . . . . . . . . . Velutina Sub-section
  a. Penicilli seldom branched below the level of the metulae; phialides not lanceolate or acuminate . . . . . . . . . . . . . . *P. citrinum* series
  b. Penicilli commonly branched below the level of the metulae.
   1′. Penicilli commonly long, with elements often loosely arranged.
    aa. Conidiophores smooth-walled; colony margin not arachnoid.
     1″. Colonies typically producing abundant yellow pigmentation in exudate and reverse . . . . . . . . . . *P. chrysogenum* series
     2″. Colonies not producing yellow pigment in exudate and reverse.
      aaa. Soil forms . . . . . . . . . . . . . . *P. oxalicum* series
      bbb. Green citrus rot . . . . . . . . . . . . *P. digitatum* series
    bb. Conidiophores rough-walled; colony margin arachnoid . . . . . . . . . . . . . . . . . . . . . . . . . . . . . . . . *P. roqueforti* series
   2′. Penicilli comparatively short, compact, with all elements compressed . . . . . . . . . . . . . . . . . . . . . . *P. brevi-compactum* series
 2. Colonies typically lanose or floccose, with conidiophores commonly long, usually arising as branches from aerial hyphae or from the substratum in marginal areas in older colonies. . . . . . . . . . . . Lanata Sub-section
  a. Colonies predominantly white and remaining so, or becoming light gray-green with the development of ripe conidia . . . . . *P. camemberti* series
  b. Colonies quickly developing some shade of green in conidial areas . . . . . . . . . . . . . . . . . . . . . . . . . . . . . . . . . *P. commune* series
 3. Colonies with surface typically ropy or funiculose from aggregation of aerial hyphae; conidial structures arising primarily from aerial hyphae or ropes of hyphae . . . . . . . . . . . . . . . . . . . . . . . . Funiculosa Sub-section
  a. Conidial areas in yellow-green, blue-green, or gray-green shades; penicilli large as in the Lanata and Fasciculata; conidia subglobose to elliptical . . . . . . . . . . . . . . . . . . . . . . . . . . . . . . *P. terrestre* series
  b. Conidial areas variously colored but never in green shades; penicilli often comparatively narrow; conidia strongly elliptical to cylindrical . . . . . . . . . . . . . . . . . . . . . . . . . . . . . . . . . . . . *P. pallidum* series
 4. Colonies with surface growth appearing mealy, tufted, fasciculate, or coremi-form due to aggregation of conidiophores into upright fascicles or bundles . . . . . . . . . . . . . . . . . . . . . . . . . . . Fasciculata Sub-section
  a. Sclerotia characteristically produced . . . . . . . . . *P. gladioli* series
  b. Sclerotia not produced.
   1′. Colonies with simple conidiophores and fascicles intermixed, but with simple conidiophores usually predominating.

**Table 4.12.** *Continued*

    aa. Conidial areas not developing true green colors in areas of ripe conidia . . . . . . . . . . . . . . . . . *P. ochraceum* series
    bb. Conidial areas typically in bright yellow-green shades, conidiophores rough. . . . . . . . . . . . . *P. viridicatum* series
    cc. Conidial areas typically in blue-green shades with the blue element predominant or at least clearly evident; conidiophores rough or smooth . . . . . . . . . . . . . . . . . . *P. cyclopium* series
    dd. Conidial areas typically in yellow-green or glaucous shades; conidiophores rough or smooth . . . . . . . . . *P. expansum* series
    ee. Conidial areas typically in pale to dull gray-green shades; conidiophores smooth-walled.
      1″. Phialides usually 8 μm or more in length. . . . *P. italicum* series
      2″. Phialides 6 μm or less in length . . . . . . . . *P. urticae* series
  2′. Colonies with most conidiophores aggregated into fascicles or definite synnemata.
    aa. Synnemata predominating but interspersed with abundant simple conidiophores . . . . . . . . . . . . . . *P. granulatum* series
    bb. Synnemata very prominent, with simple conidiophores lacking or very few in number. . . . . . . . . . . . . *P. claviforme* series

III. Penicilli characteristically biverticillate and symmetrical, but sometimes fractional in some species and strains; phialides typically lanceolate, with apices long-tapered, acuminate. . . . . . . . . . . . . . . . . . . BIVERTICILLATA-SYMMETRICA Section
  A. Colonies producing cleistothecia or sclerotia.
    1. Colonies producing soft cleistothecia upon most substrata, usually bright yellow in color. . . . . . . . . . . . . . . . . . . . . *P. luteum* series
    2. Colonies producing sclerotia or masses of thick-walled cells, commonly embedded in the substratum . . . . . . . . . . . . . . . *P. novae-zeelandiae*
                       (and scattered strains in other conidial series)
  B. Colonies not producing cleistothecia or sclerotia.
    1. Colonies regularly developing abundant, erect synnemata . . *P. duclauxi* series
    2. Colonies with surface appearing funiculose, floccose-funiculose, or occasionally somewhat tufted . . . . . . . . . . . . . . *P. funiculosum* series
    3. Colonies with ropiness absent or reduced and with surface typically velvety.
      a. Colonies usually developing an intense red or purple-red pigmentation in mycelium and reverse, with most strains growing fairly rapidly . . . . . . . . . . . . . . . . . . . . . . . . . *P. purpurogenum* series
      b. Colonies never developing an intense red pigmentation, growing very restrictedly upon Czapek and steep agars . . . . . . . *P. rugulosum* series
    4. Colonies comparatively deep, often appearing lanose; with vegetative mycelium typically in yellow-green shades and with reverse often similarly colored . . . . . . . . . . . . . . . . . . . . . . . . . . . . . *P. herquei* series
IV. Penicilli large, usually symmetrical, typically branched at three or more levels below the phialides. . . . . . . . . . . . . . . . . . . . . . . . . POLYVERTICILLATA Section

---

 [a] Reproduced and modified by permission of K. Raper and Williams & Wilkins Co. from "A Manual of the Penicillia," 1968.

260　　　　　　　　　　　　　　　　　　　　　　　　　　**4  Mould Identification**

black yeasts usually represent one morphological form or anamorph of polymorphic fungi, such as *Exophiala* and *Wangiella*. Upon subculture to potato dextrose agar, many isolates of *Phaeococcus* encountered in the clinical laboratory usually form hyphae. In most instances, these isolates can be identified as the *Phaeococcus* anamorph of *E. jeanselmei*. In my experience, no isolate of *Phaeococcus* that I have seen has turned out to be a species of *Aureobasidium* or similar fungus. The concept of *Phaeococcus* very nicely accommodates the black yeasts recovered in the clinical laboratory.

Isolates of *Phaeococcus* are occasionally recovered in the clinical laboratory. Prior to the work of de Hoog, most of these isolates were probably misidentified as *Aureobasidium* owing to the tendency of many microbiologists to "lump" all black yeasts into *A. pullulans*. De Hoog

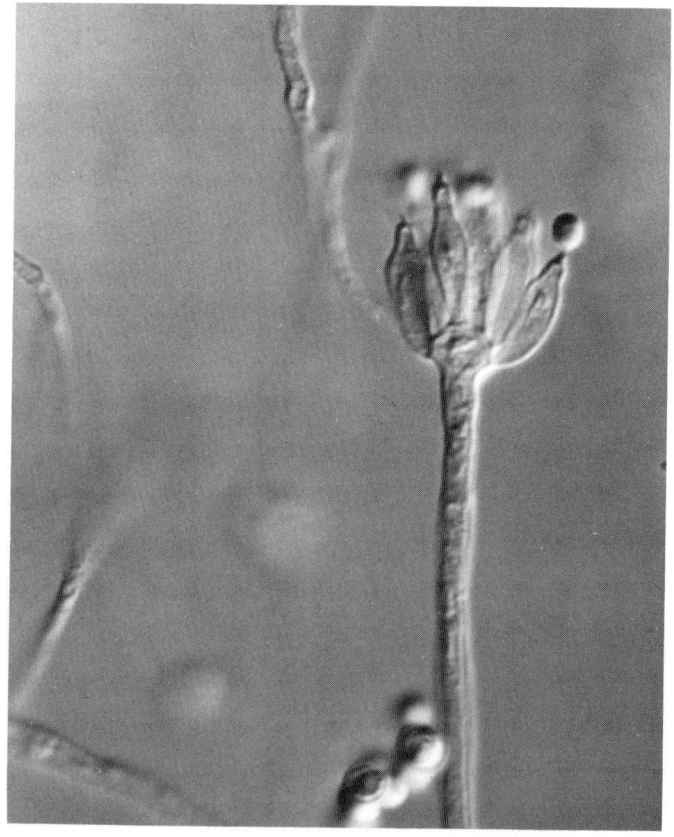

**Fig. 4.80**　*Penicillium* sp. Monoverticillate and biverticillate-symmetrically arranged heads.

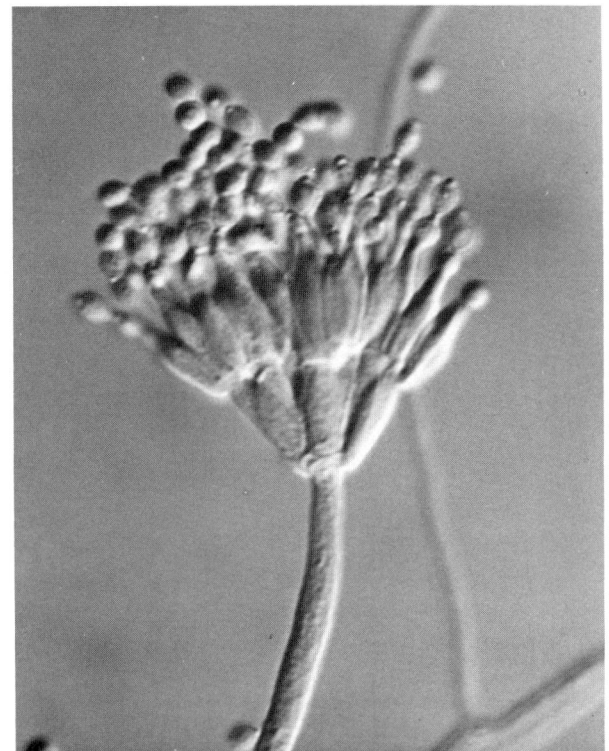

**Fig. 4.80** Continued

recognizes three species, *P. catenatus*, *P. exophialae*, and *P. nigricans*. The majority of isolates recovered in clinical laboratories are *P. exophialae*, the yeast form produced by species of *Exophiala* and *W. dermatitidis*.

*Phialophora* Medlar, 1915

Diagnostic features: Members of the genus *Phialophora* produce flask-shaped to cylindrical collarettes that gradually expand in diameter toward their apices. The phialides may arise from hyphae or on short conidiophores. Phialides may be solitary or in clusters and occasionally proliferate in a percurrent manner. The phialoconidia are hyaline to brown, 1-celled, smooth, ovoid to cylindrical, and form as a ball at the apex of the phialide.

Comments: The genus *Phialophora* was established for *P. verrucosa* (Fig. 4.82) by Medlar (146) for a new agent of chromoblastomycosis recovered

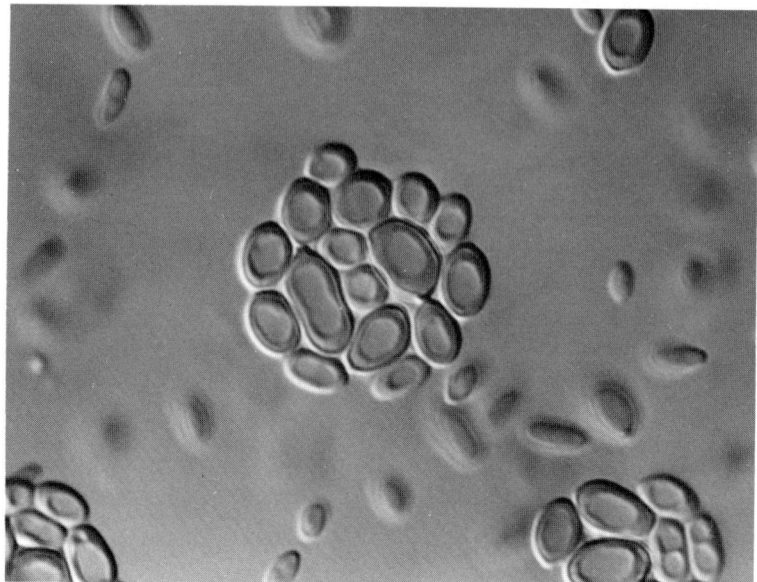

**Fig. 4.81** *Phaeococcus* anamorph of *Phialophora heteromorpha*. The dematiaceous yeast cells are typical of this genus.

in the United States. Some mycologists have incorrectly attributed the genus *Phialophora* to Dr. Thaxter. Medlar formally proposed the genus *Phialophora*, even though Thaxter did the taxonomy. Over the years, a number of medically important fungi have been incorrectly assigned to the genus *Phialophora*. *Fonsecaea pedrosoi* and *F. compacta* are two such fungi. Some medical mycologists (67) consider these two species to be members of the genus *Phialophora* because occasional isolates produce dematiaceous phialides with collarettes typical of *Phialophora*. These two species are best accommodated in *Fonsecaea* owing to their distinctive conidiogenous cells.

*Phialophora heteromorpha* has been considered by some mycologists to be a variety of *Exophiala jeanselmei* (97), or as a synonym of *Rhinocladiella mansonii* (194). These treatments of *P. heteromorpha* are unsatisfactory because this species produces phialides with distinct collarettes that fall very nicely within the concept of *Phialophora*. Another group of medically important species comprise the *P. hoffmannii* group. McGinnis (139) studied the type cultures of *P. hoffmannii*, *P. aurantiaca*, *P. luteo-viridis*, and *P. mutabilis* and concluded that they were essentially the same (Fig. 4.83). He considered the above species to be synonyms of *P. hoffmannii*. Members of this species are occasionally reported as etiologic agents of human infections. There is still some confusion surrounding the species *P. hoffmannii*

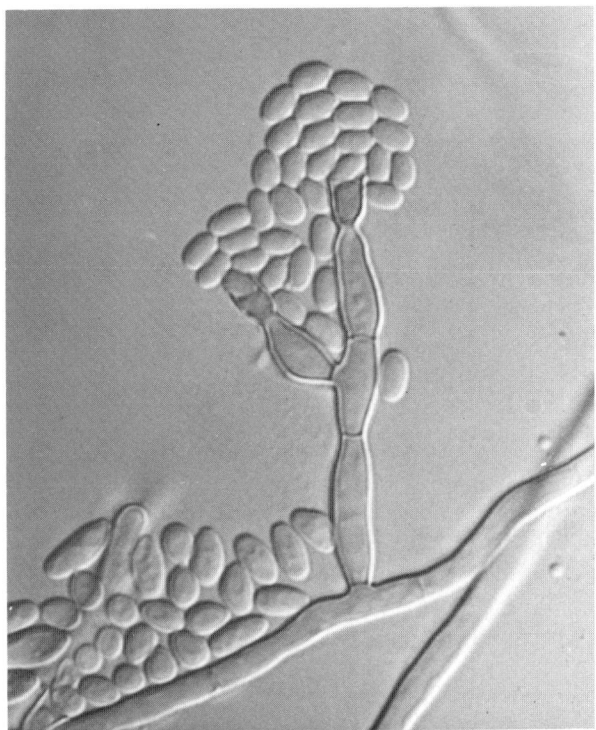

**Fig. 4.82** *Phialophora verrucosa*. The one-celled phialoconidia accumulate in balls at the apices of the phialides. The phialides have a distinct cup-shaped collarette.

and its relationship to the genera *Phialophora* and *Acremonium*. Isolates of *P. hoffmannii* are usually not dematiaceous, but are pale cream to pink. Thus, they more closely resemble species of *Acremonium* rather than *Phialophora*. If we follow Cole and Kendrick (49), this species, as well as others with cylindrical phialides and straight (parallel walls) collarettes, would be placed in the genus *Margarinomyces*. More study is needed.

*Wangiella dermatitidis* has been considered by some medical mycologists to be a species of *Phialophora* (67). Since *W. dermatitidis* does not form distinct collarettes detectable with the light microscope from its phialides, there is no reason to consider this species as *P. dermatitidis* (137). *Wangiella dermatitidis* very nicely illustrates the confusion surrounding the identification of polymorphic fungi.

Isolates of *Phialophora* are occasionally recovered in the clinical laboratory (Fig. 4.84). In addition to *P. verrucosa*, isolates of *P. hoffmannii* are not uncommon. At present, 5 species of *Phialophora* have caused documented

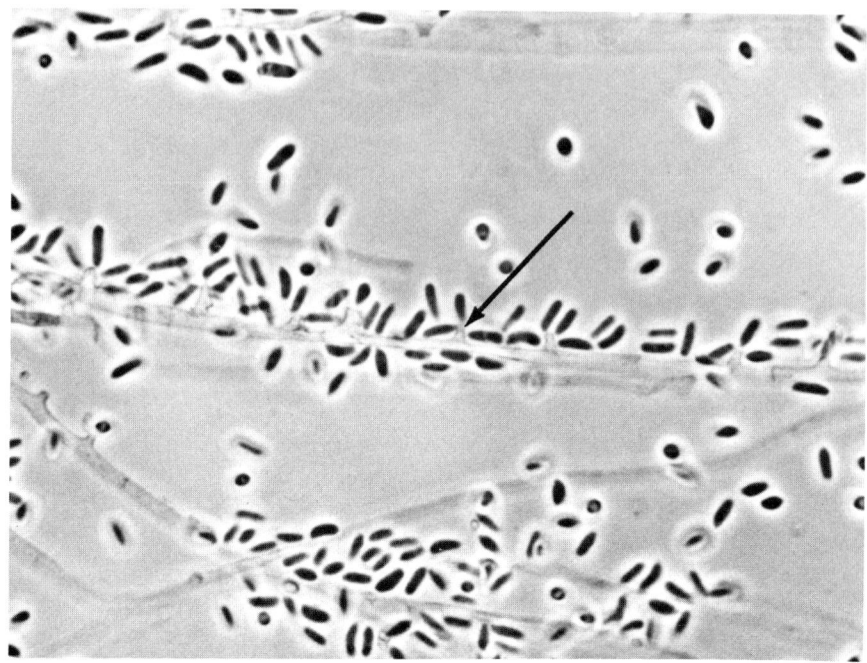

**Fig. 4.83** *Phialophora hoffmannii*. The phialides (arrow) are poorly differentiated from the vegetative hyphae.

cases of either chromoblastomycosis (*P. verrucosa* only) or phaeohyphomycosis. Ascomycetes such as *Mollisia* and *Gaeumannomyces* may form a *Phialophora* anamorph. Most species of *Phialophora* (49, 195) are associated with woody plants and soil, especially forest soils.

### Key to the Medically Important Species of *Phialophora*

1. Colonies yeastlike to cottony, cream, amber, pink to gray; phialides inconspicuous, not separated from vegetative cell by a septum; phialoconidia hyaline, cylindrical to allantoid; yeast present . . . . . . . . . . . . . . . . . . . . . . . . . . . . . . . *P. hoffmannii*

1'. Colonies velvety to cottony, gray; phialides conspicuous, distinct from vegetative hyphae, phialoconidia variable; yeast present or absent . . . . . . . . . . . . . . . . . . . 2

    2. Collarettes distinctly vase-shaped to flared . . . . . . . . . . . . . . . . . . . 3

    2'. Collarettes not distinctly vase-shaped to flared; usually continuous with cell wall of phialide (parallel walls) . . . . . . . . . . . . . . . . . . . . . . . . . . . 4

3. Collarettes vase-shaped, darkly pigmented; phialides flask-shaped; phialoconidia ovoid to ellipsoidal, hyaline, with basal scar . . . . . . . . . . . . . . . . . . . . . . *P. verrucosa*

3'. Collarettes flaring, saucer-shaped, pigmented at base; phialides flask-shaped to lageniform; phialoconidia ellipsoidal or globose, hyaline or light brown . . . . . . . *P. richardsiae*

4. Collarettes continuous, parallel walled, hyaline; phialides cylindrical to obclavate, hyaline to pale brown; phialoconidia cylindrical to allantoid hyaline; yeast usually present . . . . . . . . . . . . . . . . . . . . . . . . . . . . . . . . . . . . . . . . . . . . . . . *P. parasitica*

4'. Collarettes continuous, parallel walled, short, hyaline; phialides cylindrical to lageniform, hyaline to brown; phialoconidia cylindrical to ellipsoidal, slightly curved . . . . . *P. repens*

*Rhinocladiella* Nannfeldt, 1934

Diagnostic features: The genus *Rhinocladiella* is characterized by the development of erect, septate, pale brown, sympodial conidiophores that have distinct scars where the conidia were attached. The conidia are

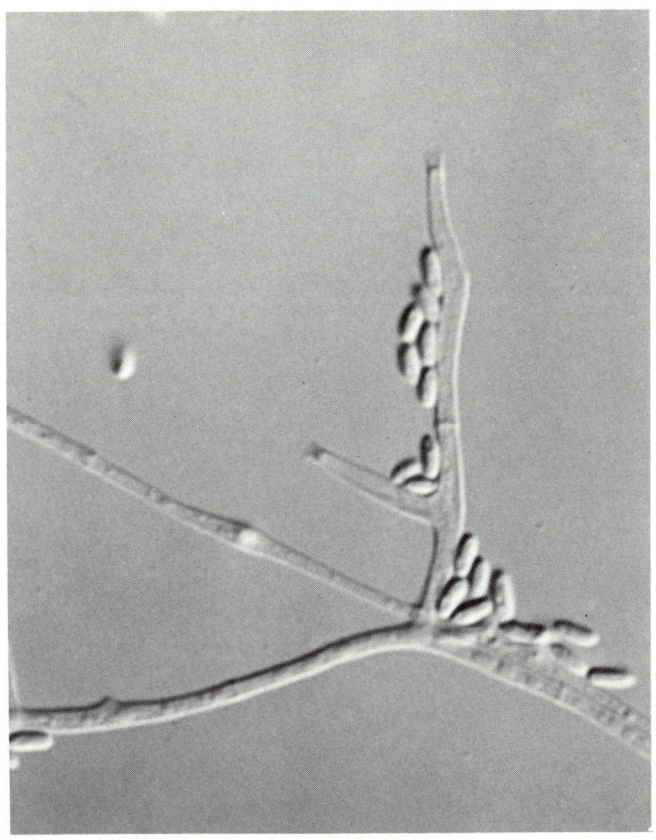

**Fig. 4.84** Variations in the phialides and phialoconidia are used to distinguish the various species of *Phialophora*. A. *P. repens*. B. *P. richardsiae*. C. *P. parasitica*. (A and C reproduced by permission from *PAHO Scientific Publ. No. 356*, pp. 37–59, 1978.)

1-celled, hyaline, and cylindrical. They occur over a large portion of the rachis in an acropleurogenous arrangement (Fig. 4.85).

Comments: The generic concept of *Rhinocladiella* has changed several times since Nannfeldt (147) first described it in 1934. Schol-Schwarz (194) expanded the concept to include, in addition to the sympodial development, a *Phialophora* (phialides with collarettes), annellide and *Cladosporium*-like types of anamorphs. With this broadened concept of *Rhinocladiella*, she considered *Exophiala jeanselmei, Phialophora heteromorpha, Wangiella dermatitidis, Cladosporium mansonii*, and *R. atrovirens* to be one and the same species, that is, *R. mansonii*. In addition, she transferred *Fonsecaea pedrosoi* and *F. compacta* to the genus *Rhinocladiella*. Few mycologists have accepted this concept.

Recently, de Hoog (97) revised the genus *Rhinocladiella*. He agrees that

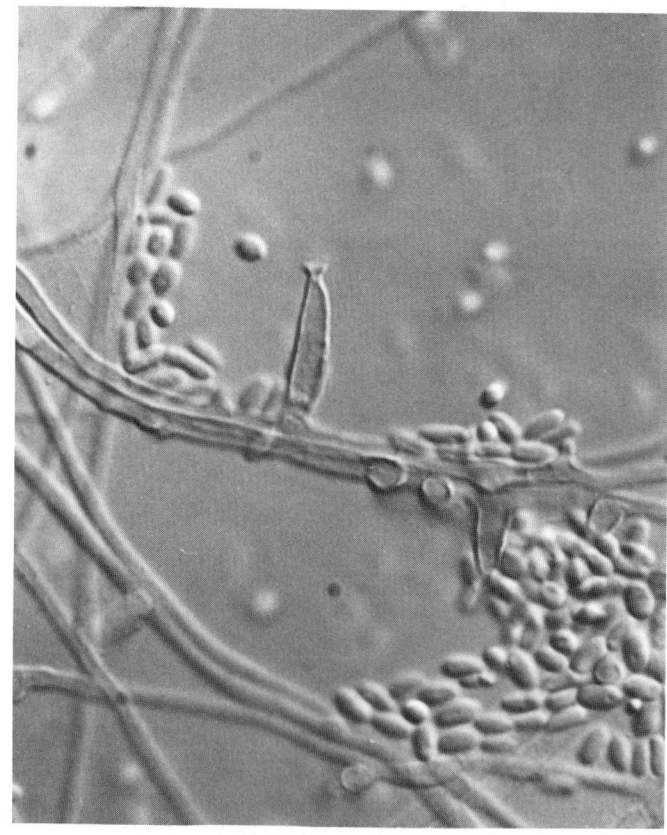

Fig. 4.84 Continued

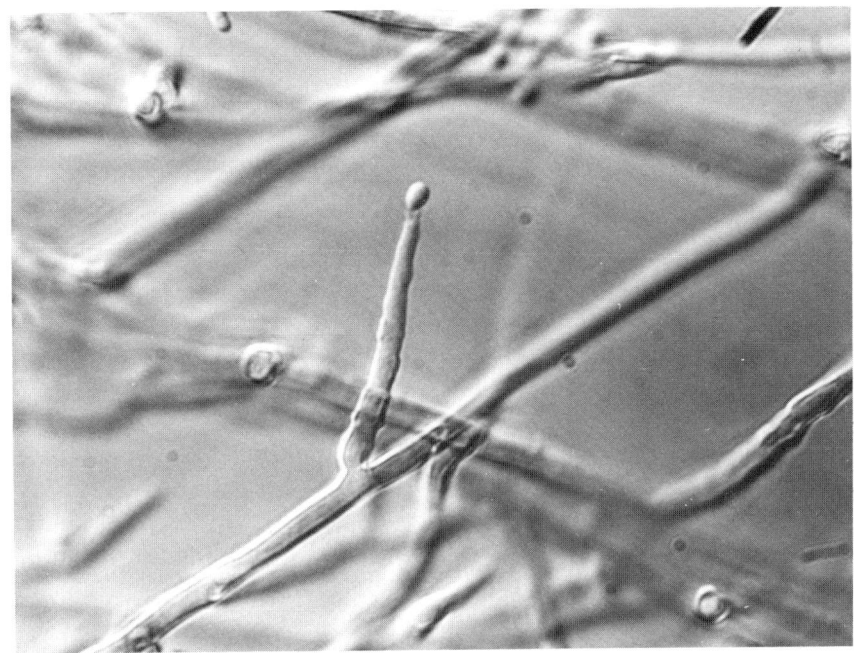

C

**Fig. 4.84** Continued

most of the species Schol-Schwarz placed in *Rhinocladiella* belong elsewhere. He supports Schol-Schwarz in part by maintaining *F. pedrosoi* and *F. compacta* in *Rhinocladiella*. In addition, de Hoog transferred *E. spinifera* to *Rhinocladiella*. This seems unnecessary since *E. spinifera* forms annellides (136), and therefore does not agree with the present sympodial concept for *Rhinocladiella*. De Hoog considers the genus *Ramichloridium* to be similar to *Rhinocladiella* and states that these two genera are "not sharply delimited." Problems arise because, according to de Hoog, one of the key characteristics of *Ramichloridium* is that they are not "pathogenic to man." Since *Ramichloridium cerophilum* (as *Acrotheca aquaspera*) (Fig. 4.86) is an agent of chromoblastomycosis, there is some question as to whether or not *Ramichloridium* is necessary. *Ramichloridium cerophilum* could be considered as a *Rhinocladiella* or *Fonsecaea*, depending upon the isolate studied; *R. pedrosoi* and *R. compacta* as members of the genus *Fonsecaea*; and *R. spinifera* as an *Exophiala*.

*Rhinocladiella* is occasionally isolated in the clinical laboratory. Members of this genus are fairly common soil fungi. Schol-Schwarz described the teleomorph for *R. mansonii* as *Dictyotrichiella mansonii*. Owing to her broad concept of *R. mansonii*, it is difficult to determine which anamorph(s) are associated with *D. mansonii*.

## *Sagrahamala* Subramanian, 1972

Diagnostic features: Members of the genus *Sagrahamala* produce long, simple, erect to flexuous, narrow, smooth, gently tapering toward the apex, simple phialides that arise from the mycelium. The phialoconidia are catenulate, hyaline, 1-celled, smooth, ovoid, cylindrical to elliptical, with both ends truncate (Fig. 4.87).

Comments: Subramanian (208) established the genus *Sagrahamala* for monophialide species of *Paecilomyces* and some isolates of *Gliomastix*. The genus is similar to *Acremonium* (see discussion under *Acremonium*).

Isolates of *Sagrahamala* are occasionally recovered in the clinical laboratory. The phialides and chains of phialoconidia are distinctive.

## *Scedosporium* Saccardo ex Castellani et Chalmers, 1919

Diagnostic features: The genus *Scedosporium* is characterized by 1-celled, pale brown to dark brown, smooth, subglobose, ovoid to elongate conidia developing upon short, denticle-like lateral hyphal outgrowths from micronematous, elongated, cylindrical conidiophores. They occur as solitary conidia or in balls at the apex of the conidiophore (Fig. 4.88).

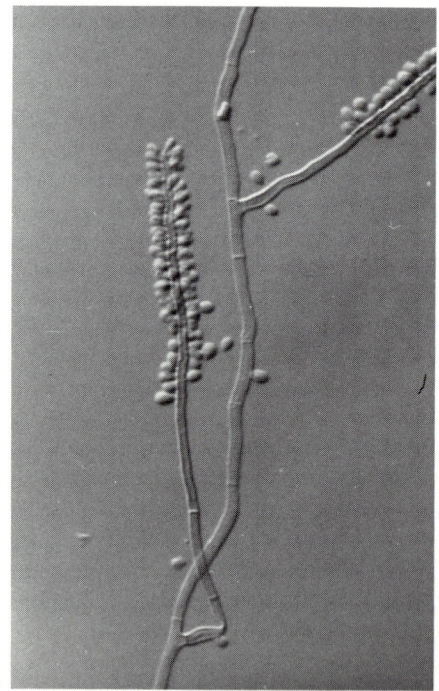

**Fig. 4.85** The one-celled conidia are produced from a sympodial conidiophore. The rachis is that portion of the conidiophore where the conidia are attached. A. *Rhinocladiella anceps*. B. *Rhinocladiella* sp.

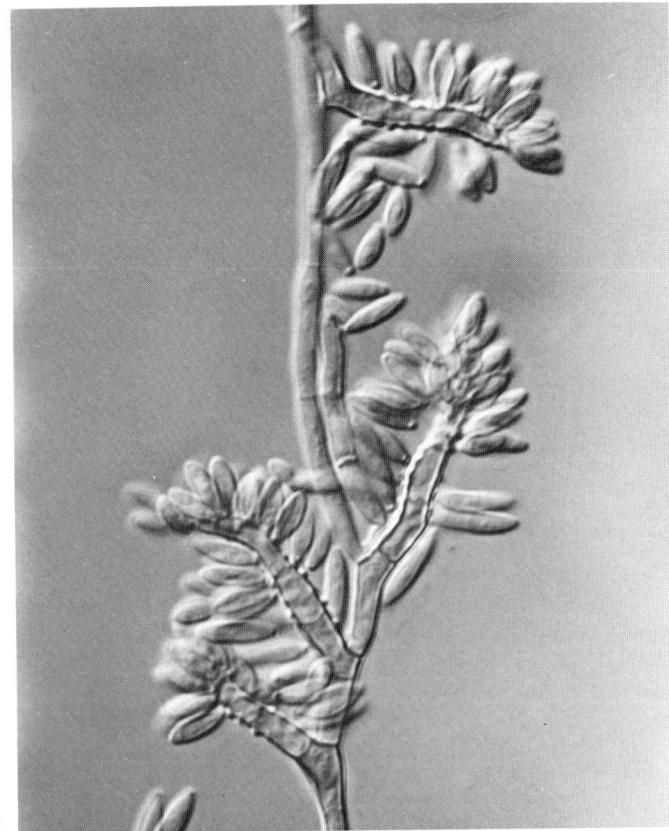

**Fig. 4.85** Continued

Conidiogenesis has not been adequately investigated in this genus; the conidiogenous cells may be annellides.

Comments: In 1911, Radaeli (169) reported the first human infection due to *Monosporium apiospermum*, a fungus that Saccardo (178) had just described as a new species. In his discussion of *M. apiospermum*, Saccardo thought that this species should be in its own genus; suggested the name *Scedosporium*; and provided a diagnosis. The name was invalidly published because Saccardo did not use it for the new species that he was describing. Article 34 of the International Code of Botanical Nomenclature states that a name is invalidly published when its author does not accept it. This conclusion is also supported in a later study in which Saccardo (179) makes no reference to the genus *Scedosporium* while discussing *M. apiospermum*. Castellani and Chalmers (46) in 1919 prepared a minimum

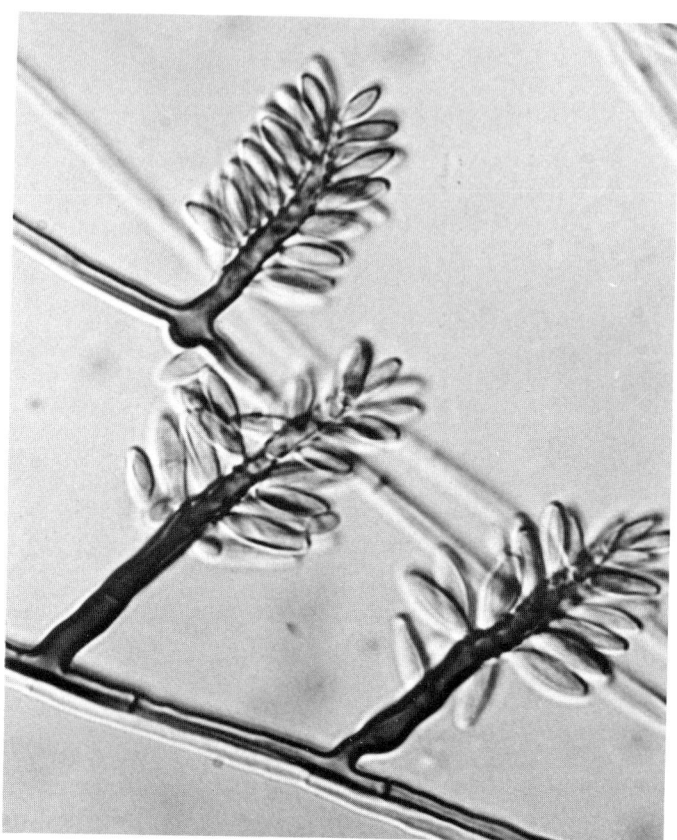

**Fig. 4.86** *Rhinocladiella* sp. The sympodial conidiophores and one-celled conidia are typical of this genus.

diagnosis for *Scedosporium* and attributed the name to Saccardo. They therefore validated the generic name *Scedosporium* and made the new combination *S. apiospermum*. Hughes (100) in 1958 pointed out that the genus *Monosporium* is illegitimate because it was included in the type species for three earlier genera. Even though the genus *Monosporium* is a *nomen illegitimum*, the epithet *apiospermum* is valid. Thus, the correct name for this fungus is *S. apiospermum* (Saccardo) Castellani et Chalmers.

Emmons (66) showed *S. apiospermum* to be the anamorph of *Petriellidium boydii* (as *Allescheria boydii*). Species of *Petriellidium*, *Petriella*, and similar genera may form a *Scedosporium* anamorph that is identical to each other. On occasion, *Scedosporium* may be associated with synnemata of the genus *Graphium*. A systemic infection in a dalmatian dog

## Part 3 Taxonomy

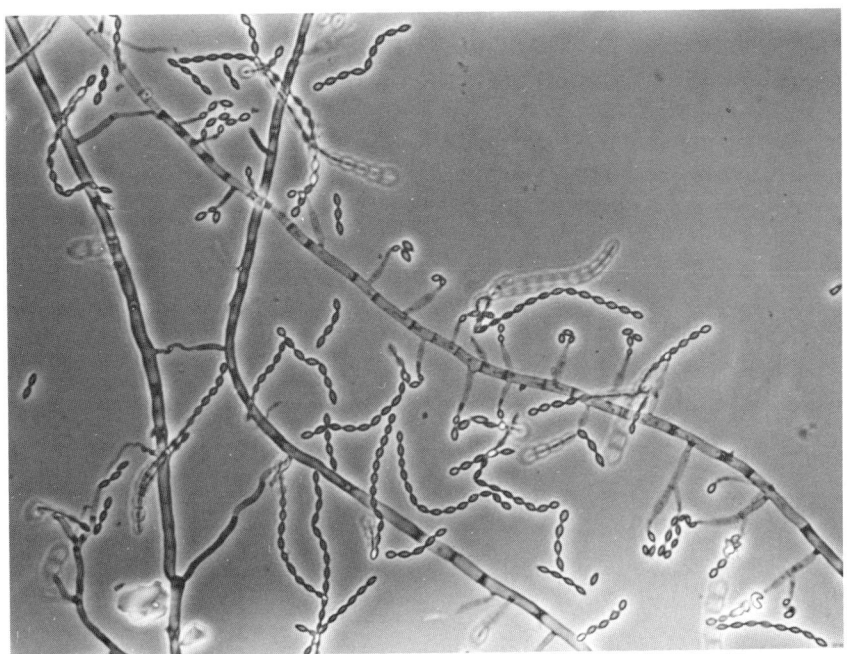

**Fig. 4.87** *Sagrahamala* sp. The hyaline conidia arise in chains from gently tapering phialides that are swollen at their bases.

caused by *G. fructicola*, a synnematous anamorph of *Scedosporium*, has been recently reported (112).

Isolates of *Scedosporium* are frequently recovered in the clinical laboratory. *Scedosporium apiospermum* may cause infections that range from mycetoma to disease of the central nervous system. *Scedosporium* is apparently a common soil fungus and is associated with Ascomycetes such as *Petriella* and *Petriellidium*.

### *Scolecobasidium* Abbott, 1927

Diagnostic features: Members of the genus *Scolecobasidium* produce hyaline to brown, 1- to several-celled, clavate to cylindrical, sympodial conidiophores. Pale brown, 2- to usually 4-celled, cylindrical to T- or Y-shaped, smooth to echinulate conidia arise from fine tubular denticles at the upper portion of the conidiophore (Fig. 4.89).

Comments: The genus *Scolecobasidium* was originally established for the two species, *S. terreum* and *S. constrictum* (1). De Hoog and von Arx (98) reviewed this genus and felt that the T- or Y-shaped conidia of *S. terreum* were distinctively different from the conidia produced by other species assigned to the genus *Scolecobasidium*. They concluded that *Scolecobasidium* should include, in essence, only T- or Y-shaped conidia, and that the other species should be transferred to *Ochroconis*. The transfer of *Scolecobasidium* species to the genus *Ochroconis* is based primarily upon conidial shape, and appears to be unnecessary. *Scolecobasidium* is similar to other genera, especially *Dactylaria* (25, 190). The distinctive conidia arising from tubular denticles help to distinguish *Scolecobasidium* from the latter genus. A number of species previously classified in the obsolete genus *Heterosporium* are now considered to be species of *Scolecobasidium*.

Isolates of *Scolecobasidium* are rarely encountered in the clinical laboratory. Species of *Scolecobasidium* (19) are commonly found in soil, especially in soils containing high amounts of organic matter.

### *Scopulariopsis* Bainier, 1907

Diagnostic features: The conidiogenous cells of *Scopulariopsis* are annellides. They may be solitary, in groups, or organized into a distinct

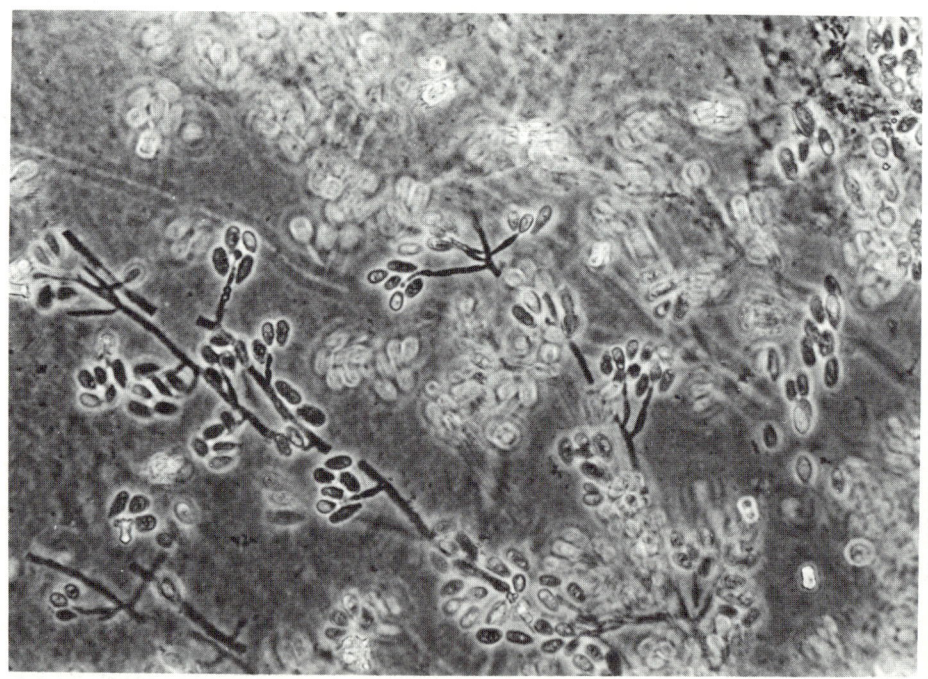

**Fig. 4.88** *Scedosporium apiospermum.* The pale brown conidia may be solitary or occur in balls.

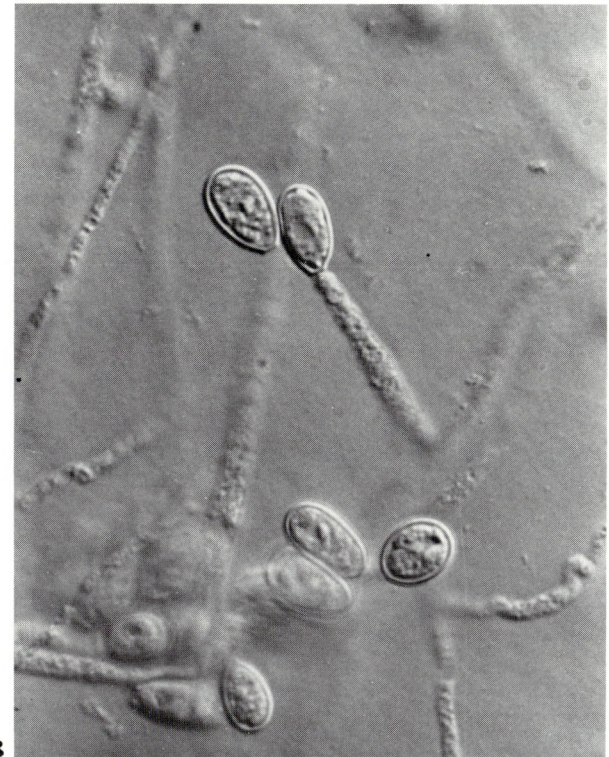

Fig. 4.88 Continued

penicillus. The annellides are variable, but usually cylindrical to slightly swollen. The annelloconidia form in chains and are globose to pyriform, usually truncate, with a rounded distal portion, smooth to rough, and hyaline to brown in color (Fig. 4.90).

Comments: *Scopulariopsis* is superficially similar to *Penicillium* and some species of *Paecilomyces*. The presence of annellides and the impression of a series of light-bulb-shaped (more common isolates) annelloconidia readily distinguish *Scopulariopsis* from *Penicillium* and *Paecilomyces*. *Scopulariopsis* may form a synnema, which is classified in the genus *Trichurus*.

*Scopulariopsis koningii* has been reported to be a pathogen of man on several occasions. Morton and Smith (150) had the opportunity to study several of these isolates. They concluded that all the isolates available to them were actually *S. brevicaulis,* not *S. koningii*. It appears that *S. koningii* may not be a pathogen, but represents a case in which *S. brevicaulis* is being incorrectly identified. *Scopulariopsis brevicaulis* is occasionally reported to cause deep tissue invasion. Most likely, this species is not invasive, but simply growing on necrotic tissue. An example of this has been seen at the North Carolina Memorial Hospital, in which *S. brevicaulis* was observed growing and producing annelloconidia on necrotic tissue behind an eye in a patient with diabetes. Viable tissue was not invaded.

Isolates of *Scopulariopsis* are frequently recovered in the clinical laboratory. In most instances, these are isolates of *S. brevicaulis*. Members of the genus *Scopulariopsis* are common soil fungi. Some species of *Chaetomium*, *Kernia*, *Microascus*, and *Petriella* may form a *Scopulariopsis* anamorph.

### *Scytalidium* Pesante, 1957

Diagnostic features: The genus *Scytalidium* is characterized by dematiaceous, intercalary, and terminal 1- to 2-celled, enlarged, smooth, subglobose to ellipsoidal arthroconidia. The arthroconidia are released by fission or fracture. A second type of fission arthroconidia, which are hyaline,

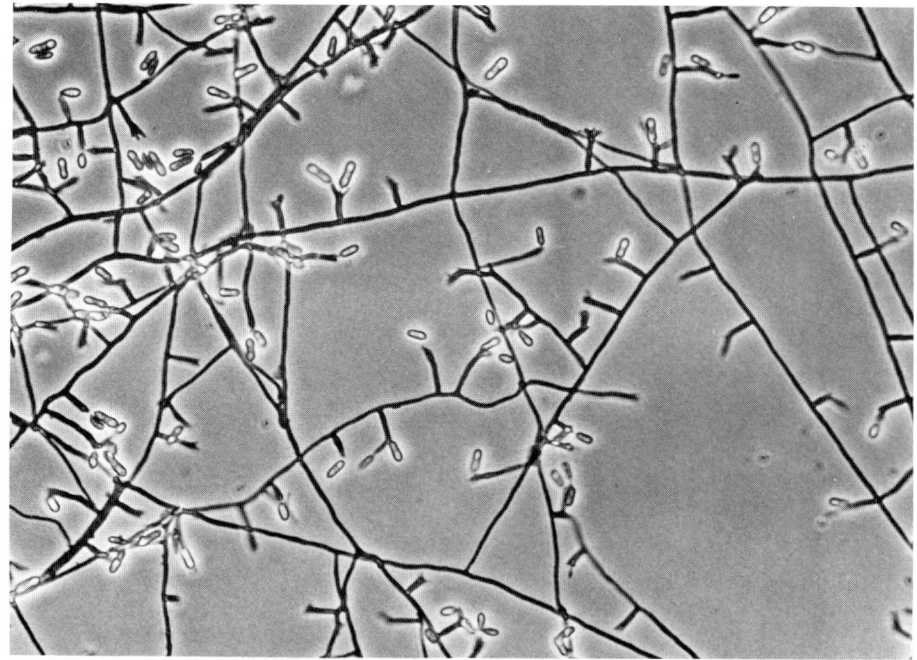

**Fig. 4.89** *Scolecobasidium humicola*. The conidia are two- to four-celled, pale brown, and develop upon fine tubular denticles from the upper portions of the conidiophores.

## Part 3  Taxonomy

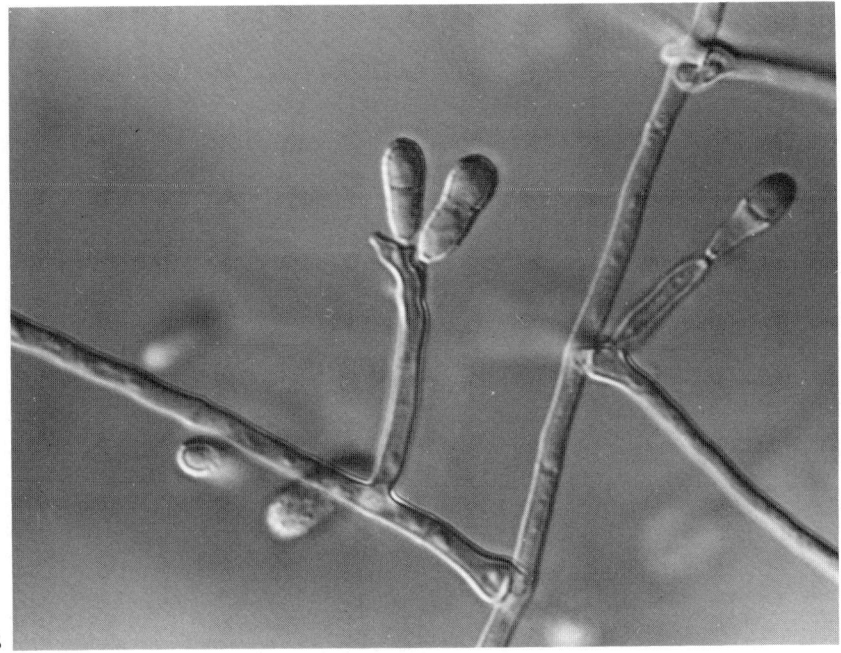

**Fig. 4.89** Continued

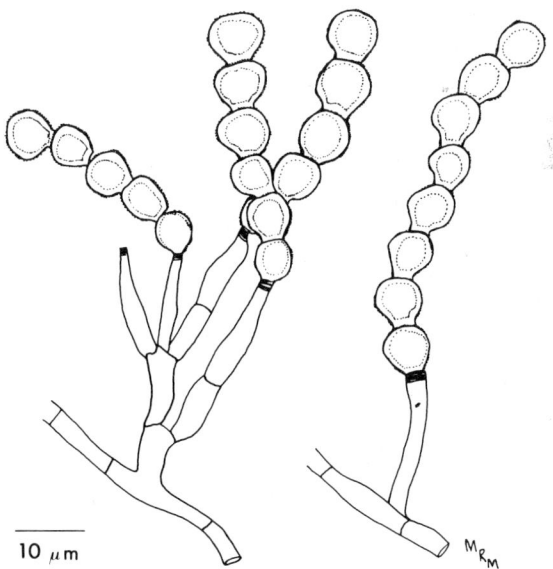

**Fig. 4.90** *Scopulariopsis brevicaulis*. The conidia arise in chains from annellides that may be solitary or in groups.

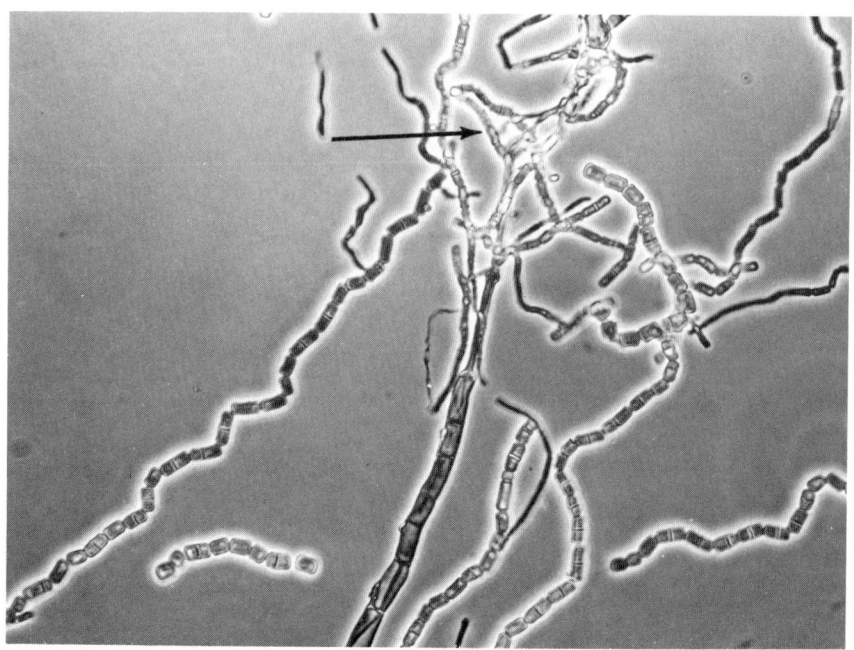

**Fig. 4.91** *Scytalidium lignicola*. This species of *Scytalidium* produces two types of arthroconidia. In addition to the one- to two-celled dark, enlarged arthroconidia, it also forms one-celled, thin-walled hyaline arthroconidia (arrow).

thin-walled, smooth, 1-celled and cylindrical, are produced in some species (Fig. 4.91).

Comments: The genus *Scytalidium* is similar to *Geotrichum*, except that the arthroconidia are pale brown to black and swollen (200). *Aureobasidium*, *Hendersonula*, and similar genera may form a *Scytalidium* anamorph. Members of this genus are primarily soil fungi and occasionally are associated with woody plant material.

## *Sepedonium* Link ex Greville, 1824

Diagnostic features: Species of *Sepedonium* produce simple to branched, hyaline, 1- to several-celled conidiophores that may be short or long. The conidia are terminal, solitary, or in clusters, 1-celled, globose to ovoid, hyaline to amber, smooth to verrucose, and usually with a thick wall (Fig. 4.92). A *Verticillium* anamorph may also be present. Microconidia are absent.

Comments: *Sepedonium* (43) is infrequently recovered in the clinical laboratory. Isolates of *Sepedonium* are extremely similar to *Histoplasma*

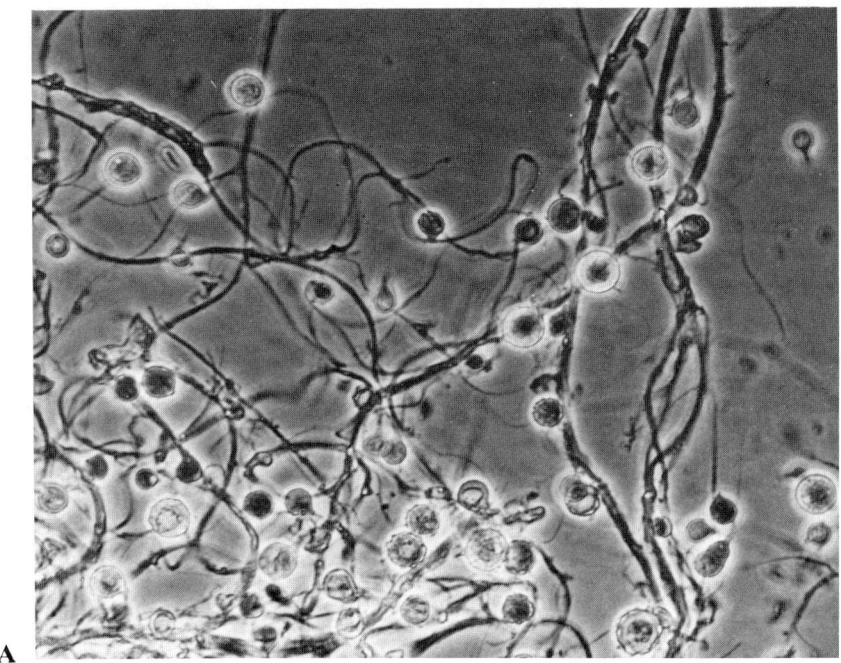

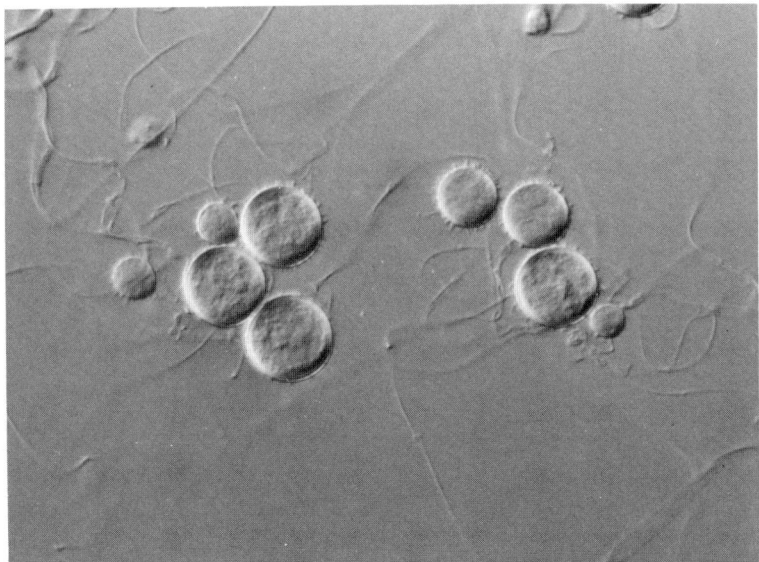

**Fig. 4.92** *Sepedonium* sp. The conidia are one-celled, amber, and usually with a thick wall. The conidia resemble those produced by members of the genus *Histoplasma*.

*capsulatum*, in that they form thick-walled, globose, verrucose, terminal conidia. Because of this similarity, the mould-to-yeast-form conversion is necessary in order to be sure that the fungus is *H. capsulatum*, not *Sepedonium*. In addition to the absence of a yeast form in *Sepedonium*, members of this genus do not form microconidia. Phialides may be present, which, of course, are not associated with *H. capsulatum*.

*Sepedonium* species are soil organisms and parasites of fleshy fungi. They are usually recognized by the presence of thick-walled, golden conidia forming in clusters. The Ascomycetes *Corynascus*, *Hypomyces*, *Peckiella*, and *Thielavia* may form a *Sepedonium* anamorph.

### *Sporothrix* Hektoen et Perkins, 1900

Diagnostic features: Conidiophores are usually present, hyaline, septate, elongate, sympodial, tapering toward the apex, and often with a swollen apical portion. The conidia are 1-celled, hyaline, globose to clavate, truncate, and arise solitarily upon distinct denticles. A second type of conidia is 1-celled, dematiaceous, thick-walled, and arises solitarily along the hyphae. These are typically seen in fresh isolates (Fig. 4. 93).

Comments: At the request of Schenck (189), E. F. Smith studied the fungus Schenck had isolated from the first case of sporotrichosis. Smith concluded that it was probably an undescribed species of *Sporotrichum*. Schenck decided to leave his fungus unclassified. Two years later in 1900, Hektoen and Perkins (85) described the second case of sporotrichosis and named their fungus *Sporothrix schenckii*. In their study of sporotrichosis in 1906, de Beurmann and Gougerot (24) transferred *S. schenckii* to the genus *Sporotrichum*. Subsequently, medical mycologists ignored the genus *Sporothrix*. Hughes (100) in 1958 chose *S. aureum* to be the lectotype for *Sporotrichum*, a genus that was described by Link in 1809. The confusion surrounding these two genera was finally resolved when Carmichael (43) clearly pointed out that *Sporothrix* produces sympodial conidiogenous cells with hyaline blastoconidia, whereas *Sporotrichum* forms ovoid, golden-brown, large conidia. *Sporotrichum* also forms large hyphae that have clamp conections. Carmichael showed that *Sporothrix* was validly published by Hektoen and Perkins.

Medical mycologists traditionally confirm the identity of *S. schenckii* by converting the mould form to the yeast form at 37°C (Fig. 4.93). Care must be exercised in using this characteristic to identify an isolate of *Sporothrix* as *S. schenckii*. For example, *S. cyanescens*, which has been recovered from cutaneous lesions (99), also produces a yeast form at 37°C. A number of species of *Ceratocystis* with a *Sporothrix* anamorph are also dimorphic and pathogenic for mice.

## Part 3  Taxonomy

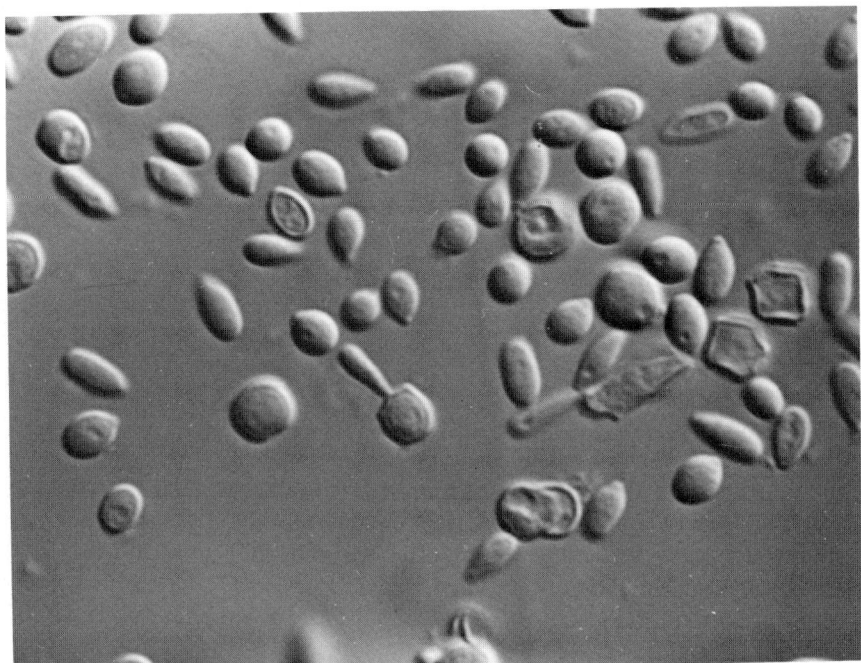

**Fig. 4.93** *Sporothrix schenckii*. A. The yeast form is produced at 37°C on enriched media such as blood agar. B. At 25°C, conidia on delicate denticles are produced directly from the hyphae as well as from sympodial conidiophores.

Isolates of *Sporothrix* are rarely encountered in the clinical laboratory unless they are associated with sporotrichosis. *Sporothrix schenckii* is associated with woody plant material. Thibaut and Ansel (213) have described the genus *Dolichoascus* as the teleomorph of *S. schenckii*. Since their genus is apparently based upon conidial structures, the genus *Dolichoascus*, which was described as an ascomycete, is in error. It has been suggested (133, 134, 160) that the teleomorph of *S. schenckii* may be *Ceratocystis stenoceras*. Species of *Sporothrix* (96) occur as anamorphs of *Ceratocystis*. De Hoog (96) has proposed that the genus *Ceratocystis* should be divided into *Ceratocystis* and *Ophiostoma*. He considers the anamorphs *Sporothrix* and *Graphium* to be associated with *Ophiostoma*, not *Ceratocystis*. This conclusion is not accepted here.

### *Sporotrichum* Link ex Gray, 1821

Diagnostic features: Members of the genus *Sporotrichum* produce 1-celled, thick-walled, golden-brown, truncate with a broad base, solitary,

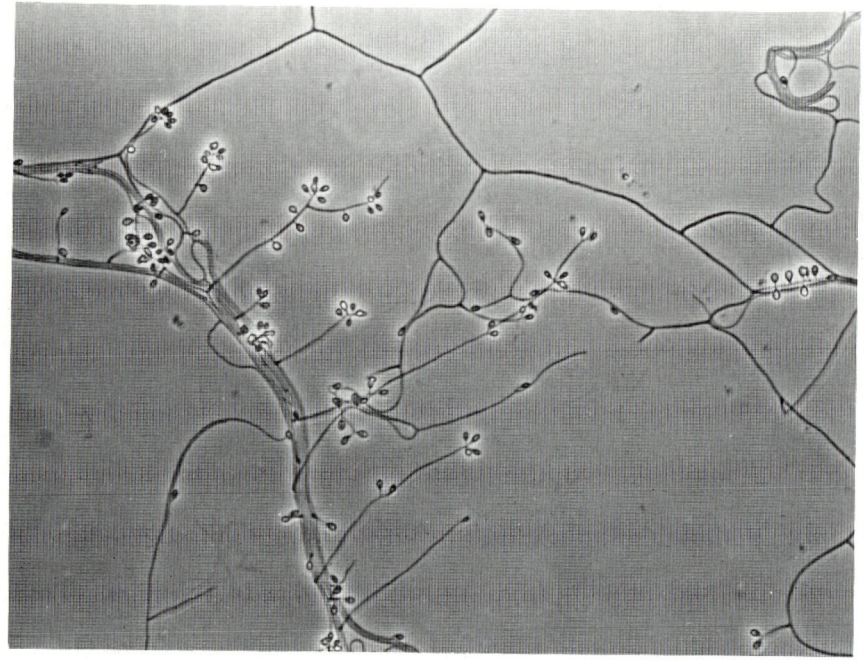

**Fig. 4.93** Continued

ovoid, holoblastic conidia that arise from the conidiophore on short, broad denticles. Upon release of the conidium, an annular frill is usually present. Clamp connections are typically present at the septa (Fig. 4.94).

Comments: A great deal of confusion has surrounded the genus *Sporotrichum* and its relationship to *Sporothrix* and *Chrysosporium*. After Hughes (100) established *S. aureum* as lectotype, the confusion surrounding this genus and *Sporothrix* was resolved by Carmichael (43). *Sporotrichum* was defined on the basis of its distinctive pigmented conidia and the presence of clamp connections, showing that it is related to the Basidiomycetes (10, 11). These characteristics clearly distinguish it from the genera *Sporothrix* (see discussion of *Sporothrix*) and *Chrysosporium*.

Species of *Sporotrichum* are rarely, if ever, recovered in the clinical laboratory. Owing to the confusion that has surrounded this genus in the past, it is essentially impossible to determine the true identity of most of the isolates previously identified as species of *Sporotrichum* (152–154). Many of these fungi (212) may belong to such genera as *Exophiala*, *Chrysosporium*, *Sporothrix*, and *Beauveria*. *Sporotrichum* species are associated with woody plants.

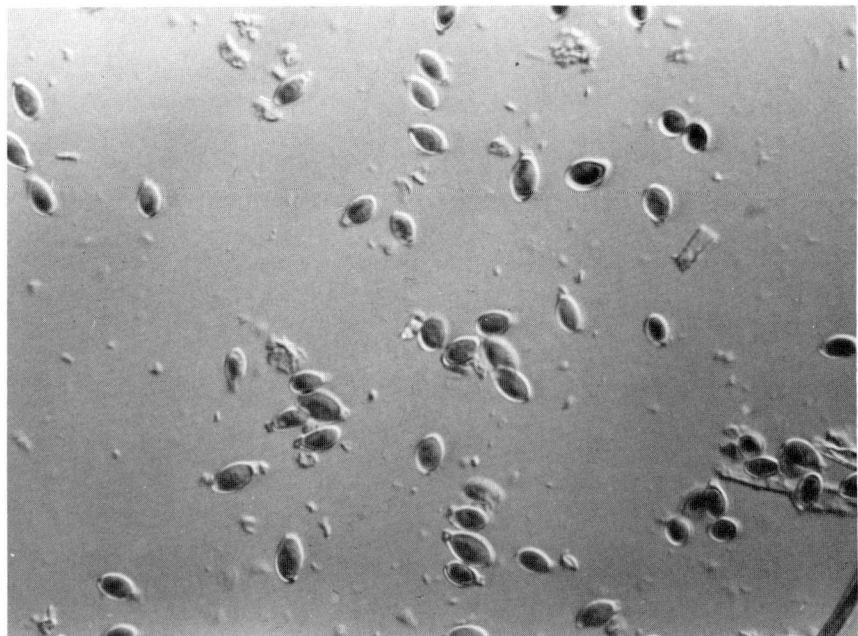

A

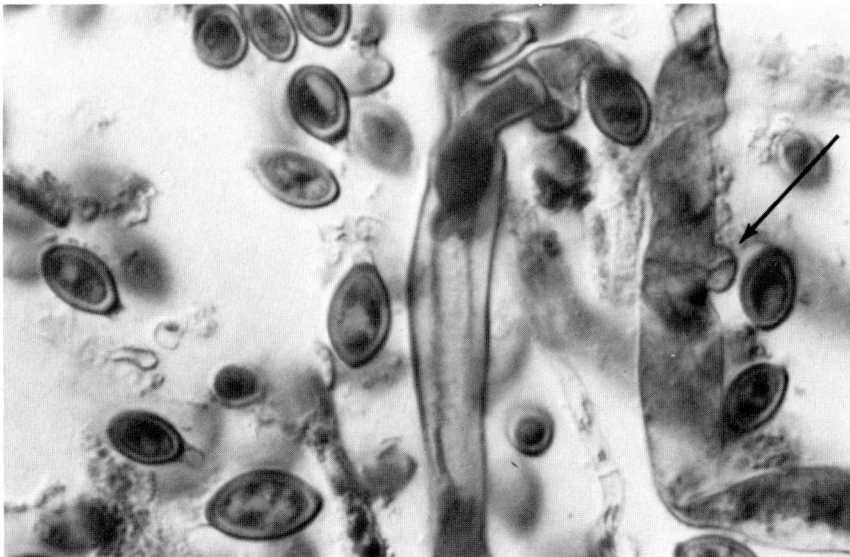

B

**Fig. 4.94** *Sporotrichum aureum*. The conidia are golden brown in color and arise from dark hyphae that have clamp connections (arrow). When the conidia separate from their conidiophores, an annular frill is usually formed.

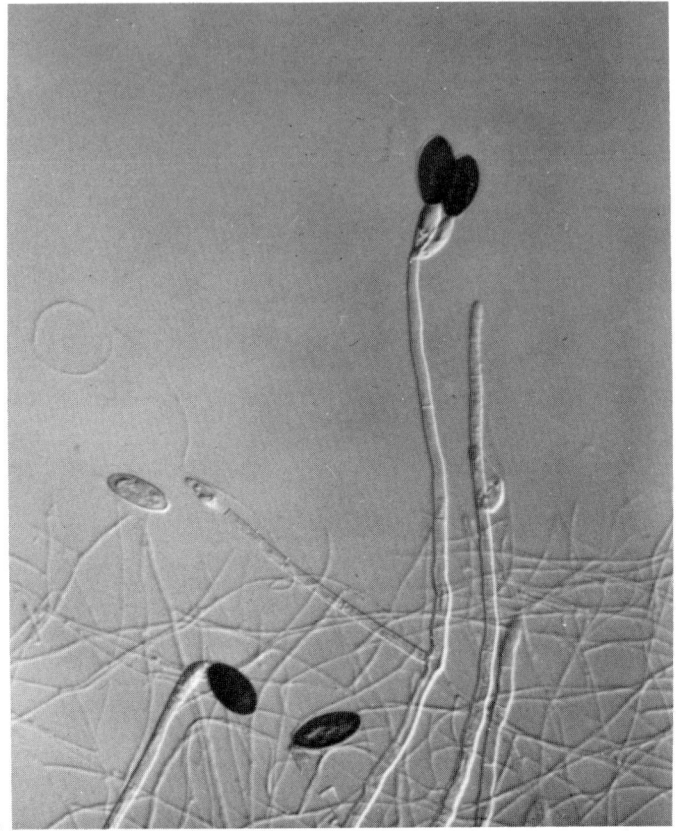

**Fig. 4.95** *Stachybotrys* sp. In species of *Stachybotrys*, dark, one-celled phialoconidia develop from phialides that are produced at the apices of erect conidiophores.

## *Stachybotrys* Corda, 1837

Diagnostic features: *Stachybotrys* species form septate, erect, smooth to rough, hyaline to brown conidiophores that arise from the vegetative hyphae. At the apex of the conidiophore, 3–10 cylindrical phialides with a swollen upper portion develop in a cluster. There is typically one central phialide with the other phialides forming around it (Fig. 4.95). The phialoconidia are hyaline to brown, 1-celled, smooth to rough, and slime down the phialides or form in chains.

Comments: The genera *Stachybotrys* and *Memnoniella* are extremely similar. Smith (202) believes that they are one and the same. Jong and Davis (110) have maintained them as separate genera based upon the ability of *Memnoniella* to form persistent chains of conidia, as well as a difference in the manner in which the phialoconidia mature.

## Part 3  Taxonomy

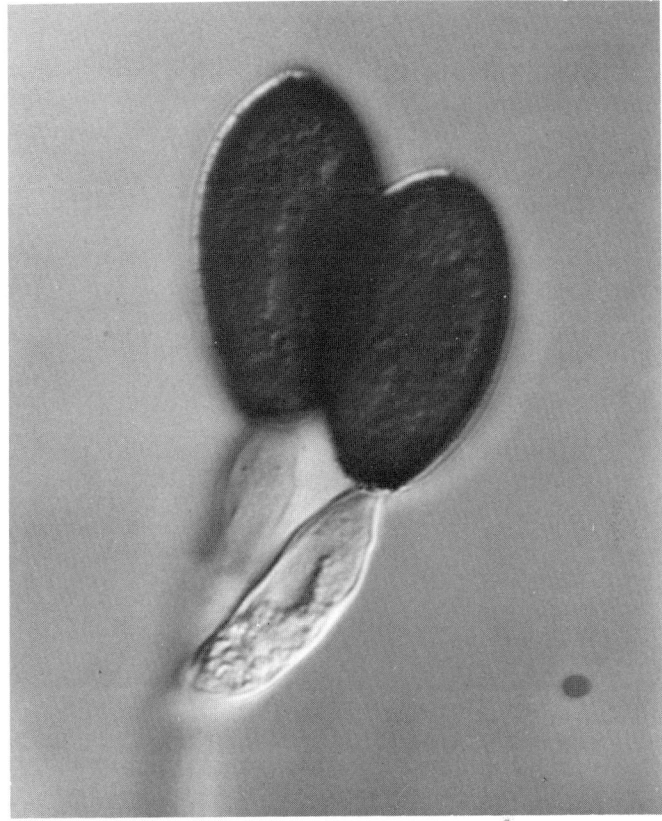

B

**Fig. 4.95** Continued

Isolates of *Stachybotrys* are infrequently encountered in the clinical laboratory. They are important in the area of veterinary medical mycology because they are the etiologic agents of stachybotryotoxicosis. The ascomycete *Melanopsamma pomiformis* produces a *Stachybotrys* anamorph.

### *Stemphylium* Wallroth, 1833

Diagnostic features: The genus *Stemphylium* is characterized by the development of simple or branched, septate, dematiaceous conidiophores with a swollen terminal portion upon which the conidia form. The conidiophore proliferates percurrently through the scar where the terminal poroconidium was formed. The conidia are solitary, muriform, pale brown to black, large, rough or smooth, and usually with a central constriction (Fig. 4.96).

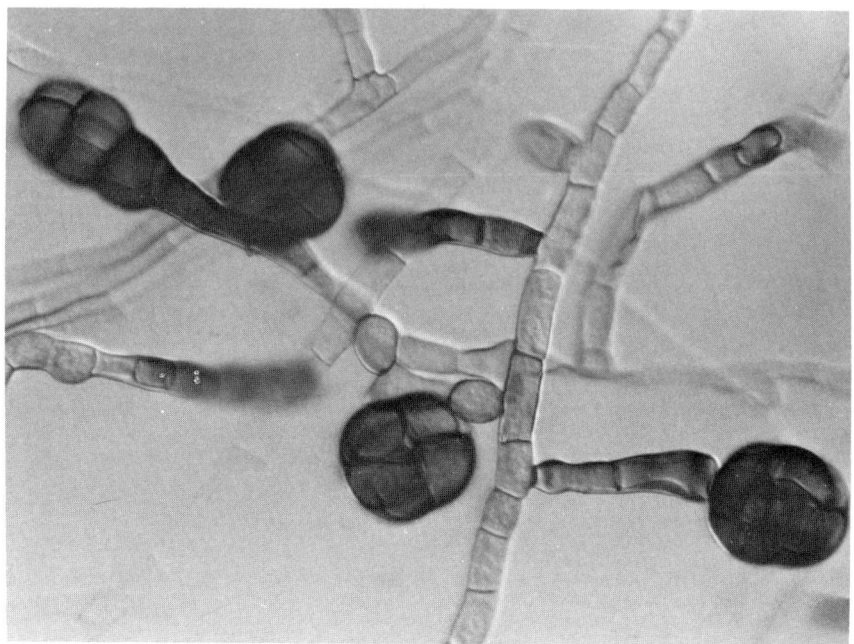

**Fig. 4.96** *Stemphylium sarcinaeforme*. The muriform conidia produced by this fungus are usually constricted in the middle. They arise from a conidiophore that proliferates percurrently.

Comments: *Stemphylium* (201) produces solitary, terminal poroconidia on a swollen conidiophore. The conidiophore increases in length by vegetatively growing through the scar where the conidium was attached. If the poroconidium is not completely broken free, it may remain attached laterally to the conidiophore as it elongates. The entire process is repeated, which results in a percurrent proliferation of the conidiophore. The conidiophore of *Stemphylium* usually has a series of swollen areas from which each conidium had originated.

Many medical mycologists have consistently confused the genera *Stemphylium* and *Ulocladium*. Isolates identified as *Stemphylium* are in nearly all instances *Ulocladium*, not *Stemphylium*. The genus *Ulocladium* produces muriform poroconidia from a sympodial conidiophore, not from a percurrent conidiogenous cell.

The isolation of *Stemphylium* in the clinical laboratory is rare. Members of the genus *Stemphylium* are primarily pathogens of higher plants, and occasionally they are associated with the soil. The ascomycete *Pleospora* may form a *Stemphylium* anamorph.

## *Stenella* Sydow, 1930

Diagnostic features: Species of *Stenella* form sympodial, simple or branched, septate, pale brown conidiophores that are straight or geniculate, with distinct conidial scars, and often a swollen apex. The blastoconidia are cylindrical to obclavate, truncate, verruculose, pale brown and 1- to 5-celled (2-celled are predominant) in loosely branching chains (Fig. 4.97).

Comments: *Stenella araguata* (= *Cladosporium castellanii*) is an etiologic agent of tinea nigra in South America. The genus *Stenella* is similar to *Cladosporium, Cercospora,* and several other fungi. *Stenella* is distinguished from these genera by its cylindrical, septate, verruculose blastoconidia arising as loosely branching chains from simple or sympodial conidiogenous cells. *Stenella araguata* is a common plant pathogen in some regions of South America. The genus is included in this handbook owing to its misidentification as *Cladosporium* in the past (145) and because *S. araguata* causes tinea nigra.

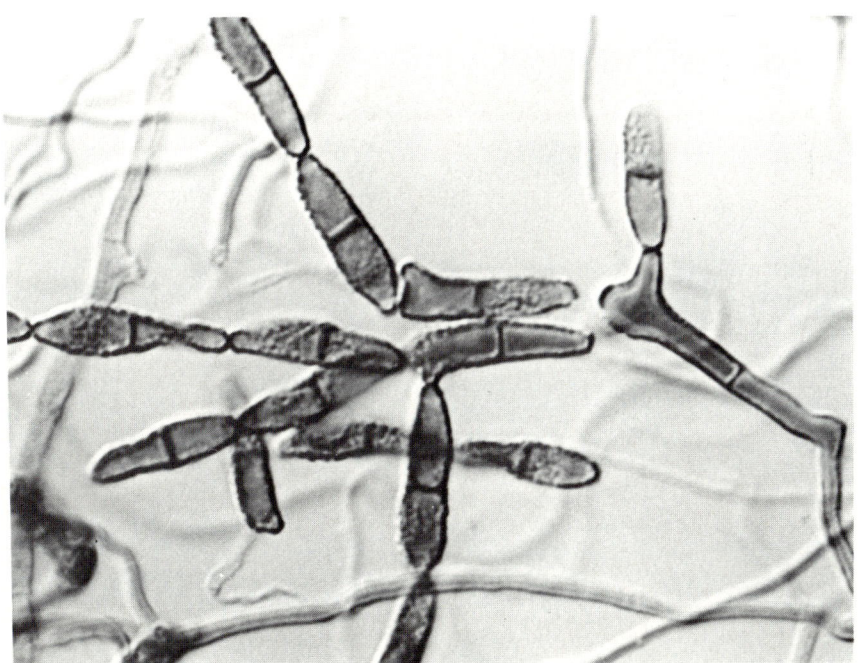

**Fig. 4.97** *Stenella araguata.* The multicelled, pale brown, verruculose blastoconidia form in loosely branching chains from sympodial conidiophores. (Reproduced by permission from *Mycotaxon* 7:415–418, 1978.)

## *Torula* Persoon ex Gray, 1821

Diagnostic features: Members of the genus *Torula* produce short, erect hyphalike conidiophores that have a swollen, subglobose apical cell. The apical cell is darkly pigmented with a thick cell wall, and functions as the conidiogenous cell. From these cells, there arise straight to curved, cylindrical, with rounded ends, 3- to 15-celled, thick-walled, pale brown to black, verrucose holoblastic conidia. Each conidium has a constriction at each septum. The terminal cell of the conidium usually functions as a conidiogenous cell, producing a second conidium. Such development results in simple to branching chains of dry conidia (Fig. 4.98).

Comments: The genus *Torula* is of special interest to medical mycologists because a number of medically important fungi have been classified in this genus at one time or another. Until the studies by Ellis and Griffiths (59) and Crane and Schoknecht (54), the mode of conidiogenesis remained confused. In the past, essentially all fungi that either formed dematiaceous toruloid hyphae or black phragmoconidia from undifferentiated hyphae were classified in *Torula* or its synonym *Hormiscium*. Reevaluation of many species assigned to the genus *Torula* has shown that they actually belong in other genera, such as *Bispora, Coniosporium, Eversia, Gliomastix,*

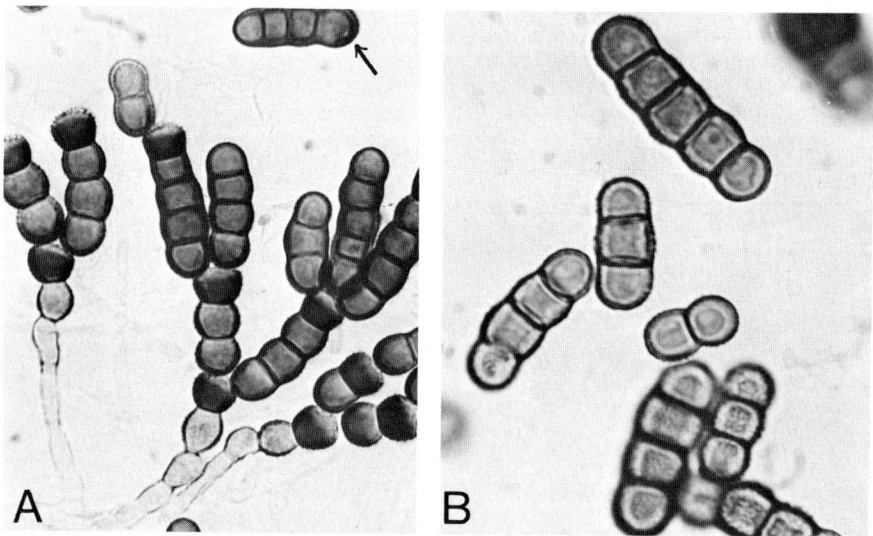

**Fig. 4.98** *Torula herbarum*. The poroconidia are produced in branching chains that break up into phragmoconidia. The pore can be seen (arrow) at the base of one of the conidia. (Reproduced by permission of G. L. Barron and Williams & Wilkins Co. from "The Genera of Hyphomycetes from Soil," 1969.)

*Papulaspora, Rutola, Xylohypha,* and others. The key characteristic of *Torula* is the darkly pigmented, thick-walled conidiogenous cells that occur at the apex of the conidiophore and conidia.

*Torula* is seldom, if ever, isolated in the clinical laboratory. Fungi such as species of *Exophiala, Eversia, Rutola, Wangiella,* and *Xylohypha* may occasionally be confused with, or misidentified as, species of *Torula*. *Torula* is associated with soil and woody plant material.

## *Torulomyces* Delitsch, 1943

Diagnostic features: *Torulomyces* species produce long, dry chains of 1-celled, hyaline to lightly pigmented, globose, smooth to echinulate phialoconidia. The phialides are cylindrical, with a swollen middle portion that gently tapers toward the apex. The phialides are solitary, arising on a distinct, short, cylindrical, hyphalike conidiophore (Fig. 4.99).

Comments: The genera *Acremonium, Monocillium, Sagrahamala,* and *Torulomyces* represent a continuum of phialides and phialoconidia. Hashmi *et al.* (83) have suggested that *Monocillium* should be considered to

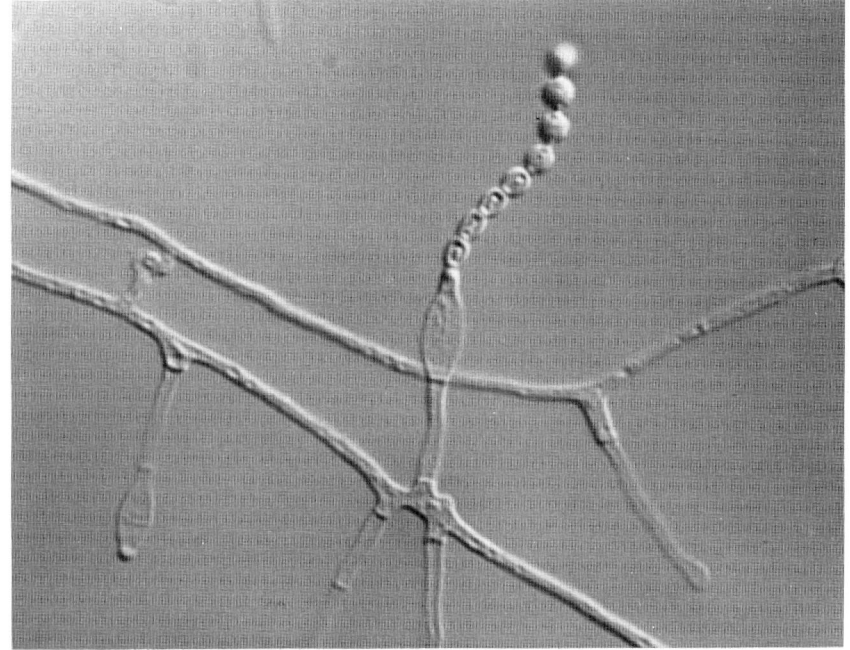

**Fig. 4.99** *Torulomyces lagena.* A and B. The phialoconidia occur in chains that arise from phialides that are swollen. Each phialide is on a hyphalike conidiophore.

be a synonym of *Torulomyces*. The ellipsoidal to obovoid phialoconidia, with truncate bases, and long, cylindrical phialides with a swollen central portion and a wavy apical region, arising directly from the hyphae without distinct conidiophores, distinguish *Monocillium* from *Torulomyces*. The shape of the phialides and production of globose phialoconidia in chains separate *Torulomyces* from *Acremonium* and *Sagrahamala*.

*Torulomyces* isolates are occasionally recovered in the clinical laboratory. Members of this genus are primarily soil fungi.

*Trichoderma* Persoon ex Gray, 1821

Diagnostic features: The colonies produced by isolates of *Trichoderma* are very distinctive. Isolates are rapid growing, at first white and flat, later

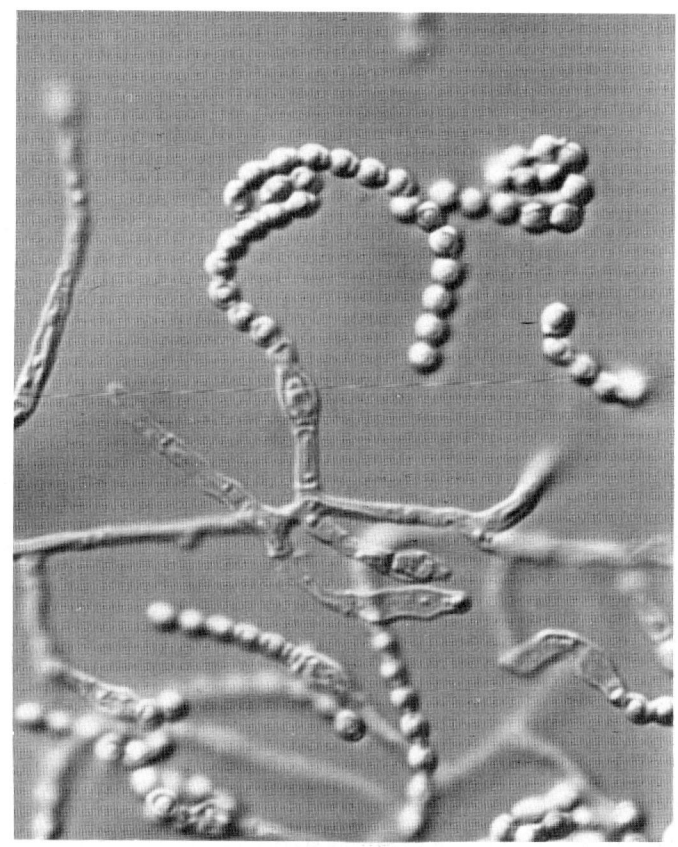

**Fig. 4.99** Continued

developing green compact tufts. The conidiophores are usually erect, solitary or in compact tufts that arise at wide angles to the hyphae, usually forming in concentric ringlike zones on the medium surface. The phialides are solitary or in clusters, hyaline, ovoid to flask-shaped, and swollen at the center portion tapering toward the apex. They arise at wide angles to each other in the clusters, as well as from the conidiophores. Phialoconidia are 1-celled, hyaline to green, subglobose to oblong, smooth to echinulate, and form in balls at the phialide apex (Fig. 4.100).

Comments: Members of the genus *Trichoderma* (175) are occasionally encountered in the clinical laboratory. *Trichoderma* is an extremely common fungus. Some species of *Hypocrea, Podostroma,* and similar genera may produce a *Trichoderma* anamorph.

## *Trichophyton* Malmsten, 1845

Diagnostic features: The genus *Trichophyton* is characterized by the development of macro- and microconidia that form at the apex of hyaline conidiophores, which usually arise at right angles to the parent hypha. The

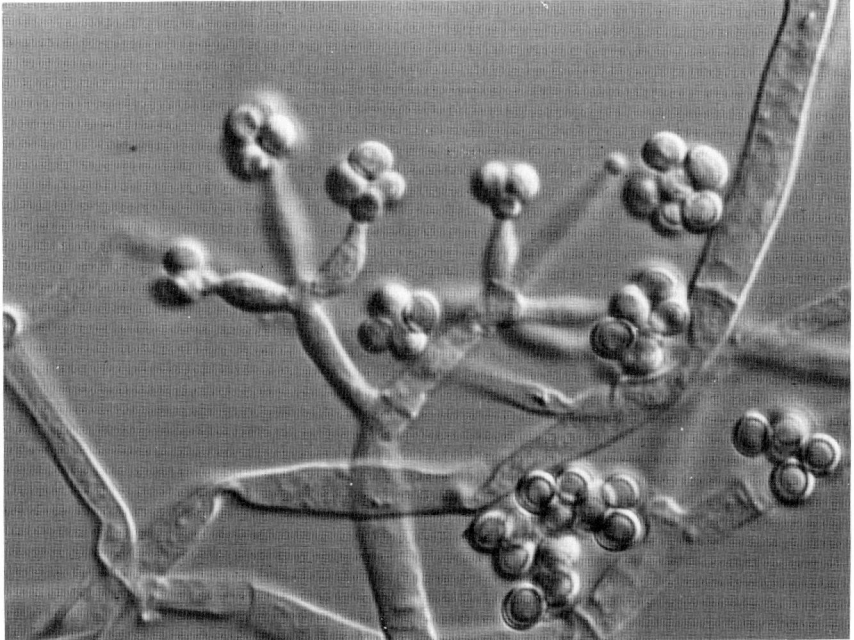

**Fig. 4.100** *Trichoderma viride.* The phialides arise at wide angles to the conidiophores. They are swollen in the central portion, tapering toward the apex. The one-celled phialoconidia accumulate in balls at the apices of the phialides.

macroconidia are usually cylindrical to clavate, several-celled, and smooth with a thin cell wall. The microconidia are typically 1-celled, but may have more than 1-cell in some species, and are smooth with a thin cell wall.

Comments: The majority of isolates of *Trichophyton* recovered from patients do not have macroconidia. As a result of this problem, medical mycologists rely upon the morphology of the microconidia for identification. This has been successful because the morphology of the microconidia is distinctive from one species to the next. When macroconidia are present, they are quite different from those produced by species of *Microsporum*.

Unlike *Microsporum*, the macroconidia of *Trichophyton* are cylindrical to clavate, and smooth with thin cell walls. *Trichophyton ajelloi* (Fig. 4.101) appears to be a transition species since it produces macroconidia that have thick cell walls like those found in some species of *Microsporum*. Owing to this characteristic, some medical mycologists in the past used the generic name *Keratinomyces* for *T. ajelloi* in order to denote that this fungus has some characteristics in common with both *Trichophyton* and *Microsporum*. The genus *Keratinomyces* is unnecessary since *T. ajelloi* can be nicely accommodated in *Trichophyton*. The genus *Trichophyton* superficially resembles the genus *Epidermophyton* but it can be distinguished from *Epi-*

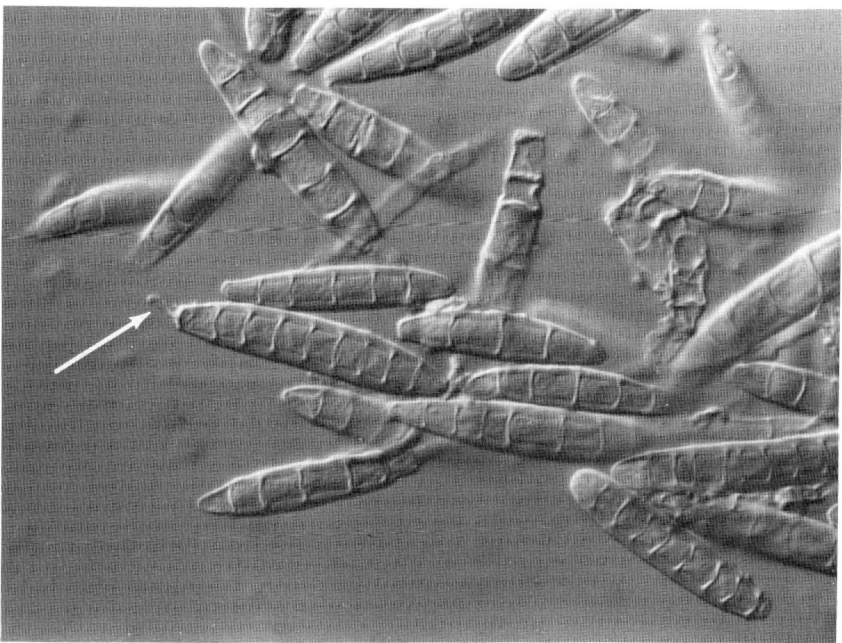

**Fig. 4.101** *Trichophyton ajelloi*. Macroconidia. An annular frill can be seen (arrow) at the base of one of the conidia.

*dermophyton* by having thin-walled macroconidia that do not occur in groups. In addition, *Epidermophyton* does not form microconidia.

Spirals, pectinate organs, nodular organs, chandeliers, racquet hyphae, and other vegetative structures are occasionally seen in some isolates of *Trichophyton*. These vegetative structures are not diagnostic for any one particular species. They are also produced by isolates of many other fungi. Colony color and morphology is a more useful characteristic for identifying dermatophytes. It is important to base colony descriptions on isolates grown on Sabouraud dextrose agar containing 4% glucose and neopeptone. This is a close approximation of the medium that the early medical mycologists used when they first described these fungi. Dermatophyte test medium (DTM) is excellent for the recovery of dermatophytes when the possibility of bacterial contamination is great, but it should be used neither for determining colony characteristics nor for microscopic morphology. Fungi on this medium are atypical.

The principal members of this genus isolated in the clinical laboratory include *T. mentagrophytes* (Fig. 4.102), *T. rubrum* (Fig. 4.103), and *T. tonsurans* (Fig. 4.104). *Trichophyton mentagrophytes* typically produces globose to subglobose microconidia that may occur either in clusters or along the hyphae, or both. Like *T. mentagrophytes, T. rubrum* produces microconidia either in clusters or along the hyphae, or both. The

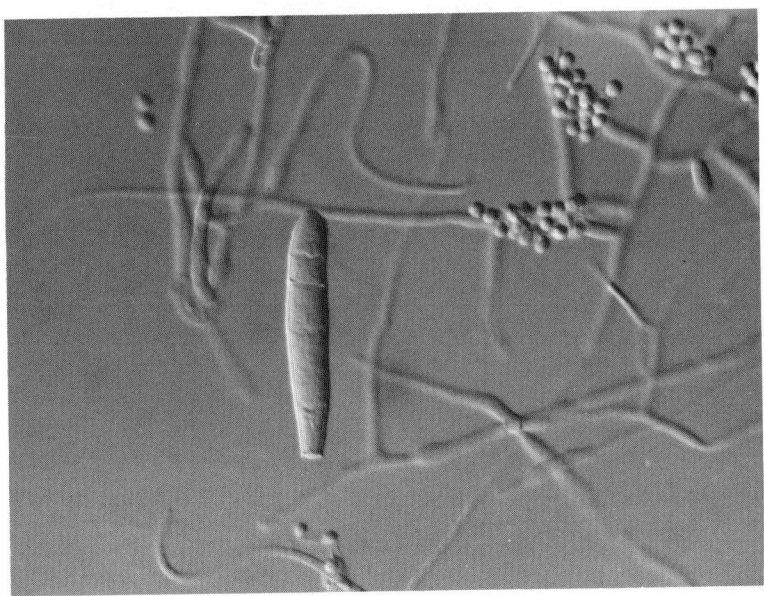

**Fig. 4.102** *Trichophyton mentagrophytes.* A. Both macro- and microconidia are formed by some isolates. B and C. The microconidia are typically globose.

microconidia of *T. rubrum* tend to be more elongate and clavate. It often becomes difficult, if not impossible on morphological grounds, to identify an isolate with subglobose to clavate microconidia. In this instance, the *in vitro* hair test becomes a valuable differential test, in which *T. mentagrophytes* is positive and *T. rubrum* is negative. Many microbiologists use a urea hydrolysis test in lieu of the *in vitro* hair test because it requires only a few days. Extreme caution must be exercised when using the production of urease within 5–7 days as a diagnostic feature of *T. mentagrophytes*. The data in Table 4.13 clearly illustrate the variability of *T. mentagrophytes* and *T. rubrum*. Both these species are readily distinguishable from *T. tonsurans*, which produces microconidia that vary from swollen, globose, balloon-like to long, narrow, and gradually tapering toward the base (resembling matchsticks). Nutritional data (75, 166) are often helpful in distinguishing some species of *Trichophyton* (Tables 4.13 and 4.14).

The colonies produced by species of *Trichophyton* are distinctive (Table 4.15). At least two basic colony types may be isolated, that is, granular and downy. The granular type of colony is associated with isolates that are

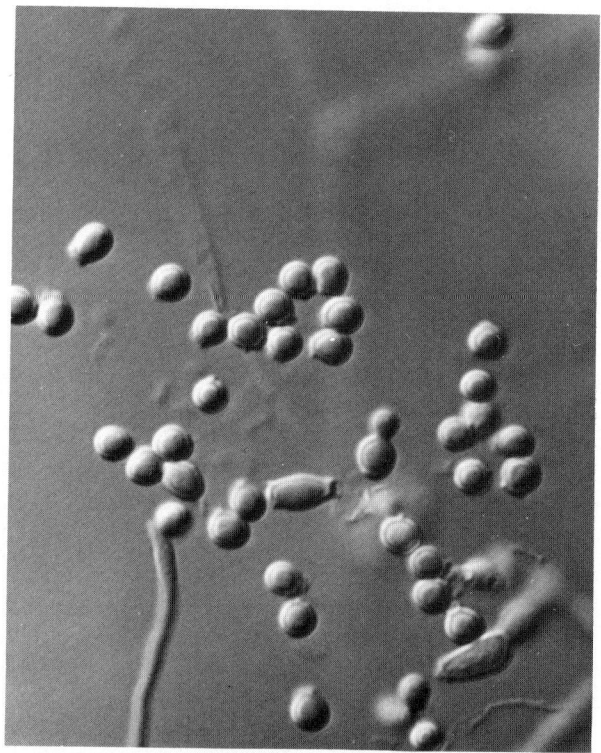

**Fig. 4.102** Continued

Part 3  Taxonomy

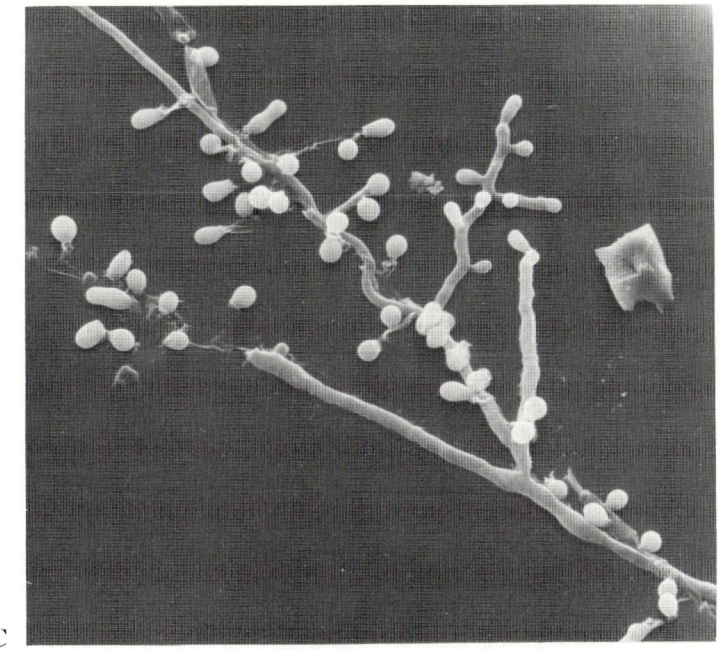

C

Fig. 4.102  Continued

producing large amounts of conidia, usually both macro- and microconidia. In contrast, downy colonies usually characterize isolates that are forming conidia sparely. The transition from a granular to sterile-downy colony is usually referred to as becoming pleomorphic.

Isolates of *Trichophyton* (2, 5, 71, 172, 215) are rarely seen in most clinical laboratories. Hair, nail, and skin specimens are typically handled by the dermatologist, not the clinical laboratory. On rare occasions, soil isolates of *Trichophyton* are recovered in the clinical laboratory. For those species of *Trichophyton* that can reproduce sexually, all have been found to produce gymnothecia characteristic of the genus *Arthroderma* (Table 4.16).

*Trichothecium* Link ex Gray, 1821

Diagnostic features: Pale rose, rapidly growing, granular colonies with alternating 2-celled conidia held together in a chain are characteristic of members of the genus *Trichothecium*. The conidiophores are indistinguishable from the vegetative hyphae until the first conidium is produced. They are erect, retrogressive, solitary or in clusters, simple or branched, hyaline,

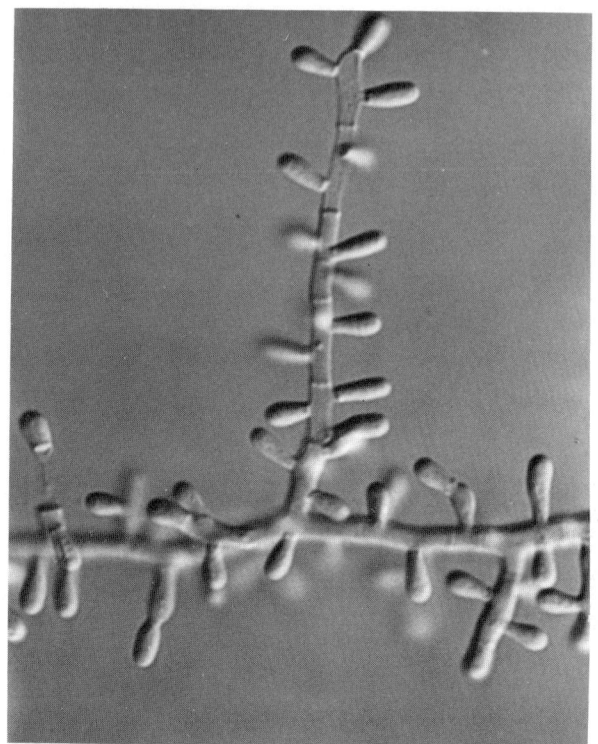

**Fig. 4.103** *Trichophyton rubrum*. The microconidia are clavate in this species.

and septate. The 2-celled, clavate to ovoid conidia are hyaline to lightly pigmented and are held together by cell wall material (Fig. 4.105).

Comments: Kendrick and Cole (115) clarified the method by which species of *Trichothecium* produced their conidia. The apex of the conidiophore swells and produces a 2-celled holoblastic conidium. Without additional elongation or growth, the conidiophore swells just below the conidium forming a second enteroblastic conidium. The process is repeated, which results in an alternate chain of conidia held together by cell wall material and a conidiophore that becomes shorter with subsequent development of conidia (retrogressive development). As conidia form, the bases of the youngest conidia are broader that the bases of the terminal, older conidia. The cell wall material connecting the conidia actually represents a collarette.

Isolates of *Trichothecium* (176) are occasionally seen in the clinical laboratory. Members of this genus are soil fungi and have been associated with the ascomycete *Hypomyces*.

Part 3 Taxonomy

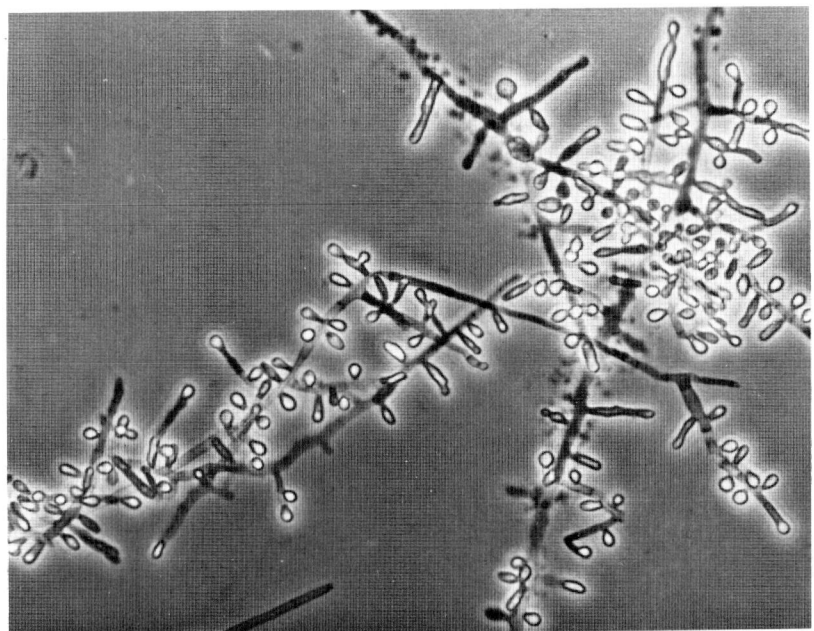

**Fig. 4.104** *Trichophyton tonsurans*. The conidia are extremely variable in size and shape. They range from subglobose to balloon-shaped to matchsticklike.

### *Trichurus* Clements et Shear, 1896

Diagnostic features: Members of the genus *Trichurus* form a synnema having a sterile stalk with the region of conidiogenesis restricted to the upper portion of the fruiting body. The conidiogenous cells are annellides. The annelloconidia are 1-celled, smooth or rough, catenulate, globose to ovoid, and usually truncate at the base. Sterile setae arise from the synnemata (Fig. 4.106).

Comments: *Trichurus* (80, 149) and *Cephalotrichum* (= *Doratomyces*) are essentially identical fungi with the exception that *Trichurus* has setae. Isolates of *Trichurus* are rarely encountered in the clinical laboratory. When they are, a *Scopulariopsis* anamorph is typically present too.

### *Tritirachium* Limber, 1940

Diagnostic features: The genus *Tritirachium* is characterized by the development of erect conidiophores that produce simple to verticillate, septate branches, upon which whorls of conidiogenous cells form. The conidiogenous cells are long, narrow, with a slight swelling at their bases, and without denticles. The geniculate rachis develops sympodially (Fig. 4.107). The conidia are 1-celled, hyaline, smooth and subglobose to ovoid.

Comments: The genera *Tritirachium* (95) and *Beauveria* are similar in that they both form delicate sympodial conidiogenous cells with a long rachis. Species of *Beauveria* are distinguished from *Tritirachium* by their sympodial cells being swollen at the base, occurring in dense clusters, and having a rachis with denticles upon which the conidia develop.

Isolates of *Tritirachium* are occasionally recovered in the clinical laboratory. Members of this genus are associated with soil and woody plant material.

## *Ulocladium* Preuss, 1851

Diagnostic features: Species of *Ulocladium* produce brown, simple to occasionally branched, septate, sympodial conidiophores that are geniculate. The poroconidia are muriform, obovoid, solitary, brown to black, smooth to rough, variable in size, and without a central constriction (Fig. 4.108).

Comments: *Ulocladium* (64, 65, 201) is important to medical mycologists because species of this genus are often misidentified as *Stemphylium*. The percurrent proliferation through the scar of the previous poroconidium at the swollen apex of the conidiophore readily distinguishes *Stemphylium* from *Ulocladium*. *Ulocladium* is somewhat similar to *Alternaria* in that both genera may form sympodial conidiogenous cells. The chains of poroconidia with distinct beaks that are formed by *Alternaria* are distinctively different from the obovoid, solitary poroconidia of *Ulocladium*.

Isolates of *Ulocladium* are occasionally recovered in the clinical laboratory. Most species of *Ulocladium* are soil fungi.

## *Verticillium* Nees ex Steudel, 1824

Diagnostic features: Members of the genus *Verticillium* produce erect conidiophores that are hyaline to lightly pigmented, simple or branched. The branching occurs at several levels, and in whorls (verticillate). Lageniform, hyaline phialides arise from the apex of the whorled branches. Phialoconidia are 1-celled, hyaline, ovoid-to-cylindrical-to-allantoid, and form in a ball at the apex of the phialide (Fig. 4.109). Chlamydospores and solitary conidia may be present.

Comments: Species of *Verticillium* (72, 105) are extremely common soil fungi. Occasionally, isolates of *Verticillium* can be confused with species of *Acremonium*. In these instances, the typical verticillate arrangement of the phialides and conidiophore branches may not be readily visible. A careful

**Table 4.13.** Nutritional Tests for the Identification of the More Common Species of *Trichophyton*[a]

A. Assimilation of carbon compounds[b]

| Species | No. of isolates tested | L-Arabinose | Dextrin | Erythritol | D-Galactose | D-Glucitol | Glycerol | Maltose | Ribitol | Ribose | Sucrose | Trehalose |
|---|---|---|---|---|---|---|---|---|---|---|---|---|
| *T. ajelloi* | 4 | 0 | 0 | 100 | 0 | 100 | 0 | 100 | 100 | 50 | 50 | 0 |
| *T. equinum* | 6 | 0 | 0 | 100 | 0 | 83 | 33 | 100 | 0 | 0 | 100 | 100 |
| *T. megninii* | 4 | 0 | 25 | 100 | 50 | 100 | 75 | 75 | 0 | 0 | 100 | 100 |
| *T. mentagrophytes* | 24 | 0 | 0 | 75 | 38 | 75 | 0 | 100 | 38 | 0 | 100 | 96 |
| *T. rubrum* | 9 | 11 | 0 | 89 | 100 | 89 | 11 | 100 | 0 | 0 | 100 | 100 |
| *T. schoenleinii* | 6 | 17 | 33 | 0 | 17 | 100 | 100 | 50 | 17 | 83 | 17 | 0 |
| *T. soudanense* | 9 | 0 | 67 | 100 | 0 | 100 | 0 | 100 | 22 | 11 | 100 | 100 |
| *T. terrestre* | 6 | 0 | 33 | 100 | 0 | 100 | 0 | 100 | 100 | 17 | 100 | 100 |
| *T. tonsurans* | 17 | 0 | 18 | 100 | 53 | 100 | 18 | 100 | 12 | 18 | 88 | 88 |
| *T. verrucosum* | 6 | 83 | 0 | 17 | 33 | 100 | 83 | 100 | 100 | 100 | 83 | 100 |
| *T. violaceum* | 6 | 17 | 67 | 0 | 17 | 100 | 67 | 17 | 17 | 0 | 0 | 100 |

*Continued*

[a] Reproduced and modified by permission of C. Philpot from *Sabouraudia* **15**:141–150, 1977.
[b] Values equal percentage positive of isolates tested.

**Table 4.13.** *Continued*

B. Hydrolysis of urea[c]

| Species | No. of isolates tested | Days to become positive | | | | | Negative |
|---|---|---|---|---|---|---|---|
| | | 0–7 | 8–10 | 11–14 | 15–21 | Over 21 | |
| T. equinum | 6 | 100 | 0 | 0 | 0 | 0 | 0 |
| T. megninii | 5 | 20 | 80 | 0 | 0 | 0 | 0 |
| T. mentagrophytes[d] | 204 | 75 | 4 | 1 | 0 | 0 | 20 |
| T. rubrum | 110 | 8 | 17 | 22 | 25 | 11 | 17 |
| T. schoenleinii | 8 | 13 | 0 | 39 | 26 | 13 | 13 |
| T. simii | 9 | 78 | 11 | 11 | 0 | 0 | 0 |
| T. soudanense | 22 | 0 | 0 | 0 | 0 | 0 | 100 |
| T. terrestre | 18 | 44 | 28 | 28 | 0 | 0 | 0 |
| T. tonsurans | 36 | 50 | 30 | 17 | 3 | 0 | 0 |
| T. verrucosum | 10 | 0 | 0 | 70 | 30 | 0 | 0 |
| T. violaceum | 7 | 0 | 0 | 0 | 43 | 43 | 14 |

[c] Values equal percentage positive of isolates tested.
[d] Includes *T. erinacei*, *T. quinckeanum*, and *T. mentagrophytes*.

Part 3  Taxonomy

**Table 4.14.** Nutritional Patterns for Groups of Similar Species of *Trichophyton*[a]

A. *T. concentricum*, *T. schoenleinii*, and *T. verrucosum*[b, c]

| Species | | Casein | Casein–inositol | Casein–thiamine | Casein–thiamine and inositol |
|---|---|---|---|---|---|
| *T. concentricum* | 50% | 4+ | 4+ | 4+ | 4+ |
|  | 50% | 2+ | 2+ | 4+ | 4+ |
| *T. schoenleinii* |  | 4+ | 4+ | 4+ | 4+ |
| *T. verrucosum* | 84% | 0 | ± | 0 | 4+ |
|  | 16% | 0 | 0 | 4+ | 4+ |

[a] Reproduced and modified by permission of L. Ajello from "Laboratory manual for medical mycology," USPHS, 1966.

[b] This is a 4-tube test incubated at 37°C and read after 7–14 days.

[c] ± Indicates a trace of submerged growth about the inoculum; 4+ indicates maximum growth for that series of tubes, growth on other tubes being judged by comparison.

B. *T. mentagrophytes*, *T. rubrum*, and *T. tonsurans*[d]

| Species | Casein | Casein–thiamine |
|---|---|---|
| *T. mentagrophytes* | 4+ | 4+ |
| *T. rubrum* | 4+ | 4+ |
| *T. tonsurans* | ± to 1+ | 4+ |

[d] This is a 2-tube test incubated at room temperature and read after 7–10 days.

C. *Microsporum gallinae* and *T. megninii*[e]

| Species | $NH_4NO_3$ | $NH_4NO_3$ + histidine |
|---|---|---|
| *M. gallinae* | 4+ | 4+ |
| *T. megninii* | 0 | 4+ |

[e] No other dermatophyte shows this regular requirement for histidine.

*(Continued)*

**Table 4.14.** *Continued*

D. *T. equinum* and *T. mentagrophytes*[f]

| Species | Casein | Casein + nicotinic acid |
|---|---|---|
| *T. equinum* | 0 | 4 + |
| *T. mentagrophytes* | 4 + | 4 + |

[f] No other dermatophyte shows this requirement for nicotinic acid.

E. *Microsporum ferrugineum* and *T. violaceum*

| Species | Casein | Casein + thiamine |
|---|---|---|
| *M. ferrugineum* | 4 + | 4 + |
| *T. violaceum* | ± | 4 + |

search of several microscope fields and observation of the colony surface with a dissecting microscope should clarify any confusion. Other hyphomycetes, such as species of *Diheterospora* and *Sepedonium*, may form a *Verticillium* anamorph.

Isolates of *Verticillium* are infrequently seen in the clinical laboratory. The ascomycete *Nectria* may form a *Verticillium* anamorph.

## *Wangiella* McGinnis, 1977

Diagnostic features: Distinct conidiophores are absent in *Wangiella*. The phialides are light brown, lageniform to flask-shaped, without collarettes, and intercalary or terminal. The phialoconidia are pale brown, 1-celled, smooth, subglobose to obovoid, and accumulating in a ball at the apex of the phialide (Fig. 4.110). Annellides may be present as an additional anamorph. Toruloid hyphae and yeast cells are typically present.

Comments: The genus *Wangiella* (137, 138) was established for the agent of phaeohyphomycosis originally described as *Hormiscium dermatitidis* (137). De Hoog (97) classified this fungus in the genus *Exophiala*, because he considered the annellides to be the most distinct conidiogenous cells. The genus *Wangiella* is preferred for *W. dermatitidis* instead of *Exophiala* because the phialides without collarettes (light microscopy), yeastlike colonies, toruloid hyphae, conspicuous yeast form, and thermotolerance are extremely stable, unique, and distinctive. Isolates of *Wangiella* can be

**Table 4.15.** Cultural Characteristics of Selected Species of *Trichophyton* on Sabouraud Dextrose Agar[a]

| Species | Macroscopic | Microscopic |
| --- | --- | --- |
| *T. equinum* | Colonies rapid growing, at first flat, becoming folded with age. White with bright yellow color near edge, becoming velvety and cream to tan in color. Reverse color bright yellow, later pink to red-brown. All isolates require nicotinic acid | Microconidia rare to abundant, pyriform to clavate. Macroconidia rare, cylindrical with rounded ends |
| *T. mentagrophytes* | Colonies rapid growing, flat, raised to irregularly folded, granular to cottony, white to cream colored, occasionally yellow. Reverse color rose-brown, occasionally yellow-orange to deep red | Microconidia numerous, globose to subglobose, in clusters, along the hyphae on short conidiophores, or both. Macroconidia rare to abundant, 2- to 5-celled, thin-walled, cylindrical to clavate. Spirals and nodular bodies may be numerous |
| *T. rubrum* | Colonies slow to rapid growing, flat to raised, granular to cottony, becoming folded. White to cream, becoming deep rose. Reverse red to purple-red, which usually disappears in subcultures. In occasional isolates, reverse color may be yellow-orange | Microconidia rare in cottony isolates, abundant in granular isolates, clavate, 1-celled, along hyphae, and in groups. Macroconidia absent to rare, common in granular isolates, cylindrical, with parallel walls, blunt ends and 3- to 8-celled |
| *T. schoenleinii* | Colonies slow growing, irregularly raised and folded, leathery, tending to crack the agar. Either white to tan, glabrous to waxy or white, granular to velvety. Some isolates largely submerged in the agar. Growth at 37°C | Microconidia absent to rare, 1-celled, clavate. Mycelium variable, chandeliers common, chlamydospores typically present |

*(Continued)*

**Table 4.15.** *Continued*

| Species | Macroscopic | Microscopic |
| --- | --- | --- |
| T. tonsurans | Colonies slow growing, raised, glabrous to granular, flat to raised, later becoming folded, often with a depressed center. Colonies are cream to tan or yellow to rose, reverse color yellow to mahogany red. Growth enhanced by thiamine | Microconidia numerous, 1- to several-celled, clavate to large and irregular with age, commonly being swollen like balloons or elongated like matchsticks. Macroconidia rare, walls somewhat thickened, poorly formed. Arthroconidia and chlamydospores may be present |
| T. verrucosum | Colonies extremely slow growing, requiring 10–14 days before new growth is visible, usually small, raised to folded, occasionally flat and disk-shaped, glabrous to waxy, later becoming powdery, white to yellow. Most isolates require thiamine and inositol, others require thiamine only. Growth more rapid at 37°C | At 25°C, irregular mycelium with chlamydospores. At 37°C, chlamydospores numerous, catenulate. Microconidia numerous on media containing thiamine, 1-celled, clavate, formed along the hyphae. Macroconidia rare, 3- to 5-celled, elongated, narrow, variable in shape and size |
| T. violaceum | Colonies extremely slow-growing, raised, granular, surface glabrous. Cream to off-white, then lavender, becoming deep purple. Old cultures may lose their purple color. Growth enhanced by thiamine | Microconidia absent to rare, when present, 1-celled, clavate. Macroconidia absent to rare, when present, poorly developed, resembling thickened hyphal branches. Conidia usually produced in the presence of thiamine |

[a] Reproduced and modified by permission of L. Ajello from "Laboratory Manual of Medical Mycology," USPHS, 1966.

Part 3  Taxonomy

Table 4.16  The Genus *Trichophyton*

| Anamorph | Teleomorph |
| --- | --- |
| *T. ajelloi* | *Arthroderma uncinatum* |
| *T. concentricum* | Unknown |
| *T. equinum* | Unknown |
| *T. fischeri* | Unknown |
| *T. flavescens* | *A. flavescens* |
| *T. georgiae* | *A. ciferrii* |
| *T. gloriae* | *A. gloriae* |
| *T. gourvilii* | Unknown |
| *T. longifusus* | Unknown |
| *T. megninii* | Unknown |
| *T. mentagrophytes* | *A. benhamiae, A. vanbreuseghemii* |
| *T. phaseoliforme* | Unknown |
| *T. rubrum* | Unknown |
| *T. schoenleinii* | Unknown |
| *T. simii* | *A. simii* |
| *T. soudanense* | Unknown |
| *T. terrestre* | *A. insingulare, A. lenticularum, A. quadrifidum* |
| *T. tonsurans* | Unknown |
| *T. vanbreuseghemii* | *A. gertleri* |
| *T. verrucosum* | Unknown |
| *T. violaceum* | Unknown |

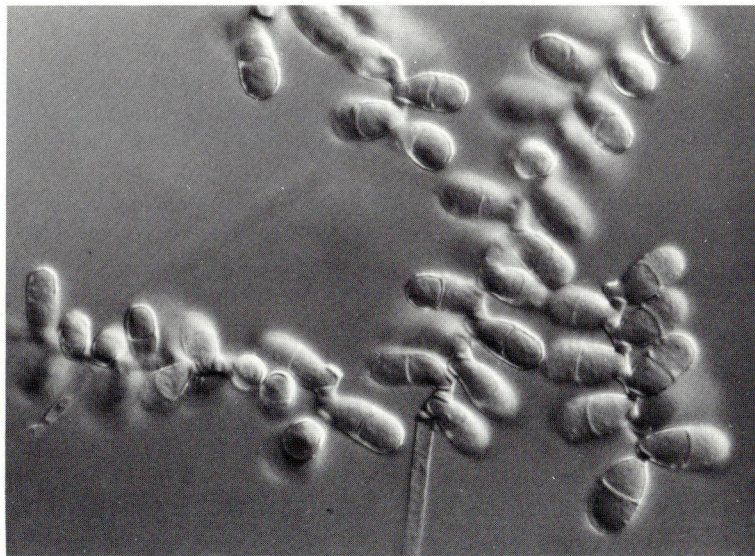

**Fig. 4.105** *Trichothecium roseum.* A and B. The alternating two-celled, clavate conidia held together at their bases are characteristic of this fungus.

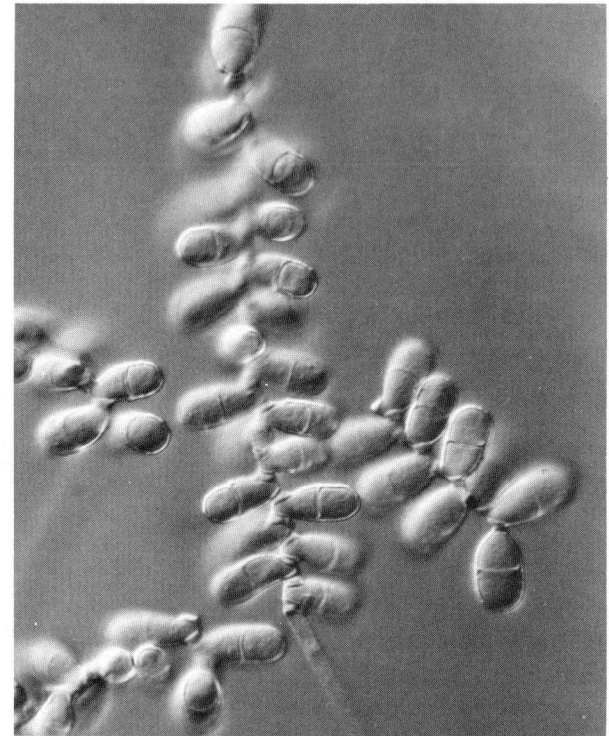

**Fig. 4.105** Continued

distinguished from similar dematiaceous hyphomycetes by their ability to grow at 40°C (165). *Wangiella* is distinguished from *Exophiala* by the production of phialides without collarettes (light microscopy). *Wangiella dermatitidis* produces a *Phaeococcus* yeast form.

Members of this genus are occasionally recovered in the clinical laboratory.

## ZYGOMYCETES

### *Absidia* van Tieghem, 1876

Diagnostic features: Members of the genus *Absidia* produce branched stolons that are curved into arches. At the node, rhizoids are typically produced. Sporangiophores arise in groups of 2 to 5 (rarely solitarily) at the internode, but never at the node. The sporangia are pyriform with a slight swelling in the sporangiophore at the point where the sporangial wall

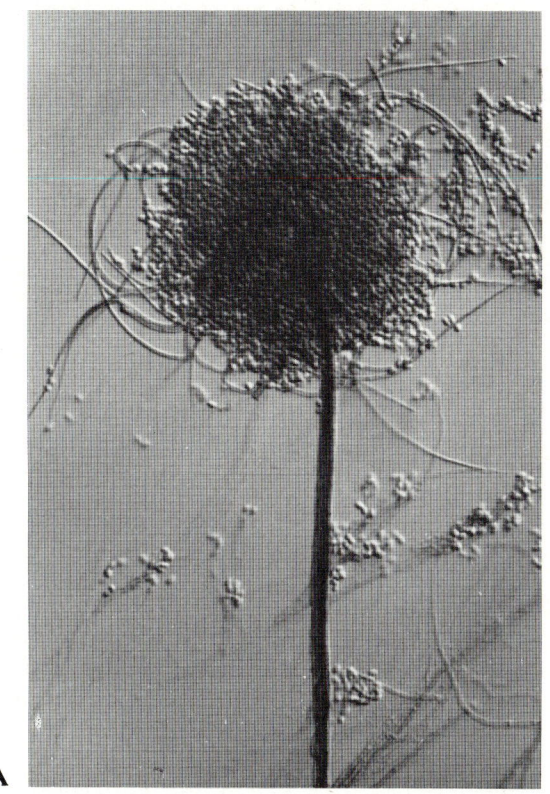

**Fig. 4.106** *Trichurus spiralis.* A and B. The synnema has sterile setae arising from among the annellides. The annelloconidia occur in chains.

originates. The swelling merges into a hemispherical to conical columella. When the sporangial wall dissolves, a short basal collarette remains at the point of attachment of the wall and the sporangiophore. The sporangiospores are 1-celled, smooth to rarely echinulate, hyaline to light black, and globose to ovoid. A septum is typically present in the sporangiophore a set distance below the sporangium (Fig. 4.111). Zygospores are formed on the stolons.

Comments: Species of *Absidia* (60, 61, 89, 90) can be distinguished from *Rhizopus*, *Rhizomucor*, and *Mucor* by their pyriform sporangia, sporangiophores arising at internodes, the swollen sporangiophores that are continuous with the columellae, and circinate appendages originating from the suspensor cells of the zygospores.

Two commonly cited species of medical interest are *A. corymbifera* and *A. ramosa.* Nottebrock *et al.* (161) studied a number of isolates of these

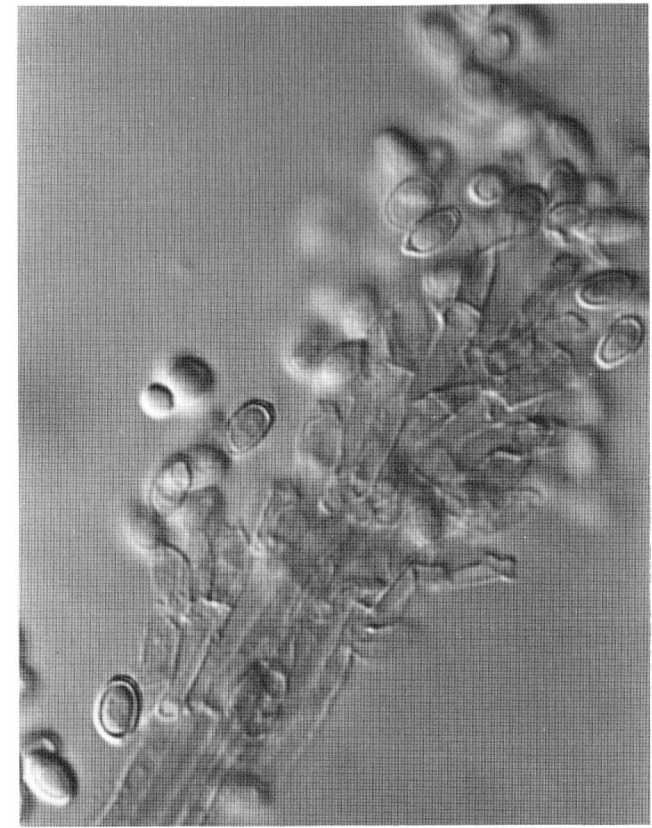

**Fig. 4.106** Continued

two species and concluded that *A. ramosa* is a synonym of *A. corymbifera*. This conclusion has been accepted by medical mycologists. *Absidia corymbifera* is the only species of *Absidia* known to cause disease in man.

Isolates of *Absidia* are occasionally recovered in the clinical laboratory. When zygomycosis is suspected, sterile bread or malt agar with chloramphenicol should be used as an additional isolation medium. Members of the genus *Absidia* are associated with the soil.

*Basidiobolus* Eidam, 1886

Diagnostic features: Members of the genus *Basidiobolus* produce two basic types of spores. The primary spores are globose, 1-celled, solitary and forcibly discharged from the sporophore. The sporophore has a distinct

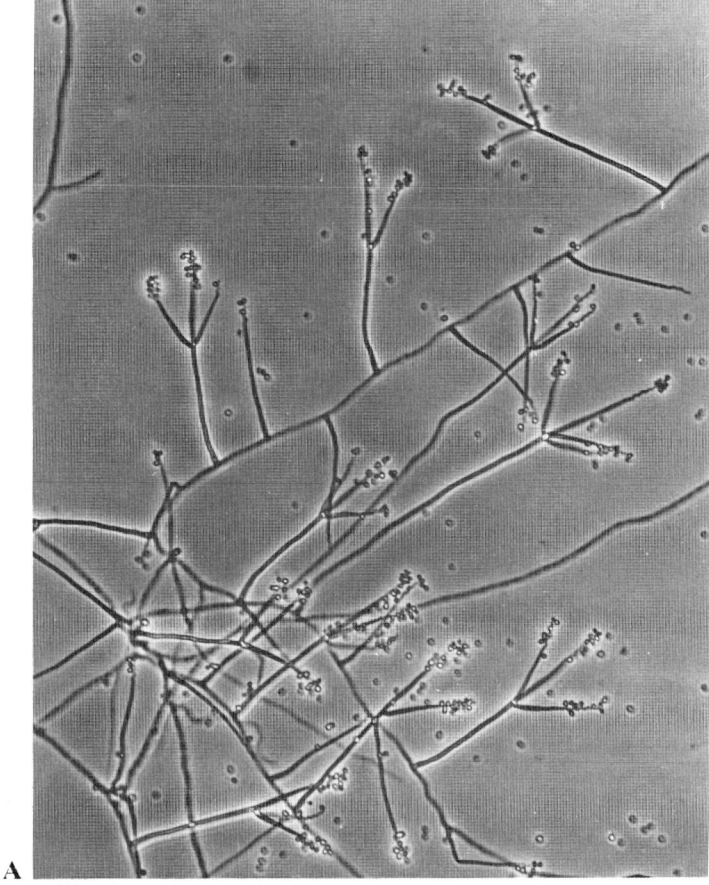

**Fig. 4.107** *Tritirachium oryzae.* A and B. The long, tapering, geniculate conidiophores produced by members of this genus occur in verticillate whorls. The one-celled conidia are attached directly to the rachis.

swollen area just below the spore that actively participates in the discharge of the spore. The second type of spore is 1-celled, clavate, and passively released from the sporophore. These sporophores are not swollen at their bases. The apex of the passively released spore has a knoblike adhesive tip. These spores may function as sporangia, producing several sporangiospores. Zygospores have two closely appressed beaklike appendages (Fig. 4.112).

Comments: *Basidiobolus ranarum* is apparently the only known human pathogen in the group. Emmons (67) originally identified *B. ranarum* as the etiologic agent of a human case of zygomycosis. The taxonomy surrounding members of the genus is complex and in a state of confusion. McGin-

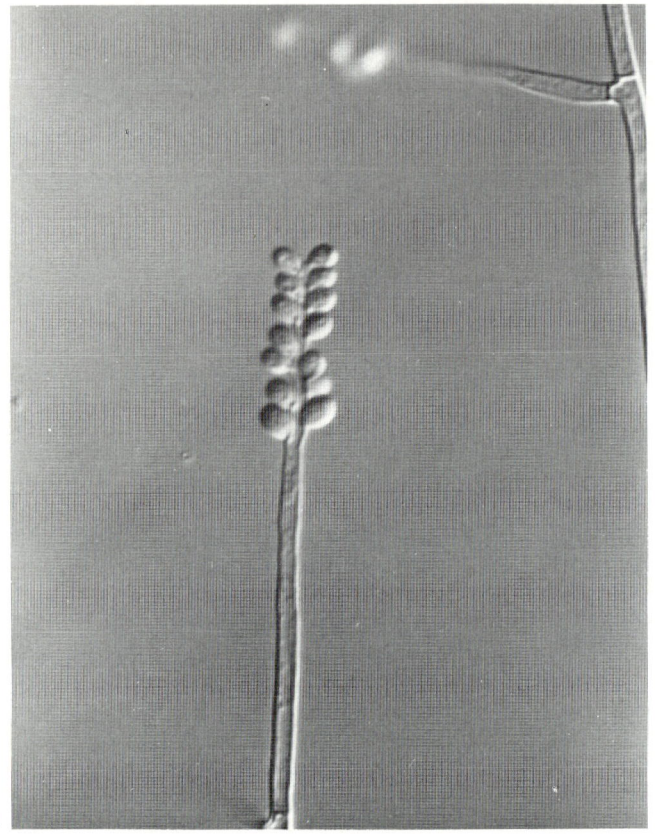

**Fig. 4.107** Continued

nis (141) has recently reviewed this problem and made several interesting conclusions. He found that most medical mycologists distinguish *B. haptosporus* (= *B. meristosporus*) from *B. ranarum* on the basis of zygospore outer cell wall topography, presence or absence of a *Streptomyces*-like odor, and differences in temperature requirements for growth. Zygospores with smooth outer cell walls, absence of a *Streptomyces*-like odor, and growth at higher temperatures distinguish *B. haptosporus* from *B. ranarum*, which has zygospores with undulating outer cell walls, a *Streptomyces*-like odor, and a lower temperature requirement for growth. The literature contains ample data showing that these characteristics are too variable to be used for distinguishing isolates in the genus *Basidiobolus*. McGinnis also noted that the original illustrations of *B. ranarum* showed that Eidam included zygospores with smooth and undulating outer cell walls in his concept of *B. ranarum*.

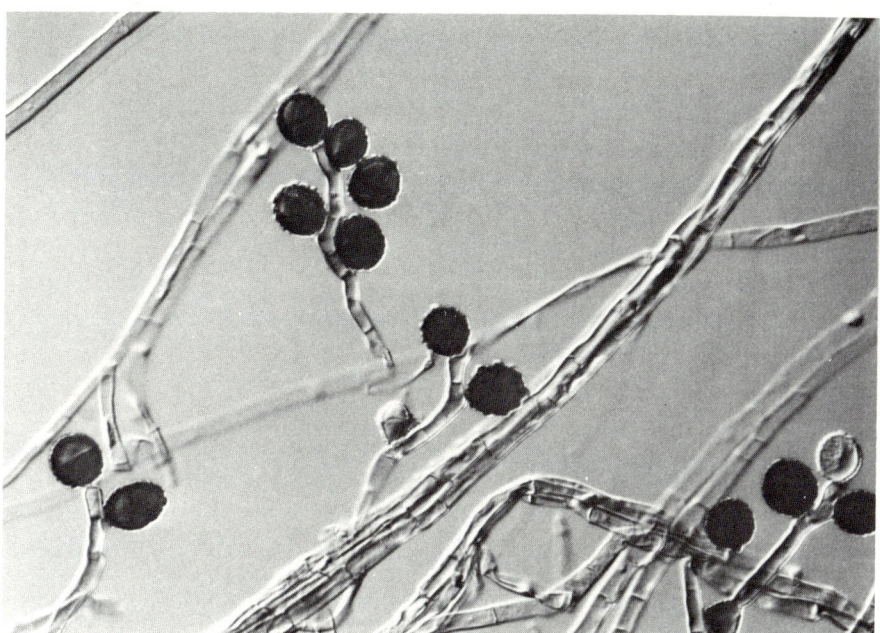

Fig. 4.108 *Ulocladium atrum*. The muriform conidia are produced by a sympodial conidiophore.

There appear to be two distinct species in the genus *Basidiobolus*, *B. microsporus* (22) and *B. ranarum*. *Basidiobolus microsporus* is readily recognized by the production of exogenous microspores. Until a taxonomic revision of the genus *Basidiobolus* is conducted, it appears best to consider *B. haptosporus*, *B. heterosporus*, *B. lacertae*, *B. magnus*, *B. meristosporus*, *B. myxophilus*, and *B. philippinensis* as synonyms of *B. ranarum* (141). If one wishes to use zygospore cell wall topography as a taxonomic characteristic, zygospores with smooth outer cell walls would be characteristic of *B. lacertae*, whereas those with undulating walls would be associated with *B. ranarum* and *B. microsporus*. *Basidiobolus haptosporus* and *B. meristosporus* produce zygospores with smooth cell walls. Based upon priority, these two species are synonyms of *B. lacertae*.

Isolates of *Basidiobolus* are rarely seen in the clinical laboratory unless they are recovered from a patient with zygomycosis.

*Circinella* van Tieghem et Le Monnier, 1873

Diagnostic features: Species of *Circinella* initially produce a nonseptate mycelium that becomes septate at maturity. The sporangiophores are erect, indeterminate, and branch in a sympodial manner. The lateral branches

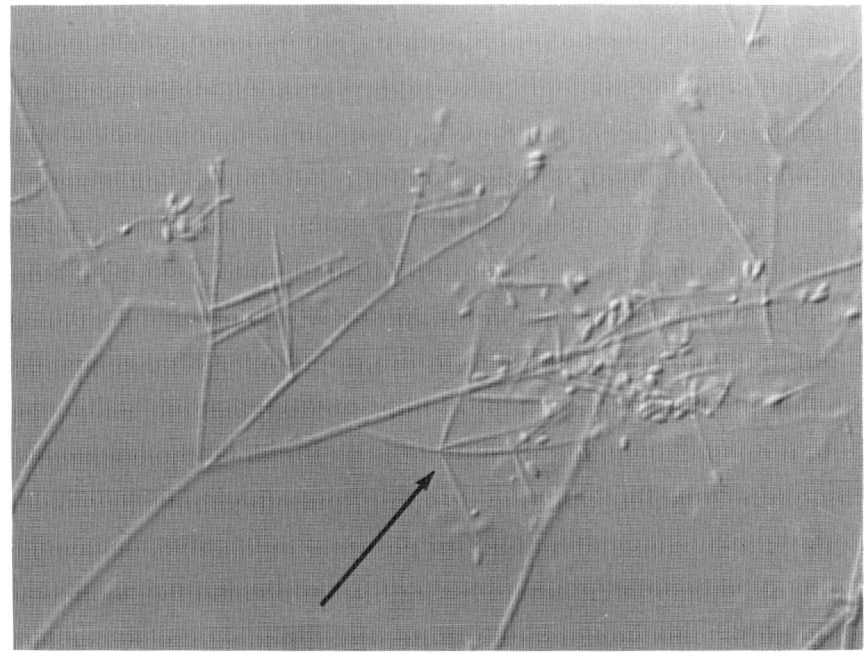

**Fig. 4.109** *Verticillium* sp. The long, narrow, tapering phialides are formed in verticils (arrow). The phialoconidia accumulate in balls at the apices of the phialides.

are solitary or in whorls, and curved, the sporangia being produced at the apices of these branches. A single sporangium is present at the apex of each branch with the exception that a sporangium is never produced at the tip of the sporangiophore (Fig. 4.113). The sporangia are globose and have walls that are incrusted with calcium oxalate crystals. The sporangial wall breaks into pieces when the sporangiospores are released and an irregular collarette remains at the base of the large columella. The sporangiospores are globose to ovoid, smooth, and blue. Zygospores are formed on erect hyphae; the suspensors do not have appendages.

Comments: Sporangia produced by species of *Circinella* (91) are extremely distinctive and delicate appearing. The sympodial development and circinate arrangement of the branches with a terminal sporangium rapidly distinguishes members of this genus from other Zygomycetes. *Circinella* is infrequently seen in the clinical laboratory.

### *Conidiobolus* Brefeld, 1884

Diagnostic features: The genus *Conidiobolus* is difficult to define adequately. King (117–119) has pointed out that collectively three hyphal

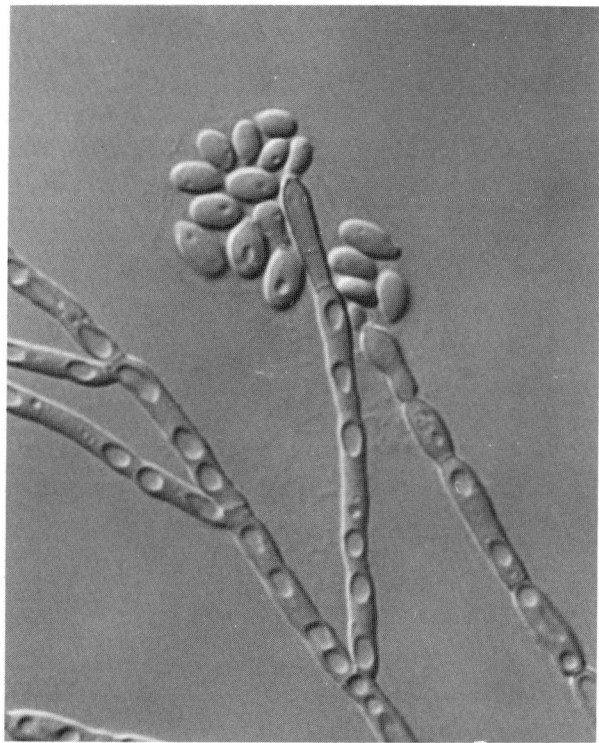

Fig. 4.110 *Wangiella dermatitidis*. The phialides without collarettes produce balls of one-celled phialoconidia. The conidia tend to slide down the conidiophores. (Reproduced by permission from *PAHO Scientific Publ. No. 356*, pp. 37–59, 1978.)

types and eight types of sporangiola (conidia) and spores are produced by the various species of *Conidiobolus*. Species of *Conidiobolus* form globose to pyriform, broadly rounded (at apex), solitary, primary spores on simple sporophores; they are forcibly discharged. These spores contain seven or more nuclei. Zygospores are usually present and are always formed within the larger of the two gametangia giving rise to them. Isolates of *Conidiobolus* grow well on routine media, such as potato dextrose agar. Spores with fine tubular appendages (villose spores) and sporangiola producing numerous secondary spores (multiplicative spores) may be present.

Comments: Many of the first reported cases due to members of this genus were identified as *Entomophthora coronata*. It was later concluded that this species belonged in the genus *Conidiobolus*, not to *Entomophthora* (20). *Conidiobolus coronatus* (Fig. 4.114), as well as the other members of *Conidiobolus*, are distinguished from species of *Entomophthora* by their globose to pyriform primary spores with seven or more nuclei per spore, good growth on mycological media, and the presence of villose spores, multiplicative spores, or both, in some isolates. The zygospores of *Entomophthora* are never formed within the larger of two gametangia. This characteristic is not helpful in identifying *C. coronatus*, since it does not produce zygospores. It is helpful with *C. incongruus* because this species does form zygospores.

Isolates of *Conidiobolus* are rarely, if ever, encountered in the clinical laboratory. The presence of ballistospores can be demonstrated with the same technique used for yeasts such as *Sporobolomyces* sp. Isolates of *Conidiobolus* can be readily obtained by placing the substrate containing them inside the lid of a Petri dish. The lid is then replaced over the bottom

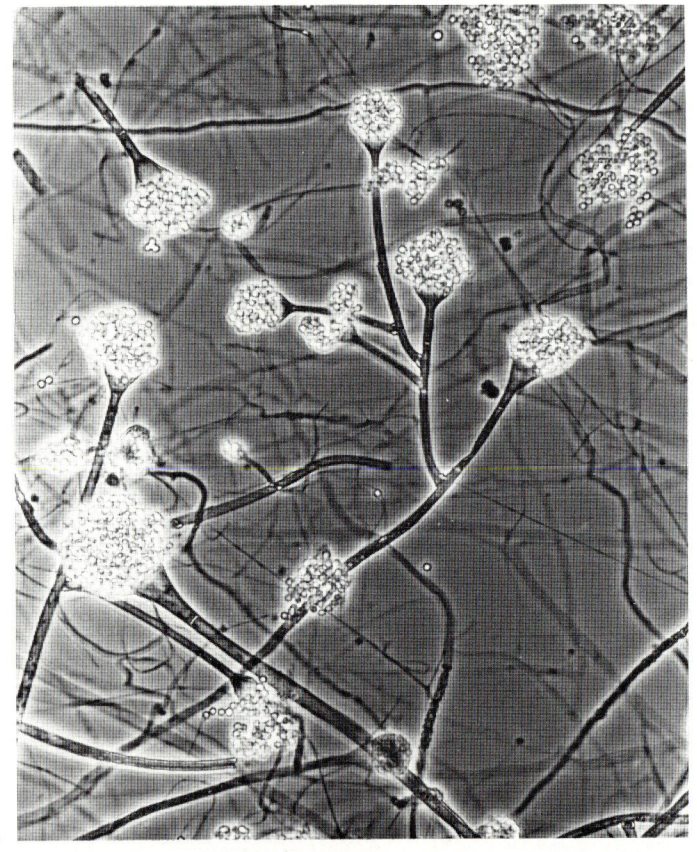

**Fig. 4.111** *Absidia* sp. The branching sporangiophores are producing terminal sporangia that have a swollen portion that merges into the columellae. A septum is usually formed in the sporangiophore just below each sporangium.

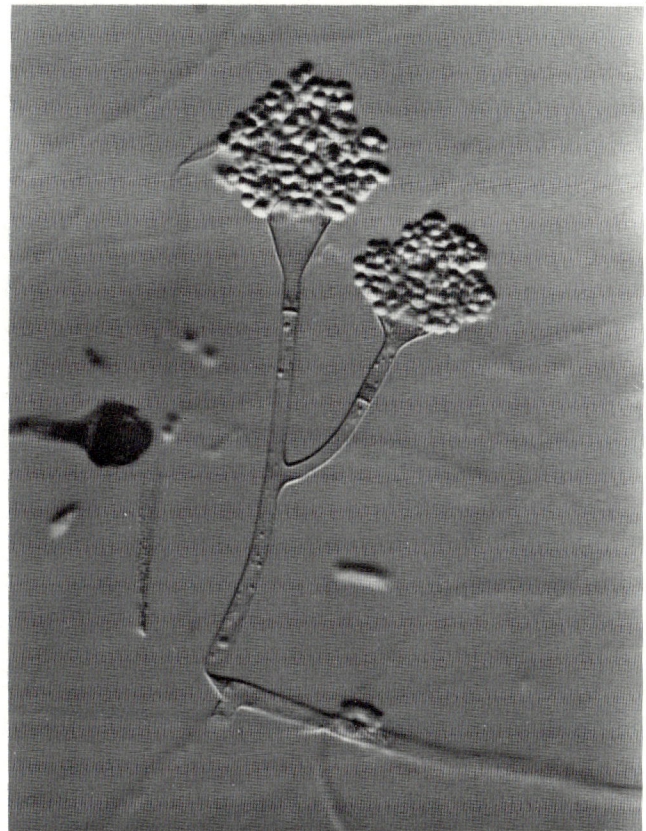

Fig. 4.111 Continued

plate containing media, such as potato dextrose agar. The forcibly discharged spores will settle on the agar surface, rapidly forming new colonies. Species of *Conidiobolus* (205) are common soil organisms.

### *Cunninghamella* Matruchot, 1903

Diagnostic features: Members of the genus *Cunninghamella* (116, 183) produce erect, straight, branching sporangiophores that are sparsely septate. The apex of the sporangiophore and its branches end in swollen vesicles. Around the vesicle, 1-celled, globose to ovoid, sporangiola develop solitarily on swollen denticles (Fig. 4.115). The walls of the sporangiola contain needlelike crystals. Chlamydospores and zygospores may be present.

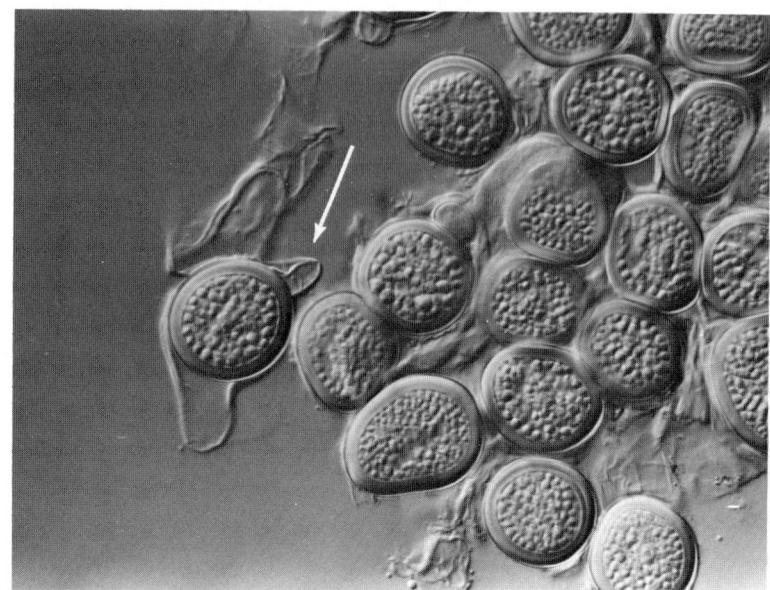

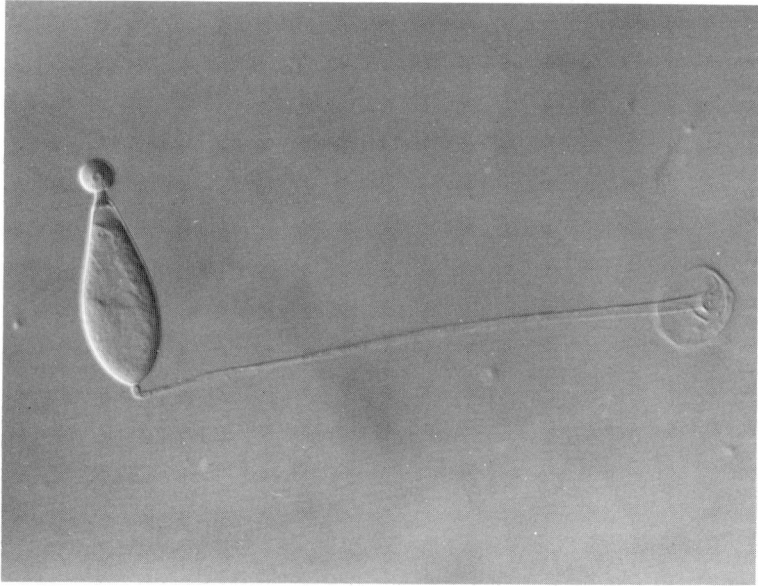

**Fig. 4.112** *Basidiobolus ranarum*. A. The zygospores have two closely appressed beaklike appendages (arrow). B. An elongate spore on a sporophore. C. A globose spore that has not been discharged from its sporophore can be seen at the edge of the preparation.

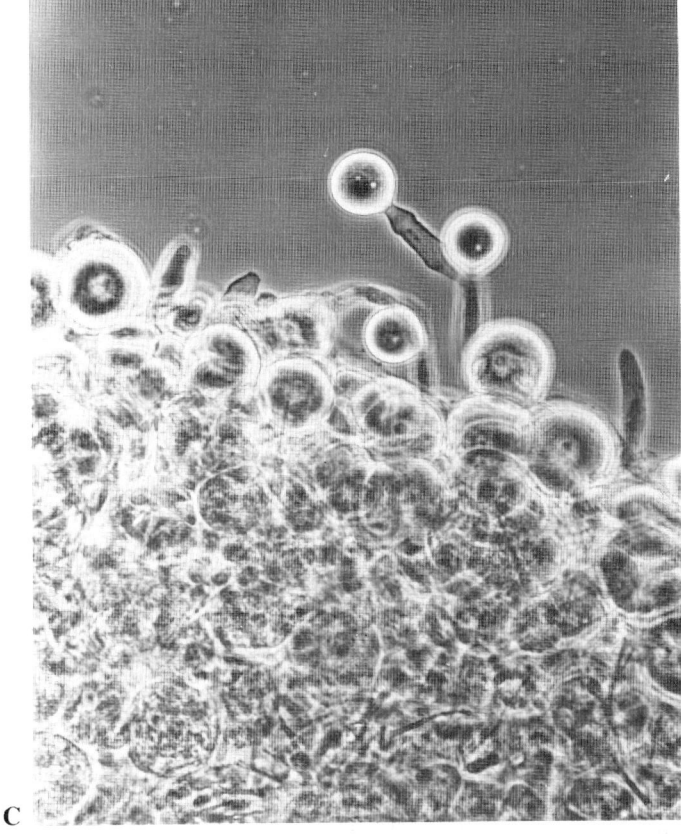

**Fig. 4.112** Continued

Comments: *Cunninghamella elegans* is the principal reported pathogenic species of *Cunninghamella*. The pathogenic isolates are actually *C. bertholletiae*, not *C. elegans* as previously believed (219). Members of this genus are occasionally isolated in the clinical laboratory.

### *Mortierella* Coemans, 1863

Diagnostic features: *Mortierella* species produce a delicate mycelium that gives rise to erect, fine, simple or branched sporangiophores that taper toward their apex. A terminal, globose sporangium without a columella (except *M. ramanniana*) develops from each sporangiophore. A collarette is typically left after the sporangial wall dissolves. The sporangiospores are globose to ellipsoidal and 1-celled (Fig. 4.116). Zygospores are globose and

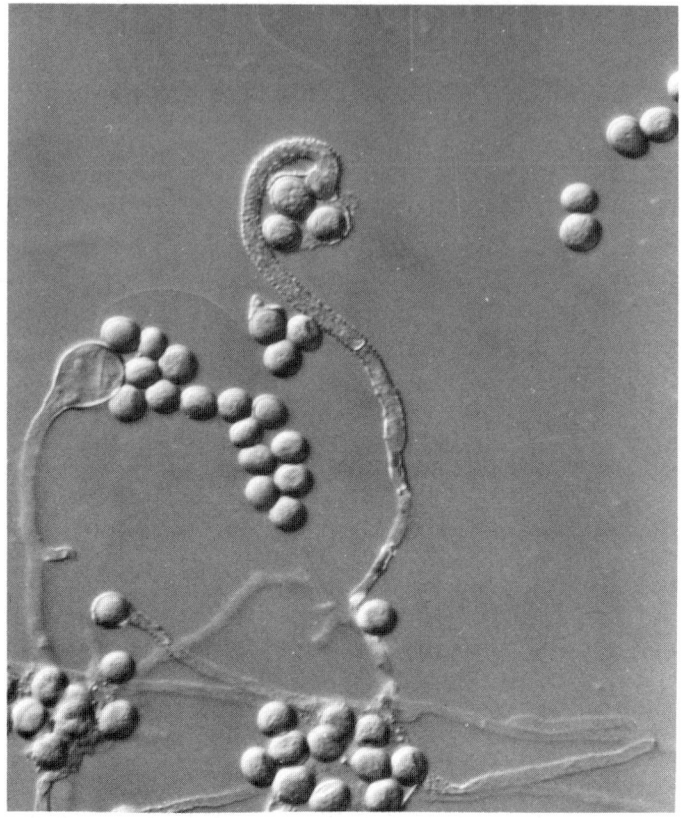

**Fig. 4.113** *Circinella* sp. The sporangia are produced at the apices of curved sporangiophores. The walls of the sporangia are encrusted with calcium oxalate crystals.

covered by a thick layer of hyphae. Globose, 1-celled, solitary spores on short side branches may be also present.

Comments: *Mortierella* sp. (73, 221) are common soil fungi that occasionally are isolated in the clinical laboratory. *Mortierella mycetomatis* (as "*mycetomi*") has been reported as an agent of mycetoma (159). There is substantial question whether or not this is a good species, and if it played a role in the disease process.

*Mucor* Micheli ex Saint-Amans, 1821

Diagnostic features: Species of *Mucor* produce erect sporangiophores directly from the mycelium; stolons and rhizoids are absent. The sporangiophores are solitary, simple or branched (in clusters or irregular),

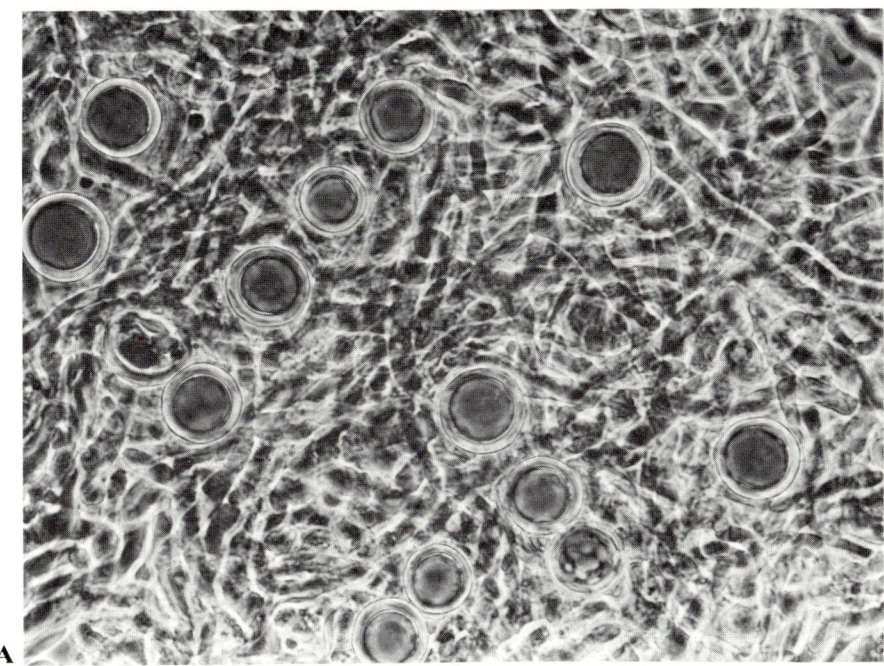

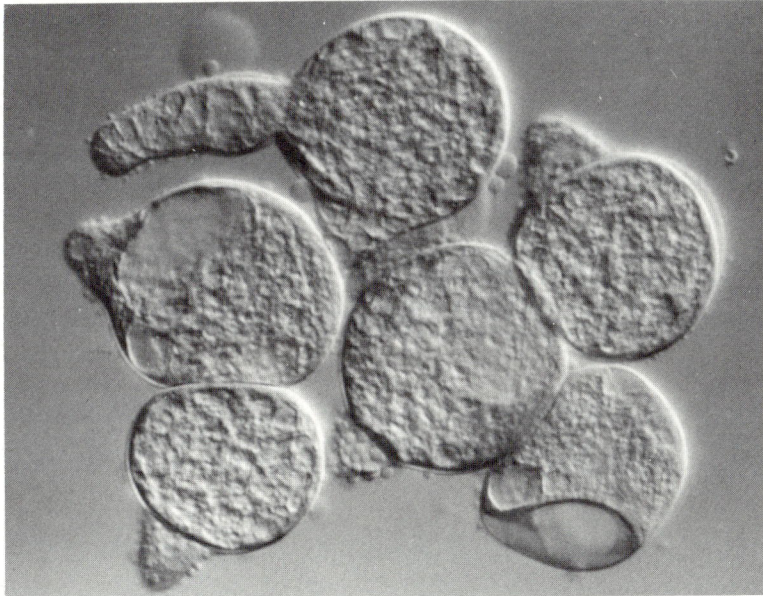

**Fig. 4.114** *Conidiobolus*. A. Zygospores of *C. incongruus*. B. Germinating spores of *C. coronatus*.

each branch forming a terminal sporangium. The sporangia are globose with walls that dissolve, thereby releasing the sporangiospores. A collarette may be present at the base of the sporangium after the spores have been released. The columella is variable in shape and hyaline to pigmented. The sporangiospores are globose to ellipsoidal and smooth (Fig. 4.117). When zygospores are present, they are naked and arise from the mycelium. Chlamydospores may be present.

Comments: The absence of rhizoids and stolons distinguishes species of *Mucor* from *Absidia, Rhizomucor*, and *Rhizopus*. *Mucor mycetomatis* (as "*mycetomi*") has been reported to be an agent of mycetoma (74). The fungus was probably a contaminant and played no role in the disease process. The description of *M. mycetomatis* is inadequate, and therefore it is impossible to determine which species of *Mucor* was actually isolated.

Several species of *Mucor* have been reported to cause zygomycosis. The most common one reported is *M. pusillus*, which has been recently trans-

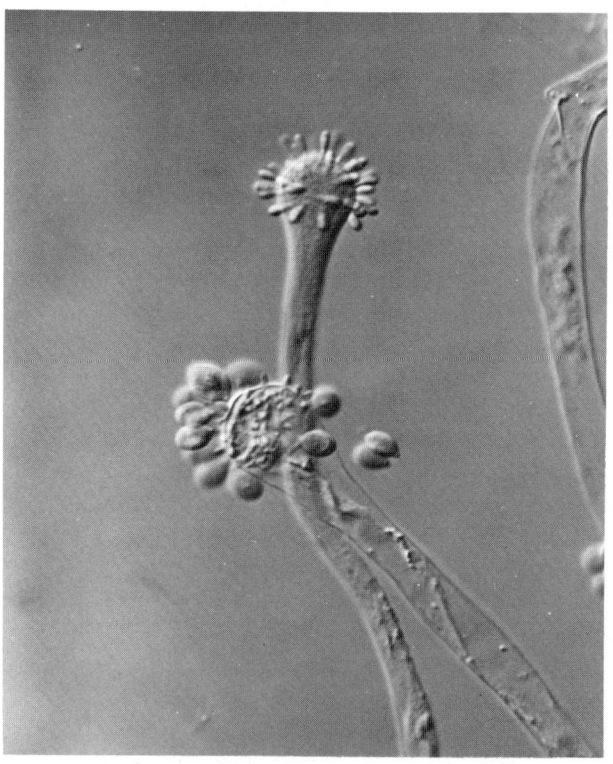

**Fig. 4.115** *Cunninghamella bertholletiae*. A. The one-spored sporangiola are developing on swollen denticles around the entire vesicle at the apex of the sporangiophore. B. A zygospore with its suspensor cells still attached.

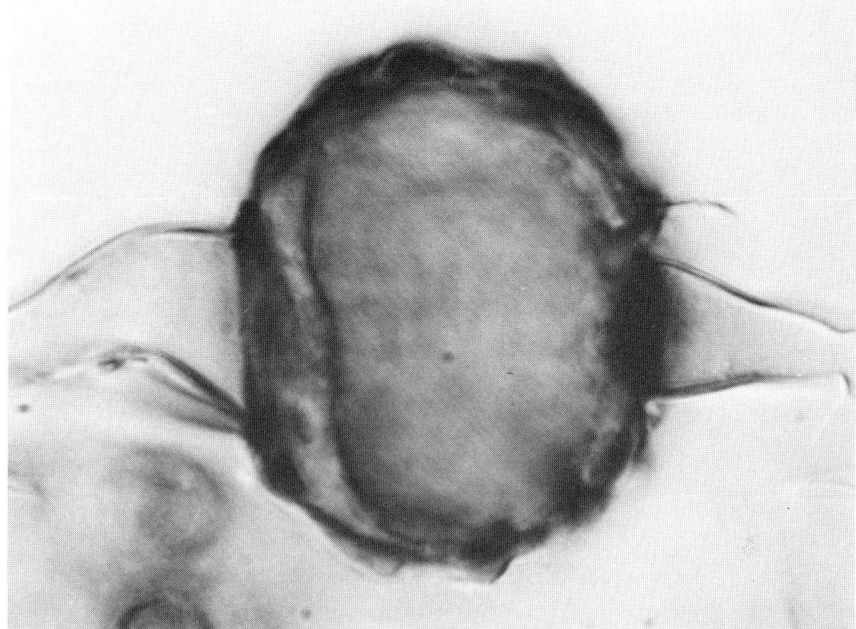

**B**

**Fig. 4.115** Continued

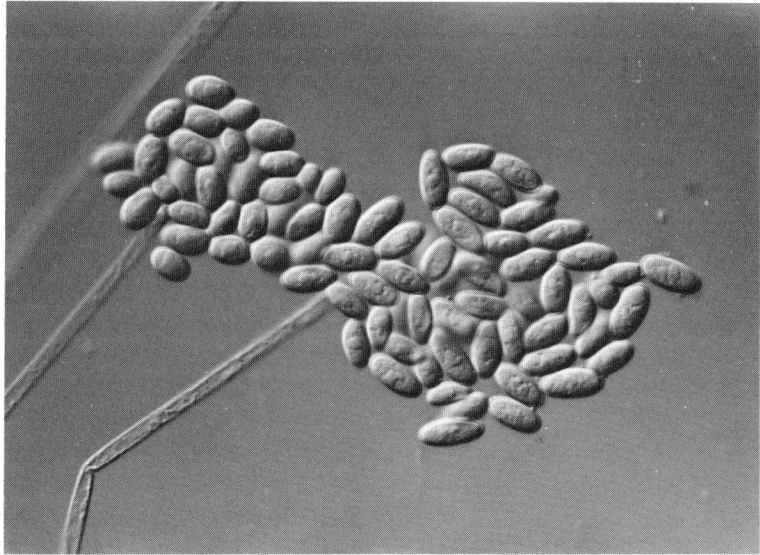

**Fig. 4.116** *Mortierella* sp. A ball of sporangiospores can be seen at the apex of the sporangiophore. Columellae are typically absent in this genus.

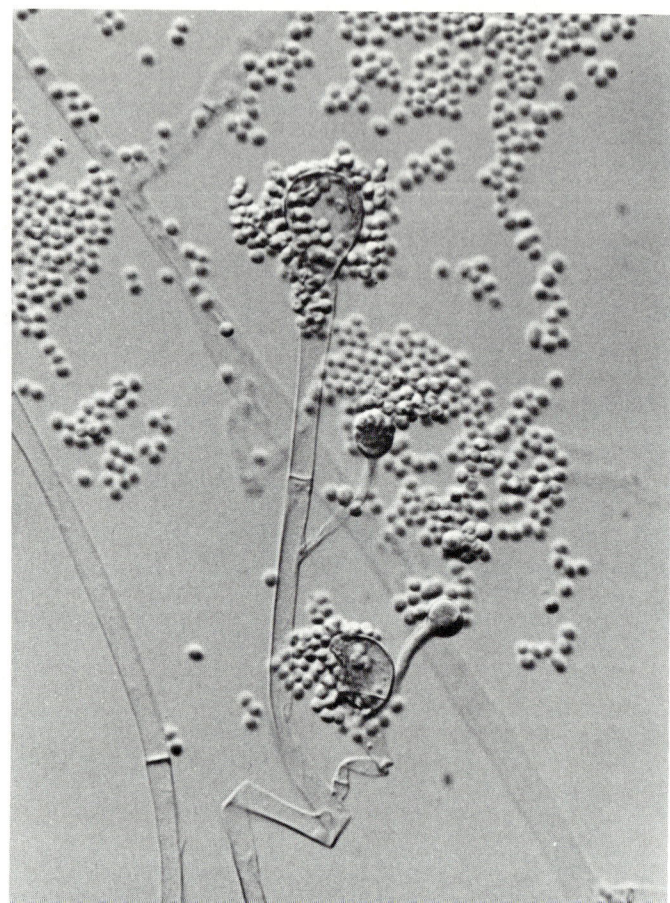

**Fig. 4.117** *Mucor* sp. The sporangial wall dissolves, thereby releasing the sporangiospores. Stolons and rhizoids are not produced by members of this genus.

ferred to the genus *Rhizomucor* (191). An agent of zygomycosis that was identified as *Rhizopus hiemalis* (156) is most likely *M. hiemalis*, which probably played no role in the disease process. Isolates of *Mucor*, as well as other of the Zygomycetes, should be kept in tubes with good aeration. The accumulation of $CO_2$ in screw cap tubes will quickly kill these fungi. For the primary isolation of *Mucor* from clinical materials, sterile bread without preservatives or malt extract agar with chloramphenicol are useful media.

Isolates of *Mucor* are occasionally recovered in the clinical laboratory, but not as often as species of *Rhizopus*. Members of this genus are soil organisms.

Part 3 Taxonomy

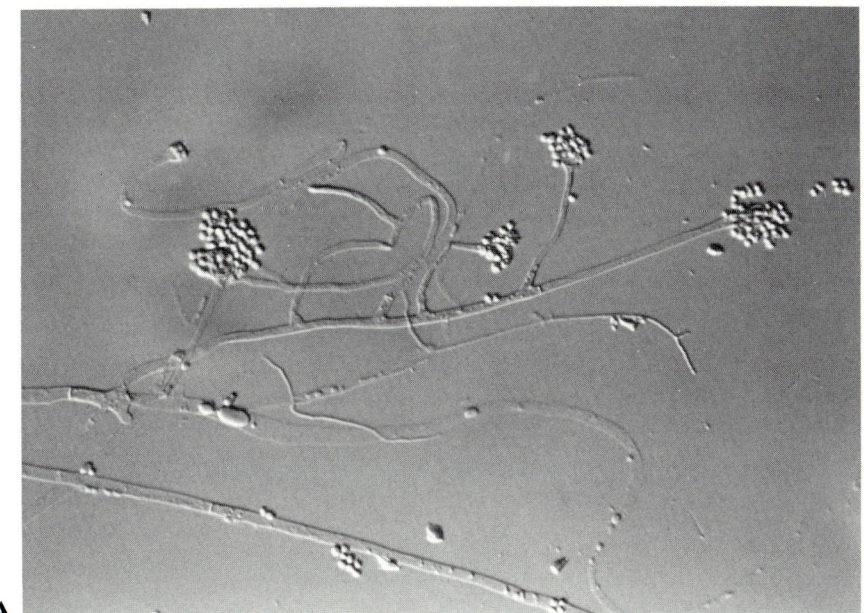

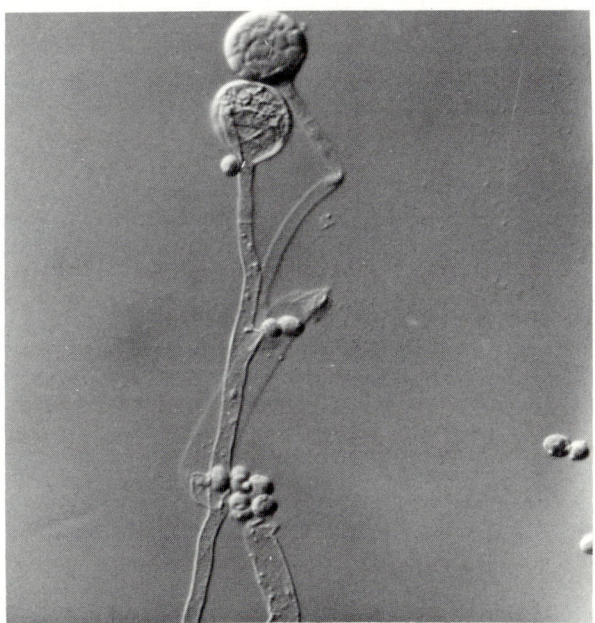

**Fig. 4.118** *Rhizomucor pusillus.* Members of this genus are intermediate between the genera *Mucor* and *Rhizopus.* A. The sporangiophores are branched; B. stolons are absent; C. primitive rhizoids are present.

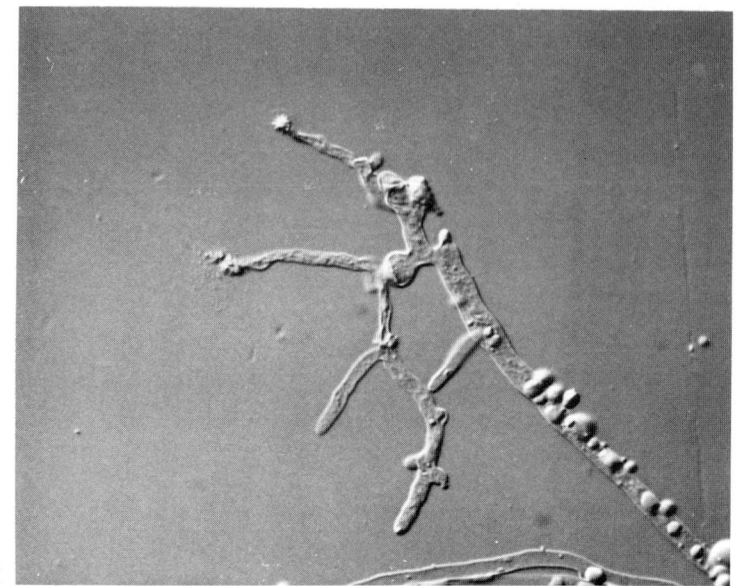

C

**Fig. 4.118** Continued

*Rhizomucor* (Lucet et Costantin) Wehmer ex Vuillemin, 1931

Diagnostic features: Members of the genus *Rhizomucor* are thermophilic. Sporangiophores develop from the aerial hyphae or stolons, with simple or weakly branched rhizoids. The sporangiophores branch repeatedly and form dark, globose sporangia with columellae. The sporangiospores are 1-celled and subglobose. Zygospores are formed in the aerial hyphae; they have blunt projections from their walls.

Comments: Members of this genus are thermophilic and are usually confused with species of *Mucor* that have globose to subglobose sporangiospores. *Rhizomucor* (Fig. 4.118) differs from species of *Mucor* by the development of stolons and rhizoids. The repeatedly branching sporangiophores distinguish it from *Rhizopus*. The pyriform sporangia and apophyses of *Absidia* readily separate it from *Rhizomucor*.

The genus *Rhizomucor* contains three species (191). *Rhizomucor pusillus*, which was previously known as *M. pusillus*, is an agent of zygomycosis in man.

The incidence of *Rhizomucor* in the clinical laboratory is unknown. Isolates of *Rhizomucor* have probably been misidentified as species of *Mucor*, or some similar zygomycete.

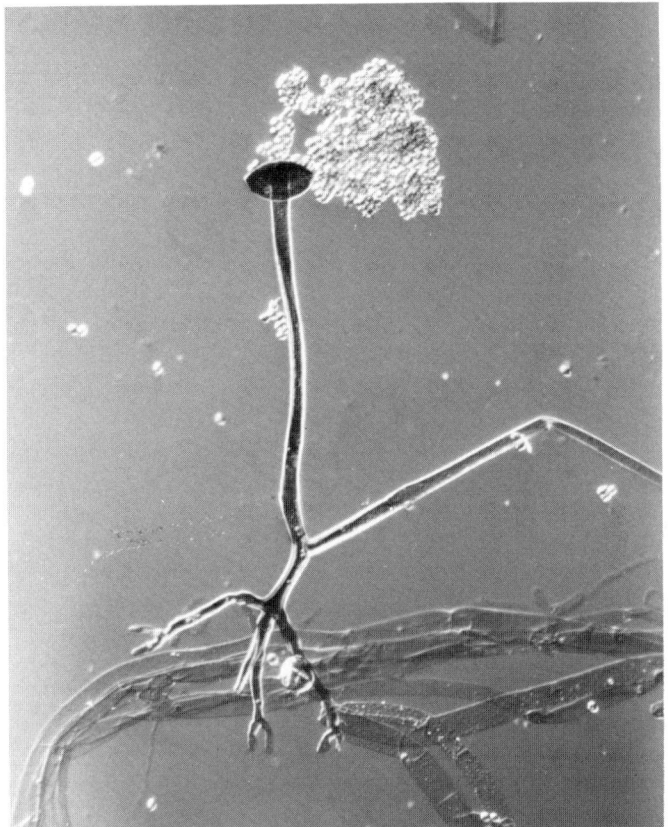

**Fig. 4.119** *Rhizopus stolonifer*. Well developed rhizoids opposite the sporangiophores, and hemispherical columellae are distinctive for members of this genus.

## *Rhizopus* Ehrenberg ex Corda, 1838

Diagnostic features: Species of *Rhizopus* form sporangiophores that are solitary, in clusters of 2, 3, or more, or both, and arise opposite the rhizoids formed at the nodes. The sporangia are globose with a flattened base. A collarette is lacking when the sporangial wall dissolves. The columellae are hemispherical. The sporangiospores are globose to ovoid, 1-celled, hyaline to brown, and smooth to striate (Fig. 4.119). The zygospores do not have appendages.

Comments: Members of the genus *Rhizopus* (104, 191) are distinguished from species of *Absidia* and *Mucor* by the development of sporangiophores that arise opposite rhizoids at the nodes, and from *Rhizomucor* by having sporangiophores that do not branch repeatedly.

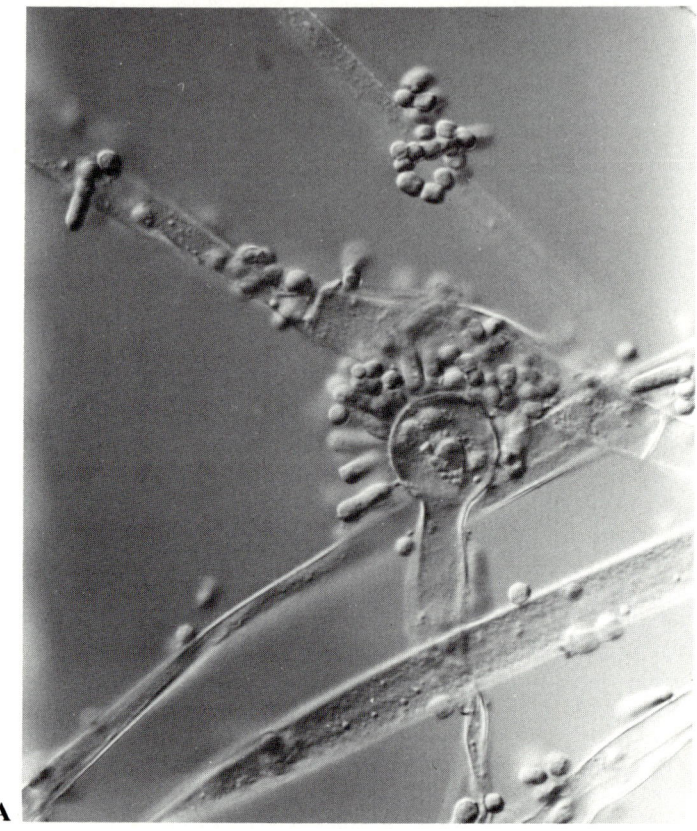

**Fig. 4.120** *Syncephalastrum racemosum*. The merosporangia arise around the entire vesicle at the apex of the sporangiophore.

Ajello (personal communication) has studied a number of isolates that were identified as *R. stolonifer* from proven cases of zygomycosis. He concluded that they were actually *R. arrhizus* and *R. oryzae*. Hesseltine (174) had the same experience with two isolates of *R. stolonifer* (as *R. nigricans*) that he reidentified as *R. arrhizus* and *R. oryzae*. In addition, *R. stolonifer* does not grow at 37°C (125). This species does not appear to be a pathogen of man. Some isolates that have been identified as *R. microsporus* are in reality *R. rhizopodiformis* (124). One of the misidentified isolates was recovered from a case of human zygomycosis.

Isolates of *Rhizopus* are recovered in the clinical laboratory. As in the case of other Zygomycetes, sterile bread is an ideal isolation medium for the recovery of members of this genus. Isolates of *Rhizopus* should be

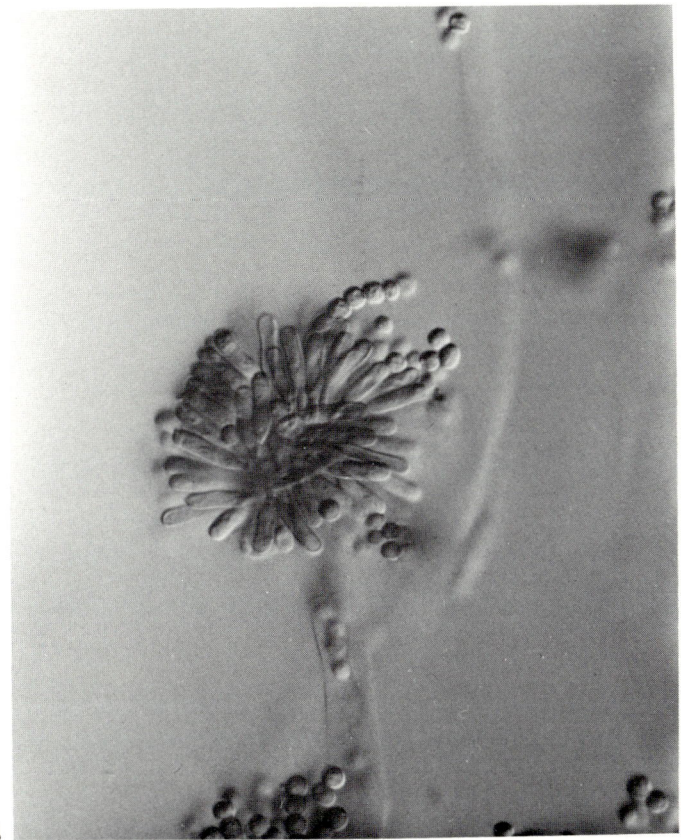

**Fig. 4.120** Continued

maintained in tubes with good aeration. Species of *Rhizopus* are associated with the soil, plant material, fruit, and similar substrates.

*Syncephalastrum* Schröter, 1886

Diagnostic features: *Syncephalastrum* species (21) produce sympodially branching sporangiophores with curved lateral branches. Each branch forms a swollen vesicle that has a septum between it and the remaining portion of the sporangiophore. Merosporangia arise directly from the vesicle, and contain several globose sporangiospores at maturity (Figs. 4.120 and 4.121). Rhizoids are usually present.

Comments: Isolates of *Syncephalastrum*, usually *S. racemosum*, are frequently encountered in the clinical laboratory. *Syncephalastrum* could be

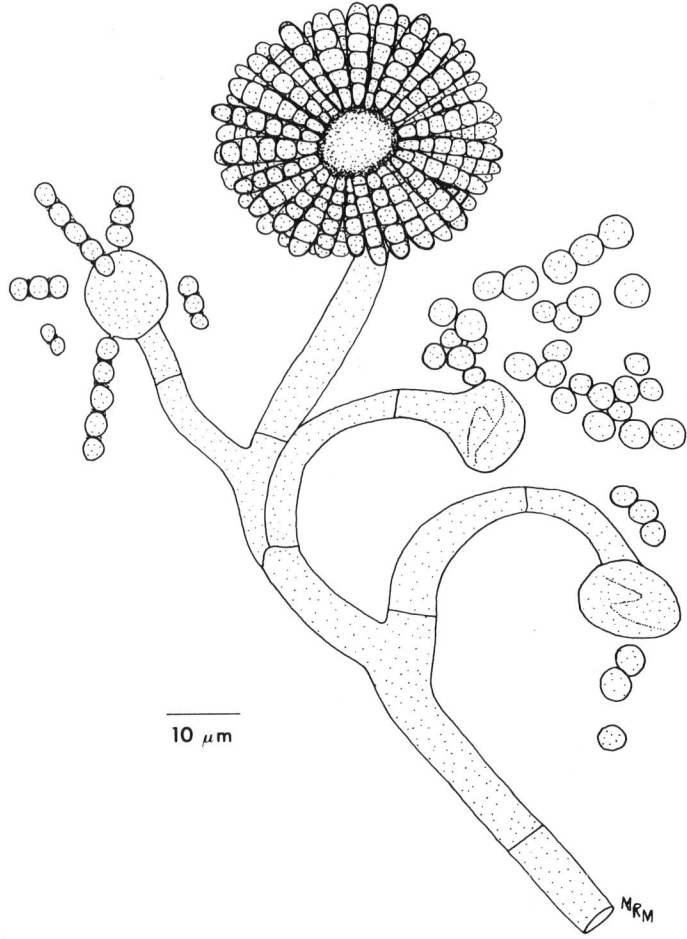

**Fig. 4.121**  *Syncephalastrum racemosum.*

confused by some microbiologists with *Aspergillus* if the isolate is not looked at carefully.

## Part 3.  General Identification References

a. Ainsworth, G. C., F. K. Sparrow, and A. S. Sussman, eds. (1973). "The Fungi: An Advanced Treatise," Vol. IVA, A Taxonomic Review with Keys: Ascomycetes and Fungi Imperfecti. Academic Press, New York.
b. Ainsworth, G. C., F. K. Sparrow, and A. S. Sussman, eds. (1973). "The Fungi: An Advanced Treatise," Vol. IVB, A Taxonomic Review with Keys: Basidiomycetes and Lower Fungi. Academic Press, New York.

c. Arx, J. A. von (1974). "The Genera of Fungi Sporulating in Pure Culture," 2nd ed. J. Cramer, Vaduz.
d. Barnett, H. L., and B. B. Hunter (1972). "Illustrated Genera of Imperfect Fungi," 3rd ed. Burgess, Minneapolis, Minnesota.
e. Barron, G. L. (1968). "The Genera of Hyphomycetes from Soil." Williams & Wilkins, Baltimore, Maryland.
f. Clements, F. E., and C. L. Shear (1931). "The Genera of Fungi." Wilson, New York.
g. Cole, G., and R. A. Samson (1979). "Patterns of Development in Conidial Fungi." Pitman, London.
h. Dennis, R. W. G. (1978). "British Ascomycetes." J. Cramer, Vaduz.
i. Ellis, M. B. (1971). "Dematiaceous Hyphomycetes." Commonwealth Mycological Institute, Kew, Surrey, England.
j. Ellis, M. B. (1976). "More Dematiaceous Hyphomycetes." Commonwealth Mycological Institute, Kew, Surrey, England.
k. Gilman, J. C. (1957). "A Manual of Soil Fungi," 2nd ed. Iowa State Univ. Press, Ames.
l. Matsushima, T. (1975). "Icones Microfungorum a Matsushima Lectorum." Published by the author, Kobe, Japan.
m. Zycha, H., R. Siepmann, and G. Linnemann (1969). "Mucorales. Eine Beschreibung aller Gattungen und Arten dieser Pilzgruppe." J. Cramer, Lehre.

## Part 3. References Cited

1. Abbott, E. V. (1927). *Scolecobasidium,* a new genus of soil fungi. *Mycologia* **19**:29–31.
2. Ajello, L. (1977). Taxonomy of the dermatophytes: a review of their imperfect and perfect states. *In* "Recent Advances in Medical and Veterinary Mycology" (K. Iwata, ed.), pp. 289–297. University Park Press, Baltimore, Maryland.
3. Ajello, L. (1977). Milestones in the history of medical mycology: the dermatophytes. *In* "Recent Advances in Medical and Veterinary Mycology" (K. Iwata, ed.), pp. 3–11. University Park Press, Baltimore, Maryland.
4. Ajello, L. (1978). The black yeasts as disease agents: historical perspective. *Proc. Int. Conf. Mycoses, 4th, PAHO Sci. Publ. No.* 356, pp. 9–16.
5. Ajello, L., L. K. Georg, W. Kaplan, and L. Kaufman (1966). "Laboratory Manual for Medical Mycology." USPHS Publ. No. 994. U.S. Government Printing Office, Washington, D.C.
6. Alasoadura, S. O. (1970). Culture studies on *Botryodiplodia theobromae* Pat. *Mycopathol. Mycol. Appl.* **42**:153–160.
7. Almeida, F. de (1930). Estudos comparativos de granuloma coccidioidico nos Estados Unidos e no Brasil. Novo genero para o parasito brasileiro. *An. Fac. Med. Univ. São Paulo* **5**:125–139.
8. Ames, L. M. (1961). "A Monograph of the Chaetomiaceae." U. S. Army Research Development Series 2, Bibliotheca Mycologica 17, reprinted 1969. J. Cramer, Lehre.
9. Arx, J. A. von (1963). Die Gattungen der Myriangiales. *Persoonia* **2**:421–475.
10. Arx, J. A. von (1971). Über die Typusart, zwei neue und einige weitere Arten der Gattung *Sporotrichum. Persoonia* **6**:179–184.
11. Arx, J. A. von (1973). Further observations on *Sporotrichum* and some similar fungi. *Persoonia* **7**:127–130.
12. Arx, J. A. von (1973). The genera *Petriellidium* and *Pithoascus* (Microascaceae). *Persoonia* **7**:367–375.
13. Arx, J. A. von (1975). On *Thielavia* and some similar genera of ascomycetes (Stud. Mycol. No. 8). Centraalbureau voor Schimmelcultures, Baarn.

14. Arx, J. A. von (1977). Notes on *Dipodascus, Endomyces* and *Geotrichum* with the description of two new species. *Antonie van Leeuwenhoek J. Microbiol. Serol.* **43**:333–340.
15. Arx, J. A. von, L. Rodrigues de Miranda, M. T. Smith, and D. Yarrow (1977). The genera of yeasts and the yeast like fungi (Stud. Mycol. No. 14). Centraalbureau voor Schimmelcultures, Baarn.
16. Barron, G. L. (1962). New species and new records of *Oidiodendron. Can. J. Bot.* **40**:589–607.
17. Barron, G. L. (1968). "The Genera of Hyphomycetes from Soil." Williams & Wilkins, Baltimore, Maryland.
18. Barron, G. L. (1977). "The Nematode-Destroying Fungi" (Top. Mycobiol. 1). Canadian Biological Publications Ltd., Guelph.
19. Barron, G. L., and L. V. Busch (1962). Studies on the soil hyphomycete *Scolecobasidium. Can. J. Bot.* **40**:77–84.
20. Batko, A. (1964). Notes on entomophthoraceous fungi in Poland. *Entomophaga Mem.* [*Hors Ser.*] **2**:129–131.
21. Benjamin, R. K. (1959). The merosporangiferous Mucorales. *Aliso* **4**:321–433.
22. Benjamin, R. K. (1962). A new *Basidiobolus* that forms microspores. *Aliso* **5**:223–233.
23. Bertoldi, M. de (1976). New species of *Humicola*: an approach to genetic and biochemical classification. *Can. J. Bot.* **54**:2755–2768.
24. Beurmann, L. de, and H. Gougerot (1906). Les sporotrichoses hypodermiques. *Ann. Dermatol. Syphiligr.* **7**:837–864, 914–922, 993–1006.
25. Bhatt, G. C., and W. B. Kendrick (1968). The generic concepts of *Diplorhinotrichum* and *Dactylaria,* and a new species of *Dactylaria* from soil. *Can. J. Bot.* **46**:1253–1257.
26. Binford, C. H., R. K. Thompson, M. E. Gorham, and C. W. Emmons (1952). Mycotic brain abscess due to *Cladosporium trichoides,* a new species. Report of a case with mycologic report. *Am. J. Clin. Pathol.* **22**:535–542.
27. Blaser, P. (1974/1975). Taxonomische und physiologische Untersuchungen über die Gattung *Eurotium* Link ex Fries. *Sydowia* **28**:1–49.
28. Boedijn, K. B., and J. Reitsma (1950). Notes on the genus *Cylindrocladium* (Fungi: Mucedinaceae). *Reinwardtia* **1**:51–60.
29. Boerema, G. H. (1976). The *Phoma* species studied in culture by Dr. R. W. G. Dennis. *Trans. Br. Mycol. Soc.* **67**:289–319.
30. Boerema, G. H., M. M. J. Dorenbosch, and H. A. van Kesteren (1977). Remarks on species of *Phoma* referred to *Peyronellaea,* V. *Kew Bull.* **31**:533–544.
31. Booth, C. (1966). The genus *Cylindrocarpon.* (Mycol. Paper No. 104). Commonwealth Mycological Institute, Kew, Surrey, England.
32. Booth, C. (1971). "The genus *Fusarium.*" Commonwealth Mycological Institute, Kew, Surrey, England.
33. Booth, C. (1977). "*Fusarium* Laboratory Guide to the Identification of the Major Species." Commonwealth Mycological Institute, Kew, Surrey, England.
34. Borelli, D. (1960). *Torula bantiana,* agente di un granuloma cerebrale. *Riv. Anat. Patol. Oncol.* **17**:615–622.
35. Borelli, D. (1964). On the importance of temperature in the pathogeny and the clinics of mycoses. *Arch. Dermatol.* **89**:504.
36. Bothast, R. J., and D. I. Fennell (1974). A medium for rapid identification and enumeration of *Aspergillus flavus* and related organisms. *Mycologia* **66**:365–369.
37. Boyd, M. F., and E. D. Cutchfield (1921). Contribution to the study of mycetoma in North America. *Am. J. Trop. Med.* **1**:215–289.
38. Brault, J. (1912). Mycétome à grains noirs observé en Algérie, isolement du *Madurella mycetomi. Ann. Dermatol. Syphiligr.* [*Ser. 5*] **3**:333–343.

39. Brown, A. H. S., and G. Smith (1957). The genus *Paecilomyces* Bainier and its perfect stage *Byssochlamys* Westling. *Trans. Br. Mycol. Soc.* **40**:17–89.
40. Brumpt, E. (1905). Sur le mycétome à grains noirs, maladie produite par une mucédinée du genre *Madurella* n.g. *C. R. Soc. Biol.* **58**:997–999.
41. Brumpt, E., Bouffard, and J. A. Chabaneix (1901). Notes sur quelques cas de paludisme et sur un cas de mycétome observés à Djibouti. *Arch. Parasitol.* **4**:564–567.
42. Carmichael, J. W. (1957). *Geotrichum candidum. Mycologia* **49**:820–830.
43. Carmichael, J. W. (1962). *Chrysosporium* and some other aleuriosporic hyphomycetes. *Can. J. Bot.* **40**:1137–1173.
44. Carmichael, J. W. (1966). Cerebral mycetoma of trout due to a *Phialophora*-like fungus. *Sabouraudia* **5**:120–123.
45. Carrión, A. L. (1940). The specific fungi of chromoblastomycosis. *P. R. J. Pub. Health Trop. Med.* **15**:340–361.
46. Castellani, A., and A. J. Chalmers (1919). "Manual of Tropical Medicine," 3rd ed. William Wood, New York.
47. Ciferri, R., and A. Montemartini (1959). Taxonomy of *Haplosporangium parvum. Mycopathol. Mycol. Appl.* **10**:303–316.
48. Cole, G. T. (1978). Conidiogenesis in the black yeasts. *Proc. Int. Conf. Mycoses, 4th, PAHO Sci. Publ. No.* 356, pp. 66–78.
49. Cole, G. T., and B. Kendrick (1973). Taxonomic studies of *Phialophora. Mycologia* **65**:661–688.
50. Cooke, R. C., and B. E. S. Godfrey (1964). A key to the nematode-destroying fungi. *Trans. Br. Mycol. Soc.* **47**:61–74.
51. Cooke, W. B. (1959). An ecological life history of *Aureobasidium pullulans* (de Bary) Arnaud. *Mycopathol. Mycol. Appl.* **12**:1–45.
52. Cooke, W. B. (1962). A taxonomic study in the "Black Yeasts." *Mycopathol. Mycol. Appl.* **17**:1–43.
53. Costantin, M., and Rolland (1888). *Blastomyces*, genre nouveau. *Bull. Soc. Mycol. Fr.* **4**:153–157.
54. Crane, J. L., and J. D. Schoknecht (1977). Revision of *Torula* species. *Rutola*, a new genus for *Torula graminis. Can. J. Bot.* **55**:3013–3019.
55. Darling, S. T. (1906). A protozoön general infection producing pseudotubercles in the lungs and focal necrosis in the liver, spleen and lymphnodes. *J. Am. Med. Assoc.* **46**:1283–1285.
56. Deighton, F. C., and J. L. Mulder (1977). *Mycocentrospora acerina* as a human pathogen. *Trans. Br. Mycol. Soc.* **69**:326–327.
57. Denton, J. F., and A. F. Di Salvo (1964). Isolation of *Blastomyces dermatitidis* from natural sites at Augusta, Georgia. *Am. J. Trop. Med. Hyg.* **13**:716–722.
58. Dickinson, C. H. (1968). *Gliomastix* Guéguen (Mycol. Paper No. 115). Commonwealth Mycological Institute, Kew, Surrey, England.
59. Ellis, D. H., and D. A. Griffiths (1975). The fine structure of conidial development in the genus *Torula*. I. *T. herbarum* (Pers.) Link ex S. F. Gray and *T. herbarum* f. *quaternella* Sacc. *Can. J. Microbiol.* **21**:1661–1675.
60. Ellis, J. J., and C. W. Hesseltine (1965). The genus *Absidia*: globose-spored species. *Mycologia* **57**:222–235.
61. Ellis, J. J., and C. W. Hesseltine (1966). Species of *Absidia* with ovoid sporangiospores. II. *Sabouraudia* **5**:59–77.
62. Ellis, M. B. (1961). Dematiaceous hyphomycetes. III (Mycol. Paper No. 82). Commonwealth Mycological Institute, Kew, Surrey, England.
63. Ellis, M. B. (1966). Dematiaceous hyphomycetes. VII: *Curvularia, Brachysporium* etc. (Mycol. Paper No. 106). Commonwealth Mycological Institute, Kew, Surrey, England.

64. Ellis, M. B. (1971). "Dematiaceous Hyphomycetes." Commonwealth Mycological Institute, Kew, Surrey, England.
65. Ellis, M. B. (1976). "More Dematiaceous Hyphomycetes." Commonwealth Mycological Institute, Kew, Surrey, England.
66. Emmons, C. W. (1944). *Allescheria boydii* and *Monosporium apiospermum. Mycologia* 36:188–193.
67. Emmons, C. W., C. H. Binford, J. P. Utz, and K. J. Kwon-Chung (1977). "Medical Mycology," 3rd ed. Lea & Febiger, Philadelphia.
68. Emmons, C. W., and W. L. Jellison (1960). *Emmonsia crescens* sp. n. and adiaspiromycosis (haplomycosis) in mammals. *Ann. N. Y. Acad. Sci.* **89**:91–101.
69. Emmons, C. W., Lie-Kian-Joe, Njo-Injo Tjoei Eng, A. Pohan, S. Kertopati, and A. van der Meulen (1957). *Basidiobolus* and *Cercospora* from human infections. *Mycologia* **49**:1–10.
70. Fennell, D. I. (1973). Plectomycetes; Eurotiales. *In* "The Fungi: An Advanced Treatise" (G. C. Ainsworth, F. K. Sparrow, and A. S. Sussman, eds.), Vol. 4A, A Taxonomic Review with Keys: Ascomycetes and Fungi Imperfecti, pp. 45–68. Academic Press, New York.
71. Galgóczy, J. (1975). Dermatophytes: conidium-ontogeny and classification. *Acta Microbiol. Acad. Sci. Hung.* **22**:105–136.
72. Gams, W. (1971). "*Cephalosporium*-artige Schimmelpilze (Hyphomycetes)." Gustav Fischer, Stuttgart.
73. Gams, W. (1977). A key to the species of *Mortierella. Persoonia* **9**:381–391.
73a. Gams, W. (1978). Connected and disconnected chains of phialoconidia and *Sagenomella* gen. nov. segregated from *Acremonium. Persoonia* **10**:97–112.
74. Gelonesi, G. (1927). Due nuovi parassiti del "piede di madura." Studio sui micetomi della Somalia Meridionale. *Ann. Med. Nav. Colon.* **33**:283–308.
75. Georg, L. K., and L. B. Camp (1957). Routine nutritional tests for the identification of dermatophytes. *J. Bacteriol.* **74**:113–121.
76. Gilchrist, T. C., and W. R. Stokes (1896). The presence of an *Oidium* in the tissues of a case of pseudo-lupus vulgaris. *Bull. Johns Hopkins Hosp.* **7**:129–133.
77. Gilchrist, T. C., and W. R. Stokes (1898). A case of pseudo-lupus vulgaris caused by a *Blastomyces. J. Exp. Med.* **3**:53–78.
78. Guého, E. (1970). Deoxyribonucleic acid base composition and taxonomy in the genus *Geotrichum. Antonie van Leeuwenhoek J. Microbiol. Serol.* **45**:199–210.
79. Haard, K. (1968). Taxonomic studies on the genus *Arthrobotrys* Corda. *Mycologia* **60**:1140–1159.
80. Hammill, T. M. (1977). Transmission electron microscopy of annellides and conidiogenesis in the synnematal hyphomycete *Trichurus spiralis. Can. J. Bot.* **55**:233–244.
81. Hanlin, R. T., ed. (1975). "The Pyrenomycetous Fungi," Lewis E. Wehmeyer, Mycologia Memoir No. 6. J. Cramer, Lehre.
82. Hardin, H. F., and D. I. Scott (1974). Blastomycosis. Occurrence of filamentous forms *in vivo. Am. J. Clin. Pathol.* **62**:104–106.
83. Hashmi, M. H., B. Kendrick, and G. Morgan-Jones (1972). Conidium ontogeny in hyphomycetes. The genera *Torulomyces* Delitsch and *Monocillium* Saksena. *Can. J. Bot.* **50**:1461–1464.
84. Hawksworth, D. L. (1979). Ascospore sculpturing and generic concepts in the Testudinaceae (syn. Zopfiaceae). *Can. J. Bot.* **57**:91–99.
85. Hektoen, L., and C. F. Perkins (1900). Refractory subcutaneous abscesses caused by *Sporothrix schenckii*. A new pathogenic fungus. *J. Exp. Med.* **5**:77–89.
86. Hennebert, G. L. (1973). *Botrytis* and *Botrytis*-like genera. *Persoonia* **7**:183–204.

87. Hennebert, G. L., and B. G. Desai (1974). *Lomentospora prolificans,* a new hyphomycete from greenhouse soil. *Mycotaxon* **1**:45–50.
88. Hermanides-Nijhof, E. J. (1977). *Aureobasidium* and allied genera. *In* The black yeasts and allied hyphomycetes (G. S. de Hoog and E. J. Hermanides-Nijhof), pp. 141–177 (Stud. Mycol. 15). Centraalbureau voor Schimmelcultures, Baarn.
89. Hesseltine, C. W., and J. J. Ellis (1964). The genus *Absidia: Gongronella* and cylindrical-spored species of *Absidia. Mycologia* **56**:568–601.
90. Hesseltine, C. W., and J. J. Ellis (1966). Species of *Absidia* with ovoid sporangiospores. I. *Mycologia* **58**:761–785.
91. Hesseltine, C. W., and D. I. Fennell (1955). The genus *Circinella. Mycologia* **47**:193.
92. Holm, L. (1952). Taxonomical notes on Ascomycetes. II. The herbicolous Swedish species of the genus *Leptosphaeria* Ces. & de Not. Sartyr. *Sven. Bot. Tidskr.* **46**:18–46.
93. Holm, L. (1957). Études taxonomiques sur les Pléosporacées. *Symb. Bot. Upsal.* **14**:1–188.
94. Holubová-Jechová, V. (1975). Problems of usage of the generic name *Oidium. Folia Geobot. Phytotax.* **10**:433–440.
95. Hoog, G. S. de (1972). The genera *Beauveria, Isaria, Tritirachium* and *Acrodontium* gen. nov. (Stud. Mycol. No. 1). Centraalbureau voor Schimmelcultures, Baarn.
96. Hoog, G. S. de (1974). The genera *Blastobotrys, Sporothrix, Calcarisporium* and *Calcarisporiella* gen. nov. (Stud. Mycol. No. 7). Centraalbureau voor Schimmelcultures, Baarn.
97. Hoog, G. S. de (1977). *Rhinocladiella* and allied genera. *In* The black yeasts and allied hyphomycetes (G. S. de Hoog and E. J. Hermanides-Nijhof), pp. 1–140 (Stud. Mycol. No. 15). Centraalbureau voor Schimmelcultures, Baarn.
98. Hoog, G. S. de, and J. A. von Arx (1973). Revision of *Scolecobasidium* and *Pleurophragmium. Kavaka* **1**:55–60.
99. Hoog, G. S. de, and G. A. de Vries (1973). Two new species of *Sporothrix* and their relation to *Blastobotrys nivea. Antonie van Leeuwenhoek J. Microbiol. Serol.* **39**:515–520.
100. Hughes, S. J. (1958). Revisiones hyphomycetum aliquot cum appendice de nominibus rejiciendis. *Can. J. Bot.* **36**:727–836.
101. Hughes, S. J., and J. Sugiyama (1972). New Zealand fungi 18. *Xylohypha* (Fr.) Mason. *N. Z. J. Bot.* **10**:447–460.
102. Hunter, B. B., and H. L. Barnett (1978). Growth and sporulation of species and isolates of *Cylindrocladium* in culture. *Mycologia* **70**:614–635.
103. Huppert, M., S. H. Sun, and E. H. Rice (1978). Specificity of exoantigens for identifying cultures of *Coccidioides immitis. J. Clin. Microbiol.* **8**:346–348.
104. Inui, T., Y. Takeda, and H. Iizuka (1965). Taxonomical studies on genus *Rhizopus. J. Gen. Appl. Microbiol. Suppl.* **11**:1–121.
105. Isaac, I. (1967). Speciation in *Verticillium. Ann. Rev. Phytopathol.* **5**:201–222.
106. Jarvis, W. R. (1977). "*Botryotinia* and *Botrytis* Species: Taxonomy, Physiology, and Pathogenicity. A Guide to the Literature." Monograph 15, Canada Department of Agriculture, Ottawa.
107. Joffe, A. Z. (1974). A modern system of *Fusarium* taxonomy. *Mycopathol. Mycol. Appl.* **53**:201–228.
108. Joly, P. (1964). Le genre *Alternaria.* Recherches Physiologiques, Biologiques et Systématiques. *Encycl. Mycol.* **33**:1–250.
109. Jones, J. P. (1976). Ultrastructure of conidium ontogeny in *Phoma pomorum, Microsphaeropsis olivaceum,* and *Coniothyrium fuckelii. Can. J. Bot.* **54**:831–851.
110. Jong, S. C., and E. E. Davis (1976). Contribution to the knowledge of *Stachybotrys* and *Memnoniella* in culture. *Mycotaxon* **3**:409–485.

111. Kamat, M. N., and V. G. Rao (1970). The genus *Curvularia* Boedijn from India. *Nova Hedwigia* **18**:597–626.
112. Käufer, I., and A. Weber (1977). *Graphium fructicola* als Ursache einer Systemmykose beim Hund. *Mykosen* **20**:39–46.
113. Kaufman, L., and P. Standard (1978). Improved version of the exoantigen test for identification of *Coccidioides immitis* and *Histoplasma capsulatum* cultures. *J. Clin. Microbiol.* **8**:42–45.
114. Kendrick, W. B., and G. T. Cole (1968). Conidium ontogeny in hyphomycetes. The sympodulae of *Beauveria* and *Curvularia*. *Can. J. Bot.* **46**:1297–1301.
115. Kendrick, W. B., and G. T. Cole (1969). Conidium ontogeny in hyphomycetes. *Trichothecium roseum* and its meristem arthrospores. *Can. J. Bot.* **47**:345–350.
116. Khan, S. R., and P. H. B. Talbot (1975). Monosporous sporangiola in *Mycotypha* and *Cunninghamella*. *Trans. Br. Mycol. Soc.* **65**:29–39.
117. King, D. S. (1976). Systematics of *Conidiobolus* (Entomophthorales) using numerical taxonomy. I. Biology and cluster analysis. *Can. J. Bot.* **54**:45–65.
118. King, D. S. (1976). Systematics of *Conidiobolus* (Entomophthorales) using numerical taxonomy. II. Taxonomic considerations. *Can. J. Bot.* **54**:1285–1296.
119. King, D. S. (1977). Systematics of *Conidiobolus* (Entomophthorales) using numerical taxonomy. III. Descriptions of recognized species. *Can. J. Bot.* **55**:718–729.
120. Kulik, M. M. (1968). "A Compilation of Descriptions of New *Penicillium* Species," U. S. Dept. Agric. Handb. 351. U. S. Government Printing Office, Washington, D.C.
121. Kwon-Chung, K. J. (1972). *Emmonsiella capsulata:* perfect state of *Histoplasma capsulatum*. *Science* **177**:368–369.
122. Laveran, M. A. (1902). Au sujet d'un cas de mycétoma à grains noirs. *Bull. Acad. Natl. Med. (Paris)* **47**:773–776.
123. Lechevalier, H., M. P. Lechevalier, D. A. Handley, B. K. Bhosh, and J. W. Carmichael (1977). Strains of fusidia which can be mistaken for actinomycetes. *Mycologia* **69**:81–95.
123a. Loeffler, W. (1976). Proposal for the conservation of the genus name *Epidermophyton* Sabouraud (1910) against *Epidermophyton* Mégnin (1881) and *Epidermophyton* Lang (1879) (Fungi: Deuteromycetes). *Taxon* **25**:208–210.
124. Lunn, J. A. (1977). CMI descriptions of pathogenic fungi and bacteria. *Rhizopus rhizopodiformis*, No. 522. Commonwealth Mycological Institute, Kew, Surrey, England.
125. Lunn, J. A. (1977). CMI descriptions of pathogenic fungi and bacteria. *Rhizopus stolonifer*, No. 524. Commonwealth Mycological Institute, Kew, Surrey, England.
126. Luttrell, E. S. (1964). Systematics of *Helminthosporium* and related genera. *Mycologia* **56**:119–132.
127. Luttrell, E. S. (1978). Biosystematics of *Helminthosporium:* Impact on Agriculture, pp. 193–209: "Biosystematics in Agriculture." Allanheld, Osmun, Montclair, New Jersey.
128. Lutz, A. (1908). Uma mycose pseudo-coccidica localizada na boca e observada no Brazil: contribuição ao conhecimento das hyphoblastomycoses americanas. *Bras. Med.* **22**:121–124, 141–144.
129. Mackinnon, J. E., L. V. Ferrada-Urzúa, and L. Montemayor (1949). *Madurella grisea* n. sp. A new species of fungus producing the black variety of maduromycosis in South America. *Mycopathol. Mycol. Appl.* **4**:384–392.
130. Malloch, D. (1970). New concepts in the Microascaceae illustrated by two new species. *Mycologia* **62**:727–740.
131. Malloch, D., and R. F. Cain (1972). New species and combinations of cleistothecial Ascomycetes. *Can. J. Bot.* **50**:61–72.
132. Malloch, D., and R. F. Cain (1973). The genus *Thielavia*. *Mycologia* **65**:1055–1077.

## Part 3 Taxonomy

133. Mariat, F. (1971). Adaptation de *Ceratocystis* à la vie parasitaire chez l'animal—Etude de l'aquisition d'un pouvoir pathogène comparable à celui de *Sporothrix schenckii*. *Sabouraudia* **9**:191–205.
134. Mariat, F. (1975). Observations sur l'écologie de *Sporothrix schenckii* et de *Ceratocystis stenoceras* en Corse et en Alsace, provinces Françaises indemnes de sporotrichose. *Sabouraudia* **13**:217–225.
135. McDonough, E. S., and A. L. Lewis (1968). The ascigerous stage of *Blastomyces dermatitidis*. *Mycologia* **60**:76–83.
136. McGinnis, M. R. (1977). *Exophiala spinifera*, a new combination for *Phialophora spinifera*. *Mycotaxon* **5**:337–340.
137. McGinnis, M. R. (1977). *Wangiella*, a new genus to accommodate *Hormiscium dermatitidis*. *Mycotaxon* **5**:353–363.
138. McGinnis, M. R. (1977). *Wangiella dermatitidis*, a correction. *Mycotaxon* **6**:367–369.
139. McGinnis, M. R. (1978). Human pathogenic species of *Exophiala*, *Phialophora*, and *Wangiella*. *Proc. Int. Conf. Mycoses*, 4th, PAHO Sci. Publ. No. 356, pp. 37–59.
140. McGinnis, M. R. (1979). Taxonomy of *Exophiala werneckii* and its relationship to *Microsporum mansonii*. *Sabouraudia* **17**:145–154.
141. McGinnis, M. R. (1980). Recent taxonomic developments and changes in medical mycology. *Annu. Rev. Microbiol.* **34** (in press).
142. McGinnis, M. R., and L. Ajello (1974). A new species of *Exophiala* isolated from channel catfish. *Mycologia* **66**:518–520.
143. McGinnis, M. R., and B. Katz (1979). *Ajellomyces* and its synonym *Emmonsiella*. *Mycotaxon* **8**:157–164.
144. McGinnis, M. R., and A. A. Padhye (1977). *Exophiala jeanselmei*, a new combination for *Phialophora jeanselmei*. *Mycotaxon* **5**:341–352.
145. McGinnis, M. R., and A. A. Padhye (1978). *Cladosporium castellanii* is a synonym of *Stenella araguata*. *Mycotaxon* **7**:415–418.
146. Medlar, E. M. (1915). A cutaneous infection caused by a new fungus, *Phialophora verrucosa*, with a study of the fungus. *J. Med. Res.* **32**:507–521.
147. Melin, E., and J. A. Nannfeldt (1934). Researches into the blueing of ground woodpulp. *Sven. Skogsvardsforen. Tidskr.* **32**:397–585.
148. Morenz, J. (1964). Taxonomische Untersuchungen zur Gattung *Geotrichum* Link. *Mykol. Schriften.* **2**:33–64.
149. Morris, E. F. (1963). "The Synnematous Genera of the Fungi Imperfecti." Ser. Biol. Sci. 3. Western Illinois Univ., Macomb, Illinois.
150. Morton, F. J., and G. Smith (1963). The genera *Scopulariopsis* Bainier, *Microascus* Zukal, and *Doratomyces* Corda (Mycol. Paper No. 86). Commonwealth Mycological Institute, Kew, Surrey, England.
151. Müller, E. (1950). Die schweizerischen Arten der Gattung *Leptosphaeria* und ihrer Verwandten. *Sydowia* [*Ser. 2*] **4**:185–319.
152. Müller, G. (1964). Die Gattung *Sporotrichum* Link. Eine taxonomische und morphologische Studie der bei Mensch und Tier vorkommenden Spezies (I. Teil). *Wiss. Z. Humboldt-Univ. Berl. Math.-Naturwiss. Reihe* **13**:611–638.
153. Müller, G. (1964). Die Gattung *Sporotrichum* Link. Eine taxonomische und morphologische Studie der bei Mensch und Tier vorkommenden Spezies (II. Teil). *Wiss. Z. Humboldt-Univ. Berl. Math-Naturwiss. Reihe* **13**:843–860.
154. Müller, G. (1965). Die Gattung *Sporotrichum* Link. Eine taxonomische und morphologische Studie der bei Mensch und Tier vorkommenden Spezies (III. Teil). *Wiss. Z. Humboldt-Univ. Berl. Math.-Naturwiss. Reihe* **14**:753–798.
155. Nag Raj, T. R., and B. Kendrick (1975). "A Monograph of *Chalara* and Allied Genera." Wilfrid Laurier Univ. Press, Waterloo, Ontario, Canada.

156. Neame, P., and D. Rayner (1960). Mucormycosis. A report of twenty-two cases. *Arch. Pathol.* **70**:261–268.
157. Negroni, P. (1936). Estudio micológico del primer caso Argentino de cromomicosis *Fonsecaea (n.g.) pedrosoi* (Brumpt, 1921). *Rev. Inst. Bacteriol., Buenos Aires* **7**:419–426.
158. Negroni, P. (1936). Estudio micológico del primer caso Argentino de cromomicosis. *Rev. Soc. Argent. Biol.* **12**:180–184.
159. Nicolau, S., and R. Evolceanu (1947). Recherches mycologiques dans un cas de "mycétome" du pied à grains noirs (*Mortierella mycetomi*). *Ann. Dermatol. Syphiligr.* [ser. 8] **7**:330–343.
160. Nicot, J., and F. Mariat (1973). Caractères morphologiques et position systématique de *Sporothrix schenckii*, agent de la sporotrichose humaine. *Mycopathol. Mycol. Appl.* **49**:53–65.
161. Nottebrock, H., H. J. Scholer, and M. Wall (1974). Taxonomy and identification of mucormycosis-causing fungi. I. Synonymity of *Absidia ramosa* with *A. corymbifera. Sabouraudia* **12**:64–74.
162. Onions, A. H. S., and G. L. Barron (1967). Monophialidic species of *Paecilomyces* (Mycol. Paper No. 107). Commonwealth Mycological Institute, Kew, Surrey, England.
163. Oorschot, C. A. N. van (1977). The genus *Myceliophthora. Persoonia* **9**:401–408.
164. Padhye, A. A., and J. W. Carmichael (1971). The genus *Arthroderma* Berkeley. *Can. J. Bot.* **49**:1525–1540.
165. Padhye, A. A., M. R. McGinnis, and L. Ajello (1978). Thermotolerance of *Wangiella dermatitidis. J. Clin. Microbiol.* **8**:424–426.
166. Philpot, C. M. (1977). The use of nutritional tests for the differentiation of dermatophytes. *Sabouraudia* **15**:141–150.
167. Punithalingam, E., and M. P. English (1975). *Pyrenochaeta unguis-hominis* sp. nov. on human toe-nails. *Trans. Br. Mycol. Soc.* **64**:539–541.
168. Punithalingam, E., and J. M. Waterston (1970). CMI descriptions of pathogenic fungi and bacteria. *Hendersonula toruloidea.* No. 274. Commonwealth Mycological Institute, Kew, Surrey, England.
169. Radaeli, F. (1911). Caso singolare di alterazione cutanea e profonda di natura probabilmente micotica in un piede (con presentazione di culture, di preparati microscopici e di microfotografie). *G. Ital. Mal. Vener. Pelle* **52**:109–116.
170. Raper, K. B., and D. I. Fennell (1965). "The Genus *Aspergillus*," Williams & Wilkins, Baltimore, Maryland.
171. Raper, K. B., and C. Thom (1949). "A Manual of the Penicillia." Williams & Wilkins, Baltimore, Maryland.
172. Rebell, G., and D. Taplin (1970). "Dermatophytes, Their Recognition and Identification," 2nd ed. Univ. of Miami Press, Coral Gables, Florida.
173. Redhead, S. A., and D. W. Malloch (1977). The Endomycetaceae: new concepts, new taxa. *Can J. Bot.* **55**:1701–1711.
174. Reinhardt, D. J., W. Kaplan, and L. Ajello (1970). Experimental cerebral zygomycosis in alloxan-diabetic rabbits. *Infect. Immun.* **2**:404–413.
175. Rifai, M. A. (1969). A revision of the genus *Trichoderma* (Mycol. Paper No. 116). Commonwealth Mycological Institute, Kew, Surrey, England.
176. Rifai, M. A., and R. C. Cooke (1966). Studies on some didymosporous genera of nematode-trapping hyphomycetes. *Trans. Br. Mycol. Soc.* **49**:147–168.
177. Rixford, E., and T. C. Gilchrist (1896). Two cases of protozoan (coccidioidal) infection of the skin and other organs. *Johns Hopkins Hosp. Rep.* **1**:209–268.
178. Saccardo, P. A. (1911). Notae mycologica. *Ann. Mycol.* **9**:249–257.
179. Saccardo, P. A. (1911). *Sylloge fungorum* **22**:1287–1288.

180. Saccardo, P. A. (1912). Notae mycologicae. I. Fungi ex Gallia, Abyssinia, Japonia, Mexico, Canada, Amer. bor. et centr. *Ann. Mycol.* **10**:310–322.
181. Saksena, S. B. (1955). A new fungus, *Monocillium indicum* gen. et sp. nov., from soil. *Indian Phytopathol.* **8**:9–12.
182. Salkin, I. F., and M. A. Gordon (1975). Evaluation of *Aspergillus* differential medium. *J. Clin. Microbiol.* **2**:74–75.
183. Samson, R. A. (1969). Revision of the genus *Cunninghamella* (Fungi, Mucorales). *Proc. Kon. Ned. Akad. Wetensch. Ser. C* **72**:322–335.
184. Samson, R. A. (1974). *Paecilomyces* and some allied hyphomycetes (Stud. Mycol. No. 6). Centraalbureau voor Schimmelcultures, Baarn.
185. Samson, R. A. (1979). A compilation of the aspergilli described since 1965 (Stud. Mycol. No. 18). Centraalbureau voor Schimmelcultures, Baarn.
186. Samson, R. A., R. Hadlok, and A. C. Stolk (1977). A taxonomic study of the *Penicillium chrysogenum* series. *Antonie van Leeuwenhoek J. Microbiol. Serol.* **43**:169–175.
187. Samson, R. A., A. C. Stolk, and R. Hadlok (1976). Revision of the subsection fasciculata of *Penicillium* and some allied species (Stud. Mycol. No. 11). Centraalbureau voor Schimmelcultures, Baarn.
188. Sarosi, G. A., and D. S. Serstock (1976). Isolation of *Blastomyces dermatitidis* from pigeon manure. *Am. Rev. Resp. Dis.* **114**:1179–1183.
189. Schenck, B. R. (1898). On refractory subcutaneous abscesses caused by a fungus possibly related to the sporotricha. *Bull. Johns Hopkins Hosp.* **9**:286–290.
190. Schenck, S., W. B. Kendrick, and D. Pramer (1977). A new nematode-trapping hyphomycete and a reevaluation of *Dactylaria* and *Arthrobotrys*. *Can J. Bot.* **55**:977–985.
191. Schipper, M. A. A. (1978). 1. On certain species of *Mucor* with a key to all accepted species. 2. On the genera *Rhizomucor* and *Parasitella* (Stud. Mycol. No. 17). Centraalbureau voor Schimmelcultures, Baarn.
192. Schneider, R. (1976). Taxonomie der Pyknidienpilzgattung *Pyrenochaeta*. *Ber. Dtsch. Bot. Ges.* **89**:507–514.
193. Schol-Schwarz, M. B. (1959). The genus *Epicoccum* Link. *Trans. Br. Mycol. Soc.* **42**:149–173.
194. Schol-Schwarz, M. B. (1968). *Rhinocladiella*, its synonym *Fonsecaea* and its relation to *Phialophora*. *Antonie van Leeuwenhoek J. Microbiol. Serol.* **34**:119–152.
195. Schol-Schwarz, M. B. (1970). Revision of the genus *Phialophora* (Moniliales). *Persoonia* **6**:59–94.
196. Segretain, G., and P. Destombes (1961). Description d'un nouvel agent de maduromycose, *Neotestudina rosatii*, n. gen., n. sp., isolé en Afrique. *C. R. Acad. Sci. (Paris)* **253**:2577–2579.
197. Seth, H. K. (1970). A monograph of the genus *Chaetomium*. *Nova Hedwigia* **37**:1–130.
198. Shear, C. L. (1922). Life history of an undescribed ascomycete isolated from a granular mycetoma of man. *Mycologia* **14**:239–243.
199. Shoemaker, R. A. (1959). Nomenclature of *Drechslera* and *Bipolaris*, grass parasites segregated from *Helminthosporium*. *Can. J. Bot.* **37**:879–887.
200. Sigler, L., and J. W. Carmichael (1976). Taxonomy of *Malbranchea* and some other hyphomycetes with arthroconidia. *Mycotaxon* **4**:349–488.
201. Simmons, E. G. (1967). Typification of *Alternaria*, *Stemphylium*, and *Ulocladium*. *Mycologia* **59**:67–92.
202. Smith, G. (1962). Some new and interesting species of micro-fungi. III. *Trans. Br. Mycol. Soc.* **45**:387–394.

203. Somal, B. S. (1976). A key to the species of *Curvularia*. *Indian J. Mycol. Plant Pathol.* **6**:59–64.
204. Splendore, A. (1912). Zymonematosi con localizzazione nella cavità della bocca, osservata in Brasile. *Bull. Soc. Pathol. Exot.* **5**:313–319.
205. Srinivasan, M. C., and M. J. Thirumalachar (1967). Evaluation of taxonomic characters in the genus *Conidiobolus*, with key to known species. *Mycologia* **59**:698–713.
206. Stockdale, P. M. (1961). *Nannizzia incurvata* gen. nov., sp. nov., a perfect state of *Microsporum gypseum* (Bodin) Guiart et Grigorakis. *Sabouraudia* **1**:41–48.
207. Stolk, A. C., and J. C. Dakin (1966). *Moniliella*, a new genus of Moniliales. *Antonie van Leeuwenhoek J. Microbiol. Serol.* **32**:399–409.
208. Subramanian, C. V., and M. Pushkaran (1975). Conidium ontogeny in some monophialidic Hyphomycetes. *Kavaka* **3**:77–99.
209. Sun, S. H., M. Huppert, and K. R. Vukovich (1976). Rapid *in vitro* conversion and identification of *Coccidioides immitis*. *J. Clin. Microbiol.* **3**:186–190.
210. Sutton, B. C. (1976). *Angiopoma* Lév., 1841, an earlier name for *Drechslera* Ito, 1930. *Mycotaxon* **3**:377–380.
211. Takashio, M., and R. Vanbreuseghem (1971). Production of ascospores by *Piedraia hortai in vitro*. *Mycologia* **63**:612–618.
212. Taylor, J. J. (1970). Further clarification of *Sporotrichum* species. *Mycologia* **62**:797–825.
213. Thibaut, M. (1972). La forme parfaite du *Sporotrichum schenckii* (Hetkoen et Perkins 1900): *Dolichoascus schenckii* Thibaut et Ansel 1970 nov. gen. *Ann. Parasitol. Hum. Comp.* **47**:431–441.
214. Trejos, A. (1954). *Cladosporium carrionii* n. sp. and the problem of Cladosporia isolated from chromoblastomycosis. *Rev. Biol. Trop.* **2**:75–112.
215. Vanbreuseghem, R., C. de Vroey, and M. Takashio (1978). "Practical Guide to Medical and Veterinary Mycology," 2nd. ed. Masson Publ. U.S.A., New York.
216. Verona, O. (1977). Considerazioni di ordine sistematico sul genere *Humicola* Traaen. *G. Bot. Ital.* **3**:85–89.
217. Vries, G. A. de (1952). Contribution to the knowledge of the genus *Cladosporium* Link ex Fr. Uitgeverij and Drukkerij Hollandia Press, Baarn.
218. Weijman, A. C. M. (1979). Carbohydrate composition and taxonomy of *Geotrichum, Trichosporon* and allied genera. *Antonie van Leeuwenhoek J. Microbiol. Serol.* **45**:119–127.
219. Weitzman, I., and M. Y. Crist (1979). Studies with clinical isolates of *Cunninghamella*. I. Mating behavior. *Mycologia* **71**:1024–1033.
220. White, W. L., and M. H. Downing (1953). *Humicola grisea*, a soil inhabiting, cellulolytic hyphomycete. *Mycologia* **45**:951–963.
221. Zycha, H., R. Siepmann, and G. Linnemann (1969). "Mucorales. Eine Beschreibung aller Gattungen und Arten dieser Pilzgruppe." J. Cramer, Lehre.

*Chapter 5*

# Yeast Identification

### Part 1. Basic Concepts

Yeasts are a heterogeneous group of fungi that superficially appear to be homogeneous. During their life cycle, yeasts grow in a conspicuous unicellular form that reproduces by fission, budding, or a combination of both. Based upon their ability, or inability, to reproduce by sexual means, yeasts have been traditionally divided into two groups. The true yeasts are those fungi that reproduce sexually, developing ascospores or basidiospores when the appropriate conditions are met. In contrast to the true yeasts, yeastlike fungi or the imperfect yeasts, reproduce only by asexual means. In the latter group of yeasts, neither ascospores nor basidiospores have been observed. In this handbook, the term yeast will encompass both imperfect and perfect yeasts. There is considerable disagreement among mycologists with respect to the classification of yeasts; thus only a superficial classification scheme will be presented. Following tradition, the black yeasts and the polymorphic and dimorphic fungi with a yeast form will be considered with the Hyphomycetes in Chapter 4. On enriched media, some members of the Mucorales, such as species of *Mycotypha*, may also develop a yeast form.

The ascomycetous yeasts are classified in the single class Hemiascomycetes of the division Ascomycota. Ascomycetes of this group are characterized by the development of free asci; that is, the asci are not formed within an ascocarp nor are ascogenous hyphae involved in the formation of the ascus. All the ascomycetous yeasts are classified within the single order Endomycetales. The various genera of ascomycetous yeasts are distinguished from each other primarily on the type of vegetative cell division (budding vs. fission, multipolar vs. bipolar budding, etc.), ascus formation, ascospore morphology, and ability to utilize nitrate as a sole source of nitrogen. Species are separated essentially by biochemical means.

Basidiomycetous yeasts are classified in the two classes Teliomycetes and Hymenomycetes of the division Basidiomycota. In addition to basidia, these yeasts usually develop hyphae with clamp connections. The basidia of basidiomycetous yeasts have been traditionally referred to as chlamydospores. This is in error since chlamydospores are asexual propagules and therefore are not derived by sexual means. Basidiospores may develop either laterally or terminally on sterigmata, or directly from the basidium itself. In contrast to popular belief, the yeast form of the basidiomycete *Ustilago* cannot be accurately identified in culture since host-specialization is a key taxonomic characteristic in the differentiation of the various species of *Ustilago* as well as other smuts. The presence of thick-walled globose cells may be an indication that a yeast is a basidiomycete.

The majority of ascomycetous and basidiomycetous yeasts isolated by medical mycologists go unrecognized because most of them are heterothallic. In order for sexual reproduction to occur, the union of two compatible mating types is necessary. In most instances, only one of these mating types is isolated at a given time. In addition, some of these yeasts will reproduce sexually only when specific mating types of the opposite mating type are present. In contrast to heterothallic yeasts, yeasts, such as some species of *Saccharomyces*, are homothallic and are able to mate with other cells of the same isolate. *Saccharomyces* is frequently recovered in the clinical laboratory.

The imperfect yeasts are classified in the class Blastomycetes of the Fungi Imperfecti. They are referred to as "imperfect" yeasts because sexual reproduction has not yet been observed. The identification of these fungi is based upon a combination of morphological and biochemical criteria. Morphology, such as the presence or absence of hyphae and pseudohyphae and the methods of asexual reproduction, are primarily used to demarcate genera, whereas biochemical data are used to differentiate the various species. Both morphological and physiological data are therefore necessary in order to accurately identify these yeasts.

The identification approach taken in this handbook is to use simple techniques that give unambiguous results in conjunction with morphological observations that can be made with the light microscope. It is felt that such an approach should minimize the confusion that normally surrounds yeast identification. Medical mycologists traditionally use a limited number of characteristics to identify the so-called "commonly encountered" 20 or so species of medical importance. In essence, the other 500 or so species of yeasts are simply disregarded, or more often misidentified. Misidentifications are due to the tendency of many laboratorians to force-fit yeasts into existing classification schemes. If a yeast is not identified accurately, it cannot be determined with a high degree of confidence whether or not a

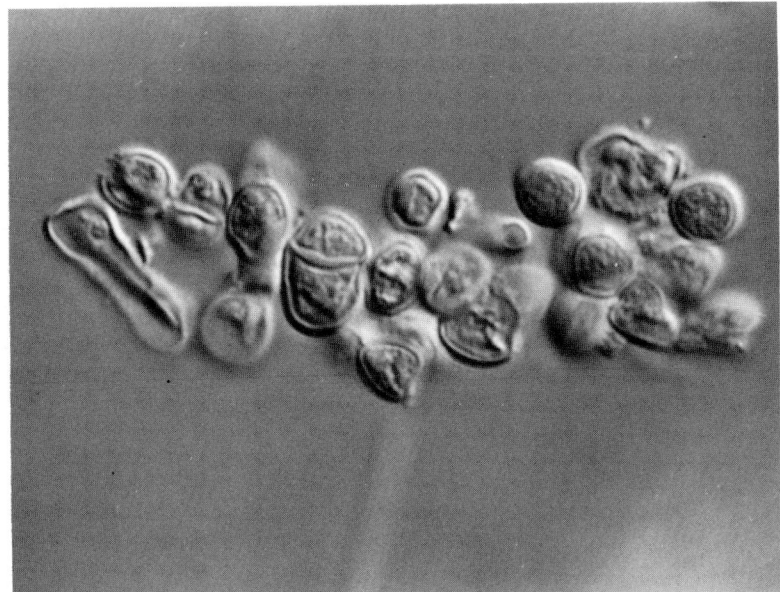

**Fig. 5.1** *Schizosaccharomyces octosporus*. The cells are dividing by fission. Note the thickened transverse septum in the center yeast cell.

second isolate recovered from another clinical specimen is the same as the first one. This is important in determining its role, if any, in the disease process.

Asexual reproduction in yeasts involves the processes of fission, or budding. Fission is typified by members of the genus *Schizosaccharomyces* (Fig. 5.1), in which the duplication of the vegetative cells occurs by the development of transverse septa and the subsequent separation of the vegetative cells into new cells by splitting transversely through the thickened septal walls. Such cells are in essence conidiogenous cells producing annelloconidia. These cells are commonly referred to as fission cells. The term blastospore, which is synonymous with budding, is extremely ambiguous. In reality, when the term blastospore is applied to yeasts, it actually encompasses annelloconidia, arthroconidia, blastoconidia, and phialoconidia.

Conidia may develop from the parent cell in several different patterns. In multipolar (multilateral) budding (Fig. 5.2), the conidia develop from numerous sites over the entire surface of the parent cell. The number of conidia that may be produced by a single parent cell is dependent upon the total surface area of the parent cell that is available for blastoconidium production. Once a site has been used for the development of a conidium,

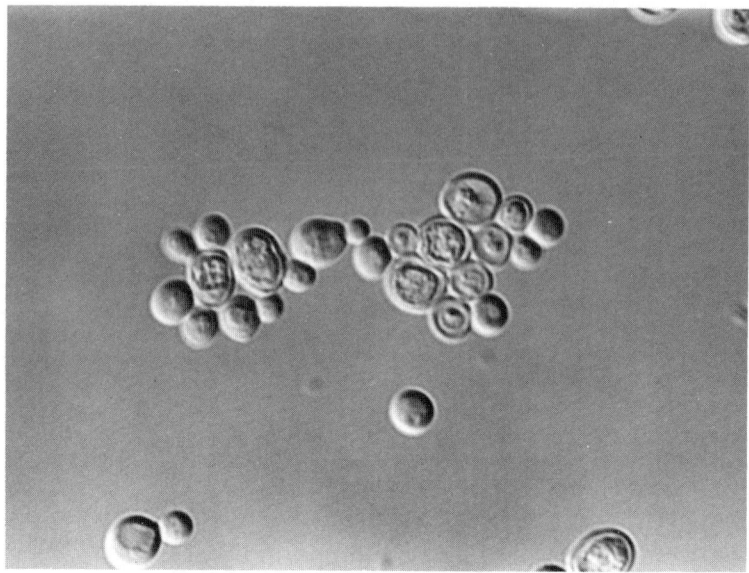

**Fig. 5.2** *Saccharomyces cerevisiae*. The blastoconidia are forming at several different sites on the yeast cells. This is an example of multipolar or multilateral budding.

it apparently is no longer available for the development of a second conidium. Multipolar development of conidia is by far the most common pattern in the yeasts (*Candida, Torulopsis,* etc.). Conidia may develop from fixed sites located at the poles of the parent cell. Bipolar budding (Fig. 5.3) has been observed in species of *Saccharomycodes, Nadsonia, Kloeckera,* and *Hanseniaspora.* In these yeasts, each new conidium develops through the scar left after the release of the preceding conidium. These conidia are in essence annelloconidia and the parent cell is an annellide. And finally, the bottle-shaped cells of *Malassezia* (Fig. 5.4) produce their conidia from a single fixed polar site (unipolar). These conidiogenous cells are phialides.

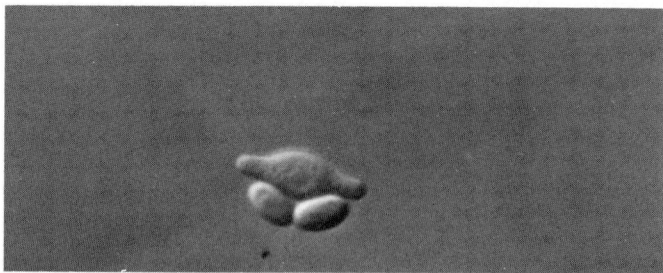

**Fig. 5.3** *Kloeckera apiculata*. The apiculate yeasts produce annelloconidia at both of their poles. This is bipolar budding.

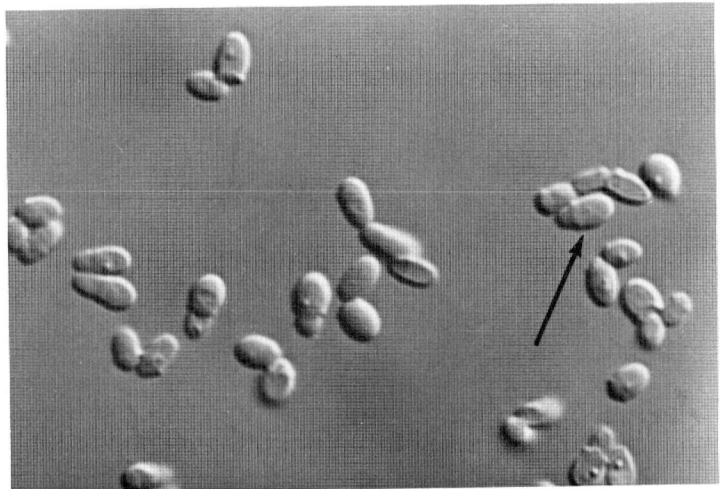

**Fig. 5.4** *Malassezia pachydermatis*. The yeast cells are producing solitary conidia. A collarette (arrow) can be seen around some of the cells. This is unipolar budding.

Yeasts, such as species of *Sporobolomyces*, produce ballistoconidia on peglike structures called denticles (Fig. 5.5). The term denticle is preferred, rather than sterigmata for these structures. Sterigmata should be restricted to the peglike structures in the Basidiomycetes upon which basidiospores develop. Ballistoconidia are forcibly discharged from the denticles by a water drop mechanism that is similar to the one in the Basidiomycetes. For this reason, some mycologists prefer to use the term sterigmata for these structures too.

In recent years, a number of organisms that are superficially yeastlike in appearance have been recovered in medical mycology laboratories. Members of the genus *Prototheca* (Fig. 5.6), which are achlorophyllous algae, are the most commonly encountered organisms. Other fungi, such as *Fissuricella* and *Sarcinosporon* (Fig. 5.7), are rarely recovered.

Yeasts have the ability to grow over a wide range of pH values and on many different media. These fungi can be maintained in the laboratory with little or no difficulty. Yeasts can be selectively recovered from clinical specimens that are heavily contaminated with bacteria by using a medium having a pH value of approximately 3.5 to 4.0. Yeast extract—malt extract agar (YM agar) and malt extract agar (ME agar) are ideal media to use for this purpose when their pH is adjusted to approximately 3.7. Media containing antibacterial agents can also be valuable, but care must be exercised in using these agents. For example, some yeasts will not grow in the presence of chloramphenicol at a concentration of 6.25 µg/ml or greater. Media containing cycloheximide must be carefully employed when

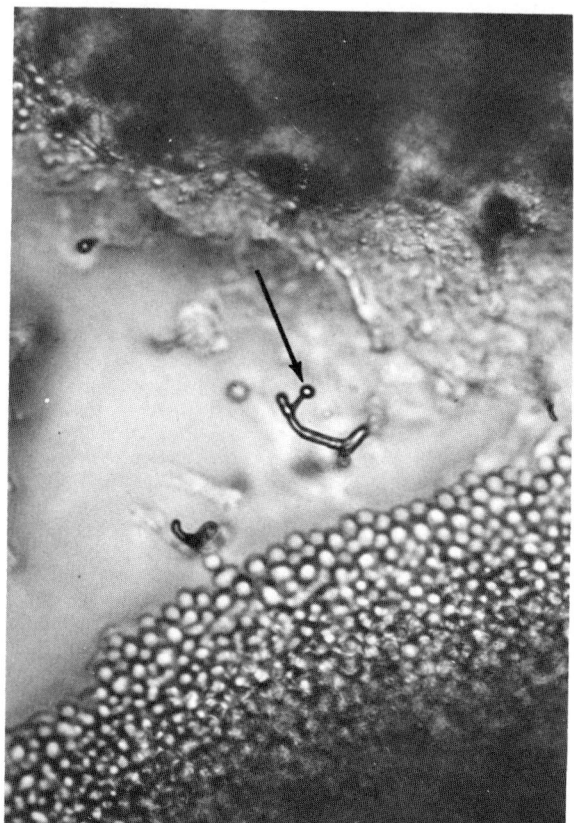

**Fig. 5.5** *Sporobolomyces salmonicolor*. A ballistoconidium (arrow) is beginning to form at the apex of a denticle. (Courtesy of C. Pinello.)

isolating yeasts because cycloheximide is inhibitory to species of *Cryptococcus*, *Saccharomyces*, and *Torulopsis*, as well as many isolates of *Candida krusei*, *C. parapsilosis*, and *C. tropicalis*.

To recover yeasts in the presence of large numbers of moulds, acidified YM broth or ME broth can be utilized. Once the mixed culture has been placed in the broth, a paraffin overlay 1 cm thick is poured over the medium surface. Since moulds do not usually grow in the absence of oxygen, the yeast can be recovered as a pure culture from the broth. Another excellent technique involves inoculating acidified broth and then incubating the broth for 1-2 days on a shaker. Moulds usually grow in the form of pellets, which can be readily separated from the yeast upon subculturing. Some isolates of *Fusarium* can be yeastlike in shake culture. Techniques for purifying mixed yeast cultures can be found elsewhere in

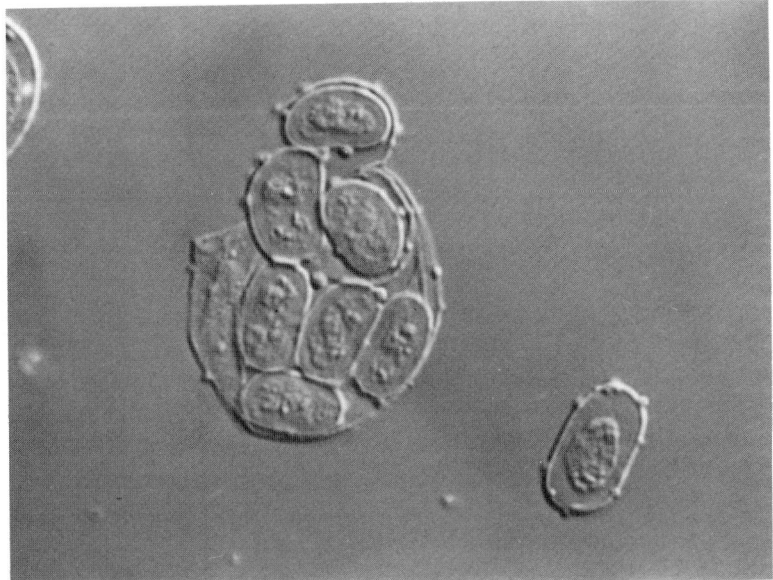

**Fig. 5.6** *Prototheca wickerhamii*. Each sporangium contains a number of sporangiospores. At maturity, the sporangiospores are released, which then develop into new sporangia.

this chapter. Various selective media such as YM agar plus 30–50% glucose, caffeic acid agar, and YM agar with lipids are helpful in isolating specific yeasts. Once a yeast has been recovered, it is purified and maintained on YM agar or ME agar. Sabouraud dextrose agar is satisfactory for the initial recovery of yeasts, but has little, if any, value thereafter. The primary value of Sabouraud dextrose agar is the isolation of fungi from clinical materials and colony descriptions of dermatophytes.

All yeast cultures should be considered contaminated or mixed upon primary isolation. The direct mount and Gram stain will tell the mycologist the condition of the isolate as well as supply valuable morphological information needed for identification. When a yeast is being subcultured to ascospore media, at least four different isolates (if available) should be inoculated together onto each tube of medium. This is necessary because only a single mating type of a heterothallic yeast may be present in each isolate. If an attempt is not made to determine whether or not ascospores can be formed, an ascomycetous yeast could be "force fitted" into a classification scheme, resulting in a misidentification. When a yeast is encountered that does not fit the classification scheme being utilized, the possibility of an ascomycetous or basidiomycetous yeast should be seriously considered, as well as the possibility that the yeast is not included in the identification table.

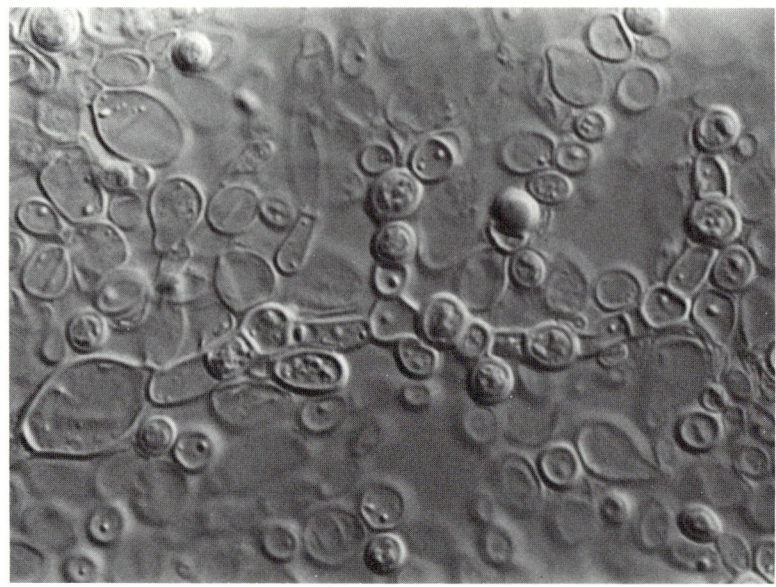

**Fig. 5.7** *Sarcinosporon inkin:* Vegetative cells.

Owing to the large number of tests and media that are available (Table 5.1), a well thought out plan for working up an unidentified yeast is necessary (Tables 5.2 and 5.3). This will greatly enhance the efficient utilization of laboratory resources. The first step is to decide which tests are critical for identification and those that are more or less only confirmatory in nature. The key tests should include direct mounts, Dalmau plates, ascospore media, assimilation and fermentation tests, nitrate utilization, temperature studies where appropriate, and urea hydrolysis. In the clinical laboratory, Wickerham's liquid medium procedure for testing assimilation and fermentation ability of different carbon sources, and nitrate utilization have restricted value because of the long incubation periods (Table 5.4) and the difficulty nonexperienced microbiologists have in reading these tests. A commercial system, or the auxanographic technique, in conjunction with the appropriate morphological and supplementary biochemical tests is the ideal approach for clinical laboratories to use for identifying yeasts to the species level.

The biochemical and flow tables for the identification of the yeasts included in this handbook were constructed so that a minimum set of carefully selected carbon sources could be used to identify the major yeasts of medical interest. The assimilation substrates and other tests are listed in the tables in the order of most useful to least useful, that is, left to right,

Part 1   Basic Concepts

**Table 5.1.** Principal Criteria and Tests for Identifying Yeasts

A. Culture characteristics
   1. Colony color, shape, and texture
B. Asexual structures
   1. Shape and size of cells
   2. Bipolar, fission, multipolar, or unipolar "budding"
   3. Absence or presence of arthroconidia, ballistoconidia, blastoconidia, clamp connections, endoconidia, germ tubes, hyphae, pseudohyphae, or sporangia and sporangiospores
C. Sexual structures
   1. Arrangement, cell wall ornamentation, number, shape, and size of ascospores or basidiospores
D. Physiological studies
   1. Assimilation
      a. Acids: citrate, lactate, and succinate
      b. α-Galactoside: melibiose
      c. β-Galactoside: lactose
      d. α-Glucosides: maltose, melezitose, α-methyl D-glucoside, raffinose, sucrose, and trehalose
      e. β-Glucosides: arbutin, cellobiose, and salicin
      f. Hexoses: D-galactose, D-glucose, L-rhamnose, and L-sorbose
      g. Pentoses: D-arabinose, L-arabinose, D-ribose, and D-xylose
      h. Polyols: erythritol, galactitol (dulcitol), D-glucitol (sorbitol), glycerol, inositol, D-mannitol, and ribitol (adonitol)
      i. Miscellaneous: ethanol, inulin, and starch
   2. Cycloheximide resistance
   3. Ester production
   4. Fat splitting
   5. Fermentation
      a. α-Galactoside: melibiose
      b. β-Galactoside: lactose
      c. α-Glucosides: maltose, raffinose, and sucrose
      d. Hexoses: D-galactose and D-glucose
   6. Gelatin liquefaction
   7. Growth in high osmotic media
   8. Growth in vitamin free media
   9. Nitrogen utilization: amino acids, amino alkanes, creatine, creatinine, and potassium nitrate
   10. Temperature studies
   11. Urea hydrolysis

respectively. The flow tables were constructed using the key substrates necessary for defining each species considered. In those instances where a test could be either positive or negative, the yeast was treated as if it had both responses. As a result, a species may be listed in the keys more than once. Once a tentative identification is obtained, the composite table

**Table 5.2.** Procedure for Identifying a Yeast Recovered from Clinical Material

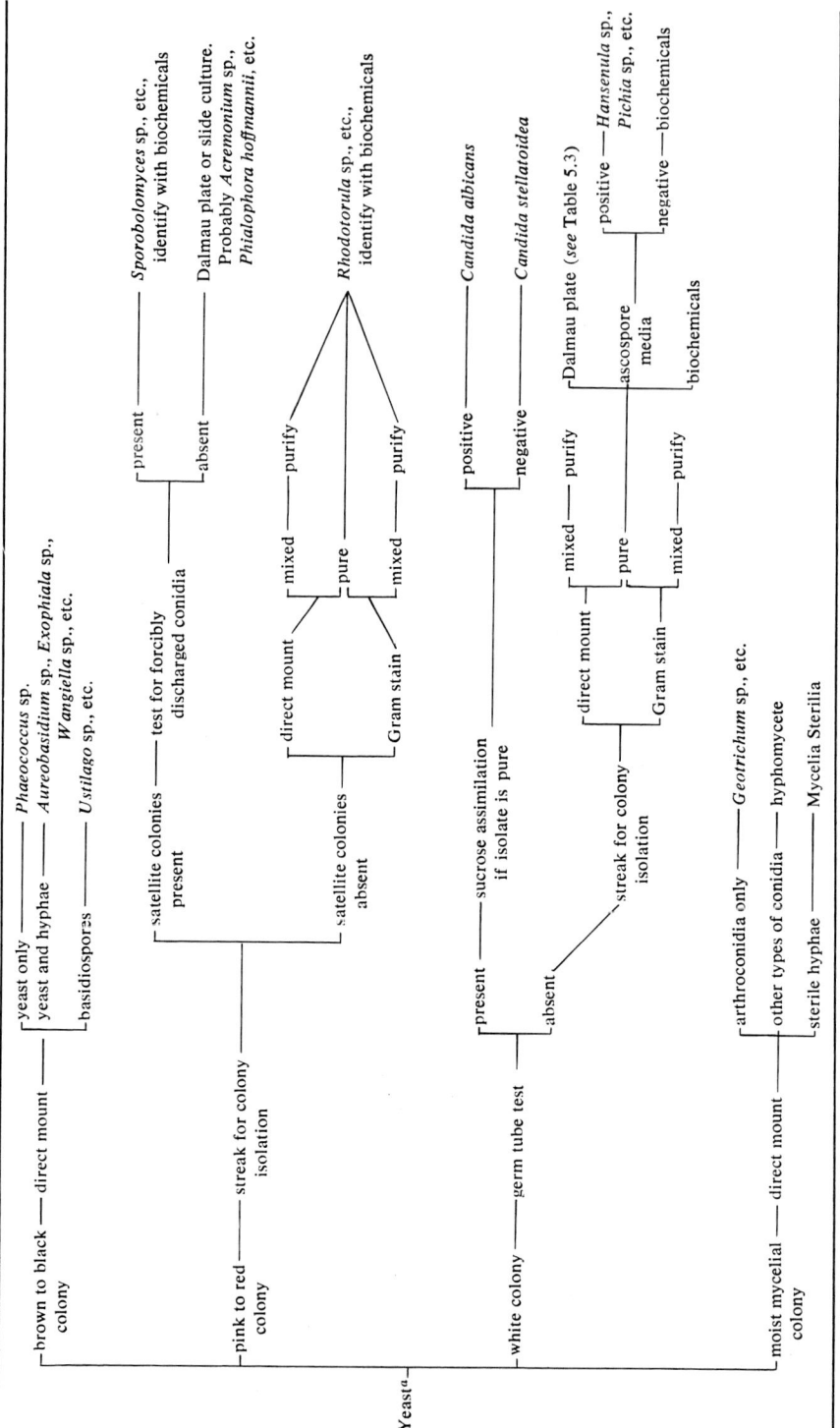

[a] If the yeast was recovered on media containing antimicrobial agents, subculture at least twice on YM agar before conducting biochemical tests.

Table 5.3. Morphology Seen on the Dalmau Plate

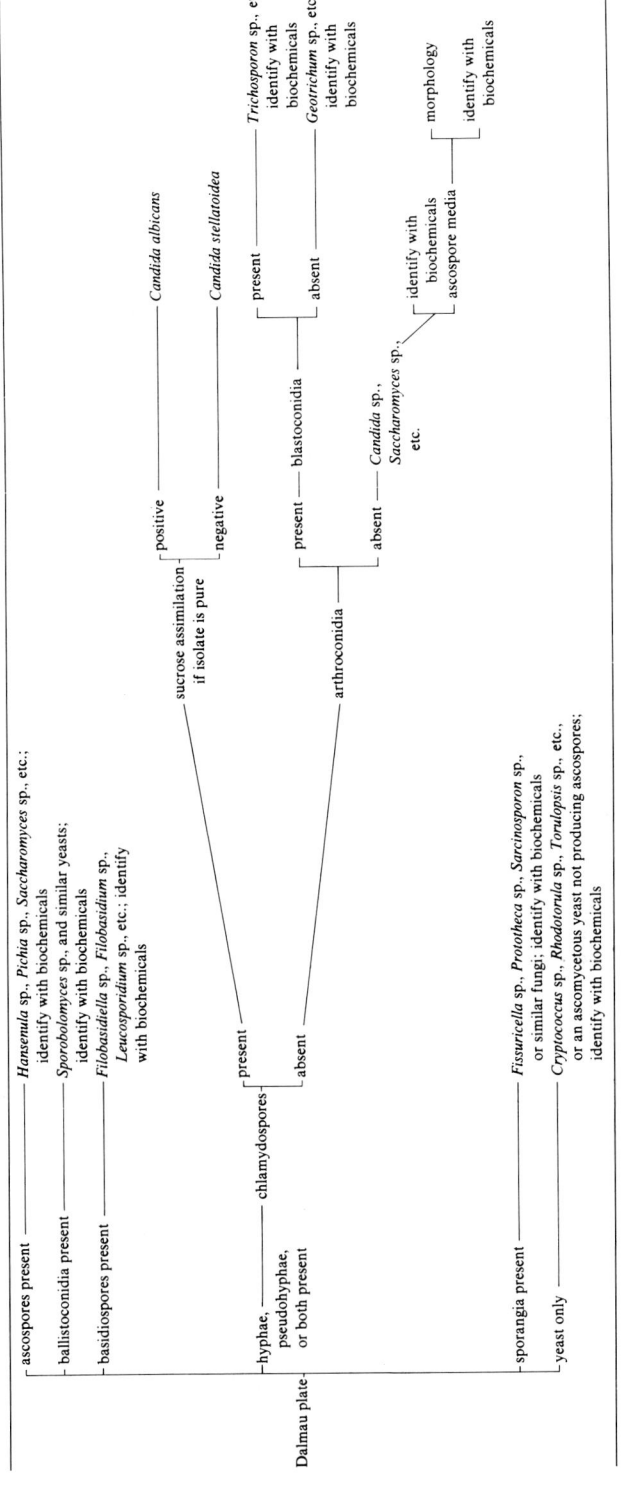

Table 5.4. Selected Methods Used in Determining Nutritional Requirements For Classifying Yeasts

| | Medium | Duration (days) before tests considered negative | Criteria for positive reaction | Comments |
|---|---|---|---|---|
| A. Assimilation | | | | |
| 1. Liquid media | | | | |
| a. Agitated tubes | YNB[a] | 10–14 | 3+ or 2[c] + growth | Good aeration, homogeneous conditions; inoculum control required |
| b. Stationary tubes | YNB | 24 | 3+ or 2+ growth | Slow test, $O_2$ and $CO_2$ variable in tube, positive reaction may be due to a mutant or autolysis; inoculum control required; not recommended for clinical labs |
| 2. Solid media | | | | |
| a. Agar slopes | YNB + arar | 24 | Presence of growth | Substrate concentration constant, inoculum on agar surface, substrate in agar; inoculum control required, some growth usually on negative control |
| b. Auxanograms | YNB + agar | 3–4 | Presence of growth | Media dehydrates rapidly, substrates must be soluble, cannot be volatile, concentration varies; inoculum in agar, substrates on agar surface |
| c. Replica plates | YNB + agar | 24 | Presence of growth | Many yeasts can be tested at one time, same as agar slopes |
| 3. Commercial systems | | | | |
| a. Analytab Products 20C | YNB + agar | 3 | Presence of growth | One-year shelf life, substrates freeze dried, identification table contains percentage values for reactions; computer identification assistance available |

348

| | | | | | |
|---|---|---|---|---|---|
| b. Uni-Yeast-Tek | | YNB + agar | 6 | Change in pH, acid reaction | Shelf life not stated, substrates in premade media; identification wheel supplied |
| B. Fermentation | | | | | |
| 1. Liquid media | | | | | |
| a. Open tubes | | Peptone–yeast extract | 24 | Production of gas bubbles | Cells grow aerobically at medium surface, fall to bottom, then grow anerobically, gas collects in inserted tubes; should not be incubated with assimilation tests |
| b. Sealed tubes | | Peptone–yeast extract | 24 | Production of gas bubbles | Large inoculum needed, limited $O_2$ used quickly, $CO_2$ does not diffuse from system, gas collects in inserted tubes |
| C. Nitrate utilization | | | | | |
| 1. Liquid media | | | | | |
| a. Stationary tubes | | YCB[b] | 21 | 3 + or 2 + growth | After 1 week, a loopful of growth is transferred to a second tube of substrate and read at 7 and 14 days; inoculum control required |
| 2. Solid media | | | | | |
| a. Agar slopes | | YCB + agar | 14 | Presence of growth | Nitrate concentration constant, nitrate in agar, inoculum placed on agar surface, some growth on negative control |
| b. Auxanograms | | YCB + agar | 3–4 | Presence of growth | Nitrate concentration variable, nitrate placed on agar surface, inoculum in agar |

[a] YNB, yeast nitrogen base.
[b] YCB, yeast carbon base.
[c] 3 + or 2 + = density of growth based upon a Wickerham card.

should be consulted to confirm the identification. Fermentation reactions are generally not necessary when identifying the yeasts included in this handbook, provided that all the assimilation substrates in the composite biochemical tables were tested.

The concept of imperfect genera and species in the yeasts is not clearly defined. Asexual structures and biochemical data are routinely used to varying degrees for distinguishing genera of ascomycetous, basidiomycetous and imperfect yeasts. In the case of ascomycetous and basidiomycetous yeasts, sexual structures are the major characteristics utilized. DNA/DNA hybridization data are being used with greater frequency to show phylogenetic relationships in both the imperfect genera and species, and perfect genera and species. The distinction between imperfect genera and species, and perfect genera and species has become vague.

## Part 1. Selected References

### General References

1. Ahearn, D. G. (1978). Medically important yeasts. *Annu. Rev. Microbiol.* **32**:59–68.
2. Arx, J. A. von, L. Rodrigues de Miranda, M. T. Smith, and D. Yarrow (1977). The genera of yeasts and the yeast-like fungi (Stud. Mycol. No. 14). Centraalbureau voor Schimmelcultures, Baarn.
3. Barnett, J. A., and R. J. Pankhurst (1974). "A New Key to the Yeasts." North-Holland Publ., Amsterdam.
4. Lodder, J. (1970). "The Yeasts: A Taxonomic Study," 2nd ed. North-Holland Publ., Amsterdam.
5. Phaff, H. J., M. W. Miller, and E. M. Mrak (1978). "The Life of Yeasts: Their Nature, Activity, Ecology, and Relation to Mankind," 2nd ed. Harvard Univ. Press, Cambridge, Massachusetts.

## Part 2. Techniques

### ASCI AND ASCOSPORES

One of the initial steps in identifying a yeast involves determining whether or not the isolate has the ability to form ascospores. Some ascomycetous yeasts readily form ascospores on the primary isolation medium, whereas others require special ascospore media. The ability to form ascospores varies from isolate to isolate and may be completely lost in older laboratory strains. Many yeasts may not develop ascospores simply because they represent only one mating type of a heterothallic yeast.

Poorly nourished cultures are very difficult to stimulate to form ascospores. The yeast must be well nourished; this may require preinoculation onto an enriched medium, if the isolate is not growing on YM agar. The inoculum is simply transferred to an ascospore medium. Ascospore media differ from other media in that they contain small amounts of carbohydrates; this restricts vegetative growth while enhancing ascospore formation. Some yeasts such as species of *Lipomyces* prefer media deficient in nitrogen. There is no single universal medium that will stimulate ascospore formation in all isolates.

Media such as Kleyn's acetate medium, Gorodkowa agar, vegetable sticks (carrots, celery, etc.), V-8 juice agar, and YM agar are good media for the stimulation of ascospore development. Several different media may have to be tried before a satisfactory medium can be found for a particular isolate. In general, YM agar is a good screening medium. A pH of 6 to 7 is optimal for most yeasts. Ascospore media must be incubated aerobically since oxygen is necessary. In the case of *Hanseniaspora* sp., a slightly reduced oxygen tension is necessary, which is achieved by placing a sterile cover glass over part of the colony. The ideal temperature for incubation of ascospore media is 20–25°C.

When inoculating ascospore media, the inoculum should consist of cells that are 2–3 days old from several different isolates of the same species. It is extremely important to inoculate cells that are young and well nourished. Most freshly isolated strains begin to form ascospores in 1–2 days. Older stock cultures usually require a longer period of time. Cultures should be examined in 3–5 days and weekly thereafter for at least 3 weeks. Some isolates may not form ascospores until 4–6 weeks. The yeast is studied by the direct mount technique in distilled water. Owing to the small size of ascospores, they should be studied under the oil immersion objective. Ascospore form, surface topography, size, color, brims, number of ascospores per ascus, and the presence or absence of inclusion bodies are characteristics used in part to identify the various species. If ascospores cannot be readily seen in the direct mount, an ascospore staining procedure should be utilized (Fig. 5.8). Since ascospores are acid-fast, an acid-fast stain can be used. An excellent procedure for staining ascospores blue-green and vegetative cells red is the Schaeffer–Fulton modified Wirtz stain.

1. Procedure for Schaeffer–Fulton modified Wirtz stain
    a. Prepare an aqueous suspension of the yeast and a control isolate, such as *Saccharomyces cerevisiae*, on a microscope slide; allow them to air dry and then heat fix.
    b. Flood the smears with 5% aqueous malachite green for 60–90 seconds.

352  5  Yeast Identification

    c. Heat to steaming 3–4 times. Add additional malachite green if necessary.
    d. Wash in running tap water for 1 minute.
    e. Counterstain with 0.5% safranin for 30 seconds.
    f. Wash off counterstain and air dry. Examine with the oil immersion objective.
2. Results
    a. Ascospores are blue-green.
    b. Vegetative cells are red.

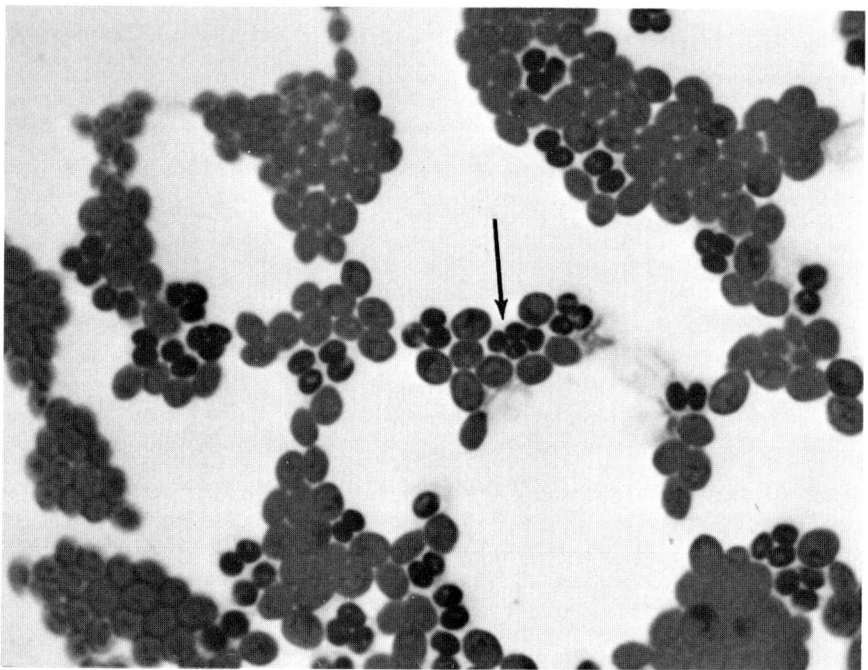

**Fig. 5.8** *Saccharomyces cerevisiae*. The ascospores (arrow) are darkly stained by the Schaeffer–Fulton modification of the Wirtz stain. Each ascus contains 1–4 ascospores. (Courtesy of C. Pinello.)

## ASSIMILATION

Assimilation is the utilization of a carbon source by a yeast in the presence of oxygen. A positive assimilation reaction is usually read either as the presence of growth or as an acid pH value in the growth medium. The aerobic oxidation (assimilation) of a sugar such as glucose results in the formation of carbon dioxide and water. The basic reaction is

$$C_6H_{12}O_6 + 6O_2 \to 6CO_2 + 6H_2O$$

In contrast to assimilation, fermentation of a carbon source by a yeast occurs in the absence of oxygen. A positive fermentation reaction is read only as the presence of gas. It is never read as an acid pH value in the growth medium. The anaerobic utilization by fermentation of a sugar such as glucose results in the formation of ethanol and carbon dioxide. The basic reaction is

$$C_6H_{12}O_6 \to 2C_2H_5OH + 2CO_2$$

Several techniques have been developed for determining the ability of a yeast to utilize various sources of carbon aerobically for energy and growth. The ability to assimilate carbon sources is tested either with a solid agar medium or in a liquid medium. Owing to the sensitivity of these techniques, only purified sugars should be used. This is necessary because lesser grade sugars may be contaminated with a second sugar. For example, maltose is commonly contaminated with small amounts of glucose. The selection of sugars to be tested depends upon the judgment of the mycologist and the genera and species of yeasts to be identified. In medical mycology, only a very small proportion of the 500 or so species of yeasts are dealt with. Thus, only a limited number of carefully chosen substrates is necessary in order to identify these selected yeasts.

The selection of substrates must be done with a great deal of thought. For example, if a yeast can assimilate cellobiose, it most likely will also utilize arbutin and salcin, with the converse holding true. Depending upon the group of yeasts to be identified, it may be wasteful to include all three of these carbohydrates in the same identification scheme. This is also the case for maltose and sucrose, and glucitol and mannitol. Of course, in some instances, all the sugars would be necessary to achieve an accurate identification. In contrast to these sugars, if raffinose is assimilated, sucrose is usually assimilated too. The converse is not true, thus both sugars would have to be included in the identification scheme because it would not be possible to predict what would happen to raffinose if the sucrose was assimilated. Other examples include inulin and sucrose, and xylose and arabinose.

The ability to assimilate different carbohydrates is valuable in distinguishing one species from another, but not usually for differentiating genera. The two most commonly employed techniques for conducting assimilation studies are the liquid medium technique designed by Wickerham and the auxanographic procedure (Table 5.4). Regardless of the method employed to study assimilation reactions, glucose is assimilated by all species of yeasts. This carbon source is included in all tests and serves as an internal quality control, ensuring that the studies are valid. Fructose is omitted from identification schemes because all yeasts have the ability to assimilate it too. Therefore, fructose is not valuable in distinguishing yeasts and would simply be a duplicate substrate for glucose. The inability of a yeast to assimilate a substrate is the result of either the substrate's not entering the yeast cell or the yeast's lacking the appropriate enzyme(s) needed to convert the substrate into an intermediate compound of a central metabolic pathway. The growth medium for assimilation studies must include vitamins and have a pH value of approximately 5.8. The vitamins are necessary for growth, but they do not support growth by themselves. The temperature of incubation is usually 25 or 28°C. In the case of medically important yeasts, 30°C is ideal since they will all grow optimally at this temperature. Assimilation studies are never incubated at 36°C because disaccharides and similar carbohydrates can be broken down into their component sugars at this temperature. Assimilation and fermentation tests should not be placed together in the same incubator. Some yeasts may be able to utilize the ethanol produced from the fermentation tests and give rise to false positive assimilation reactions.

The incubation period for the Wickerham liquid medium technique is 24 days. The tests are read at 7 days and weekly thereafter. The long incubation period is necessary because latent or adaptive enzyme systems may be involved. This is especially true for alcohols, organic acids, and pentoses. Inositol is a classic example of this problem. Most disaccharides and hexoses require much less time before the assimilation tests can be read. Some microbiologists do not feel that it is necessary to use starved inoculum in the Wickerham liquid medium technique. This is in error, since the endogenous rate of respiration is so high in nonstarved yeasts that it may actually mask any effect of the addition of an external carbon source. The rate of respiration in starved yeasts appears to be dependent upon the particular strain, composition of the medium that the yeast was grown on to include the carbon source(s), and the stage of growth in which the cells were harvested. The assimilation tests are read with a Wickerham card, which is a 3 × 5 inch white card with several black lines 0.5 mm wide. The test tube containing the liquid medium is held against the card. If the growth obliterates the lines, this is scored as 3 +. If the lines appear as indistinct bands, this is 2 +. If the lines can be clearly seen, but the edges are indistinct, this is 1 +. Distinct lines and edges are negative. Only 3 + and 2 + are considered positive in the Wickerham liquid medium technique. A 1 + is recorded as weak, but has no real importance since the small amount of growth could be due to carry-over. Growth less than 1 + is considered to be negative. Carry-over results from nutrients being accidentally transferred from the original growth medium with the inoculum to the test system, from endogenous nutrients stored within the yeast cells, or both.

Even though the Wickerham liquid medium technique is the standard method for conducting assimilation studies, it should not be used in clinical laboratories. This is because the test is often difficult to interpret unless the mycologist is constantly using this technique, and second, most clinical laboratories cannot afford to wait 24 days for an identification. For these reasons, the auxanographic procedure is much more valuable to the medical mycologist. The primary differences between the Wickerham liquid medium technique and the auxanographic technique involve time of incubation, expertise in reading the test, and the use of a solid medium instead of a liquid medium.

Auxanographic assimilation results are read within 3–4 days as the presence or the absence of growth. Some mycologists prefer to add the yeast inoculum to the medium and then place the various carbon sources on the agar surface, whereas others add the sugars to the medium and inoculate the agar surface with the yeast suspension. Most of the commercially available systems for yeast identification rely upon the auxanographic procedure. Of the various techniques for conducting assimilation studies, the oxidation–fermentation (O-F) medium should be avoided. This medium does not correlate well with standard techniques for determining assimilation ability in the yeasts. Regardless of the technique used (Table 5.4), YM agar must never be accidentally transferred with the inoculum to the test system because it can result in false-positive results.

## A. Wickerham Liquid Medium Technique

1. Preparation of inoculum
    a. Transfer the isolate to be studied 1–2 times on YM agar at 2–3 day intervals. Incubate the cultures at 25–30°C. This will result in actively growing cells.
    b. Suspend some 24- to 48-hour-old cells in 1.0 ml of the yeast starvation medium that was aseptically removed from one of the 10.0-ml tubes of this medium. The yeast starvation medium is Bacto yeast nitrogen base (YNB) containing 0.1% glucose.
    c. Pipette 0.2–0.4 ml of the suspension back into the remaining 9.0 ml of the starvation medium. Incubate at 30°C for 48 hours.
    d. Dilute the yeast starvation medium containing the yeast in YNB without a carbon source until a 2 + density is reached. This will require approximately 2 volumes of diluent for each volume of inoculum.

2. Test
   a. Aseptically transfer 0.5 ml of the YNB plus substrate to 4.5 ml of sterile distilled water. This is done for each carbon source to be tested. An additional tube without a carbon source is prepared as an inoculum control.
   b. Add 0.1 ml of the diluted inoculum to each tube.
   c. Shake the tubes and incubate at 30°C. The tubes should be shaken daily.
   d. Read the tubes for growth in 7–10 days and weekly thereafter for 24 days.
3. Results
   a. A 3+ or 2+ growth density is positive. A 1+ density is recorded as weak, and less than 1+ is considered to be negative. The YNB without substrate serves as a control for carry-over.
   b. If a pellicle is present, this should be noted on the worksheet.
   c. If a tube has a questionable positive assimilation, incubate the tube for an additional week at 30°C on a shaker and then read again.

### B. Auxanographic Technique

1. Preparation of inoculum
   a. Transfer the isolate to be studied 1–2 times on YM agar at 2- to 3-day intervals. Incubate the cultures at 25–30°C.
   b. Prepare a suspension from a 24- to 48-hour-old culture in 10.0 ml of sterile distilled water equal to a MacFarland number 5 standard.
2. Test
   a. To a 25 × 200 mm tube containing 25 ml of YNB agar held at 50°C, pipette 1.0 ml of the yeast inoculum.
   b. Mix well and pour the entire volume into a 15 × 150 mm sterile plastic Petri dish. Allow the agar to harden at room temperature.
   c. Aseptically place disks containing the various carbohydrates onto the agar surface. The pure sugar can also be placed directly onto the surface of the medium.
   d. Incubate the plates upside down at 30°C and read daily. The plates are discarded in 3–4 days.
3. Results
   a. The presence of growth around or under the disk is considered positive. The glucose-containing disk should always be read first to ensure that the inoculum was viable.
   b. If there is background growth due to carry-over, the growth around each disk must be greater than the background before it is

considered positive. Growth around a disk that is equal to the background growth is considered negative. Background growth is most frequently seen with species of *Trichosporon*.

## CHLAMYDOSPORE DEVELOPMENT (DALMAU PLATE)

The development of chlamydospores has been traditionally used by medical mycologists to tentatively identify a yeast isolated from a clinical specimen as either *Candida albicans* or *C. stellatoidea*. Approximately 90% of all clinical isolates of *C. albicans* produce chlamydospores when inoculated by the Dalmau technique on cornmeal agar supplemented with 1% Tween 80. Other yeasts such as *C. australis*, *C. claussenii*, and *C. tropicalis* may develop chlamydospores. This is especially true if *C. tropicalis* is refrigerated prior to examining it for these structures. *Trichosporon beigelii* may form chlamydospores in old cultures (approximately 3–4 weeks old), but not by the Dalmau technique. The chlamydospores formed in the Dalmau technique are thick-walled, terminal, acid-fast and typically globose (Fig. 5.9). The term chlamydospore is maintained solely for historical reasons because mature chlamydospores formed by these yeasts neither germinate nor produce blastoconidia. At maturity, they are in essence thick-walled vesicles.

The preliminary step leading to the development of chlamydospores is the formation of hyphae. Therefore, those conditions that favor formation of hyphae instead of yeast cells encourage the development of chlamydospores. Disaccharides and trisaccharides promote greater chlamydospore development than do monosaccharides, especially glucose and similar hexoses. In fact, glucose suppresses development of these structures. Other factors enhancing chlamydospore development include a slightly alkaline pH, slight anaerobism, absence of inorganic ions, use of solid medium, absence of condensation on the medium surface, decreased surface tension (by agents such as Tween 80), diluted inoculum (approximately $10^6$ cells per milliliter), young cells approximately 8 hours old as inoculum, and maintenance of the yeast in darkness.

A number of media have been used to stimulate the development of chlamydospores. The primary ones include cornmeal agar, oxgall agar, rice extract agar, starch agar, yeast morphology agar, and zein agar. Most mycologists prefer to supplement their media with 1% Tween 80, which greatly enhances chlamydospore development. Chlamydospores are usually present within 24–48 hours (maximum production 48–60 hours) when the medium is incubated at 22–26°C. Cornmeal agar with 1% Tween 80 inoculated by the Dalmau technique is the recommended procedure. The

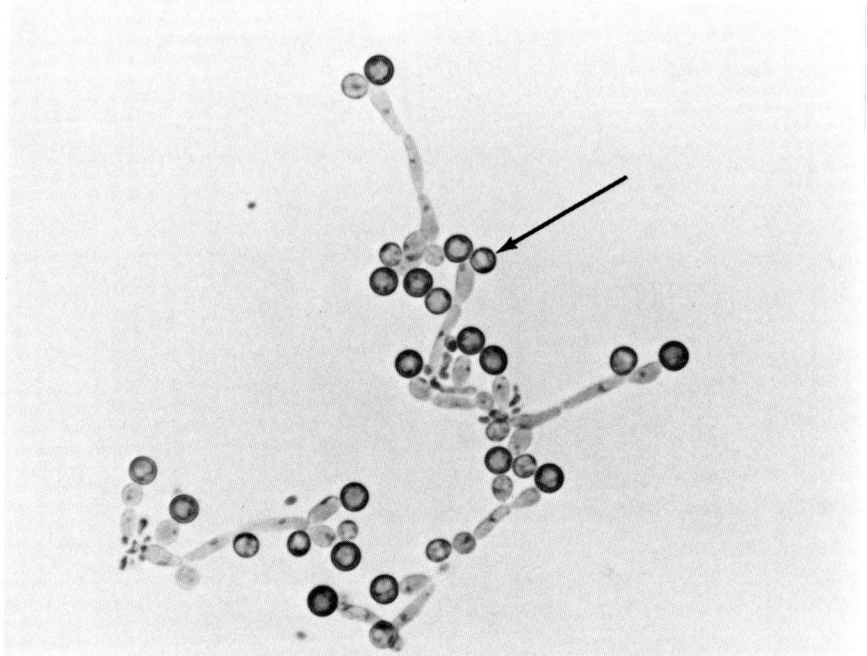

**Fig. 5.9** *Candida albicans*. The chlamydospores (arrow), pseudohyphae, and blastoconidia were formed on cornmeal agar after 48 hours at 24°C. (Reproduced by permission from *Mycopathologia Mycologia et Applicata* **45**:269–283, 1971.)

Dalmau technique consists of diluting the inoculum in the form of streak lines on the medium surface, upon which a cover glass is placed. The yeast is periodically examined through the cover glass with a microscope. A second technique for inoculating the medium that is used by some medical mycologists involves slicing or cutting through the agar with a blade containing the inoculum, and then observing the fungus through the bottom of the Petri dish with a microscope. This technique is not recommended for three reasons. First, the standard descriptions of yeasts are in part based upon observations made using the Dalmau technique. Second, some fungi can be misidentified using the cutting technique. For example, *C. humicola* and *Cryptococcus laurentii* are biochemically similar as listed in most biochemical charts. When *C. humicola* is cut into the agar, it develops as a yeast that morphologically resembles *Cryptococcus*. Thus, *C. humicola* and *Crypt. laurentii* could be confused. And third, the cover glass used in the Dalmau technique establishes an $O_2$ tension gradient permitting isolates having different gas requirements for the development of chlamydospores to produce them at some point next to or under the cover glass.

To aid in observing chlamydospores, some mycologists add 0.1 gm of trypan blue to each liter of medium. Chlamydospores tend to selectively absorb the trypan blue.

An isolate of *C. albicans* is run with each group of determinations to serve as a positive control. Only the development of chlamydospores is considered positive in this test.

1. Dalmau technique
   a. Using a marking pen, divide a Petri plate containing cornmeal agar (CMA) with 1% Tween 80 into quarters and label each quadrant on the bottom of the plate with the culture number. Each plate should be labeled with the date.
   b. With a sterile inoculating needle, lightly touch the yeast colony and then make two separate streaks approximately 3.5 cm long and 1.2 cm apart. Do not dig into the agar.
   c. Flame-sterilize the inoculating needle, allow it to cool and then streak back and forth across the two original streak lines, diluting the yeast inoculum. Do not dig into the agar.
   d. Flame-sterilize a 22-mm square cover glass; allow it to cool, then place it over the streak marks.
   e. Incubate at 22–26°C for 18–24 hours. Do not refrigerate the inoculated plates.
   f. Remove the Petri dish lid and place the dish on the microscope stage. Using low power, bring into focus the edge of the cover glass and then scan near the edge for chlamydospores and other structures (Table 5.3). Suspicious areas are examined with the high dry objective. Read the control first.
2. Results

| Observation | Tentative identification | Additional tests required |
|---|---|---|
| Chlamydospores present | *C. albicans* or *C. stellatoidea* | Sucrose assimilation |
| Chlamydospores absent | See Table 5.3 | Biochemical tests |

## DEMONSTRATION OF CAPSULES

Many yeasts, especially members of the genera *Candida, Cryptococcus, Rhodotorula, Torulopsis,* and *Trichosporon* have the ability to form mucoid capsules around their cells. In contrast to the belief of some physicians and microbiologists, the absence, presence, or amount of capsular material cannot be used to identify yeasts such as *Cryptococcus neoformans.* The

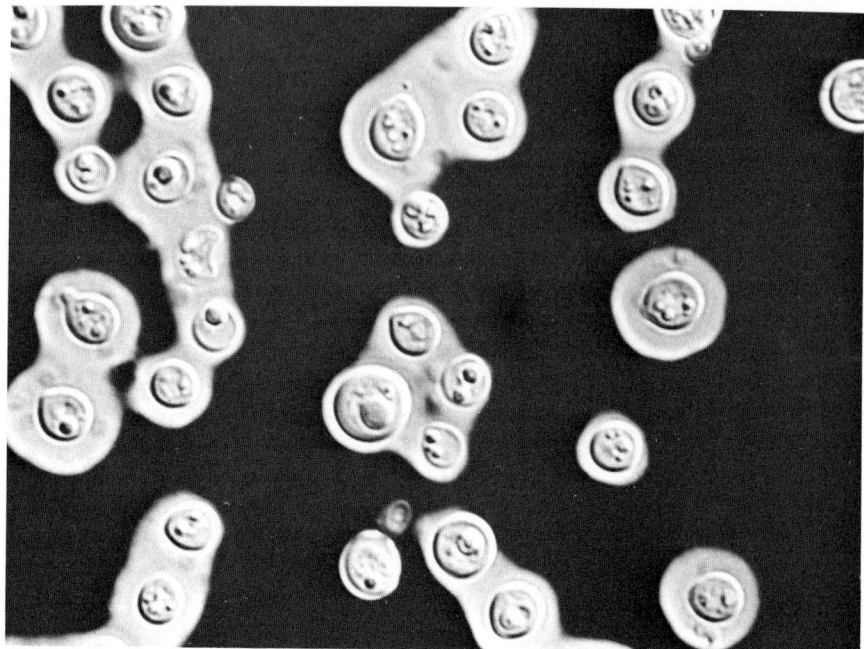

**Fig. 5.10** *Cryptococcus neoformans*. An India ink preparation is used to demonstrate the presence of capsules around yeast cells. The background is extremely dark in this photomicrograph because it was taken in Nomarski microscopy.

identification of *C. neoformans* as well as all other yeasts is based upon morphological and biochemical data. The presence or the absence of a capsule and the shape and size of the yeast cells are important to the physician in making a diagnosis of cryptococcosis, especially if the central nervous system (CNS) is involved. Because of the poor prognosis of CNS cryptococcosis if appropriate therapy is not initiated immediately, diagnosis of this infection must be prompt.

The demonstration of capsules is accomplished with an India ink preparation. Capsules can also be demonstrated by phase-contrast microscopy. The India ink does not stain the yeast, but serves as a dark background permitting the hyaline capsules to be more readily seen (Fig. 5.10). Since India ink is not a stain, internal organelles are not stained. The structures commonly seen within the yeast cells that resemble nuclei are vacuoles or similar structures that are made visible by light being reflected off of their surfaces.

1. Procedure for demonstrating capsules
    a. Ensure that there are no artifacts or agglutinating carbon particles present in the ink.

b. Place a 3-mm loopful of India ink on a clean microscope slide slightly off center.
   c. Add to the ink a 3-mm loopful of the clinical specimen (concentrate if cerebrospinal fluid) or a small portion of the yeast colony to be examined.
   d. Place a clean cover glass over the suspension. Reduce the light intensity of the microscope, then examine the preparation for the presence or the absence of capsules and note the size and shape of any yeast cells present.
2. Results

| Observation | Report |
|---|---|
| Encapsulated or nonencapsulated globose yeast 5–12 μm in diameter with blastoconidia (if present) attached by a narrow neck | Morphology suggestive of *Cryptococcus* |

## DIRECT MOUNTS

Direct mounts are made in order to study yeast morphology microscopically. This information assists in the identification of yeasts as well as in determining the purity of the isolates. Varied morphology within a single colony is usually suggestive of a mixed culture. The shape and size of arthroconidia, asci and ascospores, basidia and basidiospores, blastoconidia, hyphae, pseudohyphae, sporangia and sporangiospores, and yeast cells can be studied in the direct mount. Temporary direct mounts are prepared with distilled water because yeasts tend to settle much faster in water than in mounting media such as lactophenol cotton blue (LPCB) or lactophenol (LC). Permanent mounts can be prepared with LPCB, LP, or polyvinyl alcohol (PVA).

1. Temporary mounts
   a. Place a small drop of distilled water slightly off center on a clean glass microscope slide.
   b. Remove a small portion of the yeast colony with a long-handled inoculating needle, place it into the drop of distilled water, and then suspend the cells.
   c. Place a clean cover glass over the suspension and observe microscopically. Since water evaporates rapidly, the mount must be studied at once.
2. Permanent mounts
   a. LPCB or LP mounts
      (1) Prepare a mount as in 1a and b.

(2) Allow the preparation to air-dry and then heat-fix the cells.
  (3) Place a small drop of LPCB or LP mounting medium at the edge of the smear.
  (4) Place a clean cover glass at the edge of the drop of fluid and lower the cover glass slowly, forcing any trapped air toward the edge of the cover glass.
  (5) Remove excess LPCB or LP from the edges of the cover glass with a paper towel.
  (6) Seal the edges of the cover glass with finger nail polish ensuring that it covers the edges of the cover glass and contacts the glass slide surface. Allow to air-dry.
 b. Polyvinyl alcohol (PVA) mount
  (1) Prepare a mount as in 1a and b.
  (2) Place a small drop of PVA at the edge of the smear.
  (3) Place a clean cover glass at the edge of the fluid and cover glass gently, forcing any trapped air toward the edge of the cover glass. Trapped air not removed will be absorbed by the PVA. Allow the mount to air-dry.

## FERMENTATION

Alcoholic fermentation is the process by which a carbohydrate, such as glucose, is fermented anaerobically to form ethanol and carbon dioxide. Fermentation is read as the production of gas, not as an acid pH change. The fermentation process requires that the yeast have enzymes, such as alcohol dehydrogenase and pyruvate decarboxylase, and a transport mechanism for getting the carbohydrate across the plasma membrane under anaerobic conditions. If these are absent, the yeast will be unable to ferment the carbohydrate being tested.

If a carbohydrate can be fermented, it is also typically assimilated. The converse is not necessarily true. By comparing the assimilation and fermentation reactions, this information serves as an internal quality control ensuring that the positive fermentation reactions are valid. If fermentation occurs, glucose will always be fermented. Fermentation is usually described in terms of rapid, medium, slow, latent, etc. These descriptive expressions are based upon the time required for the gas to form and the amount of gas that is present.

The various carbohydrates to be tested are added separately to the fermentation broth (yeast extract–peptone solution). Carbohydrates are used in a final concentration of 2% except for raffinose, which is 4%. Because of the high cost of melibiose, this sugar should be tested only when it is assimilated and when raffinose is fermented. Once the tubes have been inoculated with the yeast, they are incubated in one of two manners (Table 5.4). Some mycologists prefer to use test tubes with cotton plugs. In this technique, the yeast grows aerobically at the top of the medium. With time, the cells settle to the bottom, where they grow anaerobically in the presence of a low oxygen concentration. If the yeast can ferment the carbohydrate, $CO_2$ is released and collected in the inserted tube. The second technique of incubation involves using screw cap tubes or tubes sealed with paraffin. In this procedure, a large inoculum is necessary. As the oxygen is rapidly used, the yeast begins to use the carbohydrate anaerobically, with the subsequent formation of $CO_2$. The $CO_2$ is collected in the inserted tube. In this system, it is necessary to break the seal of the tube in order to permit any $CO_2$ held in solution to escape. Escaping $CO_2$ can be detected in the solution as small bubbles rising toward the surface.

The fermentation test is never incubated at 36°C. At this temperature, disaccharides as well as other carbohydrates can be broken down into their basic sugars. These breakdown products might be fermented in lieu of the original carbohydrate being tested. Such fermentation reactions would be falsely positive, resulting in the possibility of a misidentification of the yeast.

Most mycologists prefer to use a fermentation broth that contains bromothymol blue as an indication of pH changes. The value of this indicator is primarily for quality control. A change from blue to yellow in noninoculated tubes indicates microbial contamination, carbohydrate breakdown, or both. These tubes should be discarded. The yellow color in the fermentation test (acid pH) is not read as positive for fermentation, but merely indicates that the carbohydrate has been assimilated. Too often, microbiologists fail to make this important distinction.

1. Procedure for testing fermentation ability
    a. Prepare a suspension of the yeast in 4.5 ml of sterile distilled water from a 24- to 48-hour-old culture growing on YM or ME agar. The suspension should be equal to a MacFarland number 1 standard.
    b. Pipette 0.1 ml of inoculum into each tube containing carbohydrates to be tested.
    c. Incubate the tubes at 25–30°C and shake daily. The tubes are kept 24 days before discarding them as negative.
2. Results
    a. Only the production of gas is positive. Read the tubes every 2–3 days for the first week and then weekly up to 24 days.
    b. If a sugar is fermented, it is also assimilated. There are a few exceptions if the assimilation tests are carried out in YNB. Fermentation without assimilation means that either the fermentation tube is contaminated or the inoculum in the assimilation test was not viable.

## FORCIBLY DISCHARGED CONIDIA

Occasionally, yeasts are encountered that produce forcibly discharged conidia called ballistoconidia (Fig. 5.5). The first indications that ballistoconidia are being formed by an isolate is the spontaneous development of young satellite colonies. Ballistoconidia form upon short denticles, after which they are actively discharged into the air via a water-drop mechanism. Members of the genus *Sporobolomyces* are occasionally isolated in the clinical laboratory.

A number of techniques have been developed to demonstrate the presence of ballistoconidia. The simplest technique involves pouring a layer of YM agar into both the top and bottom of a disposable plastic Petri dish. The bottom dish is inoculated with the yeast, the two dishes are put together and then inverted so that the inoculated surface is on top. After 2–3 days at 20–25°C, if ballistoconidia were formed, new growth in the form of a mirror image of the original colony will be present on the uninoculated bottom surface. This new growth resulted from ballistoconidia being discharged into the air and then settling on the surface below.

## GERM TUBE TEST

The germ tube test provides a simple, reliable and economical procedure for the tentative identification of *Candida albicans* and *C. stellatoidea*. Approximately 95% of the clinical isolates of *C. albicans* and *C. stellatoidea* produce germ tubes when they are incubated in serum at 37°C for 2.5–3 hours. Confusion may result from cultures that have developed hyphal elements during their primary isolation or subsequent incubation. The confusion surrounding germinating arthroconidia of *Geotrichum* and *Trichosporon* can be resolved by ensuring that the fungus is developing cells with blastoconidia in addition to germ tubes. Enlarged blastoconidia of *C. brumptii*, *C. tropicalis* and *C. pseudotropicalis* must be distinguished from the germ tubes of *C. albicans* and *C. stellatoidea*. Germ tubes represent the initiation of hyphal or hyphalike growth and arise directly from the yeast cell. They have parallel walls at their point of origin; they are not constricted (Fig. 5.11). The term pseudo-germ-tube has been used in the past by some medical mycologists to describe the germ tubes of *C. albicans*. Since the germ tubes of *C. albicans* are true germ tubes, the term pseudo-germ-tube is totally incorrect and should not be used.

The germ tube test may yield faulty results under some circumstances. Acidic or basic conditions result in decreased germination, while a neutral

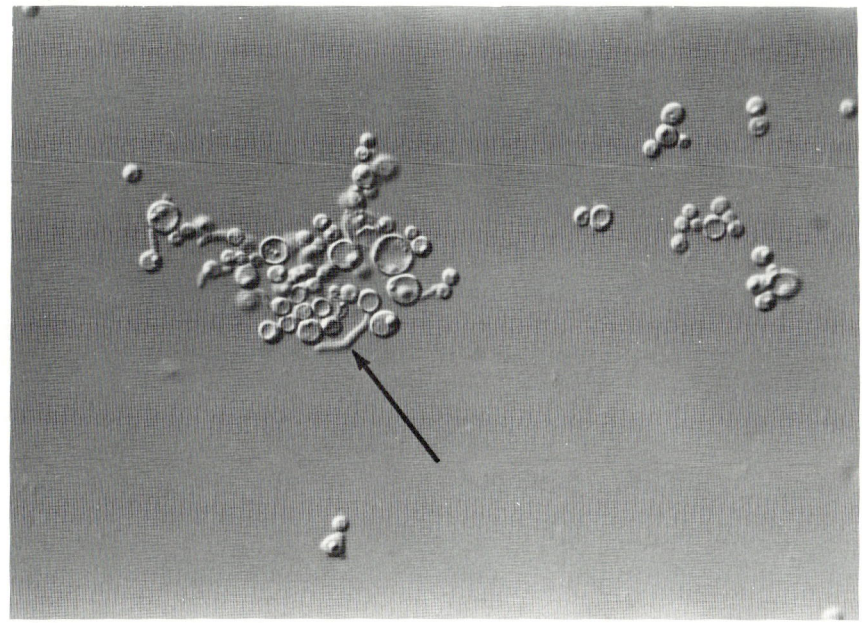

Fig. 5.11 *Candida albicans*. The germ tubes (arrow) were formed in human serum after 2.5 hours and 37°C. Germ tubes are not constricted at their point of origin from their parent cells.

pH (optimum 7.4) contributes toward maximum germ tube development. Bacterial contamination by *Escherichia, Klebsiella, Proteus, Pseudomonas, Staphylococcus, Streptococcus* sp. and others may interfere with the production of germ tubes. Antimicrobial agents that have been incorporated in the isolation media may interfere with this test. And finally, human serum often contains inhibitory factors such as ferritin (an iron–protein complex), that suppresses germ tube development.

Germ tube formation is influenced by the medium, inoculum size, temperature of incubation, concentration of simple carbohydrates, and microaerobic conditions. Media such as peptone, tissue culture medium 199, trypticase soy broth, egg whites, and sheep, rabbit, guinea pig, horse, and bovine sera are satisfactory. With reference to human sera, pooled, individual, hemolyzed, nonhemolyzed, heat-inactivated, fresh, or frozen sera work well. If these media are diluted, it must be remembered that diluted sera and physiological saline reduce the percentage of germ tubes. Most studies indicate that the maximum percentage of germ tube development occurs when $10^5$ to $10^6$ cells per milliliter are used as inoculum. The percentage of germ tubes formed decreases significantly as the concentration of inoculum increases. Thus, a faintly turbid serum suspension is ideal to enhance maximum germ tube development. Germ tube production occurs between 32 and 42°C. It is favored by small amounts of simple carbohydrates, microaerobic conditions as found in the liquid suspending medium, and inoculum from young cultures.

*Candida albicans* and *C. tropicalis* are run with each group of germ tube determinations to serve as positive and negative controls, respectively. Only the development of germ tubes is considered positive in this test.

1. Procedure for the germ tube test
    a. Remove the required number of 12 × 75 mm test tubes containing 0.3 ml of pooled human serum from the freezer and allow them to warm up to room temperature.
    b. With a clean capillary pipette, cocktail straw, or rounded wooden applicator stick, lightly touch one yeast colony that is 18–72 hours old and then place the stick into the serum. Each morphologically distinct colony is individually picked and inoculated to separate tubes of serum.
    c. Suspend the yeast in the serum leaving the wooden stick in the tube.
    d. Incubate the inoculated tests at 37°C for 2.5–3 hours.
    e. Using the wooden stick, place one drop of the yeast suspension on a clean glass microscope slide labeled with the corresponding laboratory number.
    f. Place a clean cover glass over the suspension and then examine it with a microscope using the low power objective. After locating the cells, use the high power objective to confirm the presence or absence of germ tubes.
    g. Read the controls first. If the control culture of *C. albicans* has not produced germ tubes, discard the tests. *Candida tropicalis* does not produce germ tubes under these conditions. If germ tubes are formed by *C. tropicalis,* the tests must be discarded.
2. Results

| Observation | Tentative identification | Additional tests required |
| --- | --- | --- |
| Germ tubes present | *C. albicans* or *C. stellatoidea* | Sucrose assimilation |
| Germ tubes absent | None | Dalmau plate and biochemical tests |

## MIXED CULTURES

It should be assumed that all initially isolated yeasts are mixed cultures. The Gram stain, direct mount, and subsequent streaking for colony isolation will confirm the purity of each yeast isolate. Pure cultures are mandatory if assimilation, fermentation, and other biochemical data are to be meaningful. The following techniques can be used to purify mixed cultures.

1. Bacterial contamination
   a. Colony isolation on brain heart infusion agar (BHIA)
      (1) Suspend a small portion of the yeast to be decontaminated in sterile distilled water.
      (2) Streak a loopful of the suspension for colony isolation onto two plates of BHIA.
      (3) Incubate one BHIA plate at 36°C and the second at 30°C. In 48 hours, Gram stain a portion of each colony to be selected for identification. If the colonies are not pure, further steps are necessary (1b).
   b. Colony isolation on Sabouraud dextrose (SAB) agar
      (1) Suspend a small portion of the yeast to be decontaminated in sterile distilled water.
      (2) Streak a loopful of the suspension for colony isolation onto a plate of SAB agar.
      (3) Incubate one SAB agar plate at 36°C and the second at 30°C. In 48 hours, Gram stain a portion of each colony to be selected for identification. If the colonies are not pure, further steps are necessary (1c).
   c. Colony isolation on Sabouraud dextrose agar containing chloramphenicol (SAB + C) or Sabouraud dextrose agar containing penicillin and streptomycin (SAB + P and S)
      (1) Suspend a small portion of the yeast to be decontaminated in sterile distilled water.
      (2) Streak a loopful of the suspension for colony isolation onto a plate of SAB + C or SAB + P and S.
      (3) Incubate the plate at 30° for 48 hours and then Gram stain a small portion of each colony to be identified. If the colonies are not pure, further steps are necessary (1d).
   d. Acidification of Sabouraud dextrose (SAB) broth
      (1) Suspend a small portion of the yeast to be decontaminated in sterile distilled water.

(2) To each of 4 tubes containing 10 ml of SAB broth, add 1 drop of 1 $N$ HCl to the first tube, 2 drops of 1 $N$ HCl to the second tube, 3 drops of 1 $N$ HCl to the third tube, and finally 4 drops of 1 $N$ HCl to the fourth tube.
(3) Add approximately 0.5 ml of the contaminated yeast suspension to each tube.
(4) Incubate at 30°C for 24 hours.
(5) Subculture 0.1 ml of each broth onto two plates of BHIA.
(6) Incubate the BHIA plates at 36°C and 30°C. In 48 hours Gram stain a small portion of each colony to be identified. If the colonies are not pure, the use of media containing other antibacterial agents will be required.

2. Yeast contamination
   a. Colony isolation on Sabouraud dextrose agar
      (1) Suspend a small portion of the yeast in sterile distilled water.
      (2) Streak a loopful of the suspension for colony isolation onto a plate of SAB agar.
      (3) Incubate the SAB agar at 30°C for 48 hours and then prepare direct mounts using a small portion of each colony to be identified. If the yeast is not pure, the isolate must be restreaked.
   b. Colony isolation on caffeic acid agar (CA)
      (1) Suspend a small portion of the yeast suspected to contain *Cryptococcus neoformans* in sterile distilled water.
      (2) Streak a loopful of the suspension for colony isolation onto a plate of CA agar.
      (3) Incubate the CA agar at 30°C for approximately 4 days. *Cryptococcus neoformans* produces colonies that are brown to black. Prepare a direct mount of a small portion of each colony to be identified. If the yeast is not pure, it must be restreaked.

3. Mould contamination
   a. Colony isolation on yeast malt (YM) agar
      (1) Suspend a small portion of the yeast-mould colony in sterile distilled water.
      (2) Streak a loopful of the suspension for colony isolation onto a plate of YM agar.
      (3) Incubate the YM agar plate at 30°C for approximately 4–6 days, then prepare a direct mount using a small portion of each colony to be identified. If the yeast is not pure, further steps are necessary (3b).
   b. Colony isolation in yeast malt broth (YM broth)

(1) Transfer a small portion of the yeast-mould isolate to a tube containing 10 ml of YM broth.
(2) Incubate the YM broth at 30°C for approximately 48 hours and then carefully remove a small portion of sediment with a sterile capillary pipette by slipping the pipette along the edge of the tube to the bottom without disturbing the mycelial pellicle.
(3) Streak the sediment for colony isolation onto a plate of YM agar.
(4) Incubate at 30°C for approximately 4–7 days and then prepare a direct mount using a small portion of each colony to be identified. If the yeast is not pure, further steps are necessary (3c).

c. Colony isolation in shake culture
(1) Transfer a small portion of the yeast-mould isolate to a 250-ml Erlenmeyer flask containing approximately 100 ml of YM broth.
(2) Place the flask on a rotary shaker and incubate at 30°C while shaking for 4–6 days.
(3) Carefully remove a small amount of the sediment with a sterile capillary pipette. Ensure that the balls of mycelium are not removed by accident.
(4) Streak the sediment for colony isolation onto a plate of YM agar.
(5) Incubate at 30°C for approximately 4–7 days and then prepare a direct mount using a small portion of each yeast colony to be identified. If the yeast is not pure, further procedures will be of little help.

## NITRATE UTILIZATION

Yeasts have the ability to use ammonium sulfate, asparagine, peptone, and urea (if the concentration is not toxic) aerobically as sole sources of nitrogen if adequate vitamins are provided for energy and growth. In contrast, aliphatic amines, potassium nitrate, sodium nitrate, and some amino acids are utilized selectively by different yeasts. These latter compounds are very useful in the identification of yeasts. In general, if a yeast has the ability to utilize nitrate, it can also use nitrite as a source of nitrogen. The converse is not always true; *Debaryomyces hansenii* can use nitrite, but not nitrate. The utilization of nitrate involves a series of reductase enzymes.

The ability of a yeast to use potassium nitrate as a sole source of nitrogen can be determined either by the auxanographic method or in liquid medium (Table 5.4). The auxanographic method is recommended for the clinical laboratory. The presence of growth around the potassium nitrate impregnated disk is considered positive. The absence of growth around the disk is negative. If "carry-over" is present, the growth around the disk must be greater than the amount of background growth in the agar. Yeast carbon base (YCB), a growth medium that does not contain a source of nitrogen, is used in this test.

1. Procedure for the auxanographic technique
    a. Quality control isolates
        (1) Each group of tests is controlled with *Cryptococcus albidus* (positive) and *C. neoformans* (negative).
    b. Yeast inoculum
        (1) Prepare a yeast suspension from a 24- to 48-hour-old colony on YM agar in sterile distilled water equal to a MacFarland number 1 standard.
    c. Inoculation
        (1) To each tube containing 15 ml of nitrogen assimilation medium for yeasts (YCB agar) held at 50°C in a water bath, add 1.0 ml of yeast inoculum and mix carefully.
        (2) Pour the agar-yeast suspension into a 15 × 100 mm sterile Petri dish and then allow the agar to harden at room temperature.
        (3) With a marking pen, divide the Petri dish in half. Label one side $KNO_3$ and the other side peptone.
        (4) Aseptically place disks containing $KNO_3$ and peptone on the medium surface on their corresponding halves.
        (5) Incubate the plate with its inoculated surface up at 30°C and read every other day.
    d. Results
        (1) Growth must be present around the peptone and potassium nitrate ($KNO_3$) disks in the plate inoculated with *C. albidus*. If growth is absent from around the peptone disk, the agar was too hot and the inoculum was killed.
        (2) Growth should be absent around the $KNO_3$ disk in the plate inoculated with *C. neoformans*.
        (3) Reading the test: Positive = growth around both the peptone and $KNO_3$ disks. If "carry-over" is present, growth must be greater than the background. Negative = growth around the peptone disk, but not around the $KNO_3$ disk. If "carry-over" is present, growth is equal to or less than the background.

2. Procedure for the liquid medium technique
   a. Quality control
      (1) Same as 1a.
   b. Yeast inoculum
      (1) Same as carbon asssimilation procedure.
   c. Inoculation
      (1) To each tube having 5.0 ml of 1X nitrate asssimilation medium (YCB broth) containing $KNO_3$, add 0.1 ml of yeast inoculum and mix well.
      (2) Incubate for 7 days at 30°C. If growth is present, transfer a loopful of inoculum from the tube to a second tube having 5.0 ml of 1X YCB broth containing $KNO_3$. This is necessary because the growth present may be using nitrogenous compounds that have been excreted by the inoculum, or small amounts of ammonium sulfate that was in the inoculation medium, or both.
      (3) Incubate another 1–2 weeks and then read.
   d. Results
      (1) Growth must be present in the tube containing *C. albidus* and absent in the one containing *C. neoformans*.
      (2) Reading the test: Positive = 2+ or 3+ growth on a Wickerham card. Negative = 1+ growth on a Wickerham card.
   e. Confirmation of questionable negative tests
      (1) To each questionable test, add a few drops of reagent A (sulfanilic acid) and reagent B ($\alpha$-naphthylamine) to the negative tube (nitrate reagents).
      (2) If the nitrate has been reduced to nitrite, the solution will develop a pink to red color.
      (3) To confirm that nitrate is present, add a pinch of zinc dust to the negative tube containing reagents A and B. In a few minutes the zinc will reduce all nitrate to nitrite, followed by the development of a pink to red color.

## PIGMENT FORMATION BY *CRYPTOCOCCUS NEOFORMANS*

Several years ago, it was discovered that *Cryptococcus neoformans* could produce a melanin or melaninlike pigment when it was grown on a medium containing an extract prepared from pulverized seeds of *Guizotia abyssinica* (bird seed). By use of phenol oxidase enzymes, *C. neoformans* formed melanin pigments from *o*- and *p*-diphenol compounds that were in the extract. We now know that the *o*-diphenols result in intracellular pigments whereas *p*-diphenols result in extracellular soluble pigments that diffuse into the medium. Subsequent investigations have revealed that ferric citrate stimulates the production of pigments from *p*-diphenols. Amino acids, such as asparagine, glutamine, and glycine, help stimulate pigment production.

Occasionally, other members of the genus *Cryptococcus,* that is, *C. albidus, C. laurentii, C. luteolus,* and *C. terreus,* may form pigments. This is especially true if the medium is incubated for a prolonged period of time, that is, 10 or more days. A caffeic acid medium has been developed as a replacement for "bird seed" agar. *Cryptococcus neoformans* produces a dark pigment in approximately 2–4 days on caffeic acid agar at 25–30°C. Caffeic acid agar is an excellent medium, but must be protected from the light to prevent it from becoming dark in color. This medium is used for the tentative identification of *C. neoformans.* The final identification must include the appropriate morphology and biochemical tests.

The yeast suspected to be *C. neoformans* is streaked onto caffeic acid agar in a Petri dish and then incubated in the dark for 2–4 days at 25–30°C. *Cryptococcus neoformans* turns black under these test conditions. Antimicrobial agents can be added to the caffeic acid agar if a selective isolation medium is desired. A known culture of *C. neoformans* and *C. laurentii* should be run with each group of determinations to serve as positive and negative controls, respectively.

## TEMPERATURE STUDIES

In addition to assimilation, fermentation and morphological data, the identification of some yeasts can be aided by determining whether or not they can grow at an elevated temperature. For example, *Cryptococcus neoformans* can be distinguished from most of the other members of the genus *Cryptococcus* by its ability to grow at 37°C. The ability to grow at 37°C cannot be used solely as the basis for its identification, because not all isolates of *C. neoformans* grow at this temperature.

Temperature studies are conducted by inoculating two tubes of YM agar with the isolate. One tube is incubated at 25°C and the other at 36°C. After 4–7 days, the tubes are examined for the presence of growth. Growth must be present in both tubes before it can be concluded that the yeast has the ability to grow at the elevated temperature. The tube incubated at 25°C must contain growth in order for the test to be valid, especially if growth is absent at 36°C.

## UREA HYDROLYSIS

A number of yeasts produce the enzyme urease, thereby having the capability to hydrolyze urea. The ability to produce urease is determined with Christensen's urea agar. Each group of urease determinations is controlled with *Cryptococcus albidus* (positive), *Candida albicans* (negative), and an uninoculated tube of medium. The uninoculated tube ensures that a pH change due to atmospheric gases has not occurred.

In general, the production of urease is of little value in distinguishing one species of yeast from another. When dealing with medically important yeasts, this determination is useful in distinguishing species of the genera *Cryptococcus* and *Rhodotorula,* which are urease positive, from those of *Torulopsis,* which are urease negative. Other genera of medical interest such as *Candida* and *Trichosporon* contain both urease positive and negative species.

1. Procedure for the hydrolysis of urea
    a. With a loop, inoculate a tube of Christensen's urea agar (CUA) with a small amount of the yeast colony.
    b. Incubate the slant at 30°C for 5 days.
    c. Read the control tubes first. If the tube inoculated with *Candida albicans* or the uninoculated tube has changed from yellow to pink through red, or if the tube inoculated with *C. albidus* has remained yellow, discard the test and inoculate new CUA slants with the isolates and the appropriate control organisms.
2. Read and record results: positive = pink or red color, urease was produced; negative = yellow color, urease was not produced.

### Part 2. Selected References

#### A. General References

1. Barnett, J. A., and R. J. Pankhurst (1974). "A New Key to the Yeasts." North-Holland Publ., Amsterdam.
2. Lodder, J. (1970). "The Yeasts: A Taxonomic Study," 2nd ed. North-Holland Publ., Amsterdam.

#### B. Assimilation

1. Barnett, J. A. (1968). Biochemical differentiation of taxa with special reference to the yeasts. A discussion of the biochemical basis of the nutritional tests used for classification. *In* "The Fungi: An Advanced Treatise" (G.C. Ainsworth and A. S. Sussman, eds.), Vol. III, pp. 557–595. Academic Press, New York.

2. Barnett, J. A. (1976). The utilization of sugars by yeasts. *Adv. Carbohyd. Chem. Biochem.* **32**:125–234.
3. Barnett, J. A. (1977). The nutritional tests in yeast systematics. *J. Gen. Microbiol.* **99**:183–190.

## C. Chlamydospore Development

1. Dalmau, L. M. (1929). Remarques sur la technique mycologique. *Ann. Parasitol.* **7**:536–545.
2. Hayes, A. B. (1966). Chlamydospore production in *Candida albicans. Mycopathol. Mycol. Appl.* **29**:87–96.
3. Jansons, V. K., and W. J. Nickerson (1970). Induction, morphogenesis, and germination of the chlamydospore of *Candida albicans. J. Bacteriol.* **104**:910–921.

## D. Germ Tube Test

1. Ahearn, D. G. (1974). Identification and ecology of yeasts of medical importance. In "Opportunistic Pathogens" (J. E. Prier and H. Friedman, eds.), pp. 129–146. University Park Press, Baltimore, Maryland.
2. Auger, P., and J. Joly (1977). Factors influencing germ tube production in *Candida albicans. Mycopathologica* **61**:183–186.
3. Mackenzie, D. W. R. (1962). Serum germ tube identification of *Candida albicans. J. Clin. Pathol.* **15**:563–565.

## E. Nitrate Utilization

1. Hopkins, J. M., and G. A. Land (1977). Rapid method for determining nitrate utilization by yeasts. *J. Clin. Microbiol.* **5**:497–500.

## F. Pigment Formation by Cryptococcus neoformans

1. Chaskes, S., and R. L. Tyndall (1978). Pigment production by *Cryptococcus neoformans* and other *Cryptococcus* species from aminophenols and diaminobenzenes. *J. Clin. Microbiol.* **7**:146–152.
2. Hopfer, R. L., and F. Blank (1975). Caffeic acid-containing medium for identification of *Cryptococcus neoformans. J. Clin. Microbiol.* **2**:115–120.
3. Wang, H. S., R. T. Zeimis, and G. D. Roberts (1977). Evaluation of a caffeic acid–ferric citrate test for rapid identification of *Cryptococcus neoformans. J. Clin. Microbiol.* **6**:445–449.

## G. Urea Hydrolysis

1. Roberts, G. D., C. D. Horstmeier, G. A. Land, and J. H. Foxworth. (1978). Rapid urea broth test for yeasts. *J. Clin. Microbiol.* **7**:584–588.
2. Zimmer, B. L., and G. D. Roberts (1979). Rapid selective urease test for presumptive identification of *Cryptococcus neoformans. J. Clin. Microbiol.* **10**:380–381.

## Part 3. Taxonomy

## ASCOMYCETOUS YEASTS

### Key to the Principal Groups of Yeasts

1. Asci and ascospores present . . . . . . . . . . . . . . . . . . . . . Ascomycetous yeast
1'. Asci and ascospores absent . . . . . . . . . . . . . . . . . . . . . . . . . . . . . . 2
    2. Basidia or teliospores present . . . . . . . . . . . . . . . . Basidiomycetous yeast
    2'. Basidia or teliospores absent . . . . . . . . . . . . . . . . . . . . . . Imperfect yeast

### Key to the More Commonly Encountered Ascomycetous Yeasts

1. Ascospores fusiform with a whiplike appendage; ascospores in 2 bundles of 4 within each ascus . . . . . . . . . . . . . . . . . . . . . . . . . . . . . . . . . . . . . . . . . *Nematospora*
1'. Ascospores not fusiform, whiplike appendage absent . . . . . . . . . . . . . . . . 2
    2. Ascus resulting from conjugation of two vegetative cells that resulted from fission; 4–8 ascospores per ascus . . . . . . . . . . . . . . . . . . . . . . . . *Schizosaccharomyces*
    2'. Vegetative cells resulting from fission absent . . . . . . . . . . . . . . . . . . . 3
3. Bipolar budding; ascospores globose to hat-shaped; 2 or 4 per ascus . . . . *Hanseniaspora*
3'. Multipolar budding . . . . . . . . . . . . . . . . . . . . . . . . . . . . . . . . . 4
    4. Ascospores ellipsoidal to reniform, tending to agglutinate; 1 to numerous per ascus . . . . . . . . . . . . . . . . . . . . . . . . . . . . . . . . . . . . . . . . *Kluyveromyces*
    4'. Ascospores globose to hat-shaped . . . . . . . . . . . . . . . . . . . . . . . . 5
5. Ascospores subglobose to hat-shaped, smooth, usually with a ledge . . . . . . . . . . 6
5'. Ascospores globose to ovate, without ledge . . . . . . . . . . . . . . . . . . . . . 7
    6. Nitrate assimilated . . . . . . . . . . . . . . . . . . . . . . . . . . . . *Hansenula*
    6'. Nitrate not assimilate . . . . . . . . . . . . . . . . . . . . . . . . . . . . *Pichia*
7. Asci without protuberances; 1–4 ascospores, ascospores smooth . . . . . . *Saccharomyces*
7'. Asci usually with protuberances; 1–4 ascospores, ascospores usually verrucose . . . . . . . . . . . . . . . . . . . . . . . . . . . . . . . . . . . . . . . . . . . . . . *Debaryomyces*

### *Debaryomyces* Klöcker, 1909

Diagnostic features: *Debaryomyces* produces 1 or 2 (or up to 4), globose to ovoid, verrucose ascospores in each ascus (Fig. 5.12). Vegetative cells are variable in shape with multipolar blastoconidia. Pseudohyphae are rudimentary to well developed, nitrate is not utilized, and fermentation is slow to absent. The anamorphs are species of *Torulopsis* (16).

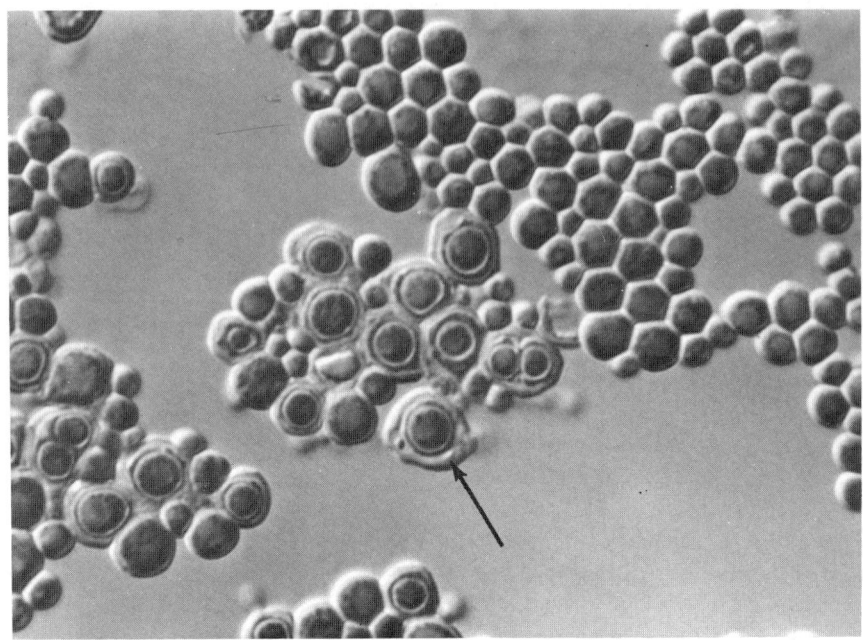

**Fig. 5.12** *Debaryomyces hansenii.* Each ascus typically contains a single globose ascospore. Occasionally, two ascospores may form in an ascus.

Comments: There has been considerable debate concerning *Debaryomyces* and its relationship to *Torulaspora* (20). Current feelings are that these two genera are probably different.

*Debaryomyces hansenii* and similar yeasts can be differentiated by the key assimilation reactions in Table 5.5. Isolates of *Debaryomyces* are occasionally seen in the mycology laboratory.

### *Hanseniaspora* Zikes, 1911

Diagnostic features: The asci typically contain either 2 or 4 hat-shaped ascospores (Fig. 5.13) that are rapidly released at maturity, or 1 or 2 globose (sometimes verrucose), ascospores with an indistinct equatorial to subequatorial ledge in each ascus, which are not released at maturity. The vegetative cells are ovoid to elongate, apiculate, bipolar, and form annelloconidia. Pseudohyphae are usually absent, but may be rudimentary to well developed. Hyphae are absent, nitrate is not utilized, fermentation is positive, and all species have an absolute requirement for inositol and pantothenate. The anamorphs are species of *Kloeckera* (16).

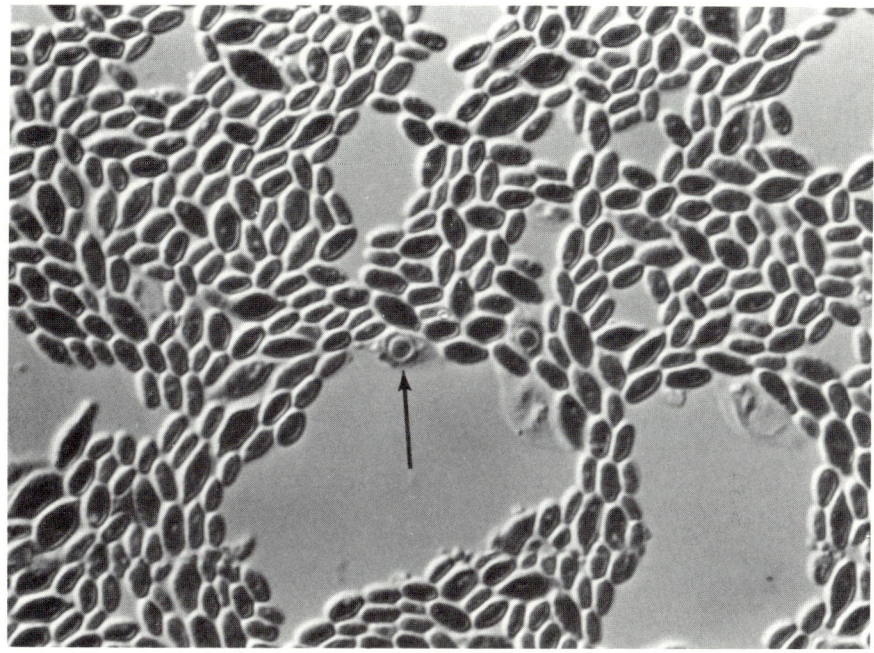

**Fig. 5.13** *Hanseniaspora uvarum*. Each ascus typically contains a single ascospore (arrow). Apiculate conidiogenous cells can be seen surrounding some of the asci.

Comments: Isolates of *Hanseniaspora* are rarely seen in the clinical laboratory.

*Hansenula* H. Sydow et P. Sydow, 1919

Diagnostic features: Asci are shaped like the vegetative cells; that is, they are globose to elongate. The 1–4 ascospores in each ascus are globose to hat- to Saturn-shaped, and usually smooth (Fig. 5.14). Pseudohyphae and true hyphae may be present, nitrate is utilized and fermentation is variable. The anamorphs are species of *Candida* and *Torulopsis* (16).

Comments: The more commonly isolated species can be differentiated with the key assimilation reactions in Table 5.5. Isolates of *Hansenula* are rarely seen in the clinical laboratory.

*Kluyveromyces* van der Walt emend. van der Walt, 1965

Diagnostic features: The ascospores are globose to crescent-shaped, smooth, 1 to many per ascus (Fig. 5.15), and tend to agglutinate after being

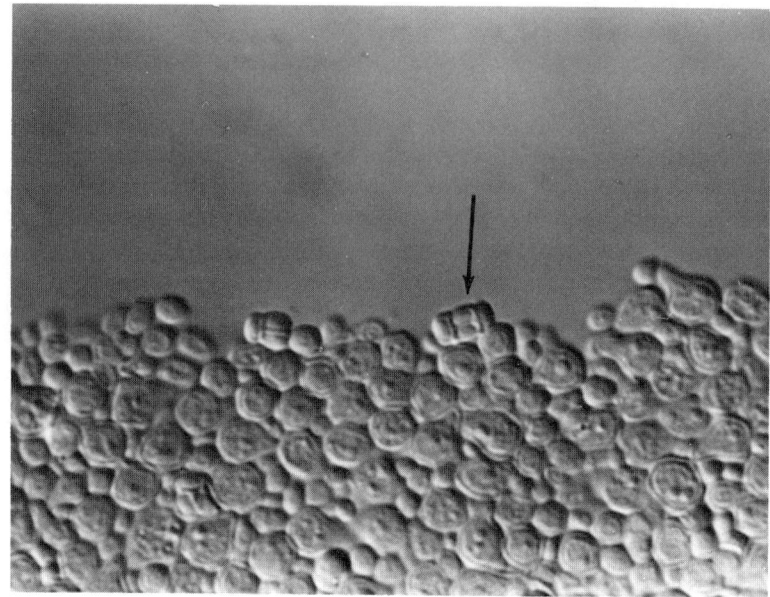

**Fig. 5.14** *Hansenula polymorpha*. Each ascus contains 1–4 ascospores (arrow). There is a brim around each ascospore that turns downward.

released at maturity. The vegetative cells are globose to elongate, pseudohyphae may be produced, true hyphae are absent, nitrate is not utilized, fermentation is variable, and a red pigment may be formed. The anamorphs are species of *Candida* and *Torulopsis* (16).

Comments: Isolates of *Kluyveromyces* are rarely seen in the clinical laboratory.

## *Nematospora* Peglion, 1897

Diagnostic features: Ascospores are long and narrow with a whiplike appendage. The elongated ascus contains 8 ascospores that are in two bundles of 4 (Fig. 5.16). The vegetative cells are variable in shape, and produce multipolar blastoconidia. Pseudohyphae and true hyphae are produced, nitrate is not utilized, and fermentation is positive (16).

Comments: Isolates of *Nematospora* are rarely seen in the clinical laboratory.

## *Pichia* Hansen, 1904

Diagnostic features: Ascospores are globose to hat- to Saturn-shaped, usually smooth, but occasionally verrucose, usually with an oil drop, and

# Part 3 Taxonomy

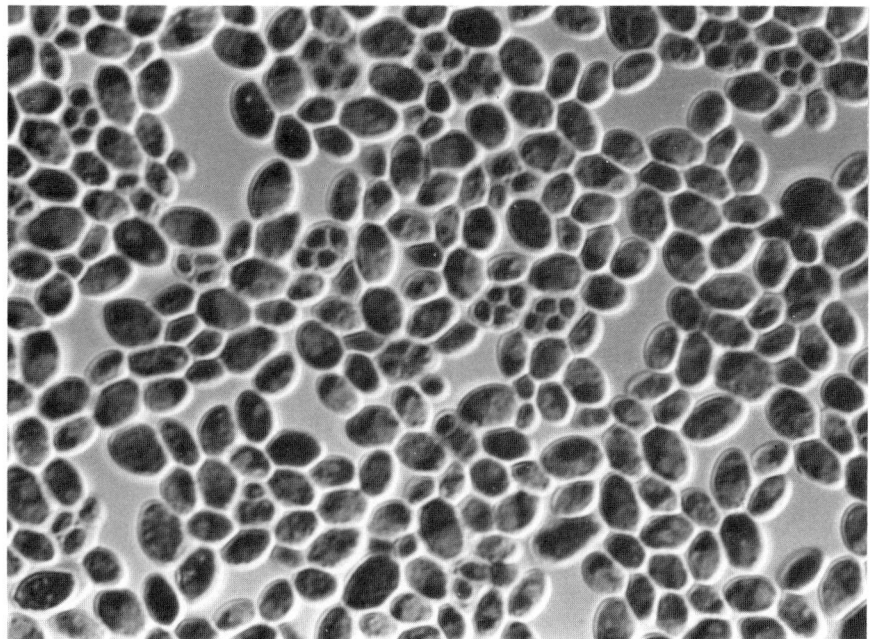

**Fig. 5.15** *Kluyveromyces marxianus*. Each ascus contains 1–4 ascospores that tend to agglutinate after they are released from the asci.

there are 1–4 ascospores per ascus (Fig. 5.17). The vegetative cells are variable in shape with multipolar blastoconidia. Pseudohyphae generally are present, true hyphae may be produced, nitrate is not utilized and fermentation is variable. The anamorphs are species of *Candida* (16).

Comments: *Pichia farinosa* and similar yeasts can be differentiated with the key assimilation reactions in Table 5.5. Isolates of *Pichia* are occasionally recovered in the clinical laboratory.

## *Saccharomyces* Meyen ex Hansen, 1883

Diagnostic features: The genus *Saccharomyces* is characterized by 1–4, globose to ellipsoidal ascospores per ascus, which do not rupture at maturity (Fig. 5.18). The vegetative cells are globose to elongate with multipolar blastoconidia. Pseudohyphae may be formed, true hyphae are absent, nitrate is not utilized, lactose is not assimilated, and fermentation is positive. The anamorphs are species of *Candida* and *Torulopsis* (16).

Comments: *Saccharomyces cerevisiae* and similar yeasts can be differentiated with the key assimilation reactions in Table 5.5. Isolates of *S. cerevisiae* are frequently isolated in the clinical laboratory.

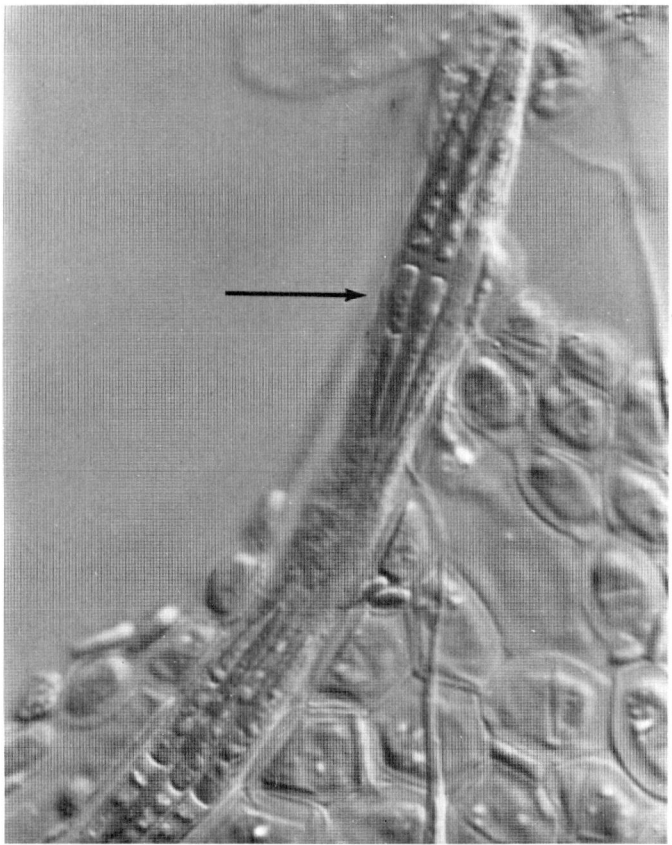

**Fig. 5.16** *Nematospora coryli*. Each ascus typically contains two groups of four ascospores (arrow).

## *Schizosaccharomyces* Lindner, 1893

Diagnostic features: The asci of *Schizosaccharomyces* are elongate and contain 4–8 globose to ovoid, thin-walled ascospores, which swell during their development (Fig. 5.19). The vegetative cells are globose to cylindrical and divide by fission. The vegetative cells are actually annellides. True hyphae may be present, which may form arthroconidia. Fermentation is positive, nitrate is not utilized (16).

Comments: Isolates of *Schizosaccharomyces* are rarely seen in the clinical laboratory.

### Key to the Major Basidiomycetous Yeasts

1. Swollen basidia at apex of sporophores present . . . . . . . . . . . . . . . . . . . 2

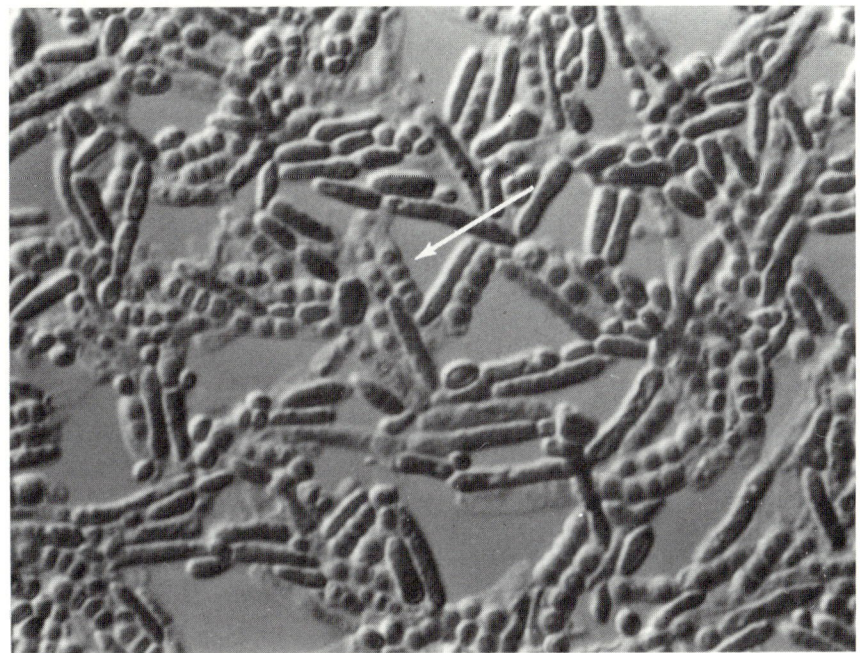

**Fig. 5.17**  *Pichia farinosa*. Each ascus contains 1–4 ascospores (arrow).

1'. Swollen basidia absent; thick-walled teliospores present . . . . . . . . . . . . . . . . 3

    2. Basidiospores forming chains . . . . . . . . . . . . . . . . . . . . . . *Filobasidiella*

    2'. Basidiospores single, formed synchronously · . . . . . . . . . . . . . *Filobasidium*

3. Carotenoid pigments present; anamorphs are species of *Rhodotorula* . . . *Rhodosporidium*

3'. Carotenoid pigments absent; anamorphs are species of *Candida* . . . . . *Leucosporidium*

## BASIDIOMYCETOUS YEASTS

### *Filobasidiella* Kwon-Chung, 1975

Diagnostic features: *Filobasidiella* forms a swollen basidium at the apex of a sporophore, upon which 4 chains of 1-celled basidiospores develop (Fig. 5.20). The hyphae have clamp connections. The anamorph is *Cryptococcus neoformans* (12).

Comments: The formation of the sexual state of *F. neoformans* can be enhanced on YNB agar containing 0.5% uracil. The fungus is heterothallic, thus the appropriate mating types are necessary for sexual reproduction to occur. A second species, *F. bacillispora* (13) has been described, which

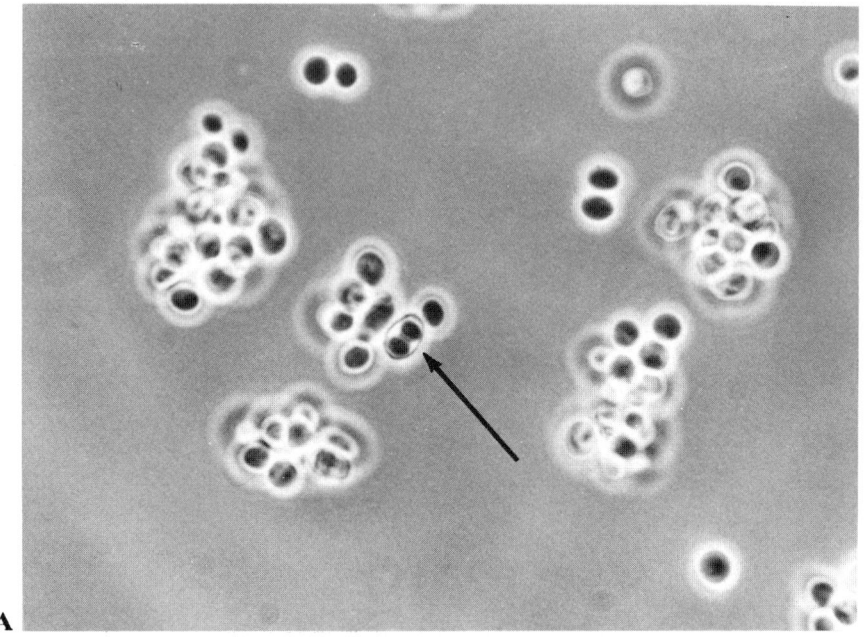

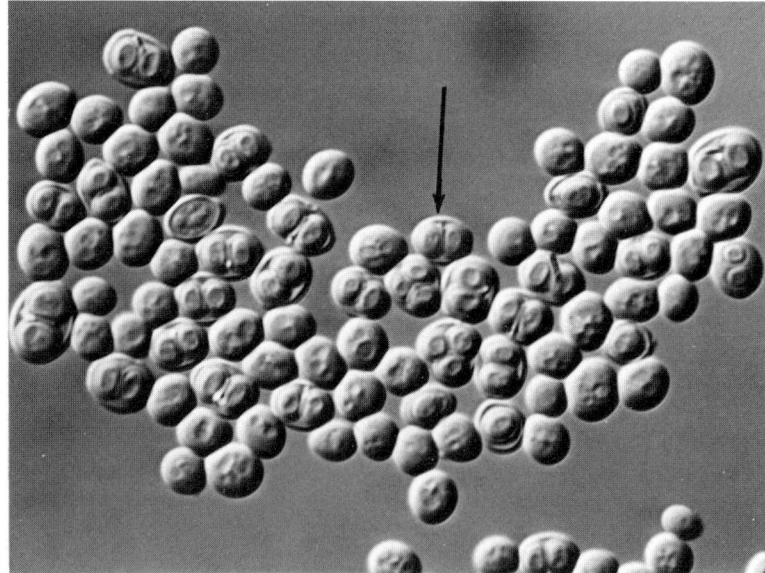

**Fig. 5.18** *Saccharomyces cerevisiae*. Each ascus in this yeast contains 1–4 ascospores (arrows). The preparations are seen in phase-contrast and Nomarski microscopy, respectively.

Part 3  Taxonomy 383

Table 5.5. Key Characteristics of Selected Genera and Species of Ascomycetous and Other yeasts

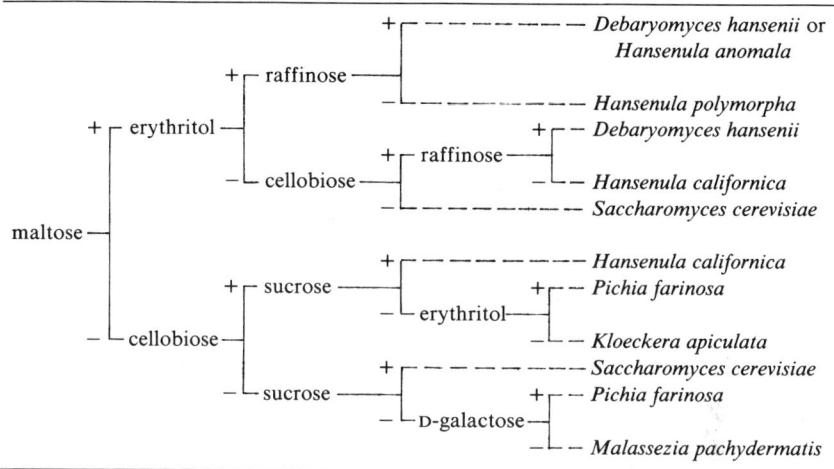

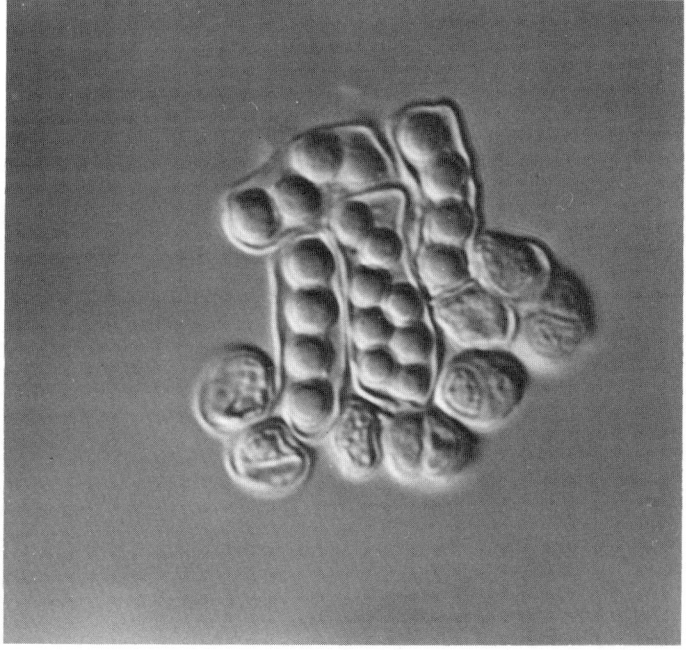

**Fig. 5.19** *Schizosaccharomyces octosporus*. Each of the mature asci contain eight ascospores.

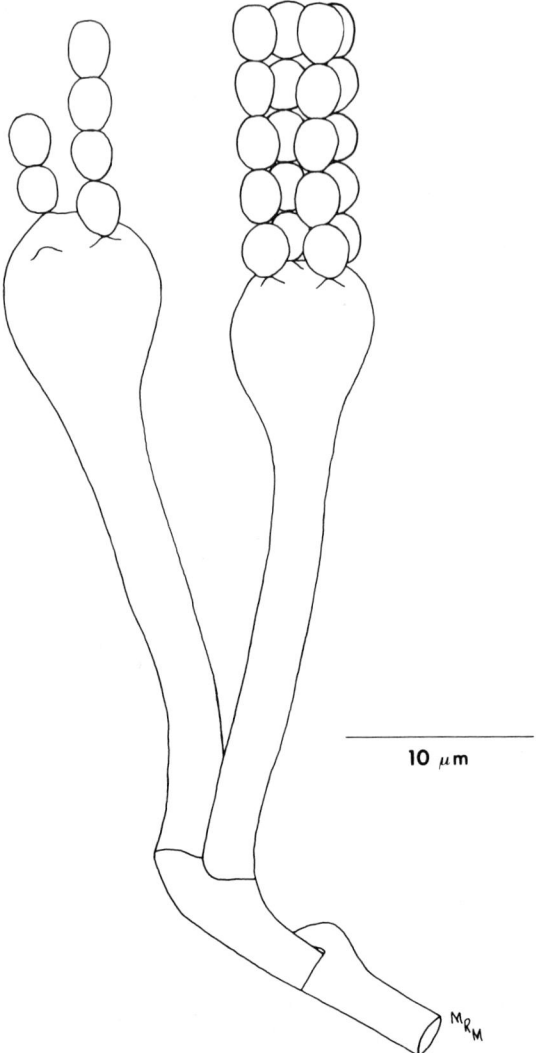

**Fig. 5.20** *Filobasidiella neoformans*. The one-celled basidiospores arise in four chains from the upper portion of each of the basidia.

could be considered as a synonym of *F. neoformans*. The genus apparently contains only two species, *F. arachnophila* and *F. neoformans*. *Filobasidiella* is differentiated from *Filobasidium* (17) by the development of basidiospores in a chain. There is some question whether or not the genera *Filobasidium* and *Filobasidiella* are congeneric. This genus is not seen in the clinical laboratory unless mating studies are conducted.

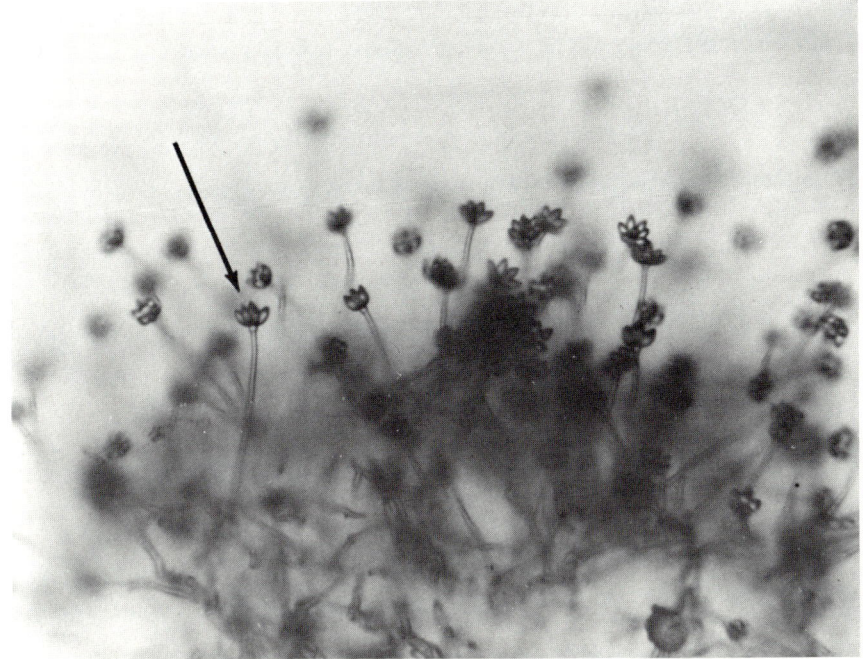

**Fig. 5.21** *Filobasidium floriforme*. The solitary basidiospores (arrow) can be seen at the apices of the basidia. (Reproduced by permission of L. Olive from *Journal of the Elisha Mitchell Scientific Society* **84**:261–266, 1968.)

## *Filobasidium* Olive, 1968

Diagnostic features: The genus *Filobasidium* produces a slightly swollen basidium at the apex of a sporophore, upon which 4–7 basidiospores form synchronously (Fig. 5.21). The hyphae have clamp connections. The morphs are species of *Cryptococcus* and *Torulopsis* (3, 17).

Comments: Isolates of *Filobasidium* are not typically seen in the clinical laboratory.

## *Leucosporidium* Fell, Statzell, Hunter et Phaff, 1969

Diagnostic features: The teliospores are intercalary or terminal, with a thick granular appearing wall. The basidiospores develop laterally and terminally from the promycelium. The hyphae have clamp connections, and the colonies do not produce carotenoid pigments. The anamorphs are species of *Candida* (8).

Comments: *Leucosporidium* (8) was established to accommodate yeasts that were similar to *Rhodosporidium* (4), but produced *Candida* anamorphs and colonies without carotenoid pigments. Colonies with carotenoid pigments are characteristic of the genus *Rhodosporidium* and its anamorph *Rhodotorula* (6). Isolates of *Leucosporidium* are not seen in the clinical laboratory.

### *Rhodosporidium* Banno, 1967

Diagnostic features: The teliospores of *Rhodosporidium* are intercalary or terminal, with a distinctly thick wall. The basidiospores develop laterally and terminally from the promycelium. The hyphae have clamp connections, and the colonies form carotenoid pigments. The anamorphs are species of *Rhodotorula* (4).

Comments: *Rhodosporidium* (4) was established for the sexual stages produced by species of *Rhodotorula*. The carotenoid pigments and *Rhodotorula* anamorph are used to distinguish this genus from *Leucosporidium* (6, 8). Members of this genus are not seen in the clinical laboratory.

### *Ustilago* (Persoon) Roussel, 1806

Diagnostic features: On artificial media *Ustilago* produces a profuse blastoconidial form (Fig. 5.22) in the agar. Thick-walled, round teliospores and hyphae may be present (1, 19).

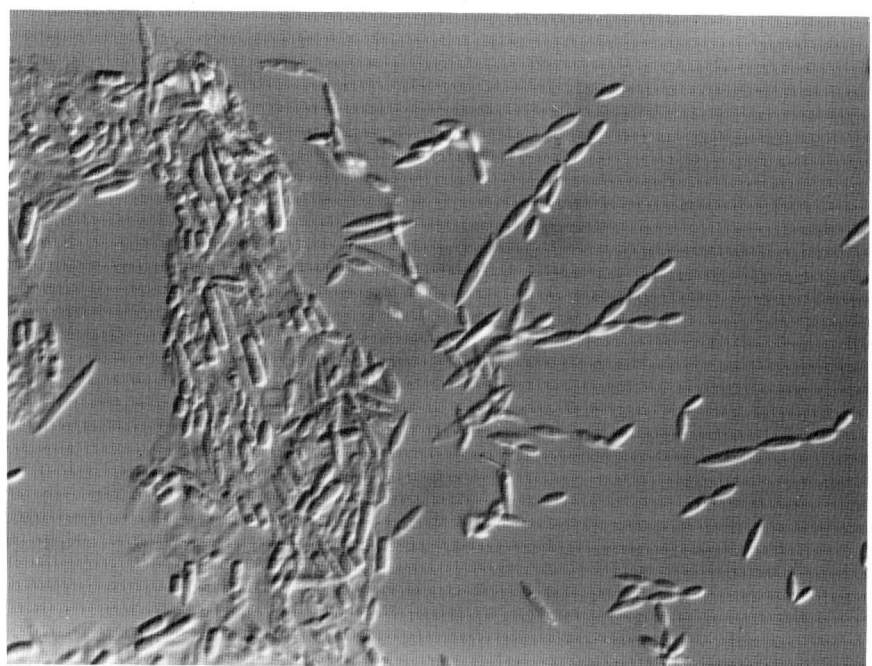

**Fig. 5.22** *Ustilago violaceum*. The hyphae, pseudohyphae, and blastoconidia are not distinctive for any particular species of smut.

Comments: Species of *Ustilago* and similar smuts do not form diagnostic characteristics in culture that can be used for identification. In general, they develop as budding yeasts. Teliospore production can be enhanced with enriched media such as malt or oatmeal agar if the appropriate mating types are present (19). It is difficult to determine the true frequency of *Ustilago* in the medical mycology laboratory.

## IMPERFECT YEASTS

### Key to the More Commonly Encountered Imperfect Yeasts and Similar Fungi

1. Mycelium predominant; arthroconidia present . . . . . . . . . . . . . . . . . . 2

1'. Mycelium usually absent; if present, arthroconidia absent; pseudomycelium absent, rudimentary, or well developed . . . . . . . . . . . . . . . . . . . . . . . . . 3

    2. Blastoconidia absent . . . . . . . . *Geotrichum* (see the Hyphomycetes in Chapter 4)

    2'. Blastoconidia present; pseudomycelium typically present . . . . . . . *Trichosporon*

3. Ballistoconidia absent . . . . . . . . . . . . . . . . . . . . . . . . . . . 4

3'. Ballistoconidia present; satellite colonies usually present; colonies red to salmon in color
. . . . . . . . . . . . . . . . . . . . . . . . . . . . . . . . . . . *Sporobolomyces*

    4. Sporangia and sporangiospores absent . . . . . . . . . . . . . . . . . . . 5

    4'. Sporangia and sporangiospores present; blastoconidia, pseudomycelium, and mycelium absent . . . . . . . . . . . . . . . . . . . . . . . . . . . . *Prototheca**

5. Unipolar or bipolar budding present; conidia attached by a broad base . . . . . . . . 6

5'. Multipolar budding present; conidia attached either by a broad or a narrow base . . . . 7

    6. Vegetative cells lemon-shaped and apiculate; conidiogenous cells annellides . *Kloeckera*

    6'. Vegetative cells globose to ellipsoidal; conidiogenous cells phialides . . . *Malassezia*

7. On YM agar, young colonies pink to red; inositol assimilation negative; fermentation absent; urease positive . . . . . . . . . . . . . . . . . . . . . . . . *Rhodotorula*

7'. On YM agar, young colonies not pink to red . . . . . . . . . . . . . . . . . . 8

    8. Pseudomycelium always present; true mycelium may occur . . . . . . . . *Candida*

    8'. Pseudomycelium absent, rudimentary if present . . . . . . . . . . . . . . . 9

9. Inositol assimilation positive; fermentation absent; vegetative cells usually globose and encapsulated; urease positive . . . . . . . . . . . . . . . . . . . . *Cryptococcus*

9'. Inositol assimilation negative; fermentation may occur; vegetative cells globose to ovoid; urease negative . . . . . . . . . . . . . . . . . . . . . . . . . *Torulopsis*

*Candida* Berkhout, 1923 *nom. cons.*

Diagnostic features: Members of the genus *Candida* are characterized by globose to elongate vegetative cells (Fig. 5.23) that typically produce multipolar blastoconidia, well developed pseudohyphae, and occasionally

* *Prototheca* sp. are achlorophyllus algae.

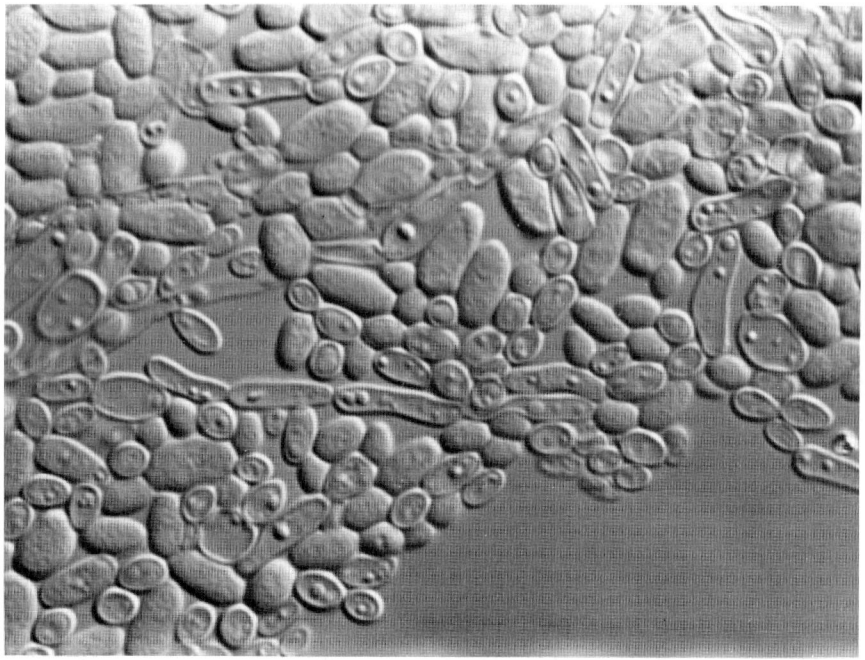

**Fig. 5.23** *Candida sorbosa*. Pseudohyphae and yeast cells producing blastoconidia are typical of this genus.

true hyphae. Arthroconidia, ballistoconidia, and colony pigmentation are always absent (16).

Comments: In the past, many medical mycologists and physicians have incorrectly referred to members of the genus *Candida* as *Monilia* species. *Monilia* is the anamorph of *Monilinia* or *Neurospora* (2), and is characterized by hyaline branching chains of blastoconidia that arise from a distinct conidiophore. As a result of this error, the term moniliasis was unfortunately proposed and used. The term moniliasis is obviously unacceptable and should be avoided when referring to diseases caused by species of *Candida*. Owing to common usage, candidiasis is the preferred name for infections caused by *Candida* species, even though candidosis is also etymologically correct.

There is often considerable difficulty in separating the genera *Candida* and *Torulopsis* from each other. In essence, the distinguishing feature is the presence or the absence of pseudohyphae, which unfortunately are not always distinct. Some mycologists believe that the genera *Candida* and *Torulopsis* should be merged into the single genus *Candida* (23). Such a merger would result in a genus of enormous size and complexity. In addition, a great deal of confusion would result in distinguishing the genus *Cryptococcus* from the broadened concept of *Candida*. For these reasons, *Candida* and *Torulopsis* are maintained as separate genera in this handbook, even though their separation is occasionally difficult.

Some members of the genus *Candida* are known to reproduce sexually. The more commonly encountered species that have been observed to produce ascospores include *C. guilliermondii (Pichia guilliermondii), C. krusei (P. kudriavzevii), C. lambica (P. fermentans), C. macedoniensis (Kluyveromyces marxianus)*, and *C. pseudotropicalis (K. marxianus)*. Clinical isolates of these species do not usually form asci without extensive study. Some mycologists (7) consider *C. albicans* and *C. stellatoidea* to be one species, even though biochemical (16) and DNA–RNA hybridization (15) data do not necessarily support this conclusion. Stenderup and Leth Bak (18) using percentage GC data maintained these as separate species. These two species are maintained as separate species in this handbook. It has been suggested (21) that the genus *Syringospora* contains the sexual stage of *C. albicans, C. claussenii*, and *C. stellatoidea*. There is some doubt concerning these species and their ability to reproduce sexually. In addition, the name *Candida* was specifically conserved against the generic name *Syringospora* Quinq., 1868, which was based upon asexual structures.

The more commonly encountered clinically important species of *Candida* can be distinguished from each other by using the key biochemical data in Table 5.6. Other species of *Candida* can be recovered; thus this key should be used only as an aid in distinguishing species, the final identification being based upon the reactions recorded in the composite table of assimilation and fermentation reactions. In the past, the species epithet *membranifaciens* has been incorrectly spelled *membranaefaciens*. The latter spelling is incorrect because the connecting vowel "i" is required in order to combine the two root words into *membranifaciens* (making membranes).

### *Cryptococcus* Kützing emend. Phaff et Spencer, 1969

Diagnostic features: Species of *Cryptococcus* produce globose to ovoid vegetative cells with multipolar blastoconidia that are attached by a narrow neck (Fig. 5.24). The cells are usually encapsulated by a heteropolysaccharide and may form rudimentary pseudohyphae. Neither the presence or absence of capsular material nor the size of the capsule when present is related to the virulence of the isolate (5). All species of *Cryptococcus* assimilate inositol, are nonpigmented when young on YM agar, and lack fermentative ability. *Cryptococcus neoformans* is considered to be the only pathogen in the genus (16).

**Table 5.6. Key Characteristics of Selected Species of *Candida***

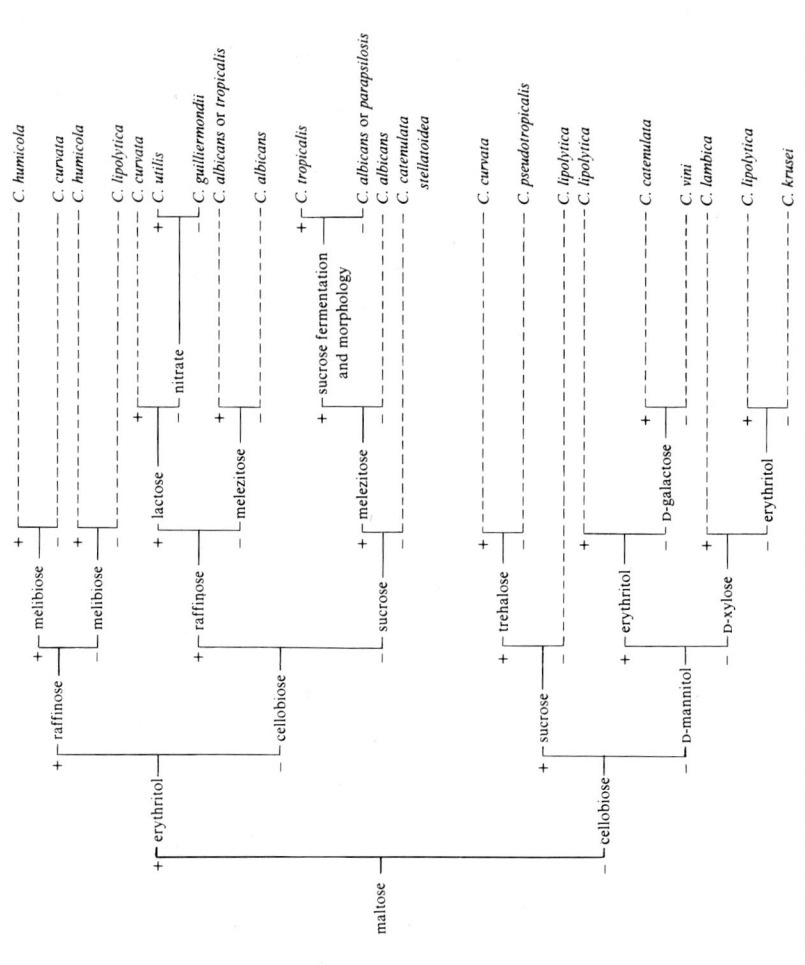

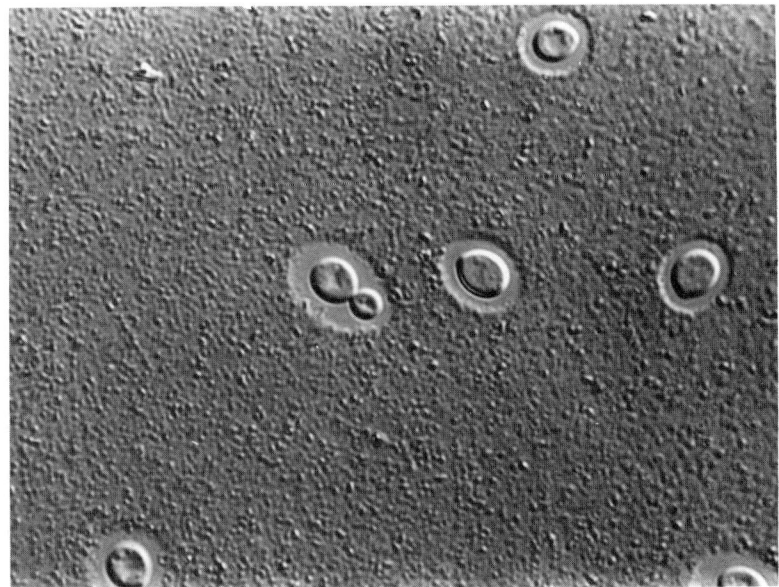

**Fig. 5.24** *Cryptococcus laurentii.* An India ink preparation is used to demonstrate the presence of capsules around the yeast cells.

Comments: *Cryptococcus* and *Rhodotorula* are very similar in morphology and physiology. Species of both genera may form capsules, produce a yellow to red colony, form globose to ovoid vegetative cells, and lack fermentative ability. Inositol assimilation is the key test used to distinguish these two genera. In contrast to *Cryptococcus,* species of *Rhodotorula* cannot assimilate inositol as a sole carbon source. This characteristic is also extremely valuable in distinguishing species of *Torulopsis* from *Cryptococcus,* since *Torulopsis* species are unable to assimilate inositol. Occasional isolates of *Torulopsis* have fermentative ability, which is another helpful characteristic in separating these two genera.

Some members of the genus *Cryptococcus* have the ability to reproduce sexually. These include *C. albidus (Filobasidium floriforme), C. infirmo-miniatus (Rhodosporidium infirmo-miniatum), C. neoformans (Filobasidiella neoformans)* and *C. uniguttulatus (Filobasidium uniguttulatum).*

*Cryptococcus neoformans* has been recently divided by Kwon-Chung and Bennett (14) into two species, *C. neoformans* and *C. bacillisporus.* There seems to be little reason to maintain these as separate species. Thus, *Cryptococcus bacillisporus* is considered to be a synonym of *C. neoformans* in this handbook.

The commonly encountered species of *Cryptococcus* can be differentiated with the key assimilation reactions in Table 5.7.

**Table 5.7.** Key Characteristics of Selected Species of *Cryptococcus*

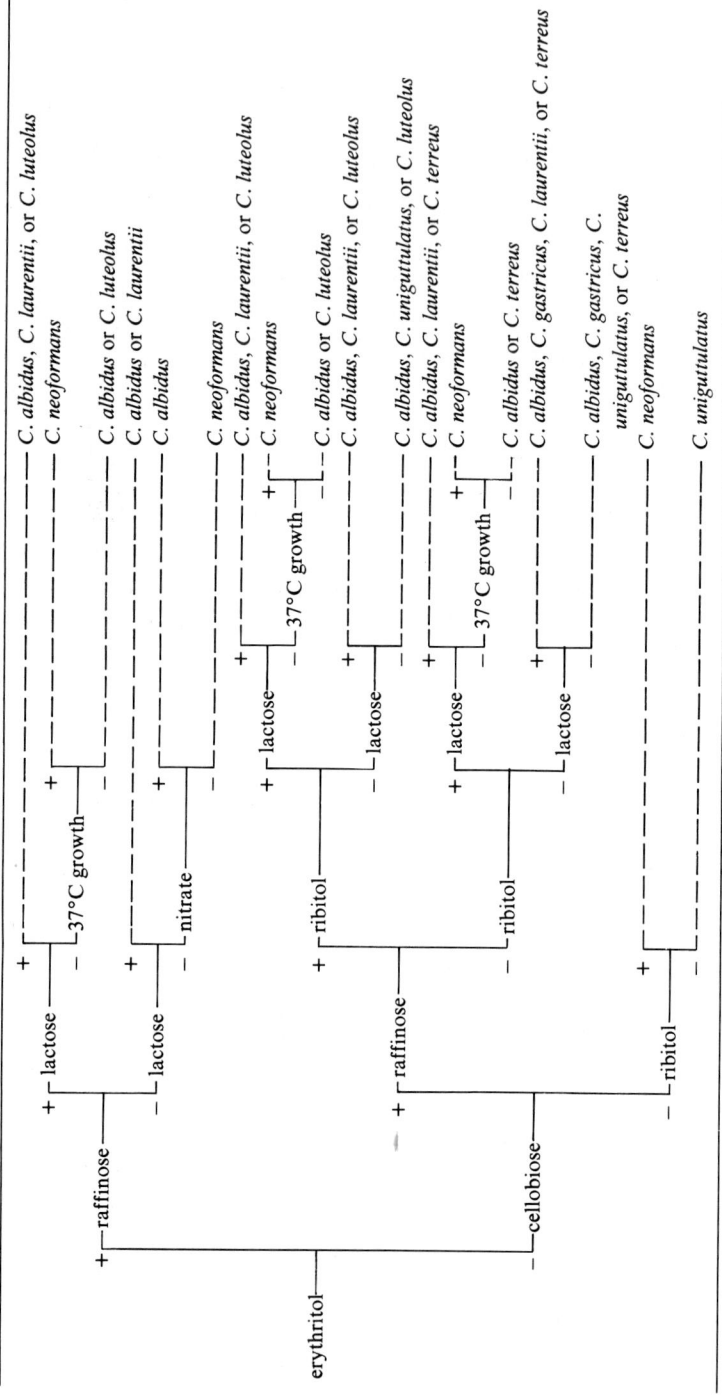

## *Kloeckera* Janke, 1923

Diagnostic features: The genus *Kloeckera* is characterized by ovoid to elongate apiculate vegetative cells, and the development of bipolar annelloconidia (Fig. 5.25). Pseudohyphae are usually absent, but they may be rudimentary to well developed, depending upon the isolate. Nitrate is not assimilated, and all members of this genus have an absolute requirement for inositol and pantothenic acid. If an isolate forms asci and ascospores, it is classified in the ascomycetous genus *Hanseniaspora* (16).

Comments: *Kloeckera apiculata* and similar yeasts can be differentiated with the key assimilation reactions in Table 5.5. Isolates of *Kloeckera* are occasionally isolated in the clinical laboratory.

## *Malassezia* Baillon, 1889

Diagnostic features: The vegetative cells of the genus *Malassezia* are globose to ellipsoidal, and produce unipolar conidia (Fig. 5.26). The conidiogenous cells are in essence phialides with small collarettes. Pseudohyphae and true hyphae are usually absent, but if present, they are usually sparse. The growth of *Malassezia* species is greatly enhanced

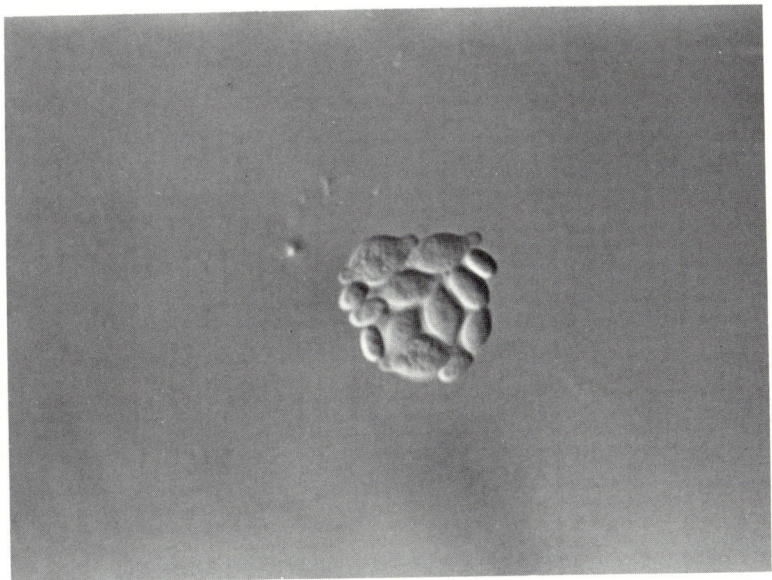

**Fig. 5.25** *Kloeckera apiculata*. The apiculate cells are annellides that are forming annelloconidia at both ends.

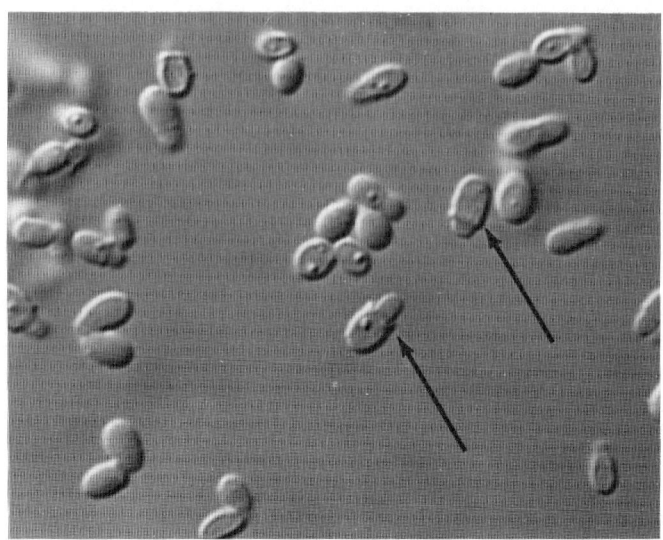

**Fig. 5.26** *Malassezia pachydermatis*. The yeast cells are producing conidia at one end. A delicate collarette can be seen around some of the yeast cells (arrows).

by natural oils and fatty substances. All members of the genus lack fermentative ability (16).

Comments: The genus *Pityrosporum* was originally described to accommodate yeasts isolated from the scalp. Following the isolation of *P. orbiculare* from scales of pityriasis versicolor, it was conclusively demonstrated that the genera *Malassezia* and *Pityrosporum* are one and the same. Since *Malassezia* was validly described 15 years prior to *Pityrosporum*, *Malassezia* is the correct generic name for these yeasts (16).

*Malassezia furfur* is the etiologic agent of pityriasis versicolor. Owing to its lipophilic nature, it is typically not recovered in the clinical laboratory unless special media and techniques are employed. *Malassezia pachydermatis* is occasionally recovered in the clinical laboratory and can be easily recognized by its bottle shape and unipolar conidia attached by a broad base.

*Malassezia pachydermatis* and similar yeasts can be differentiated with the key assimilation reactions in Table 5.5. This species is occasionally seen in the clinical laboratory.

### *Prototheca* Krüger, 1894

Diagnostic features: The genus *Prototheca* is included in this chapter because it is often mistaken for a yeast. *Prototheca* is an achlorophyllous alga that is similar to *Chlorella*. The colonies are yeastlike and white. Reproduction occurs solely by the development of sporangia and sporangiospores (Fig. 5.27). Mycelium and conidia are absent. The sporangia are unique in that there is usually a central sporangiospore surrounded by several other sporangiospores. Upon rupture of the sporangium, the sporangiospores are released. They increase in size and then themselves function as sporangia (9).

Comments: *Prototheca* species are occasionally recovered in the clinical laboratory, the most common ones being *P. wickerhamii* and *P. zopfii*.

## *Rhodotorula* Harrison, 1927

Diagnostic features: Members of the genus *Rhodotorula* are usually readily recognized by their distinctive yellow to red colony color. The vegetative cells are round to elongate, and the blastoconidia are multipolar (Fig. 5.28). Pseudohyphae are absent, rudimentary or well developed; true hyphae are rarely produced. All species of *Rhodotorula* lack the ability to assimilate inositol and to ferment carbon sources. A capsule may or may not be formed (16).

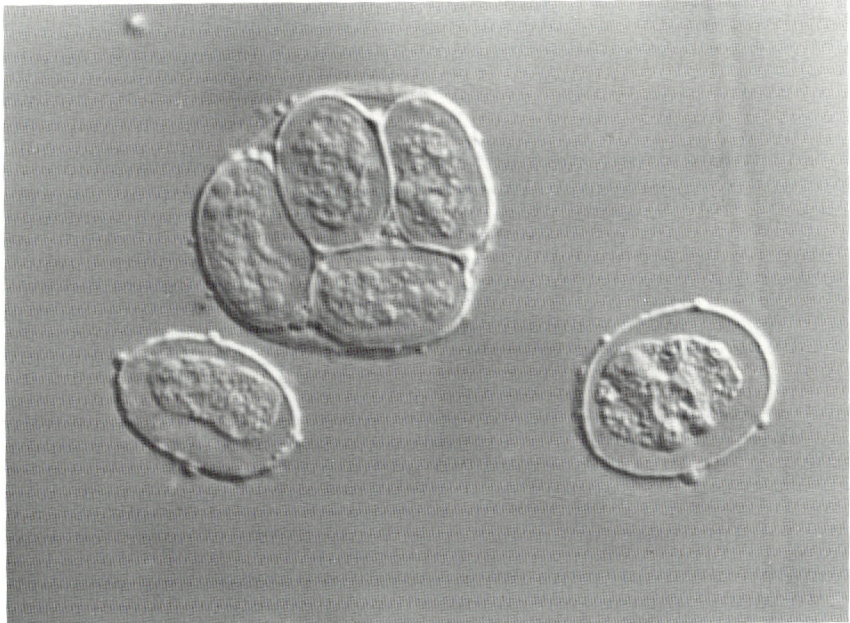

**Fig. 5.27** *Prototheca wickerhamii*. This organism only produces sporangia and sporangiospores.

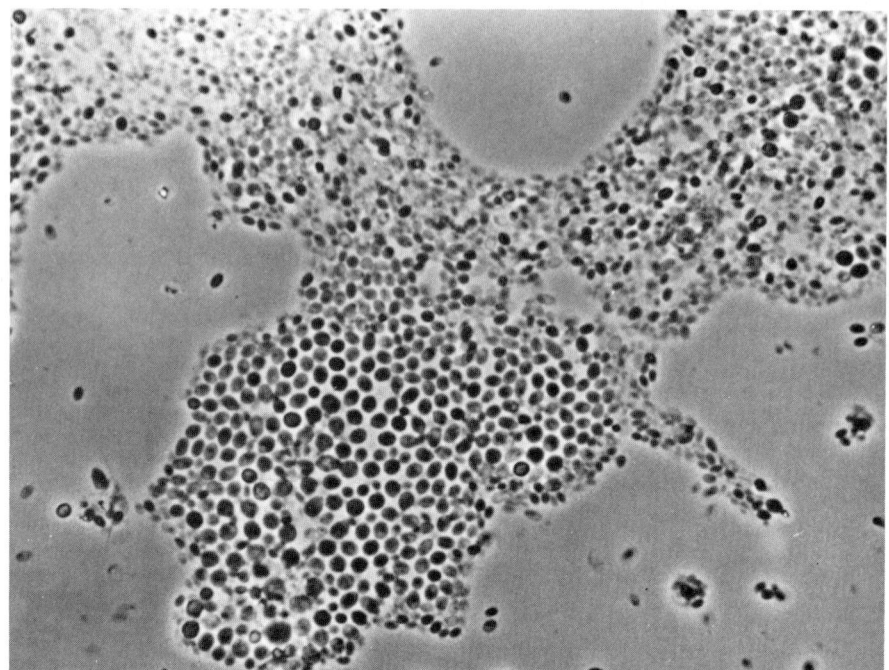

**Fig. 5.28** *Rhodotorula glutinis*. The globose yeast cells are producing blastoconidia.

Comments: *Rhodotorula* is very similar to *Cryptococcus* in that both genera can form globose, encapsulated cells with blastoconidia attached by a narrow base. *Rhodotorula* sp. are characterized by forming a distinctive red pigment on YM agar. Occasional isolates of *Cryptococcus* may form a light yellow to pink color on YM agar. Species of these two genera can be readily distinguished from each other by the inositol assimilation test. *Rhodotorula* is similar to *Torulopsis* in that neither group can assimilate inositol. The distinctive red pigmentation, lack of fermentative ability, and the large globose encapsulated cells of *Rhodotorula* help distinguish it from the genus *Torulopsis*.

Some species of *Rhodotorula* have the ability to produce basidia and basidiospores. To date, the sexual forms have been placed in the genus *Rhodosporidium* (4). *Rhodotorula* species with teleomorphs include *R. glutinis* (*Rhod. diobovatum*, *Rhod. sphaerocarpum*, and *Rhod. toruloides*), *R. graminis* (*Rhod. malvinellum*), *R. minuta* (*Rhod. dacryoidum*), and *R. pallida* (*Rhod. dacryoidum*).

The more commonly encountered clinically important species of *Rhodotorula* can be distinguished from each other using the biochemical data in Table 5.8.

Table 5.8. Key Characteristics of Selected Species of *Rhodotorula*

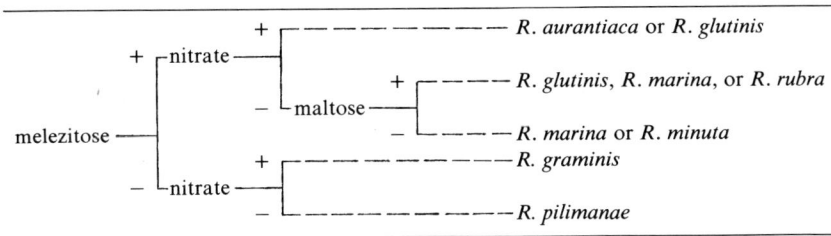

## *Sporobolomyces* Kluyver et van Niel, 1924

Diagnostic features: *Sporobolomyces* is characterized by the development of ballistoconidia on denticles. The ballistoconidia are forcibly discharged by a water-drop mechanism. The vegetative cells are ovoid to elongate (Fig. 5.29), and pseudohyphae and true hyphae are usually present. The colonies are typically red to salmon pink.

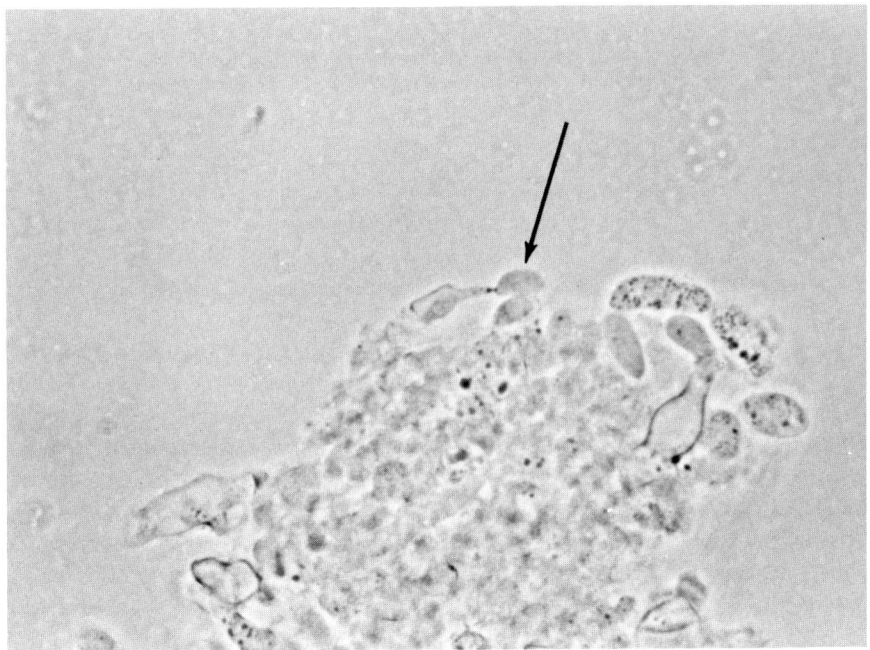

**Fig. 5.29** *Sporobolomyces salmonicolor*. Members of this genus produce ballistoconidia (arrow) upon denticles in addition to nonforcibly discharged conidia. The ballistoconidia of this species are reniform.

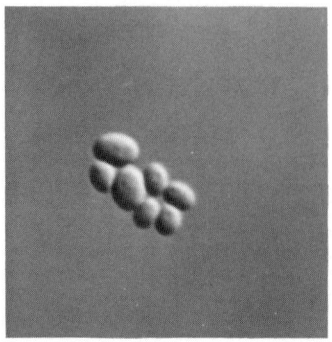

**Fig. 5.30** *Torulopsis glabrata*. This small yeast produces blastoconidia.

Comments: *Sporobolomyces* and *Bullera* are extremely similar to each other in that they both form ballistoconidia. *Bullera* species are distinguished from those of *Sporobolomyces* by their symmetrical, globose ballistoconidia and the absence of a distinct reddish color. *Sporobolomyces* and *Bullera* typically form small satellite colonies around the main colony. *Sporobolomyces salmonicolor* is most frequently recovered, but other species may be found in clinical specimens (3, 16).

*Sporobolomyces salmonicolor* forms a teleomorph consisting of basidia and basidiospores. The teleomorph is *Aessosporon salmonicolor*.

### *Torulopsis* Berlese, 1894

Diagnostic features: The genus *Torulopsis* contains yeasts that form globose to ovoid (rarely elongate) small vegetative cells with multipolar blastoconidia (Fig. 5.30). Pseudohyphae may be either absent or rudimentary. As in *Candida*, arthroconidia and ballistoconidia are absent. Species of *Torulopsis* do not assimilate inositol (16).

Comments: A substantial amount of confusion surrounds *Torulopsis* and its relationship to *Candida*. These two genera are traditionally distinguished from each other by the presence or the absence of pseudohyphae. Unfortunately, this characteristic is not always clear, a situation that has resulted in the arbitrary placement of some species into one genus rather than the other. Because of this and an additional taxonomic problem, Yarrow and Meyer (23) have merged *Torulopsis* into the genus *Candida*, which under their concept now contains an extremely large number of species. This was accomplished by emending the description of the genus *Candida* to read in part "pseudohyphae absent, rudimentary or well developed." With this broadened concept of *Candida*, members of the genus *Cryptococcus* could also be logically transferred to *Candida*. It is felt by this author that, at least for the present, *Torulopsis* and *Candida* should

## Part 3  Taxonomy

be maintained as separate genera. The emended concept of *Candida* appears to be too broad. It must be remembered that variation is the rule, not the exception. If these two genera are united on. taxonomic grounds, *Torulopsis* is the correct name, not *Candida*. *Torulopsis* was described before *Candida*.

Several members of the genus *Torulopsis* produce asci and ascospores, but none of these are of medical interest. The various sexual forms have been assigned to the genera *Debaryomyces, Entelexis, Kluyveromyces, Saccharomyces,* and *Wickerhamiella*.

### *Trichosporon* Behrend, 1890

Diagnostic features: The genus *Trichosporon* is characterized by the development of hyaline arthroconidia, blastoconidia, hyphae, and pseudohyphae (Fig. 5.31). The colonies are usually raised and have a waxy appearance (11).

Comments: *Trichosporon* is similar to *Aciculoconidium* (10), but can be distinguished by the formation of blastoconidia that are not partly needle-shpaed. Recently, von Arx *et al.* (3) slightly modified the concepts of

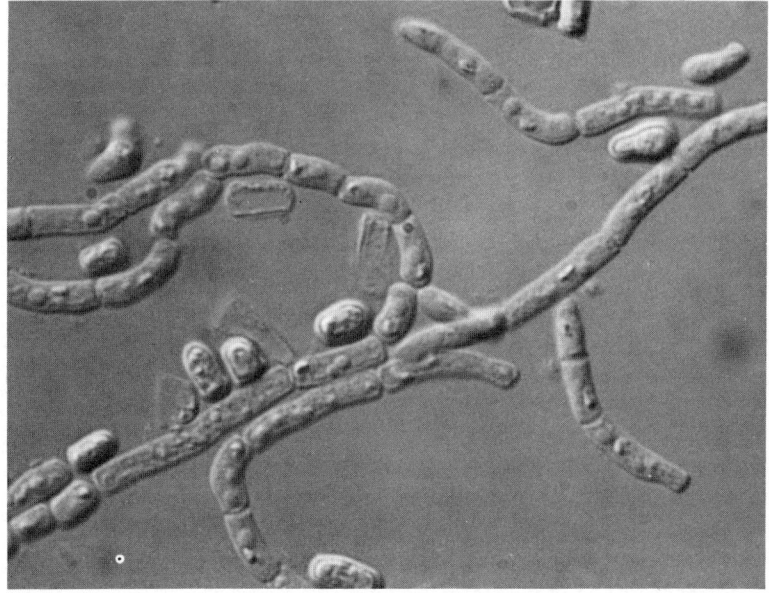

**Fig. 5.31** *Trichosporon beigelii*. A and B. The presence of hyphae, arthroconidia, and blastoconidia (arrow) are characteristic of the genus *Trichosporon*.

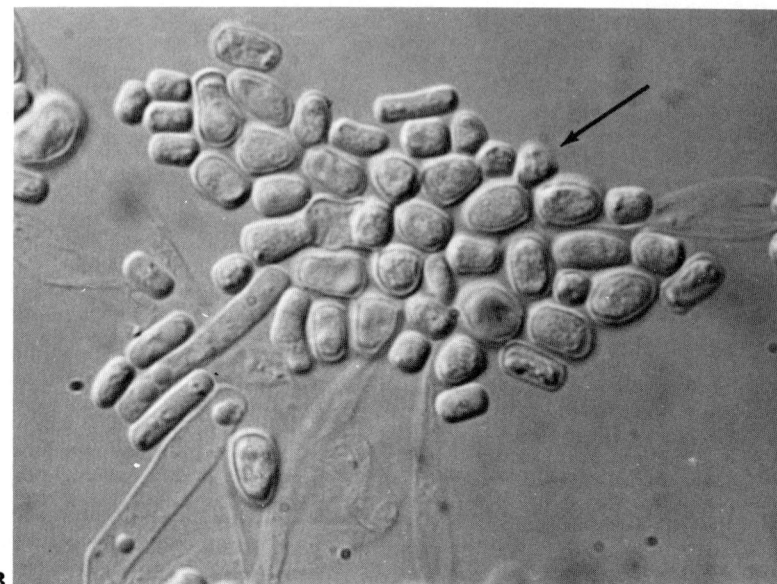

**Fig. 5.31** Continued

*Trichosporon* and *Geotrichum*. With reference to *Trichosporon* they remarked in their key to the genera of the Torulopsidales, "blastoconidia usually present" and, in the case of *Geotrichum,* "blastoconidia usually absent." They proposed that *T. capitatum, T. fermentans,* and *T. penicillatum* should be considered as *G. capitatum, G. fermentans,* and *G. penicillatum,* respectively. The transfer of *T. capitatum* and *T. fermentans* to *Geotrichum* does not seem necessary. Without doubt, *Geotrichum* is the proper genus for *G. penicillatum.* The genus *Geotrichum* is being defined along ascomycetous affinities, whereas *Trichosporon* is being associated only with Basidiomycetes (22).

Some mycologists feel that *T. beigelii* and *T. cutaneum* are separate species. This assumption is based upon the belief that the type of disease and *in vivo* morphology are valuable characteristics for distinguishing species of fungi. The use of diseases and tissue morphology are unacceptable taxonomic characteristics, and therefore should not be used to distinguish one species from another. Since *T. beigelii* was described several years prior to *T. cutaneum, T. beigelii* is the correct name for this fungus (11).

The commonly encountered species of *Trichosporon* can be differentiated with the key reactions in Table 5.9.

Part 3  Taxonomy

**Table 5.9.** Key Characteristics of Selected Species of *Trichosporon*

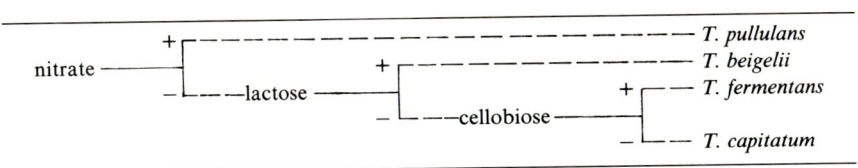

## CHARACTERISTICS OF MEDICALLY IMPORTANT YEASTS

Fermentation and assimilation characteristics and size of vegetative cells for various medically important yeasts are summarized in the following tabulations (Tables 5.10 to 5.16).

**Table 5.10.** Characteristics of Some Medically Important Yeasts in the Genus *Candida*

| | Fermentations[a] | | | | | | | | | | | |
|---|---|---|---|---|---|---|---|---|---|---|---|---|
| | D-Glucose | D-Galactose | Sucrose | Maltose | Cellobiose | Trehalose | Lactose | Raffinose | D-Glucose | D-Galactose | L-Sorbose | Sucrose |
| C. albicans | + | v | − | + | − | v | − | − | + | + | v | + |
| C. catenulata | + | − | − | − | − | − | − | − | + | + | − | − |
| C. claussenii | + | + | − | + | − | − | − | − | + | + | − | + |
| C. curvata | − | − | − | − | − | − | − | − | + | + | v | + |
| C. guilliermondii | + | v | v | − | − | v | − | v | + | + | + | + |
| C. humicola | − | − | − | − | − | − | − | − | + | v | v | + |
| C. ingens | − | − | − | − | − | − | − | − | + | + | v | − |
| C. kefyr | + | + | + | − | − | − | + | v | + | + | − | + |
| C. krusei | + | − | − | − | − | − | − | − | + | − | − | − |
| C. lambica | + | − | − | − | − | − | − | − | + | − | − | − |
| C. lipolytica | − | − | − | − | − | − | − | − | + | − | v | − |
| C. lusitaniae | + | + | v | − | + | v | − | − | + | + | + | + |
| C. macedoniensis | + | + | + | − | − | − | − | v | + | + | − | + |
| C. membranifaciens | v | v | v | − | − | v | − | v | + | + | + | + |
| C. norvegensis | v | − | − | − | v | − | − | − | + | − | − | − |
| C. parapsilosis | + | v | − | − | − | − | − | − | + | + | v | + |
| C. pseudotropicalis | + | + | + | − | − | − | + | v | + | + | − | + |
| C. rugosa | − | − | − | − | − | − | − | − | + | + | v | − |
| C. sake | v | v | v | v | − | v | − | − | + | + | v | + |
| C. sorbosa | + | − | − | − | − | − | − | − | + | − | + | − |
| C. stellatoidea | + | − | − | + | − | − | − | − | + | + | − | − |
| C. tropicalis | + | v | + | + | − | v | − | − | + | + | v | + |
| C. utilis | + | − | + | − | − | − | − | + | + | − | − | + |
| C. valida | v | − | − | − | − | − | − | − | + | − | − | − |
| C. veronae | + | v | − | − | − | v | − | − | + | + | − | + |
| C. vini | − | − | − | − | − | − | − | − | + | − | − | − |
| C. viswanathii | + | v | − | + | − | + | − | − | + | + | v | + |
| C. zeylanoides | v | − | − | − | − | − | − | − | + | v | + | − |

[a] + = positive; − = negative; v = variable.

# Part 3  Taxonomy

| Cellobiose | Trehalose | Lactose | Melibiose | Raffinose | Melezitose | D-Xylose | L-Arabinose | Erythritol | Ribitol | D-Mannitol | Methyl α-D-glucoside | Inositol | Nitrate | Vegetative cells (sizes in μm) |
|---|---|---|---|---|---|---|---|---|---|---|---|---|---|---|
| v | + | − | − | − | v | + | v | − | v | + | v | − | − | Globose to ovoid; 3.5–6 × 6–10 |
| − | + | − | − | − | − | v | − | − | − | + | − | − | − | Ovoid to cylindrical; 1.5–4 × 5–10 |
| − | + | − | − | − | + | + | v | − | v | + | + | − | − | Ovoid to cylindrical; 4.5–6 × 6–12 |
| + | + | + | − | + | v | + | v | v | v | v | v | v | − | Ovoid to allantoid; 2–3 × 6–10 |
| + | + | − | + | + | v | + | + | − | + | + | + | − | − | Ovoid; 2–4.5 × 2.5–7 |
| v | + | v | + | v | v | + | v | + | v | + | + | v | − | Ovoid to cylindrical; 3.5–5 × 8–30 |
| v | − | − | − | − | − | − | − | − | − | − | − | − | − | Ovoid to cylindrical; 4–8 × 8–16 |
| v | − | + | − | + | − | − | v | − | − | − | − | − | − | Ovoid; 3.5–9 × 6–14 |
| − | − | − | − | − | − | − | − | − | − | − | − | − | − | Ovoid to cylindrical; 3–5 × 6–20 |
| − | − | − | − | − | − | + | − | − | − | − | − | − | − | Ovoid; 3.5–6 × 5–12 |
| v | − | − | − | − | − | − | − | + | − | v | − | − | − | Ovoid to cylindrical; 3–5 × 5–11 |
| + | + | − | − | − | + | + | v | − | + | + | v | − | − | Subglobose to ovoid; 1.5–6 × 2.5–10 |
| + | − | + | − | + | − | + | + | − | v | v | − | − | − | Ovoid; 2.5–6 × 4.5–9 |
| + | + | − | + | + | + | + | + | + | + | + | + | + | − | Globose to ovoid; 3–6 × 3.5–7 |
| + | − | − | − | − | − | − | − | − | − | − | − | − | − | Ovoid to cylindrical; 2–8 × 5–13 |
| − | + | − | − | − | + | + | v | − | + | + | + | − | − | Ovoid; 2.5–4 × 2.5–9 |
| + | − | + | − | + | − | + | + | − | − | v | − | − | − | Ovoid; 2.5–5 × 5–10 |
| − | − | − | − | − | + | + | − | − | − | v | − | − | − | Ovoid to allantoid; 2.5–4 × 7–15 |
| v | + | − | − | − | + | v | v | − | v | + | v | − | − | Globose to ovoid; 1.5–5 × 4–10 |
| − | − | − | − | − | − | − | − | − | − | − | − | − | − | Ovoid to cylindrical; 2–4 × 4–15 |
| − | + | − | − | − | − | + | v | − | − | + | v | − | − | Ovoid; 4–8 × 5–10 |
| − | + | − | − | − | + | + | v | − | + | + | + | − | − | Globose to ovoid; 4–8 × 5–11 |
| − | v | − | − | + | + | v | − | − | − | v | v | − | + | Ovoid to cylindrical; 3.5–4.5 × 7–13 |
| − | − | − | − | − | − | v | − | − | − | − | − | − | − | Ovoid to cylindrical; 2–4 × 4–10 |
| − | + | − | − | − | + | + | + | + | + | + | + | − | − | Ovoid to cylindrical; 2–5 × 4–10 |
| − | − | − | − | − | − | − | − | − | − | + | − | − | − | Ovoid to cylindrical; 2–5 × 3–9 |
| − | + | − | − | − | + | + | v | − | + | + | + | − | − | Globose to cylindrical; 2.5–7 × 4–12 |
| − | + | − | − | − | − | − | − | − | − | v | + | − | − | Ovoid; 1.5–5 × 4–10 |

**Table 5.11.** Characteristics of Some Medically Important Yeasts in the Genus *Cryptococcus*

|  | Fermentations[a] | | | | | | | | | | | | |
|---|---|---|---|---|---|---|---|---|---|---|---|---|---|
|  | D-Glucose | D-Galactose | Sucrose | Maltose | Cellobiose | Trehalose | Lactose | Raffinose | D-Glucose | D-Galactose | L-Sorbose | Sucrose | Maltose |
| *C. albidus* | − | − | − | − | − | − | − | − | + | v | v | + | + |
| *C. gastricus* | − | − | − | − | − | − | − | − | + | + | − | v | + |
| *C. laurentii* | − | − | − | − | − | − | − | − | + | + | v | + | + |
| *C. luteolus* | − | − | − | − | − | − | − | − | + | + | v | + | + |
| *C. neoformans* | − | − | − | − | − | − | − | − | + | + | v | + | + |
| *C. terreus* | − | − | − | − | − | − | − | − | + | v | + | − | v |
| *C. uniguttulatus* | − | − | − | − | − | − | − | − | + | v | − | + | + |

[a] + = Positive; − = negative; v = variable.

**Table 5.12.** Characteristics of Some Medically Important Yeasts in the Genus *Hansenula*

|  | Fermentations[a] | | | | | | | | | | | | |
|---|---|---|---|---|---|---|---|---|---|---|---|---|---|
|  | D-Glucose | D-Galactose | Sucrose | Maltose | Cellobiose | Trehalose | Lactose | Raffinose | D-Glucose | D-Galactose | L-Sorbose | Sucrose | Maltose |
| *H. anomala* | + | v | + | v | v | v | − | + | + | v | − | + | + |
| *H. californica* | + | − | − | − | v | v | − | − | + | − | + | + | v |
| *H. polymorpha* | + | − | − | − | v | v | − | − | + | v | v | + | + |

[a] + = Positive; − = negative; v = variable.

| Trehalose | Lactose | Melibiose | Raffinose | Melezitose | D-Xylose | L-Arabinose | Erythritol | Ribitol | D-Mannitol | Methyl α-D-glucoside | Inositol | Nitrate | Vegative cells (sizes in μm) |
|---|---|---|---|---|---|---|---|---|---|---|---|---|---|
| v | v | v | v | v | + | + | v | v | v | v | + | + | Globose to ovoid; 3–8.8 × 3.5 × 10.2 |
| + | v | – | – | + | + | + | – | – | v | – | + | – | Globose to ovoid; 3–7 × 3.5–9.5 |
| v | + | v | v | + | + | + | v | v | v | v | + | – | Ovoid to elongate; 2–5.5 × 3–7 |
| + | v | v | + | + | + | + | v | v | + | + | + | – | Ovoid to elongate; 3.1–6 × 5.5–9 |
| + | – | – | v | + | + | v | v | + | + | + | + | – | Globose; 3–7.5 |
| v | v | – | – | v | + | + | – | v | + | – | + | + | Globose to ovoid; 3.5–6.5 × 4–6.5 |
| v | – | – | v | + | + | + | – | – | v | v | + | – | Globose to ovoid; 3–5.2 × 3.5–7 |

| Trehalose | Lactose | Melibiose | Raffinose | Melezitose | D-Xylose | L-Arabinose | Erythritol | Ribitol | D-Mannitol | Methyl α-D-glucoside | Inositol | Nitrate | Vegetative cells (sizes in μm) |
|---|---|---|---|---|---|---|---|---|---|---|---|---|---|
| + | – | – | + | + | v | v | + | v | + | + | – | + | Globose to ellipsoidal; 2–4.8 × 2.6–5.2 |
| v | – | – | – | – | + | – | – | – | + | + | – | + | Globose to ellipsoidal; 2–4.8 × 2.6–5.2 |
| + | – | – | – | + | v | – | + | + | + | v | – | + | Globose to cylindrical; 1–3.4 × 2.1–5.2 |

**Table 5.13.** Characteristics of Some Medically Important Yeasts in the Genus *Rhodotorula*

|  | Fermentations[a] | | | | | | | | | | | | |
|---|---|---|---|---|---|---|---|---|---|---|---|---|---|
|  | D-Glucose | D-Galactose | Sucrose | Maltose | Cellobiose | Trehalose | Lactose | Raffinose | D-Glucose | D-Galactose | L-Sorbose | Sucrose | Maltose |
| R. aurantiaca | − | − | − | − | − | − | − | − | + | v | v | + | v |
| R. glutinis   | − | − | − | − | − | − | − | − | + | v | v | + | + |
| R. graminis   | − | − | − | − | − | − | − | − | + | + | v | + | v |
| R. marina     | − | − | − | − | − | − | − | − | + | + | v | + | v |
| R. minuta     | − | − | − | − | − | − | − | − | + | v | v | + | − |
| R. pilimanae  | − | − | − | − | − | − | − | − | + | v | + | + | − |
| R. rubra      | − | − | − | − | − | − | − | − | + | v | v | + | + |

[a] + = Positive; − = negative; v = variable.

**Table 5.14.** Characteristics of Some Medically Important Yeasts in the Genus *Torulopsis*

|  | Fermentations[a] | | | | | | | | | | | | |
|---|---|---|---|---|---|---|---|---|---|---|---|---|---|
|  | D-Glucose | D-Galactose | Sucrose | Maltose | Cellobiose | Trehalose | Lactose | Raffinose | D-Glucose | D-Galactose | L-Sorbose | Sucrose | Maltose |
| T. candida       | v | − | v | − | − | v | − | v | + | + | v | + | + |
| T. glabrata      | + | − | − | − | − | v | − | − | + | − | − | − | − |
| T. inconspicua[b] | − | − | − | − | − | − | − | − | + | − | − | − | − |
| T. magnoliae     | + | − | + | − | − | − | − | − | + | v | v | + | − |
| T. maris         | − | − | − | − | − | − | − | − | + | + | − | − | − |
| T. pintolopesii[b] | v | − | − | − | − | − | − | − | + | − | − | − | − |

[a] + = Positive; − = negative; v = variable.
[b] *T. inconspicua* is lactate positive; *T. pintolopesii* is lactate negative.

| Cellobiose | Trehalose | Lactose | Melibiose | Raffinose | Melezitose | D-Xylose | L-Arabinose | Erythritol | Ribitol | D-Mannitol | Methyl α-D-glucoside | Inositol | Nitrate | Vegetative cells (sizes in μm) |
|---|---|---|---|---|---|---|---|---|---|---|---|---|---|---|
| | v | v | − | − | + | + | v | − | v | + | − | − | + | Ovoid to cylindrical; 3–5 × 6–13 |
| | + | − | − | v | + | v | v | − | v | v | v | − | v | Globose to ovoid; 2.3–5.0 × 4–10 |
| | + | − | − | + | − | v | v | − | v | v | v | − | + | Globose to ovoid; 2.5–4 × 4–8 |
| − | v | v | − | v | + | + | + | − | v | + | v | − | − | Globose to ellipsoidal; 2.5–5 × 3–12 |
| | + | v | − | − | + | + | + | − | v | v | − | − | − | Globose to ovoid; 2.3–4.5 × 3.5–11 |
| | + | − | − | v | − | + | + | − | v | + | − | − | − | Globose to ovoid; 2.3–5.2 × 3.5–7 |
| | + | − | − | + | + | + | v | − | v | v | v | − | − | Ovate to cylindrical; 2–5.5 × 4.5–14 |

Assimilations[a]

| Cellobiose | Trehalose | Lactose | Melibiose | Raffinose | Melezitose | D-Xylose | L-Arabinose | Erythritol | Ribitol | D-Mannitol | Methyl α-D-glucoside | Inositol | Nitrate | Vegetative cells (sizes in μm) |
|---|---|---|---|---|---|---|---|---|---|---|---|---|---|---|
| | + | v | v | + | v | + | + | v | + | + | + | − | − | Globose to ovoid; 2.5–7 × 3–8.5 |
| | + | − | − | − | − | − | − | − | − | − | − | − | − | Ovoid; 2.5–4.5 × 4–6 |
| | − | − | − | − | − | − | − | − | − | − | − | − | − | Ovoid; 1.5–5.5 × 3–7.5 |
| | − | − | − | v | − | − | − | − | + | − | − | − | + | Globose to ovoid; 1.5–5 × 2–5 |
| | − | − | − | − | − | + | − | − | + | + | − | − | − | Globose; 3–4.5 |
| | − | − | − | − | − | − | − | − | − | − | − | − | − | Ovoid; 2.5–3 × 3–5 |

**Table 5.15.** Characteristics of Some Medically Important Yeasts in the Genus *Trichosporon*

|  | Fermentations[a] | | | | | | | | | | | | |
|---|---|---|---|---|---|---|---|---|---|---|---|---|---|
|  | D-Glucose | D-Galactose | Sucrose | Maltose | Cellobiose | Trehalose | Lactose | Raffinose | D-Glucose | D-Galactose | L-Sorbose | Sucrose | Maltose |
| T. beigelii | − | − | − | − | − | − | − | − | + | v | v | v | v |
| T. capitatum | − | − | − | − | − | − | − | − | + | v | v | − | − |
| T. fermentans | v | v | − | − | v | − | − | − | + | + | + | − | − |
| T. pullulans | − | − | − | − | − | − | − | − | + | + | v | + | + |

[a] + = Positive; − = negative; v = variable.

**Table 5.16.** Characteristics of Some Medically Important Yeasts

|  | Fermentations[a] | | | | | | | | | | | | |
|---|---|---|---|---|---|---|---|---|---|---|---|---|---|
|  | D-Glucose | D-Galactose | Sucrose | Maltose | Cellobiose | Trehalose | Lactose | Raffinose | D-Glucose | D-Galactose | L-Sorbose | Sucrose | Maltose |
| Debaryomyces hansenii | v | v | v | v | v | v | − | v | + | + | v | + | + |
| Kloeckera apiculata | v | − | − | − | v | − | − | − | + | − | − | − | − |
| Malassezia pachydermatis | − | − | − | − | − | − | − | − | + | − | − | − | − |
| Pichia farinosa | + | v | − | − | v | v | − | v | + | + | v | − | − |
| Saccharomyces hansenii | + | v | + | v | − | v | − | + | + | v | − | + | v |

[a] + = Positive; − = negative; v = variable.

| Cellobiose | Trehalose | Lactose | Melibiose | Raffinose | Melezitose | D-Xylose | L-Arabinose | Erythritol | Ribitol | D-Mannitol | Methyl α-D-glucoside | Inositol | Nitrate | Vegetative cells (sizes in μm) |
|---|---|---|---|---|---|---|---|---|---|---|---|---|---|---|
| | v | + | v | v | v | + | v | v | v | v | v | v | − | Ovoid to ellipsoidal; 3.5–7 × 3.5–14 |
| | − | − | − | − | − | − | − | − | − | − | − | − | − | Ellipsoidal; 3.5–6.7 × 7.4–12.3 |
| | − | − | − | − | − | + | v | − | + | + | − | − | − | Ovoid to ellipsoidal; 3.9–7 × 7–17.5 |
| | + | v | + | + | + | v | v | + | v | + | + | v | + | Ovoid to cylindrical; 3.5–7 × 5.3–21 |

| Trehalose | Lactose | Melibiose | Raffinose | Melezitose | D-Xylose | L-Arabinose | Erythritol | Ribitol | D-Mannitol | Methyl α-D-glucoside | Inositol | Nitrate | Vegetative cells (sizes in μm) |
|---|---|---|---|---|---|---|---|---|---|---|---|---|---|
| + | v | v | + | + | + | + | v | + | + | + | − | − | Globose to ovoid; 2–5 × 2–7 |
| − | − | − | − | − | − | − | − | − | − | − | − | − | Ovoid to elongate, apiculate; 1.4–5.3 × 2.6–12.2 |
| − | − | − | − | − | − | − | − | + | − | − | − | − | Globose to ellipsoidal; 2.5–6 × 2.6–7 |
| v | v | − | − | − | v | v | + | + | + | − | − | − | Ovoid to cylindrical; 1.5–7 × 3–21 |
| v | − | − | + | v | − | v | − | − | v | v | − | − | Globose to cylindrical; 3–8 × 4–19 |

## Part 3. References Cited

1. Ainsworth, G. C., and K. Sampson (1950). "The British Smut Fungi (Ustilaginales)." Commonwealth Mycological Institute, Kew, Surrey, England.
2. Arx, J. A. von (1974). "The Genera of Fungi Sporulating in Pure Culture," 2nd ed. J. Cramer, Lehre.
3. Arx, J. A. von, L. Rodrigues de Miranda, M. T. Smith, and D. Yarrow (1977). The genera of yeasts and the yeast-like fungi (*Stud. Mycol.* No. 14). Centraalbureau voor Schimmelcultures, Baarn.
4. Banno, I. (1967). Studies on the sexuality of *Rhodotorula. J. Gen. Appl. Microbiol.* **13**:167–196.
5. Dykstra, M. A., L. Friedman, and J. W. Murphy (1977). Capsule size of *Cryptococcus neoformans:* control and relationship to virulence. *Infect. Immun.* **16**:129–135.
6. Fell, J. (1974). Heterobasidiomycetous yeasts *Leucosporidium* and *Rhodosporidium.* Their systematics and sexual incompatibility systems. *Trans. Mycol. Soc. Jpn.* **15**:316–323.
7. Fell, J. W., and S. A. Meyer (1967). Systematics of yeast species in the *Candida parapsilosis* group. *Mycopathol. Mycol. Appl.* **32**:177–193.
8. Fell, J. W., A. C. Statzell, I. L. Hunter, and H. J. Phaff (1969). *Leucosporidium* gen. n., the heterobasidiomycetous stage of several yeasts of the genus *Candida. Antonie van Leeuwenhoek J. Microbiol. Serol.* **35**:433–462.
9. Kaplan, W. (1978). Protothecosis and infections caused by morphologically similar green algae. *Proc. Int. Conf. Mycoses, 4th, PAHO Sci. Publ. No. 356,* pp. 218–232.
10. King, D. S., and S. C. Jong (1976). *Aciculoconidium*: a new hyphomycetous genus to accommodate *Trichosporon aculeatum. Mycotaxon* **3**:401–408.
11. King, D. S., and S. C. Jong (1977). A contribution to the genus *Trichosporon. Mycotaxon* **6**:391–417.
12. Kwon-Chung, K. J. (1975). A new genus, *Filobasidiella,* the perfect state of *Cryptococcus neoformans. Mycologia* **67**:1197–1200.
13. Kwon-Chung, K. J. (1976). A new species of *Filobasidiella,* the sexual state of *Cryptococcus neoformans* B and C serotypes. *Mycologia* **68**:942–946.
14. Kwon-Chung, K. J., J. E. Bennett, and T. S. Theodore (1978). *Cryptococcus bacillisporus* sp. nov.: serotype B-C of *Cryptococcus neoformans. Int. J. Syst. Bacteriol.* **28**:616–620.
15. Leth Bak, A., and A. Stenderup (1969). Deoxyribonucleic acid homology in yeasts. Genetic relatedness within the genus *Candida. J. Gen. Microbiol.* **59**:21–30.
16. Lodder, J. (1970). "The Yeasts. A Taxonomic Study," 2nd ed. North Holland Publ., Amsterdam.
17. Olive, L. S. (1968). An unusual new heterobasidiomycete with *Tilletia*-like basidia. *J. Elisha Mitchell Sci. Soc.* **84**:261–266.
18. Stenderup, A., and A. Leth Bak (1968). Deoxyribonucleic acid base composition of some species within the genus *Candida. J. Gen. Microbiol.* **52**:231–236.
19. Stevens, R. B., ed. (1974). "Mycology Guidebook." Univ. of Washington Press, Seattle.
20. Walt, J. P. van der, and E. Johannsen (1975). The genus *Torulaspora. CSIR Res. Rep. (Pretoria)* **325**, 23 pp.
21. Walt, J. P. van der (1969). The genus *Syringospora* Quinquad emend. *Antonie van Leeuwenhoek J. Microbiol. Serol.* **35**:A1–A2.
22. Weijman, A. C. M. (1979). Carbohydrate composition and taxonomy of *Geotrichum, Trichosporon,* and allied genera. *Antonie van Leeuwenhoek J. Microbiol. Ser.* **45**:119–127.
23. Yarrow, D., and S. A. Meyer (1978). Proposal for amendment of the diagnosis of the genus *Candida* Berkhout nom. cons. *Int. J. Syst. Bacteriol.* **28**:611–615.

*Chapter 6*

# Susceptibility Testing and Bioassay Procedures

The treatment of mycotic infections is a perplexing problem since fungi are eukaryotic organisms with a structure and metabolism that is similar to those of their eukaryotic hosts. For this reason the antimicrobial agents presently available for the treatment of fungal infections can damage the host as well as destroy the fungal pathogen. Unlike many antibacterial agents that work intracellularly, most of the antifungal drugs exhibit a restricted spectrum of action because they work at the level of the cell membrane. Contributing to this perplexity is the fact that most of the antimycotic agents are relatively unstable and insoluble in biological fluids.

The major antimycotic agents can be conveniently divided into true antimicrobials or secondary metabolites isolated from living organisms, and synthetic compounds produced chemically within the laboratory. Ambruticin, amphotericin B, griseofulvin, nystatin, and pimaricin are examples of natural antimicrobics, whereas clotrimazole, econazole, ketoconazole (R41,400), miconazole, 5-fluorocytosine (5-FC), haloprogen, tolnaftate, and similar compounds are synthetic. Laboratory susceptibility testing is warranted for amphotericin B, 5-fluorocytosine, and miconazole under some circumstances, but in general, not for the other agents listed above. As more clinical data for such compounds as ambruticin and ketoconazole become available, testing of these agents will probably become necessary.

Interpretation of susceptibility data is an estimate of the potential value of the drug based upon clinical experience. *In vitro* data are expressed either as the minimal inhibitory concentration (MIC) or minimal fungicidal concentration (MFC). Both these values are reported in $\mu g/ml$

(mcg/ml). The MIC is the least concentration of drug under standard test conditions that will inhibit the growth of a fungus, and the MFC is the least concentration of drug that under standard test conditions will kill the fungus. With amphotericin B, the MIC and MFC values are usually within twofold dilutions of each other; this may not always be the case with 5-FC, especially with respect to the filamentous fungi.

Many different techniques have been published for determining the MIC and MFC levels of the major antimycotic agents. The more common ones include broth dilution, drug impregnated disks, filter paper disks, microtiter technique, semisolid agar, solid agar, and radiometric procedures. The techniques included in this handbook were selected because they represent proven procedures that give reproducible results. If one problem with laboratory susceptibility testing can be singled out, it is the lack of standardization in conducting the tests and reading their end points. Temperature and length of incubation, inoculum concentration, and composition of medium are all critical parameters that must be controlled from one test to the next if the results obtained are going to be meaningful.

## In Vitro SUSCEPTIBILITY TESTING

### A. Amphotericin B (Fungizone)

Amphotericin B is a polyene antimycotic agent with a molecular weight of 924 and chemical formula of $C_{47}H_{73}NO_{17}$ that was originally derived from the aerobic actinomycete *Streptomyces nodosus*. The molecule consists of a macrolide ring containing seven double-bond carbon atoms with clearly demarcated hydrophilic and hydrophobic regions. The amphipathic property of amphotericin B is important in its mode of action. Amphotericin B is insoluble in water, unstable at 37°C, and affected by exposure to light (absorption maxima 298 nm). Its half-life is approximately 36 hours at 0.8 µg/ml in culture media.

Amphotericin B alters cell membrane permeability, resulting in a leakage of cellular constitutents and ultimate lysis and death of the cells. It has been suggested that the polyenes interact with the membrane sterols, resulting in rearrangement of the lipids and fragmentation of the cell membrane due to the presence or formation of polyene–sterol complexes. Amphotericin B actively interacts with ergosterol, the major sterol component of fungal cell membranes. It has been demonstrated that the sterol content as related to the phospholipids is important in determining susceptibility to amphotericin B. Susceptible organisms contain sterols in their cell membranes.

Resistant isolates are infrequently recovered in the clinical laboratory. These usually consist of species of *Aspergillus*, various Zygomycetes such as *Rhizopus* and *Mucor* species, and several species of dematiaceous hyphomycetes. Most MIC values for susceptible fungi are usually 0.05–1.0 µg/ml. Because of drug inactivation, slow growing fungi may show false levels of resistance if the test is read beyond 24 hours. In the case of *Histoplasma capsulatum*, the yeast form is less sensitive than the mould form. Amphotericin B is fungicidal at high concentrations, but at most clinically achievable levels it is fungistatic.

*In vitro* susceptibility testing may be necessary with amphotericin B for mycoses involving the central nervous system; in patients with severe renal disease; in order to explain treatment failure or relapse; and, when unusual opportunistic pathogens, especially the dematiaceous hyphomycetes, are involved. Since the yeasts and dimorphic fungi are, for the most part, susceptible to amphotericin B, testing may not be necessary in all instances. One clinical interpretation with normal therapy for MIC values is

Serum: susceptible = 0.1–1 µg/ml, intermediate = 2–4 µg/ml, resistant = greater than 4 µg/ml
CSF: susceptible = 0.1–0.2 µg/ml

1. Preparation of the stock amphotericin B solution.

   The amphotericin B used in susceptibility testing is pure assayed powder that is commercially available. Amphotericin B for patient use is not recommended because the actual concentration may vary slightly from one bottle or lot to the next. If medicinal amphotericin B is to be used, two to three bottles should be combined for each test. The potency of amphotericin B powder varies from one lot to the next and is usually expressed in terms of actual activity, or actual milligrams per 1000 mg. For example, a potency of 90% is equal to 900 mg of active drug in 1000 mg of the powder. Each time a portion of drug is used to prepare a new stock solution, its weight must be recorded in a weight log book. This will permit rechecking of concentrations, if necessary. The dried powder is kept in a desiccator at $-70°C$ in order to retard decay of the amphotericin B.

   To prepare a stock solution with a concentration of 10,000 µg/ml of amphotericin B in a volume of 5.0 ml, the following formula can be used:

   $$\frac{10{,}000\ \mu g/ml}{\text{potency of the amphotericin B}} \times 5.0\ ml = \text{mg of amphotericin to be weighed}$$

   a. To prepare the stock drug solution
      (1) Remove the dimethyl sulfoxide (DMSO) from the refrigerator at least 1 hour prior to its use and allow it to warm up to

room temperature. This is necessary to ensure that the volume of DMSO used is correct.
(2) Pour a small amount of DMSO into a clean sterile 5.0-ml volumetric flask. USE THE CHEMICAL FUME HOOD.
(3) Add the proper amount of amphotericin B to the 5.0-ml volumetric flask to achieve a final concentration of 10,000 µg of amphotericin B per milliliter.
(4) Wash any drug residue from the weighing paper into the volumetric flask with DMSO.
(5) Bring the volume up to 5.0 ml with DMSO.
(6) Allow the stock drug solution to sit at room temperature for 30 minutes prior to its use. This permits self-sterilization of the amphotericin B by the DMSO. Amphotericin B cannot be sterilized by filtration, as it will not pass through membranes with pore sizes of approximately 0.22 µg or less.

The stock amphotericin B solution containing 10,000 µg/ml is dispensed in 1.5-ml aliquots into good quality glass screw-cap tubes, which are then placed at −70°C until needed. The stock solutions should be discarded after 1 month. When an aliquot of the stock solution is needed, a tube is transferred from the freezer to a refrigerator. This solution is discarded after 1 week.

The working solution of amphotericin B contains 1000 µg/ml. This solution is prepared (to be discussed later) from the stock amphotericin B solution. It can be kept for 1 week in a refrigerator prior to being discarded.

2. Control isolate

The control isolate must be run with each set of tests. For this purpose, *Saccharomyces cerevisiae* (ATCC 36375) is an ideal isolate since it has reproducible MIC (0.1 µg/ml) and MFC (0.2 µg/ml) values. Other control isolates could include *Candida albicans* (Squibb 1539), *C. tropicalis* (ATCC 13803), and *S. cerevisiae* (ATCC 2601 and 9763). The latter two strains of *S. cerevisiae* are also recognized by the FDA for nystatin and amphotericin B susceptibility testing, respectively. Any yeast isolate can be used as long as it has been evaluated thoroughly and gives consistent results from one test to the next. A stock culture of this isolate should be kept in the culture collection.

3. Preparation of inocula

a. Using sterile, distilled water with or without 0.05% Tween 80, wash the growth from the sporulating mould colony grown on Sabouraud dextrose agar (2% dextrose). Mycelial growth can be broken up with sterile glass beads. If a yeast is being tested, use sterile distilled water without 0.05% Tween 80. Some mycologists

prefer to use saline instead of distilled water. The yeast is simply transferred to the water with an inoculating loop. Inoculum from the control isolate is transferred from a 48-hour-old culture on Sabouraud dextrose agar to sterile distilled water without 0.05% Tween 80. Approximately 5.0 ml of inoculum are required for each organism.
    b. Using a spectrophotometer set at 530 nm, adjust the suspension to 90% T. Record the % T. This will result in approximately $10^6$ colony-forming units/ml.

4. Preparation of inoculum control
    a. Pipette 2.0 ml of inoculum into a sterile 12 × 75 mm tube.
    b. Label this "inoculum control."

5. Incubation of the test
    a. Incubate the tests at 30°C and read at 24 and 48 hours.

6. Reading the test
    a. The end point is that dilution in which two of the three tubes or both of the plates show no growth.
    b. Growth should be present in the medium and DMSO controls.
    c. Growth should be minimal in the inoculum control. If slight growth is present, this indicates carry-over.
    d. The control isolate must be read first. The test is valid only if the control isolate gives an MIC of 0.1–0.39 µg/ml. Variation extending over two dilutions is considered acceptable for these techniques. An obvious button, or a film in the bottom of a tube is considered positive. A clear tube is negative.

7. The final concentrations

| Tube or plate number | Concentration of amphotericin B (µg/ml) |
|---|---|
| 1 | 100 |
| 2 | 50 |
| 3 | 25 |
| 4 | 12.5 |
| 5 | 6.25 |
| 6 | 3.13 |
| 7 | 1.56 |
| 8 | 0.78 |
| 9 | 0.39 |
| 10 | 0.20 |
| 11 | 0.10 |
| 12 | 0.05 |
| 13 | 0.025 |
| Medium Control | 0.0 |
| DMSO Control | 0.0 |
| Inoculum Control | 0.0 |

(A) *Broth Technique for Yeasts or Moulds to Determine MIC Values*

1. Preparation of working stock drug solution
   a. Dispense 0.5 ml of stock amphotericin B solution (10,000 µg/ml) into 4.5 ml of antibiotic medium 3 FDA (M-3 broth). The final concentration is 1000 µg/ml.
2. Preparation of amphotericin B dilutions
   a. Remove the working stock drug solution from the refrigerator (1000 µg/ml).
   b. Pipette 2.0 ml of the 1000 µg/ml dilution into a tube containing 18.0 ml of M-3 broth. The final concentration is 100 µg/ml. This is tube No. 1.
   c. Prepare twofold dilutions in 7.0-ml volumes of M-3 broth until a concentration of 0.025 µg/ml is reached. Label each tube from 2 through 13 to correspond to each serial dilution.
   d. Dispense 1.0-ml aliquots of each dilution into each of six sterile 12 × 75 mm tubes.
3. Preparation of medium control
   a. Dispense 1.0 ml aliquots of M-3 broth into each of six sterile 12 × 75 mm tubes.
   b. Label these "medium control."
4. Preparation of DMSO control
   a. Add 0.1 ml of DMSO to 7.0 ml of M-3 broth.
   b. Pipette 1.0-ml aliquots into each of six sterile 12 × 75 mm tubes.
   c. Label these "DMSO control."
5. Inoculation of media
   a. Using a pipettor with calibrated tips to deliver 0.05 ml, inoculate three tubes with the unknown and three tubes with the control strain. Start with the control tubes, working from 0.025 to 100 µg/ml.
   b. Incubate the test at 30°C.

(B) *Semisolid Agar Technique to Determine MIC Values for Moulds or Yeasts*

1. Preparation of working stock drug solution
   a. Pipette 1.0 ml of the stock solution (10,000 µg/ml) into 9.0 ml of M-3 broth. The final concentration is 1000 µg/ml.
2. Preparation of amphotericin B dilutions
   a. Remove one tube of the working stock drug solution from the refrigerator (1000 µg/ml).
   b. Pipette 4.0 ml of the working stock drug solution into 6.0 ml of sterile M-3 broth. The final concentration is 400 µg/ml.

# In Vitro Susceptibility Testing 417

  c. Pipette 7.5 ml of the M-3 broth containing 400 µg/ml into 7.5 ml of M-3 broth and label 200 µg/ml. This is tube 1.
  d. Continue preparing twofold dilutions in 7.5 ml volumes of M-3 broth until an amphotericin B concentration of 0.05 µg/ml is reached. Label each tube from 2 through 13 to correspond to each serial dilution.
  e. To each of the M-3 broth dilutions containing amphotericin B (one at a time) add 7.5 ml of M-3 agar maintained at 50–52°C. Mix the medium well and then immediately pipette 2.0-ml aliquots into each of six sterile 12 × 75 mm snap-cap test tubes. Stand the test tubes vertically while the medium hardens. The final twofold concentrations of amphotericin B are 100 to 0.025 µg/ml (that is, tubes 1 through 13, respectively).
3. Preparation of medium control
  a. Mix 7.5 ml of M-3 broth and 7.5 ml of M-3 agar together.
  b. Dispense in 2.0-ml aliquots into sterile 12 × 75 mm snap-cap test tubes. Stand the test tubes vertically until the medium hardens.
  c. Label these "medium control."
4. Preparation of DMSO control
  a. Add 0.2 ml of DMSO to 7.3 ml of M-3 broth.
  b. Add the 7.5 ml of M-3 broth containing DMSO to 7.5 ml of M-3 agar maintained at 50–52°C.
  c. Pipette 2.0-ml aliquots into each of six sterile 12 × 75 mm tubes. Stand the test tubes vertically while the medium hardens.
  d. Label these "DMSO control."
5. Inoculation of media
  a. Using a pipettor with calibrated tips to deliver 0.05 ml, inoculate three tubes with the unknown and three tubes with the control isolate. Start with the control tubes working from 0.025 to 100 µg/ml.
  b. Make sure that the inoculum neither runs down the side of the tube nor splashes when it is placed on the agar surface.
  c. Incubate the test tubes at 30°C.

(C) *Solid Agar Technique for Moulds or Yeasts to Determine MIC Values*

1. Preparation of working stock drug solution
  a. Pipette 2.0 ml of the stock solution (10,000 µg/ml) into 18.0 ml of M-3 broth. The final concentration is 1000 µg/ml.
2. Preparation of amphotericin B dilutions
  a. Remove one tube of the working stock drug solution from the refrigerator (1000 µg/ml). This is tube 1.

b.  Pipette 7.0 ml of the working stock drug solution into 7.0 ml of sterile M-3 broth. The final concentration is 500 µg/ml. This is tube 2. Pipette 7.0 ml of the M-3 broth containing 500 µg/ml of amphotericin B into 7.0 ml of M-3 broth.
c.  Continue preparing twofold dilutions in 7.0 ml volumes of M-3 broth until an amphotericin B concentration of 0.05 µg/ml is reached. Label each tube from 3 through 13 to correspond to each serial dilution.
d.  From each M-3 broth dilution, one at a time, pipette 3.0 ml of the M-3 broth with amphotericin B into each of two tubes containing 27.0 ml of M-3 agar (2%) maintained at 50–52°C in a water bath. Mix the medium well and then pour each 30.0-ml volume into separate 10 × 10 cm Integrid Petri dishes. Allow the medium to harden. The final twofold concentrations of amphotericin B are 100 to 0.025 µg/ml (that is, tubes 1 to 13, respectively).

3.  Preparation of medium control
    a.  Pipette 3.0 ml of M-3 broth into each of two tubes containing 27.0 ml of M-3 agar maintained at 50–52°C in a water bath. Mix the medium well and then pour each 30.0 ml volume into separate 10 × 10 cm Integrid Petri dishes. Allow the medium to harden.
    b.  Label as "medium control."

4.  Preparation of DMSO control
    a.  Add 0.65 ml of DMSO to 7.0 ml of M-3 broth.
    b.  Pipette 3.0 ml of the M-3 broth containing DMSO into each of two tubes containing 27.0 ml of M-3 agar maintained at 50–52°C in a water bath. Mix the medium well and then pour each 30.0 ml volume into separate 10 × 10 cm Integrid Petri dishes. Allow the medium to harden.
    c.  Label as "DMSO control."

5.  Inoculation of media
    a.  Using a pipettor with calibrated tips to deliver 0.05 ml, inoculate 0.05 ml of inoculum on the surface of each Integrid Petri dish. Start with the control tubes working from 0.025 to 100 µg/ml.
    b.  Leave the plates undisturbed to permit the inoculum to be absorbed into the medium surface. Place no more than seven moulds and the control isolate on one plate.
    c.  Incubate the test at 30°C.

(D) *MFC Determinations from the Broth, Semisolid, and Solid Agar Techniques*

1.  Procedure

a. With a marking pen, divide an SAB plate into several pie-shaped portions.
b. Label the pie-shaped portions with the appropriate drug dilutions. The last drug dilution showing growth and all the dilutions showing no growth must be streaked on SAB.
c. Broth technique: Agitate each tube to be sampled. With a sterile 0.01-mm calibrated loop, remove a loopful of the broth. Semisolid agar technique: With a sterile 0.01-mm calibrated loop (loop portion bent at a right angle to the shaft), lightly touch the surface of the medium where the inoculum was placed without digging into it. The loop must be full. Solid agar technique: With a sterile 0.01-mm calibrated loop, lightly touch the surface of the medium where the inoculum was placed without digging into it. The loop must be full.
d. Streak the inoculum in the appropriately labeled pie-shaped area on the SAB plate. Repeat for each dilution.
e. Incubate the SAB plates at 30°C.
2. Results
a. Read the control isolate first. It should have an MFC of 0.2 $\mu$g/ml ± one dilution. The MFC is the last dilution with 3 or fewer colonies present from two of the three tubes or both of the plates.
b. Read the other isolate(s) and record the results.

### B. 5-Fluorocytosine (Ancobon, Flucytosine)

5-Fluorocytosine is a synthetic antimycotic agent with a molecular weight of 129.1 and the chemical formula $C_4H_4N_3OF$. The molecule is a fluorinated pyrimidine that is approximately 1.2% soluble in water at 25°C and stable for nearly 5 years at 14–31°C when protected from the light.

Upon active transport by permease enzymes into the fungal cell, deaminase enzymes convert 5-fluorocytosine into 5-fluorouracil, which is eventually incorporated as 5-fluorouracil into RNA as fluorouracil riboside. This interferes with nucleotide metabolism and subsequent protein synthesis. 5-Fluorocytosine susceptibility in the aspergilli also may be related to a block of thymidylate synthetase, the end effect being inhibition of DNA synthesis. Cytosine, purines, pyrimidines, and nucleosides are antagonistic to 5-fluorocytosine. Media used for susceptibility testing should not contain these materials if the results are to be meaningful.

Many yeasts and dematiaceous hyphomycetes are usually susceptible to

5-fluorocytosine. The agent is ineffective against the dimorphic fungi Most isolates of *Cryptococcus neoformans* have an initial MIC range of 0.46 to 7.8 µg/ml. During therapy, resistance rapidly develops in many isolates. Depending upon the yeast, resistance may vary from a few isolates to nearly all the isolates within a particular species. If resistance is associated with the permease enzymes, synergism may be achievable when 5-fluorocytosine is used in conjunction with other membrane-active drugs such as amphotericin B. 5-Fluorocytosine is fungistatic for most filamentous fungi, but may be fungicidal for yeasts at clinically achievable concentrations.

*In vitro* susceptibility testing with 5-fluorocytosine is appropriate for mycoses involving the central nervous system; for patients with severe renal disease; in order to explain treatment failure or relapse; to monitor for emerging resistance (especially in the yeasts); and, when infections are due to yeasts, for species of *Aspergillus* and the dematiaceous hyphomycetes. While a patient is on 5-fluorocytosine therapy, the isolates recovered must be monitored periodically for resistance. CSF levels of 5-fluorocytosine approximate 75–80% of concurrent serum levels. One clinical interpretation with normal therapy for MIC values is

Serum or CSF: susceptible = 1–8 µg/ml, intermediate = 16–64 µg/ml, resistant = 100 > µg/ml

1. Preparation of the stock 5-fluorocytosine solution
   5-Fluorocytosine (5-FC) used in the *in vitro* assay system is pure assayed powder. The potency is 100% when the drug is used in this form. Each time a portion of drug is used to prepare a new stock solution, the amount of drug weighed must be recorded in the weight log book. The dried powder is kept in a desiccator at −70°C.
   a. To prepare the stock drug solution
      (1) Pour a small amount of distilled water into a clean 5.0-ml volumetric flask.
      (2) Add 50.0 mg of 5-fluorocytosine powder.
      (3) Wash any drug residue on the weighing paper into the volumetric flask with distilled water.
      (4) Bring the volume up to the 5.0-ml mark with distilled water (final concentration is 10,000 µg/ml).
      (5) Place the suspension in a water bath set at 52°C until the suspension goes into solution. Agitate when necessary.
      (6) Sterilize by filtration through a 0.22 µm membrane filter.

The stock 5-FC solution containing 10,000 µg/ml of 5-FC is dispensed in 1.5-ml aliquots into good quality glass screw-cap tubes, which are then placed at −70°C until needed. The stock solutions should be discarded after one year. When an aliquot of the stock solution is needed, it is simply taken from the −70°C storage conditions and kept in the refrigerator. Solutions kept in the refrigerator are discarded after one year.

2. Control isolate

   A control isolate must be run with each set of tests. *Saccharomyces cerevisiae* (ATCC 36375) is an ideal isolate, since it has reproducible MIC (0.05 μg/ml) and MFC (0.05 μg/ml) values. Any isolate can be used as long as it has been evaluated thoroughly and gives consistent values from one test to the next. The stock culture of this isolate should be kept in the culture collection.

3. Preparation of inoculum

   a. Using sterile distilled water with or without 0.05% Tween 80, wash the growth from the sporulating mould colony grown on Sabouraud dextrose agar (2% dextrose). Care must be exercised to ensure that medium is not transferred with the inoculum. Various peptones, etc., may bind the 5-FC in the test system. Mycelial growth can be broken up with sterile glass beads. If a yeast is being tested, use sterile distilled water without 0.05% Tween 80. The yeast is simply transferred to the water with an inoculating loop. The inoculum from the control isolate is transferred from a 48-hour-old culture on Sabouraud dextrose agar to sterile distilled water without 0.05% Tween 80. Approximately 5.0 ml of inoculum are required for each organism.

   b. Using a spectrophotometer set at 530 nm, adjust the suspension to 90% T. Record the % T. This should result in approximately $10^6$ colony-forming units/ml.

4. Preparation of inoculum control

   a. Pipette 2.0 ml of inoculum into a sterile 12 × 75 mm tube.
   b. Label this "inoculum control."

5. Reading the test

   a. The end point is that dilution in which two of the three tubes, or both of the plates, show no growth. Read at 24 and 48 hours.
   b. Growth should be present in the medium controls.
   c. Growth should be absent in the inoculum control. If slight growth is present, this indicates carry-over.
   d. The control isolate must be read first. The test is valid if the control isolate gives an MIC of 0.05 μg/ml. A variation of one dilution is considered acceptable for these techniques. A button or a film in the bottom of a tube is considered positive. A clear tube is negative.

6. The final concentrations

| Tube or plate number | Concentration of 5-FC ($\mu g/ml$) |
| --- | --- |
| 1 | 100 |
| 2 | 50 |
| 3 | 25 |
| 4 | 12.5 |
| 5 | 6.25 |
| 6 | 3.13 |
| 7 | 1.56 |
| 8 | 0.78 |
| 9 | 0.39 |
| 10 | 0.20 |
| 11 | 0.10 |
| 12 | 0.05 |
| 13 | 0.025 |
| Medium Control | 0.0 |
| DMSO Control | 0.0 |
| Inoculum Control | 0.0 |

*(A) Broth Technique for Yeasts or Moulds to Determine MIC Values*

1. Preparation of working stock drug solution
   a. Dispense 0.5 ml of the stock 5-FC solution (10,000 $\mu g/ml$) into 4.5 ml of 1 × yeast nitrogen base (YNB). The final concentration is 1000 $\mu g/ml$.
2. Preparation of 5-fluorocytosine dilutions
   a. Remove the working stock drug solution from the refrigerator (1000 $\mu g/ml$).
   b. Pipette 1.0 ml of the 1000 $\mu g/ml$ dilution into the tube containing 9.0 ml of 1 × YNB. The final concentration is 100 $\mu g/ml$. This is tube No. 1.
   c. Prepare twofold dilutions in 7.0-ml volumes of 1 × YNB until a concentration of 0.025 $\mu g/ml$ is reached. Label each tube from 2 through 13 to correspond to each serial dilution.
   d. Dispense 1.0-ml aliquots of each dilution into each of six sterile 12 × 75 mm tubes.
3. Preparation of medium control
   a. Dispense 1.0-ml aliquots of 1 × YNB into each of six sterile 12 × 75 mm tubes.
   b. Label this "medium control."
4. Inoculation of media

a. Using a pipettor with calibrated tips to deliver 0.05 ml, inoculate three tubes with the unknown and three tubes with the control isolate. Start with the control tubes working from 0.025 to 100 $\mu g/ml$.
　　b. Incubate the test at 30°C.

(B) *Semisolid Agar Technique for Moulds or Yeasts to Determine MIC Values*

1. Preparation of working stock drug solution
　　a. Pipette 1.0 ml of the stock solution (10,000 $\mu g/ml$) into 9.0 ml of $1 \times$ YNB. The final concentration is 1000 $\mu g/ml$.
2. Preparation of 5-fluorocytosine dilutions
　　a. Remove one tube of the working stock drug solution from the refrigerator (1000 $\mu g/ml$).
　　b. Pipette 4.0 ml of the working stock drug solution into 6.0 ml of sterile $1 \times$ YNB (final concentration is 400 $\mu g/ml$).
　　c. Pipette 7.5 ml of the $1 \times$ YNB containing 400 $\mu g/ml$ into 7.5 ml of $1 \times$ YNB and label 200 $\mu g/ml$. This is tube No. 1.
　　d. Continue preparing twofold dilutions in 7.5 ml volumes of $1 \times$ YNB until a concentration of 0.05 $\mu g/ml$ 5-FC is reached. Label each tube from 2 through 13 to correspond to each serial dilution.
　　e. To each of the $1 \times$ YNB dilutions containing 5-FC (one at a time), add 7.5 ml of $1 \times$ YNB agar maintained at 50–52°C. Mix the medium well and then immediately pipette 2.0 ml-aliquots into each of six sterile $12 \times 75$ mm snap-cap test tubes. Stand the test tubes vertically while the medium hardens. The final twofold concentrations of 5-FC are 100 to 0.025 $\mu g/ml$ (that is, tubes 1 to 13, respectively).
3. Preparation of medium control
　　a. Mix 7.5 ml of $1 \times$ YNB and 7.5 ml of $1 \times$ YNB agar together.
　　b. Dispense 2.0-ml aliquots into sterile $12 \times 75$ mm snap-cap test tubes. Stand the test tubes vertically while the medium hardens.
　　c. Label these "medium control."
4. Inoculation of media
　　a. Using a pipettor with calibrated tips to deliver 0.05 ml, inoculate three tubes with the unknown and three tubes with the control isolate. Start with the control tubes working from 0.025 to 100 $\mu g/ml$.
　　b. Make sure that the inoculum neither runs down the side of the tube nor splashes when it is placed on the agar surface.
　　c. Incubate the test tubes at 30°C.

*(C) Solid Agar Technique for Moulds or Yeasts to Determine MIC Values*

1. Preparation of working stock drug solution
   a. Pipette 2.0 ml of the stock solution (10,000 µg/ml) into 18.0 ml of 10 × YNB. The final concentration is 1000 µg/ml.
2. Preparation of 5-fluorocytosine dilutions
   a. Remove one tube of the working stock drug solution from the refrigerator (1000 µg/ml). This is tube No. 1.
   b. Pipette 7.0 ml of the working stock drug solution into 7.0 ml of sterile 10 × YNB. The final concentration is 500 µg/ml. This is tube No. 2. Pipette 7.0 ml of the 10 × YNB broth containing 500 µg/ml of 5-FC into 7.0 ml of 10 × YNB.
   c. Continue preparing twofold dilutions in 7.0-ml volumes of 10 × YNB until a 5-FC concentration of 0.05 µg/ml is reached. Label each tube from 3 through 13 to correspond to each serial dilution.
   d. From each 10 × YNB dilution, one at a time, pipette 3.0 ml of the 10 × YNB with 5-FC into each of two tubes containing 27.0 ml of 2% water agar maintained at 50–52°C in a water bath. Mix the medium well and then immediately pour each 30.0-ml volume into separate 10 × 10 cm Integrid Petri dishes. Let the medium harden. The final twofold concentrations of 5-FC are 100 to 0.025 µg/ml (that is, tubes 1 to 13, respectively).
3. Preparation of medium control
   a. Pipette 3.0 ml of 10 × YNB into each of two tubes containing 27.0 ml of 2% water agar maintained at 50–52°C in a water bath. Mix the medium well and then pour each 30.0-ml volume into separate 10 × 10 cm Integrid Petri dishes. Let the medium harden.
   b. Label as "medium control."
4. Inoculation of media
   a. Using a pipettor with calibrated tips to deliver 0.05 ml, inoculate 0.05 ml of inoculum on the surface of each Integrid Petri dish. Start with the control tubes working from 0.025 to 100 µg/ml.
   b. Allow the plates to sit undisturbed to permit the inoculum to be absorbed onto the medium surface. Place no more than seven moulds and the control strain on one plate. Thirty-six yeasts can be tested on one plate.
   c. Incubate the test at 30°C.

*(D) MFC Determinations from the Broth, Semisolid, and Solid Agar Techniques*

1. Procedure

a. With a marking pen, divide an SAB plate into several pie-shaped portions.
b. Label the pie-shaped portions with the appropriate drug dilutions. The last drug dilution showing growth and all the dilutions showing no growth must be streaked on SAB.
c. Broth technique: Agitate each tube to be sampled. With a sterile 0.01 mm calibrated loop, remove a loopful of the broth. Semisolid agar technique: With a sterile 0.01-mm calibrated loop (loop portion bent at a right angle to the shaft), lightly touch the surface of the medium where the inoculum was placed without digging into it. The loop must be full. Solid agar technique: With a sterile 0.01 mm calibrated loop, lightly touch the surface of the medium where the inoculum was placed without digging into it. The loop must be full.
d. Streak the inoculum in the appropriately labeled pie-shaped area on the SAB plate. Repeat for each dilution.
e. Incubate the SAB plates at 30°C.
2. Results
a. Read the control isolate first. It should have an MFC of 0.05 μg/ml ± one dilution. The MFC is the last dilution with three or fewer colonies present from two of the three tubes or both of the plates.
b. Read the other strain(s) and record their results.

### C. Miconazole

Miconazole nitrate is a synthetic antimycotic agent with a molecular weight of 479.16 and chemical formula of $C_{18}H_{14}Cl_4N_2O \cdot NHO_3$. This compound is a phenethyl imidazole derivative that is slightly soluble in water. It is stable at room temperature.

Miconazole interacts with the cell membrane and cell wall resulting in the leakage of cytoplasmic cations, amino acids, and proteins. It has been recently postulated that fungal cell death results from miconazole inhibiting the peroxidative enzymes cytochrome $c$ peroxidase and catalase, which results in peroxide accumulation. Miconazole may also decrease the uptake of purines and glutamine.

Yeasts, dermatophytes, species of *Aspergillus*, and several dimorphic fungi are susceptible to miconazole in a range of 0.1–10 μg/ml. Most isolates are susceptible at approximately 2 μg/ml. In susceptibility testing, the medium and the concentration of inoculum are especially critical. *In vitro* testing is appropriate for mycoses involving the central nervous system; for unusual opportunistic pathogens; and when indicated by the clinical status of the patient.

1. Preparation of the stock miconazole nitrate solution
    The miconazole used in susceptibility testing is pure assayed powder (miconazole nitrate). The potency of miconazole nitrate is 100%. Each time a portion of drug is used to prepare a new stock solution, its weight must be recorded in the weight log book. This will permit rechecking of concentrations if necessary. The dried powder is kept in a desiccator at $-70°C$.
    a. To prepare the stock drug solution
        (1) Remove the dimethyl sulfoxide (DMSO) from the refrigerator at least 1 hour prior to its use and allow it to warm up to room temperature.
        (2) Pour a small amount of DMSO into a clean sterile 5.0-ml volumetric flask. USE THE CHEMICAL FUME HOOD.
        (3) Add 50.0 mg of miconazole nitrate to the 5.0 ml volumetric flask to achieve a final miconazole concentration of 10,000 $\mu g/ml$.
        (4) Wash any drug residue from the weighing paper into the volumetric flask with DMSO.
        (5) Bring the volume up to 5.0 ml with DMSO.
        (6) Allow the stock solution to sit at room temperature for 30 minutes prior to its use. This permits self-sterilization of the miconazole by the DMSO.

    The stock miconazole solution containing 10,000 $\mu g/ml$ is dispensed in 1.5-ml aliquots into good quality glass screw-cap tubes, which are then placed at $-70°C$ until needed. The stock solutions should be discarded after 1 year. When an aliquot of the stock solution is needed, a tube is transferred from the freezer to a refrigerator. This solution is discarded after 1 year.

2. Control isolate
    A control isolate must be run with each set of tests. *Candida stellatoidea* (ATCC 36232) is an ideal isolate to use since it has reproducible MIC (0.39 $\mu g/ml$) and MFC (0.39 $\mu g/ml$) values. Any isolate can be used as long as it has been evaluated thoroughly and it gives consistent results from one test to the next. The stock culture of this isolate should be kept in the culture collection.

3. Preparation of inoculum
    a. Broth technique

# In Vitro Susceptibility Testing

      (1) Transfer growth from a 24- to 48-hour-old SAB slant into sterile distilled water. Approximately 5.0 ml of inoculum will be needed for each yeast.
      (2) With a spectrophotometer set at 530 nm, adjust the suspension to 95–98% T. Record the % T.
      (3) Add 0.1 ml of the suspension to 9.9 ml of sterile distilled water. The final concentration should be approximately $5 \times 10^4$ colony-forming units/ml.
  b. Semisolid and solid agar techniques
      (1) Using sterile distilled water with or without 0.05% Tween 80, wash the growth from the sporulating mould colony grown on Sabouraud dextrose agar (2% dextrose). Mycelial growth can be broken up with sterile glass beads. If a yeast is being tested, use sterile distilled water without 0.05% Tween 80. The yeast is simply transferred to the water with an inoculating loop. The inoculum from the control isolate is transferred from a 48-hour-old culture on Sabouraud dextrose agar to sterile distilled water without 0.05% Tween 80. Approximately 5.0 ml of inoculum are required for each organism.
      (2) Using a spectrophotometer set at 530 nm, adjust the suspension to 95 to 98% T. Record the % T.
      (3) Add 0.1 ml of the suspension to 9.9 ml of sterile distilled water.
      (4) Add 1.0 ml of the new suspension to 9.0 ml of sterile distilled water. The final concentration is approximately $5 \times 10^3$ colony-forming units/ml.
4. Preparation of inoculum control
  a. Pipette 2.0 ml of inoculum into a sterile $12 \times 75$ mm tube.
  b. Label this "inoculum control."
5. Reading the test
  a. The end point is that dilution in which two of the three tubes or both of the plates show no growth. Read at 24 and 48 hours.
  b. Growth should be present in the medium and DMSO controls.
  c. Growth should be absent in the inoculum control. If there is slight growth present, this indicates carry-over.
  d. The control isolate must be read first. The test is valid if the control isolate gives an MIC of 0.39 $\mu$g/ml. A variation of one dilution is considered acceptable for these techniques. A button or a film in the bottom of a tube is considered positive. A clear tube is negative.
6. The final concentrations

| Tube or plate number | Concentration of miconazole ($\mu g/ml$) |
|---|---|
| 1 | 100 |
| 2 | 50 |
| 3 | 25 |
| 4 | 12.5 |
| 5 | 6.25 |
| 6 | 3.13 |
| 7 | 1.56 |
| 8 | 0.78 |
| 9 | 0.39 |
| 10 | 0.20 |
| 11 | 0.10 |
| 12 | 0.05 |
| 13 | 0.025 |
| Medium Control | 0.0 |
| DMSO Control | 0.0 |
| Inoculum Control | 0.0 |

*(A) Broth Technique for Yeasts to Determine MIC Values*

1. Preparation of working stock drug solution
   a. Dispense 0.5 ml of the stock miconazole solution (10,000 $\mu g/ml$) into 4.5 ml of casitone broth. The final concentration is 1000 $\mu g/ml$.
2. Preparation of miconazole dilutions
   a. Remove the working stock drug solution from the refrigerator (1000 $\mu g/ml$).
   b. Pipette 2.0 ml of the 1000 $\mu g/ml$ dilution into the tube containing 18.0 ml of casitone broth. The final concentration is 100 $\mu g/ml$. This is tube No. 1.
   c. Prepare twofold dilutions in 7.0 ml volumes of casitone broth until a concentration of 0.025 $\mu g/ml$ is reached. Label each tube from 2 through 13 to correspond to each serial dilution.
   d. Dispense a 1.0-ml aliquot of each dilution into each of six sterile 12 × 75 mm tubes.
3. Preparation of medium control
   a. Dispense a 1.0-ml aliquot of casitone broth into each of six sterile 12 × 75 mm tubes.
   b. Label these "medium control."
4. Preparation of DMSO control
   a. Add 0.1 ml of DMSO to 7.0 ml of casitone broth.
   b. Pipette a 1.0-ml aliquot into each of six sterile 12 × 75 mm tubes.
   c. Label these "DMSO control."

5. Inoculation of media
   a. Using a pipettor with calibrated tips to deliver 0.05 ml, inoculate three tubes with the unknown and three tubes with the control isolate. Start with the control tubes working from 0.025 to 100 μg/ml.
   b. Incubate the test at 30°C.

*(B) Semisolid Agar Technique for Moulds or Yeasts to Determine MIC Values*

1. Preparation of working stock drug solution
   a. Pipette 1.0 ml of the stock solution (10,000 μg/ml) into 9.0 ml of casitone broth. The final concentration is 1000 μg/ml.
2. Preparation of miconazole dilutions
   a. Remove one tube of the working stock drug solution from the refrigerator (1000 μg/ml).
   b. Pipette 4.0 ml of the working solution into 6.0 ml of sterile casitone broth. The final concentration is 400 μg/ml.
   c. Pipette 7.5 ml of the casitone broth containing 400 μg/ml into 7.5 ml of casitone broth and label 200 μg/ml. This is tube No. 1.
   d. Continue preparing twofold dilutions in 7.5-ml volumes of casitone broth until a miconazole concentration of 0.05 μg/ml is reached. Label each tube from 2 through 13 to correspond to each serial dilution.
   e. To each of the casitone broth dilutions containing miconazole (one at a time), add 7.5 ml of casitone agar maintained at 50–52°C. Mix the medium well and then immediately pipette a 2.0-ml aliquot into each of six sterile 12 × 75 mm snap-cap test tubes. Stand the test tubes vertically while the medium hardens. The final twofold concentrations of miconazole are 100 to 0.025 μg/ml (that is, tubes 1 to 13, respectively).
3. Preparation of medium control
   a. Mix 7.5 ml of casitone broth and 7.5 ml of casitone agar together.
   b. Dispense in 2.0-ml aliquots into sterile 12 × 75 mm snap cap test tubes. Stand the test tubes vertically while the medium hardens.
   c. Label these "medium control."
4. Preparation of DMSO control
   a. Add 0.2 ml of DMSO to 7.3 ml of casitone broth.
   b. Add the 7.5 ml of casitone broth containing DMSO to 7.5 ml of casitone agar maintained at 50–52°C.
   c. Pipette a 2.0-ml aliquot into each of six sterile 12 × 75 mm tubes. Stand the test tubes vertically while the medium hardens.
   d. Label these "DMSO control."

5. Inoculation of media
   a. Using a pipettor with calibrated tips to deliver 0.05 ml, inoculate three tubes with the unknown and three tubes with the control isolate. Start with the control tubes working from 0.025 to 100 µg/ml.
   b. Make sure that the inoculum neither runs down the side of the tube nor splashes when it is placed on the agar surface.
   c. Incubate the test at 30°C.

*(C) Solid Agar Technique for Moulds or Yeasts to Determine MIC Values*

1. Preparation of working stock drug solution
   a. Pipette 2.0 ml of the stock solution (10,000 µg/ml) into 18.0 ml of casitone broth. The final concentration is 1000 µg/ml.
2. Preparation of miconazole dilutions
   a. Remove one tube of the working stock drug solution from the refrigerator (1000 µg/ml). This is tube No. 1.
   b. Pipette 7.0 ml of the working stock drug solution into 7.0 ml of sterile casitone broth. The final concentration is 500 µg/ml. This is tube No. 2. Pipette 7.0 ml of the casitone broth containing 500 µg/ml of miconazole into 7.0 ml of casitone broth.
   c. Continue preparing twofold dilutions in 7.0-ml volumes of casitone broth until a concentration of 0.05 µg/ml is reached. Label each tube from 3 through 13 to correspond to each serial dilution.
   d. From each casitone broth dilution, one at a time, pipette 3.0 ml of the casitone broth with miconazole into each of two tubes containing 27.0 ml of casitone agar (2%) maintained at 50–52°C in a water bath. Mix the medium well and then immediately pour each 30.0-ml volume into separate 10 × 10 cm Integrid Petri dishes. Allow the medium to harden. The final twofold concentrations of miconazole are 100 to 0.025 µg/ml (that is, tubes 1 to 13, respectively).
3. Preparation of medium control
   a. Pipette 3.0 ml of casitone broth into each of two tubes containing 27.0 ml of casitone agar maintained at 50–52°C in a water bath. Mix the medium well and then pour each 30.0-ml volume into separate 10 × 10 cm Integrid Petri dishes. Allow the medium to harden.
   b. Label these "medium control."

# In Vitro Susceptibility Testing

4. Preparation of DMSO control
   a. Add 0.65 ml of DMSO to 7.0 ml of casitone broth.
   b. Pipette 3.0 ml of the casitone broth containing DMSO into each of two tubes containing 27.0 ml of casitone agar maintained at 50–52°C in a water bath. Mix the medium well and then immediately pour each 30.0-ml volume into separate 10 × 10 cm Integrid Petri dishes. Allow the medium to harden.
   c. Label as "DMSO control."
5. Inoculation of media
   a. Using a pipettor with calibrated tips to deliver 0.05 ml, inoculate 0.05 ml of inoculum on the surface of each Integrid Petri dish. Start with the control tubes working from 0.025 to 100 µg/ml.
   b. Allow the plates to sit undisturbed to permit the inoculum to be absorbed into the medium surface. Place no more than seven moulds and the control isolate on one plate.
   c. Incubate the test at 30°C.

*(D) MFC Determinations for the Broth, Semisolid, and Solid Agar Techniques*

1. Procedure
   a. With a marking pen, divide the bottom of an SAB plate into several pie-shaped portions.
   b. Label the pie-shaped portions with the appropriate drug dilutions. The last dilution showing growth and all the dilutions showing no growth must be streaked on SAB.
   c. Broth technique: Agitate each tube to be sampled. With a sterile 0.01-mm calibrated loop, remove one loopful of the broth. Semisolid agar technique: With a sterile 0.01-mm calibrated loop (loop portion bent at a right angle to the shaft), lightly touch the surface of the medium where the inoculum was placed without digging into it. The loop must be full.
   Solid agar technique: With a sterile 0.01-mm calibrated loop, lightly touch the surface of the medium where the inoculum was placed without digging into it. The loop must be full.
2. Results
   a. Incubate at 30°C. Read the control isolate first. It should have an MFC of 0.39 µg/ml ± one dilution. The MFC is the last dilution with three or fewer colonies present from two of the three tubes or both the plates.
   b. Read the other isolate(s) and record results.

# BIOASSAY TO DETERMINE DRUG LEVELS IN BODY FLUIDS

The determination of drug concentrations in body fluids, such as serum and cerebral spinal fluid (CSF), is a great aid in adjusting chemotherapy. There are a number of methods available to determine drug levels in body fluids. The major reported techniques involve bioassay using micro- and macrotechniques, gas–liquid chromatography, high pressure liquid chromatography, measurement of an efflux of rubidium ions, and radiometric procedures. Because of its accuracy, reference value, and reproducibility, the bioassay technique will be presented in this handbook.

### A.  Amphotericin B Body Fluid Level Determination

1. Preparation of the working amphotericin B solution
   a. Pipette 1.0 ml of the stock solution containing 10,000 $\mu$g/ml into a tube containing 9.0 ml of distilled water to give a 1000 $\mu$g/ml solution. This solution can be stored at $-70°C$ for 1 month.
   b. Add 1.0 ml of the 1000 $\mu$g/ml solution to 19.0 ml of sterile distilled water to give a 50 $\mu$g/ml solution. This solution can be stored in the refrigerator for 1 week.
2. Preparation of inoculum
   a. *Paecilomyces variotii* (ATCC 36257) is grown at 30°C on slants of Sabouraud dextrose agar for 48–72 hours. The conidia are harvested by washing the slants with sterile water. The suspension of conidia and hyphal fragments is adjusted to 85 to 90% T at 360 nm with a spectrophotometer. This suspension will remain viable for 5 days at 4°C. Approximately 2.0 ml of inoculum will be needed for each determination. The inoculum contains approximately $10^6$ colony-forming units/ml.
3. Preparation of medium
   a. Antibiotic medium 12 FDA (Nystatin Assay Agar) is prepared in 100-ml quantities. After autoclaving, it is cooled to 50°C and each 100-ml quantity is inoculated with 1.0 ml of the mould suspension. One of the 100-ml volumes is required for each determination.
   b. The inoculated medium is dispensed in 25-ml aliquots with a serological pipette into sterile 15 × 150 mm plastic Petri dishes. After hardening on a level surface, the plates are refrigerated at 4°C for at least 1 hour and then dried at 37°C for 10 minutes to remove surface moisture. Sixteen evenly spaced wells are then cut into the agar and removed using a sterile 5-mm cork borer at-

tached to a vacuum flask. Two plates are needed for each determination.
4. Preparation of drug dilutions and dose response curve
   a. The 50 µg/ml solution of amphotericin B is diluted 1:10 (1.0 ml in 9.0 ml of serum) in pooled sterile normal human serum (filtered and heat inactivated) to give a 5 µg/ml solution.
   b. The 5 µg/ml solution is then diluted twofold in 2.0-ml volumes of normal serum from 2.5 to 0.078 µg/ml.
   c. Two wells are filled with 100 µl (0.1 ml) of each drug dilution. Wells are filled using a micropipettor fitted with sterile, disposable tips calibrated to deliver 100 µl.
   d. Plates are incubated at 30°C for 24 hours.
   e. Zones of inhibition are measured in two diameters using a vernier caliper.
   f. The dose response curve is obtained by plotting the concentration of drug in µg/ml as the ordinate and the zone diameter in millimeters as the abscissa on 2- or 3-cycle semilog graph paper. The points are joined to give the best-fit straight line. The line can be calculated by the formula on the worksheet.
5. Preparation of patient's fluids for assay and measurement of unknown concentration
   a. Two wells are filled with 100 µl of the patient's undiluted serum.
   b. The drug concentration is measured by plotting the patient's zone of inhibition against the dose response curve.
6. Serum control
   a. Two wells are filled with 100 µl of normal human serum that has been heat inactivated for 1 hour at 56°C (1:10 dilution in sterile distilled water).
   b. There should be no zones of inhibition. If one is present, the test is invalid and must be repeated.
7. DMSO control
   a. Two wells are filled with 100 µl of DMSO in distilled water prepared by the same method as the drug (without amphotericin B).
   b. There should be no zones of inhibition. If one is present, the test is invalid and must be repeated.
8. Internal standard
   a. Two wells are filled with 100 µl of a randomly chosen internal standard.
   b. The drug concentration is measured by plotting the zone of inhibition against the dose response curve.

### B. Bioassay for Amphotericin B in the Presence of 5-Fluorocytosine

To assay amphotericin B in the presence of 5-fluorocytosine, the latter must be inactivated.

1. Prepare a stock 10,000 µg/ml solution of cytosine in normal saline. Sterilize by filtration.
2. Add 1.0 ml of the stock solution to 6.0 ml of sterile distilled water.
3. Add 1.0 ml of this solution to the 100 ml of media cooled to 48–50°C. This will give a final concentration of approximately 10 µg/ml of cytosine.
4. The assay organism is *Chrysosporium pruinosum* (ATCC 36374), which is resistant to 5-fluorocytosine.
5. Serum is assayed as outlined in the procedure for the amphotericin B bioassay.
6. Internal standards
   a. Prepare a set of standards as in the bioassay protocol for amphotericin B.
   b. Dispense the standards in 2.0 ml volumes and label as follows: A = 1.25 µg/ml, B = 0.078 µg/ml, C = 0.312 µg/ml, D = 0.625 µg/ml, E = 5 µg/ml, F = 0.156 µg/ml, G = 2.5 µg/ml
   c. Freeze at −70°C and discard in 1 month.

The data can be plotted directly onto 2- or 3-cycle semilog paper, or a best-fit line representing the data can be calculated using the linear regression equation. Some mycologists prefer to handle the data in the form of logarithms to base 2. This results in much smaller numbers in the various calculations.

1. Linear regression equation

$$Y = b_0 + b_1 X$$

2. Calculations ($n = 7$)

$$b_1 = \frac{\Sigma XY - [(\Sigma X)(\Sigma Y)]/n}{\Sigma X^2 - (\Sigma X)^2/n}$$

$$b_0 = \frac{1}{n}(\Sigma Y - b_1 \Sigma X)$$

3. To plot the line (2- or 3-cycle semilog paper), select the extreme zone diameters (that is, $X$) and plug these values into the linear regression equation. Locate the two points on the graph paper and connect them with a straight line ($y$ axis is vertical, $x$ axis is horizontal).

**Drug Levels in Body Fluids**

| Amphotericin B Work Sheet for Calculations | | | | | |
|---|---|---|---|---|---|
| | Well 1 measurements | | Well 2 measurements | | Average diameter (mm) |
| | 1 | 2 | 1 | 2 | |
| 5.0 | ___ | ___ | ___ | ___ | ___ |
| 2.5 | ___ | ___ | ___ | ___ | ___ |
| 1.25 | ___ | ___ | ___ | ___ | ___ |
| 0.625 | ___ | ___ | ___ | ___ | ___ |
| 0.312 | ___ | ___ | ___ | ___ | ___ |
| 0.156 | ___ | ___ | ___ | ___ | ___ |
| 0.078 | ___ | ___ | ___ | ___ | ___ |
| Patient's fluid | ___ | ___ | ___ | ___ | |
| Serum control | ___ | ___ | ___ | ___ | If not zero, test is invalid. Repeat. |
| DMSO conrol | ___ | ___ | ___ | ___ | If not zero, test is invalid. Repeat. |
| Internal Standard | ___ | ___ | ___ | ___ | ___ |
| $Y$ (conc.) | $X$ (Zone diam.) | | $XY$ | $X^2$ | |
| 5.0 | ___ | | ___ | ___ | |
| 2.5 | ___ | | ___ | ___ | |
| 1.25 | ___ | | ___ | ___ | |
| 0.625 | ___ | | ___ | ___ | |
| 0.312 | ___ | | ___ | ___ | |
| 0.156 | ___ | | ___ | ___ | |
| 0.078 | ___ | | ___ | ___ | |
| Totals 9.921 Summation ($\Sigma$) | ___ | | ___ | ___ | |

4. The unknown fluid and internal standards can now be read off the straight line. Find the zone size on the $X$ axis, read up to the straight line, and then read over to the $Y$ axis, recording the concentration.
5. The concentration can also be calculated directly by using the formula

$$Y_1 = b_0 + b_1 X_1$$

### C. 5-Fluorocytosine Body Fluid Level Determination

1. Preparation of the working 5-fluorocytosine solution
   a. Pipette 1.0 ml of the stock solution containing 10,000 $\mu g/ml$ into a tube containing 9.0 ml of distilled water to give a 1000 $\mu g/ml$ solution.

b. Add 1.0 ml of the 1000 µg/ml solution to 9.0 ml of pooled normal human serum to give a 100 µg/ml solution. This solution can be kept in the refrigerator for 1 year.
2. Preparation of inoculum
   a. *Saccharomyces cerevisiae* (ATCC 36375) is grown at 30°C on slants of Sabouraud dextrose agar for 48–72 hours. A suspension of the yeast cells in sterile distilled water is then adjusted to 65–70% T at 530 nm with a spectrophotometer. Approximately 2.0 ml of inoculum will be needed for each determination. The inoculum contains approximately $10^6$ colony-forming units/ml.
3. Preparation of medium
   a. Yeast morphology agar is prepared in 100-ml volumes. After autoclaving, it is cooled to 50°C and each 100-ml volume is inoculated with 1.0 ml of the yeast suspension. One 100 ml volume is required for each determination.
   b. The inoculated medium is dispensed in 25.0-ml aliquots with a serological pipette into sterile 15 × 150 mm plastic Petri dishes. After hardening on a level surface, the plates are refrigerated at 4°C for at least 1 hour and then dried at 37°C for 10 minutes to remove surface moisture. Six evenly spaced wells are then aseptically cut into the agar and removed using a sterile 5-mm cork borer attached to a vacuum flask. Three plates are needed for each determination.
4. Preparation of drug dilutions and dose–response curve
   a. Of the 100 µg/ml solution, 8.0 ml is mixed with 2.0 ml of sterile pooled normal human serum (heat-inactivated for 1 hour at 56°C) to make a 80 µg/ml solution. This solution is then diluted twofold in 2.0-ml volumes of normal serum from 40 to 2.5 µg/ml.
   b. Each of the six wells is filled with 100 µl (0.1 ml) of each of the six standards. Two plates are needed to assay the standards in duplicate. Wells are filled using a micropipettor calibrated to deliver 100 µl and fitted with sterile disposable tips.
   c. Plates are incubated at 30°C for 24 hours.
   d. Zones of inhibition are measured in two diameters using a vernier caliper.
   e. The dose response curve is obtained by plotting the concentration of drug in µg/ml as the ordinate and the zone diameter in millimeters as the abscissa on 2- or 3-cycle semilog graph paper. The points are joined to give the best-fit straight line. The line can be calculated by the formula on the work sheet.
5. Preparation of the patient's fluids for assay and measurement of unknown concentration

a. Three wells for each dilution are filled with 100 µl of the patient's serum that has been diluted 1:5 and 1:10. 5-FC levels above 100 µg/ml in undiluted serum are inaccurate.
   b. The drug concentration is measured by plotting the patient's zone of inhibition against the dose-response curve.
6. Serum control
   a. Two wells are filled with 100 µl of diluted pooled normal human serum (1:10 dilution in sterile distilled water).
   b. There should be no zones of inhibition. If one is present, the test is invalid and must be repeated.
7. Internal standard
   a. Two wells are filled with 100 µl of a randomly chosen internal standard.
   b. The drug concentration is measured by plotting the zone of inhibition against the dose response curve.

### D. Bioassay for 5-Fluorocytosine in the Presence of Amphotericin B

To assay 5-FC in the sera of patients treated with both amphotericin B and 5-fluorocytosine, the former must be inactivated.

1. The patient's serum is heated at 100°C for 45 minutes to destroy the amphotericin B. This is achieved by using flowing steam at 0 psi in a manually operated autoclave set to run between "sterilize" and "exhaust." This procedure must be closely monitored; if the temperature falls below 100°C the setting should be moved closer to "sterilize"; if the pressure should rise above 0 psi, the setting should be moved closer to "exhaust."
2. Serum is then assayed as outlined in the procedure for the 5-fluorocytosine bioassay.
3. Internal Standards
   a. Prepare a set of standards as in the bioassay protocol in pooled sterile heat-inactivated serum.
   b. Dispense the standards in 2.0-ml volumes and label as follows: 1 = 5.0 µg/ml, 2 = 80 µg/ml, 3 = 10 µg/ml, 4 = 2.5 µg/ml, 5 = 40 µg/ml, 6 = 20 µg/ml
   c. Freeze at $-70°C$ and discard after 1 year.

The data can be plotted directly onto 2- or 3-cycle semilog paper, or a best-fit line representing the data can be calculated using the linear

## 6 Susceptibility Testing and Bioassay Procedures

| 5-Fluorocytosine Work Sheet for Calculations | | | | | | | |
|---|---|---|---|---|---|---|---|
| | Well 1 measurements | | Well 2 measurements | | Well 3 measurements | | Average diameter (mm) |
| | 1 | 2 | 1 | 2 | 1 | 2 | |
| 80.0 | —— | —— | —— | —— | —— | —— | —— |
| 40.0 | —— | —— | —— | —— | —— | —— | —— |
| 20.0 | —— | —— | —— | —— | —— | —— | —— |
| 10.0 | —— | —— | —— | —— | —— | —— | —— |
| 5.0 | —— | —— | —— | —— | —— | —— | —— |
| 2.5 | —— | —— | —— | —— | —— | —— | —— |
| Patient's fluid | —— | —— | —— | —— | | | |
| Serum control | —— | —— | —— | —— | | | If not zero, test is invalid. Repeat. |
| Internal standard | —— | —— | —— | —— | | | —— |

| $Y$ (conc.) | $X$ (zone diam.) | $XY$ | $X^2$ |
|---|---|---|---|
| 80 | ———— | —— | —— |
| 40 | ———— | —— | —— |
| 20 | ———— | —— | —— |
| 10 | ———— | —— | —— |
| 5 | ———— | —— | —— |
| 2.5 | ———— | —— | —— |
| Totals 157.5 Summation ($\Sigma$) | ———— | —— | —— |

regression equation. Some mycologists prefer to handle the data in the form of logarithms to base 2. This results in much smaller numbers in the various calculations.

1. Linear regression equation

$$Y = b_0 + b_1 X$$

2. Calculations ($n = 6$)

$$b_1 = \frac{\Sigma XY - [(\Sigma X)(\Sigma Y)]/n}{\Sigma X^2 - (\Sigma X)^2/n}$$

$$b_0 = \frac{1}{n}(\Sigma Y - b_1 \Sigma X)$$

3. To plot the line (2- or 3-cycle semilog paper), select the extreme zone diameters (that is, $X$) and plug these values into the linear regression

equation. Locate the two points on the graph paper and connect them with a straight line ($y$ axis is vertical, $x$ axis is horizontal).
4. The unknown fluid and internal standards can now be read off the straight line. Find the zone size on the $x$ axis, read up to the straight line, and then read over to the $y$ axis, recording the concentration.
5. The concentration can also be calculated directly by using the formula

$$Y_1 = b_0 + b_1 X_1$$

### E. Miconazole Body Fluid Level Determination

1. Preparation of the working miconazole solution
   a. For bioassay, the form of miconazole prepared for intravenous administration is used rather than the pure drug.
   b. Dilute 1.0 ml of the intravenous preparation of miconazole (10,000 µg/ml) with 1.0 ml of sterile isopropyl alcohol to give a 5000 µg/ml solution.
   c. Add 1.0 ml of the 5000 µg/ml solution to 49.0 ml of normal human serum to give a 100-µg/ml solution. This solution can be stored in the refrigerator for 1 year.
2. Preparation of inoculum
   a. *Candida stellatoidea* (ATCC 36232) is grown at 30°C on slants of Sabouraud dextrose agar for 24–48 hours. A suspension of the yeast cells in sterile distilled water is then adjusted to 70% T at 570 nm with a spectrophotometer. Approximately 2.0 ml of inoculum will be needed for each determination.
3. Preparation of medium
   a. Sabouraud dextrose agar (Difco) is prepared in 100-ml volumes. After autoclaving, it is cooled to 50°C and each 100-ml volume is inoculated with 1.0 ml of the yeast suspension.
   b. The inoculated medium is dispensed in 25.0-ml aliquots with a serological pipette into sterile 15 × 150 ml plastic Petri dishes and allowed to harden on a level surface. After hardening, the plates are refrigerated at 4°C for at least 1 hour and then dried at 37°C for 10 minutes to remove surface moisture. Fourteen evenly spaced wells are cut into the agar and removed using a sterile 5-mm cork borer attached to a vacuum flask. Two plates are needed for each determination.
4. Preparation of drug dilutions and the dose response curve
   a. Of the 100 µg/ml solution of miconazole, 8.0 ml is mixed with 2.0 ml of serum to give a 80 µg/ml solution.
   b. Of the 80 µg/ml solution, 1.0 ml is added to 4.0 ml of normal human serum to give a 16 µg/ml solution.

c. The 16 μg/ml solution is then diluted twofold in 2.0 ml volumes of normal serum from 8.0 to 0.5 μg/ml.
d. Two wells are filled with each of the dilutions and with the patient's undiluted serum. Wells are filled using a micropipettor calibrated to deliver 100 μl (0.1 ml) and fitted with sterile disposable tips.
e. Plates are incubated at 30°C for 24 hours.
f. Zones of inhibition are measured in two diameters using a vernier caliper.
g. The dose-response curve is obtained by plotting the concentration of drug in μg/ml as the ordinate and the zone diameter in millimeters as the abscissa on 2- or 3-cycle semilog graph paper. The points are joined to give the best-fit straight line. The line can be calculated by the formula on the work sheet.

5. Preparation of the patient's fluids for assay and measurement of unknown concentration
   a. Two wells are filled with 100 μl of the patient's undiluted serum.
   b. The drug concentration is measured by plotting the patient's zone of inhibition against the dose-response control.

6. Serum control
   a. Two wells are filled with 100 μl of normal human serum that has been heat inactivated for 1 hour at 56°C (1:10 dilution in sterile distilled water).
   b. There should be no zones of inhibition. If one is present, the test is invalid and must be repeated.

7. Placebo/isopropyl alcohol control
   a. Two wells are filled with 100 μl of placebo/isopropyl alcohol prepared in the same method as the drug (without miconazole).
   b. There should be no zones of inhibition. If one is present, the test is invalid and must be repeated.

8. Internal standard
   a. Two wells are filled with 100 μl of a randomly chosen internal standard.
   b. The drug concentration is measured by plotting the zone of inhibition against the dose-response curve.

9. Internal standards
   a. Prepare a set of standards as in the bioassay protocol for miconazole.
   b. Dispense the standards in 2.0-ml volumes and label as follows: A1 = 0.5 μg/ml, A2 = 8 μg/ml, A3 = 2 μg/ml, A4 = 4 μg/ml, A5 = 1 μg/ml
   c. Freeze at −70°C and discard after 1 year.

# Drug Levels in Body Fluids

| Miconazole Work Sheet for Calculations | | | | | |
|---|---|---|---|---|---|
| | Well 1 measurements | | Well 2 measurements | | Average diameter |
| | 1 | 2 | 1 | 2 | (mm) |
| 8.0 | ___ | ___ | ___ | ___ | ___ |
| 4.0 | ___ | ___ | ___ | ___ | ___ |
| 2.0 | ___ | ___ | ___ | ___ | ___ |
| 1.0 | ___ | ___ | ___ | ___ | ___ |
| 0.5 | ___ | ___ | ___ | ___ | ___ |
| Placebo | ___ | ___ | ___ | ___ | |
| Patient's fluid | ___ | ___ | ___ | ___ | ___ |
| Serum control | ___ | ___ | ___ | ___ | If not zero, test is invalid. Repeat. |
| Internal standard | ___ | ___ | ___ | ___ | ___ |

| Y (conc.) | X (zone diam.) | XY | $X^2$ |
|---|---|---|---|
| 8 | ___ | ___ | ___ |
| 4 | ___ | ___ | ___ |
| 2 | ___ | ___ | ___ |
| 1 | ___ | ___ | ___ |
| 0.5 | ___ | ___ | ___ |
| Totals 15.5 Summation ($\Sigma$) | ___ | ___ | ___ |

The data can be plotted directly onto 2- or 3-cycle semilog paper, or a best-fit line representing the data can be calculated using the linear regression equation. Some mycologists prefer to handle the data in the form of logarithms to base 2. This results in much smaller numbers in the various calculations.

1. Linear regression equation

$$Y = b_0 + b_1 X$$

2. Calculations ($n = 5$)

$$b_1 = \frac{\Sigma XY - [(\Sigma X)(\Sigma Y)]/n}{\Sigma X^2 - (\Sigma X)^2/n}$$

$$b_0 = \frac{1}{n}(\Sigma Y - b_1 \Sigma X)$$

3. To plot the line (2- or 3-cycle semilog paper), select the extreme zone diameters (that is, $X$) and plug these values into the linear regression

equation. Locate the two points on the graph paper and connect them with a straight line ($y$ axis is vertical, $x$ axis is horizontal).
4. The unknown fluid and internal standards can now be read off the straight line. Find the zone size on the $x$ axis, read up to the straight line, and then read over to the $y$ axis, recording the concentration.
5. The concentration can also be calculated directly by using the formula

$$Y_1 = b_0 + b_1 X_1$$

## SYNERGISM STUDIES

Amphotericin B is often used in combination with other antimycotic agents, especially 5-fluorocytosine. Synergism, or at least potentiation, has been observed for amphotericin B and 5-fluorocytosine, rifampin, or tetracycline, and for 5-fluorocytosine with nystatin or rifampin. Amphotericin B in combined therapy promotes the uptake of the second drug into the cells. Second, it either stimulates or suppresses components of the host's immune system. The combined effect varies from one fungus to the next. Thus, laboratory studies are helpful in determining the potential benefit of using two drugs together. Occasionally, the combined use of drugs may result in an increased toxic effect. Increased bone marrow toxicity has been noted with combined amphotericin B and 5-fluorocytosine therapy.

Synergism can be defined as a fourfold or greater reduction in the MIC of one agent in the presence of a subinhibitory concentration of a second antimicrobial agent. If the reduction is twofold, this indicates possible potentiation. In contrast to synergism, if there is a twofold or greater increase in the MIC, the two agents are antagonistic. Synergism studies with amphotericin B and 5-fluorocytosine are appropriate when the MIC of 5-fluorocytosine is approximately 8–25 µg/ml. Therefore, MIC values for both drugs must be known prior to conducting synergism studies.

### A. Amphotericin B and 5-Fluorocytosine

1. Preparation of stock drug solutions
   a. Prepare stock drug solutions as outlined in the susceptibility testing procedures for amphotericin B and 5-fluorocytosine (5-FC).
2. Preparation of inoculum
   a. Prepare inoculum as outlined in the susceptibility testing procedure for amphotericin B. The inoculum should contain approximately $10^6$ colony-forming units/ml.
3. Preparation of drug dilutions
   Buffered yeast nitrogen base is used to avoid inactivation of the

amphotericin B. 5-FC is titrated from 100 to 0.05 µg/ml in twofold increments in the presence and in the absence of amphotericin B. Amphotericin B is used in concentrations of 1.0, 0.5, 0.1, 0.05, and 0.025 µg/ml. The test is conducted using the classical checkerboard scheme.
- a. Prepare twofold dilutions of amphotericin B in buffered yeast nitrogen base from 2.0 µg/ml to 0.05 µg/ml. Use the procedure outlined in the *in vitro* broth susceptibility testing protocol for amphotericin B.
- b. Prepare twofold dilutions of 5-FC in buffered yeast nitrogen base from 200 to 0.1 µg/ml. Use the procedure outlined in the *in vitro* broth susceptibility testing protocol for 5-FC.
- c. Arrange two 78 hole test tube racks containing 12 × 75 mm sterile snap-cap test tubes as in Fig. 6.1.
- d. Starting with row 13, pipette 0.5 ml of the 5-FC 200 µg/ml dilution from A through F.
- e. Starting with row 12, pipette 0.5 ml of the 5-FC 100 µg/ml dilution from A through F. Continue pipetting 0.5 ml volumes in descending order of 5-FC concentrations as above until the 0.05 µg/ml dilution has been pipetted in row 2, A through F.
- f. Starting with row F, pipette 0.5 ml of the amphotericin B 2.0 µg/ml dilution from 2 through 13.
- g. Starting with row E, pipette 0.5 ml of the amphotericin B 1.0 µg/ml dilution from 2 through 13. Continue pipetting 0.05-ml volumes in descending order of amphotericin B concentrations as above until the 0.05 µg/ml dilution has been pipetted in row b, 2 through 13.
- h. Add 0.5 ml of buffered yeast nitrogen base to each tube in row 1, B through F, and in row A, 2 through 13. Each tube now contains a total of 1.0 ml with the final concentrations indicated in Fig. 6.1.
- i. Repeat a–h using the second rack of 12 × 75 snap-cap test tubes. This set of tubes is the duplicate synergism study. Incubate the study at 30°C and read at 24 and 48 hours.
4. Controls
    - a. The MIC values for 5-FC and amphotericin B should be within one dilution of those previously determined for the isolate. The MIC values are read from row 1, 2 through 13 for 5-FC and row 1, B through F for amphotericin B. The end point is the same as outlined in the *in vitro* broth susceptibility testing protocols for amphotericin B and 5-FC.
    - b. DMSO, inoculum and medium controls are prepared and read in the same manner as outlined in the *in vitro* broth susceptibility testing protocols.

444                             6  Susceptibility Testing and Bioassay Procedures

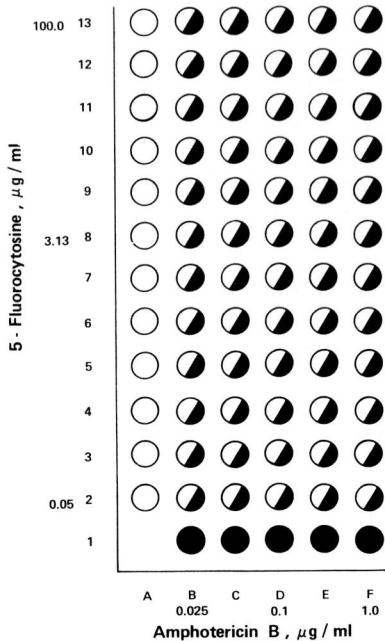

Fig. 6.1  Schematic representation of combined 5-fluorocystosine and Amphotericin B synergism study. ○, tube containing 5-fluorocytosine; ●, tube containing Amphotericin B; ◐, tube containing 5-fluorocytosine and Amphotericin B.

5. Reading the test
   a. Orient the tests as shown in Fig. 6.1.
   b. Label a 12 × 12 paper grid with the antimycotic agents and concentrations tested along the vertical and horizontal margins. The grid should be identical to the inoculated tubes.
   c. In boxes corresponding to each tube, indicate the presence of growth (button) by a plus sign and the absence of growth by a minus sign.
   d. Plot the results of the synergism study on graph paper having 10 squares to the inch.
      (1) On the vertical and horizontal axes of the graph, list the concentration of each drug.
      (2) Plot the inhibitory concentrations of each drug for each row.
      (3) Connect the plotted points.
6. Interpretation
   a. There must be a sharp fourfold decrease in the 5-FC MIC with the addition of a subinhibitory level of amphotericin B (Fig. 6.2).
   b. Report results as "Combination of amphotericin B and 5-fluorocytosine is (antagonistic, additive, or synergistic) against (name of fungus) from (patient's name and culture number)."
   c. The graph and isobologram are kept as a record of the synergism study.

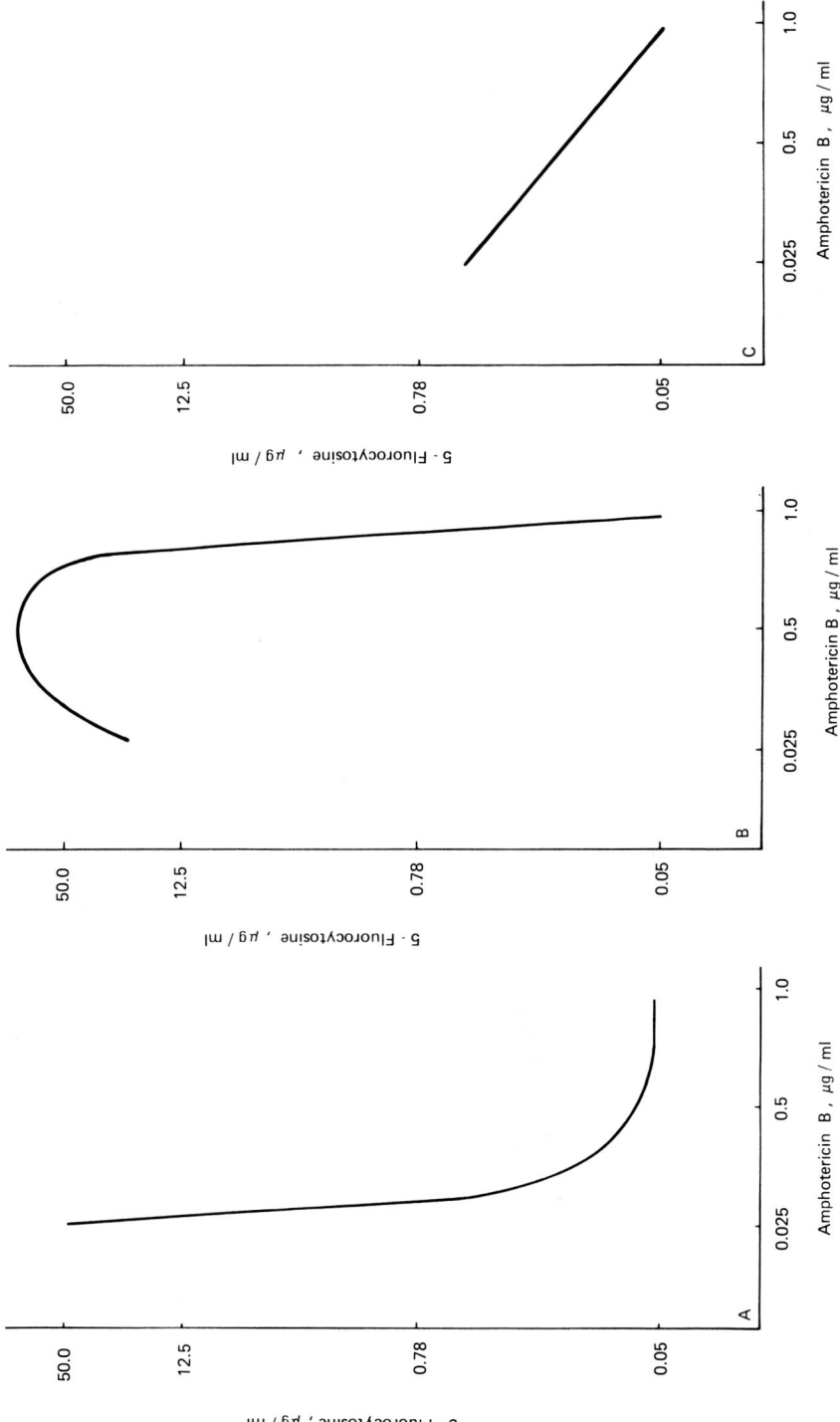

**Fig. 6.2** Schematic examples of isobolograms showing synergistic, antagonistic, and additive combined effects of 5-fluorocytosine and Amphotericin B.

*Selected References*

## A. General

1. Grove, D. C., and W. A. Randall (1955). "Assay Methods of Antibiotics, a Laboratory Manual." Antibiotics Monograph 2. Medical Encyclopedia, Inc., New York.
2. Haley, L. D., and C. S. Callaway (1978). "Laboratory Methods in Medical Mycology," DHEW Publ. No. (CDC) 78-8361. U. S. Government Printing Office, Washington, D.C.
3. Hamilton-Miller, J. M. T. (1973). Chemistry and biology of the polyene macrolide antibiotics. *Bacteriol. Rev.* **37**:166–196.
4. Hoeprich, P. D. (1978). Chemotherapy of systemic fungal diseases. *Annu. Rev. Pharmacol. Toxicol.* **18**:205–231.
5. Kobayashi, G. S., and G. Medoff (1977). Antifungal agents: recent developments. *Annu. Rev. Microbiol.* **31**:291–308.
6. Shadomy, S., and A. Espinel-Ingroff (1974). Susceptibility testing of antifungal agents. *In* "Manual of Clinical Microbiology," (E. H. Lennette, E. H. Spaulding, and J. P. Truant, eds.), 2nd ed., pp. 569–574. American Society for Microbiology, Washington, D.C.

## B. Susceptibility Testing

1. Bossche, H. Van Den, G. Willemsens, and J. M. Van Cutsem (1975). The action of miconazole on the growth of *Candida albicans*. *Sabouraudia* **13**:63–73.
2. Espinel-Ingroff, A., S. Shadomy, and J. F. Fisher (1977). Bioassay for miconazole. *Antimicrob. Agents Chemother.* **11**:365–368.
3. Kauffman, C. A., J. A. Carleton, and P. T. Frame (1976). Simple assay for 5-fluorocytosine in the presence of amphotericin B. *Antimicrob. Agents Chemother.* **9**:381–383.
4. Kitahara, M., V. K. Seth, G. Medoff, and G.S. Kobayashi (1976). Antimicrobial susceptibility testing of six clinical isolates of *Aspergillus*. *Antimicrob. Agents Chemother.* **9**:908–914.
5. Saubolle, M. A., and P. D. Hoeprich (1978). Disk agar diffusion susceptibility testing of yeasts. *Antimicrob. Agents Chemother.* **14**:517–530.
6. Shadomy, S. (1969). *In vitro* studies with 5-fluorocytosine. *Appl. Microbiol.* **17**:871–877.

## C. Synergism Studies

1. Arroyo, J., G. Medoff, and G. S. Kobayashi (1977). Therapy of murine aspergillosis with amphotericin B in combination with rifampin or 5-fluorocytosine. *Antimicrob. Agents Chemother.* **11**:21–25.
2. Dougherty, P. F., D. W. Yotter, and T. R. Matthews (1977). Microdilution transfer plate technique for determining *in vitro* synergy of antimicrobial agents. *Antimicrob. Agents Chemother.* **11**:225–228.
3. Polak, A. (1978). Synergism of polyene antibiotics with 5-fluorocytosine. *Chemotherapy* **24**:2–16.
4. Shadomy, S., G. Wagner, A. Espinel-Ingroff, and B. A. Davis. (1975). *In vitro* studies with combinations of 5-fluorocytosine and amphotericin B. *Antimicrob. Agents Chemother.* **8**:117–121.

*Chapter 7*

# Culture Collection

The culture collection, whether it consists of a few isolates or thousands of fungi, is an invaluable resource for the medical mycologist. The collection is a permanent home for reference isolates, atypical strains, quality control isolates, teaching cultures, isolates of epidemiological importance, and cultures that serve as a mycological history of a patient's infection. The absence in the past of culture collections for medically important fungi clearly accounts for much of the taxonomic confusion we are experiencing in contemporary medical mycology. The medical mycological culture collection in essence represents the primary bridge spanning the past, present, and future.

Upon receiving a new isolate to be deposited in the culture collection, it should be assumed that the culture is mixed. This assumption is made regardless of whether the culture originated in the institution's own laboratory or from an outside laboratory. Cultures can become contaminated with bacteria or fungi during subculturing, while in transit, or at some other time.

The value of the collection is directly proportional to the accuracy and completeness of the records maintained for each isolate. Isolates without their corresponding collection data are for all practical purposes worthless. Most mycologists maintain either a permanently bound accession book with each fungus listed in numerical order or a file folder system containing all the pertinent information regarding the isolate.

## CULTURE RECORDS

To maintain a uniform system of record keeping, all the information recorded should be done in an identical manner. When assigning accession or culture numbers, a number is used only once. If an isolate dies, its accession number dies too. The following information should be placed in the accession book in a consistent format.

1. Accession number, name of the fungus, and the date entered into the book.
2. When the fungus was isolated; where; by whom. For clinical isolates, a clinical summary is helpful.
3. When isolate was sent; who sent it.
4. The name used for the fungus when it was received. This name may or may not be the correct name for the fungus.
5. Any collection numbers, diagnostic numbers, or other accession numbers for the isolate.

A more elaborate system can be established utilizing file folders. The collection data for each new isolate is placed on a culture collection data sheet (Form 7.1), which is then placed in a file folder. The folders are kept in numerical order based upon the accession number. The file folder may also contain clinical summaries, drawings, photographs, laboratory data, and other information germane to the isolate.

Regardless of the method of indexing the isolate into the culture collection, a cross-index system filed by scientific name is necessary in order to locate a specific isolate. As the collection grows, other mycologists will probably request subcultures of the various fungi. Since these mycologists also need the collection data for each isolate requested, this information can be transferred to a culture collection data sheet (Form 7.2) and sent along with the isolate. Dangerous fungi should not be given to high school and undergraduate level students. Care must be exercised when sending cultures to other laboratories and training programs. The distribution of dangerous fungi should be recorded on the culture collection data sheet or in the accession book.

## RECEIVING NEW ISOLATES

Upon receiving a culture for deposit in the culture collection, the following steps should be taken.

1. Immediately fill out a culture collection data sheet or log the isolate into the accession book. Record the name of the fungus in pencil until its identity has been confirmed. If any portion of the required data is missing, request it from the sender.
2. Prepare a tease mount to ensure that the culture is properly identified. If the fungus is a yeast, biochemical tests will be necessary for confirmation of the identification.
3. Streak the original culture on a plate of PDA to ensure that the culture

| **Form 7.1.** Culture Collection Data Sheet |
|---|

1. Name of fungus: _____

   ACCESSION NUMBER _____

2. Sender _____
   name

   _____
   address

   _____
   date

3. I.D. confirmed _____  _____
                    date              by whom

4. Purity confirmed _____  _____
                    date              by whom

5. Collection data (source, etc.): _____

6. Additional accession numbers: _____
   _____
   _____

7. Storage _____  _____
           date              by whom

8. Distribution of subcultures:

| name | address | by whom |
|---|---|---|
| name | address | by whom |
| name | address | by whom |
| name | address | by whom |

is pure. If the culture is a yeast, set up the complete battery of biochemical tests and record the results.

4. Once the purity and identification have been confirmed, assign the culture an accession number and label all plates and slants with this number.

5. From the streaked-out-PDA plate, prepare a slide culture using PDA, a permanent mount labeled with the accession number, and then place these in the culture collection.

| Form 7.2. Information on Cultures ||||||||
| Name of the Institution<br>Address of the Institution ||||||||
| IDENTITY |||| ISOLATION DATA ||||
| No. | Your No. | NAME | DETERMINED BY | SUBSTRATE | LOCATION | ISOLATED BY | DATE |
|  |  |  |  |  |  |  |  |

6. From the streaked-out-PDA plate, prepare 5 subcultures on PDA. Label the tubes with the accession number.
7. Check the cultures at 7-day intervals until good sporulation has developed.
8. Preserve the subcultures as follows:
   a. Use one slant to prepare a water culture.
   b. Place two slants at $-70°C$.
   c. Cover two slants with a sterile mineral oil overlay.
9. Record all missing data on the culture collection data sheet.

## RECONSTITUTING LYOPHILIZED CULTURES

On occasion, laboratories will receive freeze-dried or lyophilized cultures. These cultures are either in single or double vials (one inside another), depending upon the sender. Lyophilized cultures are prepared in skim milk, human serum, or some other medium, and then freeze-dried. To reconstitute a lyophilized culture, the following steps are taken.

1. Have ready a nutrient broth, such as Sabouraud dextrose broth, or distilled water to reconstitute the lyophilized material; culture media, such as Sabouraud dextrose agar; and Pasteur pipettes.
2. With a sharp triangular metal file, score the vial containing the lyophilized material. Be sure to leave room at both ends of the vial so that it can be held safely.
3. Wipe the outside of the vial with a gauze soaked in 70% ethanol.
4. Holding the vial with the alcohol-soaked gauze, snap the vial in two at the score mark.
5. Aseptically pipette a few drops (0.2–0.3 ml) of broth or water into the portion of the vial containing the lyophilized material.
6. Suspend all the particles completely in the broth or water. This may require 15–30 minutes.
7. Pipette all the reconstituted material to a plate of nutrient agar. Some mycologists prefer to transfer the reconstituted material to broth instead of agar. Both techniques work well. Fungal growth should be present within 2–3 weeks. Approximately twice their normal growth time is required when isolates are first reconstituted from lyophilization.

## STORAGE TECHNIQUES

Many methods have been proposed and used effectively for maintaining culture collections. The more common techniques include dispersal in sterile soil, sterile mineral oil overlay, deep freezing, ultralow freezing, water culture, and lyophilization. Some of these techniques involve substantial amounts of time and expensive equipment. Four simple and inexpensive techniques are outlined below.

1. Water culture technique
   The water culture is probably the simplest technique to maintain fungal isolates. Most isolates stored in sterile water will remain viable for years.
   a. Procedure for setup of water cultures
      (1) To an actively sporulating culture on PDA, aseptically add approximately 2 ml of sterile distilled water.
      (2) Dislodge the conidia with a sterile long-handled inoculating wire or a rubber policeman without digging into the agar.
      (3) With a sterile capillary pipette, remove the suspension and transfer it to a sterile 1-dram vial labeled with the accession number. If the isolate is a yeast, transfer a small portion of the colony with a long-handled inoculating loop directly to a

sterile 1-dram vial containing approximately 2–3 ml of sterile distilled water.
- (4) If the volume of water is less than 3–4 ml, add additional sterile distilled water.
- (5) Screw the cap down tightly and then store at room temperature.
- (6) Additional sterile distilled water may be added at any time.

b. Procedure for preparing subcultures from water cultures
- (1) Wipe off the neck and cap of the vial with 70% ethanol.
- (2) Shake the water culture to resuspend the fungus.
- (3) Open the vial, flame the mouth, and aseptically transfer with a pipette approximately 0.2–0.5 ml to the suspension to a plate of PDA labeled with the accession number.
- (4) Tighten the cap on the vial and then return it to storage at room temperature.
- (5) Incubate the PDA plate at 25–30°C until growth appears.
- (6) Prepare a tease mount and confirm the identity of the isolate.
- (7) Prepare subcultures as needed.

2. Freezing Technique

One of the easiest techniques for preserving fungi is to freeze the cultures. This technique requires no special equipment.

a. Procedure for preparing frozen cultures
- (1) Tighten the cap of a test tube (made of good quality glass) containing an actively sporulating culture on PDA.
- (2) Place the slant, labeled with its accession number, into the freezer set at minus 70°C.

b. Procedure for preparing subcultures
- (1) Remove the tube from the freezer, open the tube and "chip" a small amount of the colony from the frozen agar with a long-handled inoculating needle. Recap the tube and immediately return it to the freezer. If the agar begins to thaw, do not return the slant to the freezer. If the culture thaws, prepare a new stock culture.
- (2) Spread out the inoculum on a plate of PDA labeled with the accession number.
- (3) Incubate at 30°C until growth appears.
- (4) Prepare a tease mount and confirm the identity of the isolate.
- (5) Prepare subcultures as needed.

3. Periodic transfer and refrigerator storage techniques

Many mycology laboratories maintain their culture collections by periodically transferring each isolate. This procedure is not recommended, as it is very time consuming and hyphae instead of conidia are usually transferred. An alternative solution to continuous transferring of cultures is to place freshly transferred isolates into a refrigerator set at 5°C. In general, the fungi need only be transferred at approximately 6-month intervals. Sensitive isolates will have to be subcultured more frequently.

The cultures are transferred once or twice each year if they are maintained in screw-cap tubes. Unfortunately, screw-cap tubes are unsatisfactory for the maintenance of the Mucorales because the tubes permit the accumulation of carbon dioxide, which is toxic to some members of this group of fungi. When tubes with cotton plugs are used, these cultures must be subcultured every 4 to 6 months owing to the rapid rate of dehydration of the medium. In addition to the dehydration problem, cotton-plugged tubes are readily pregnable to mite invasion, hence special precautions must be taken to prevent such an infestation.

4. Sterile mineral oil overlay technique

The sterile mineral oil technique is one of the more traditional methods of maintaining culture collections. Its major disadvantage involves working with messy mineral oil.

   a. Procedure for preparing mineral oil overlays

      (1) To an actively sporulating culture on a PDA slant labeled with the accession number, aseptically pour sterile mineral oil over the entire slant. Ensure that the mineral oil reaches only approximately 1 cm below the lip of the screw-cap tube. If the oil reaches the lip, it then becomes difficult and messy to remove the fungus at a later date.

      (2) Tighten the cap and store the tube at room temperature.

   b. Procedure for preparing subcultures

      (1) Wipe off the neck and cap of the slant with 70% ethanol.

      (2) Open the tube, flame the mouth, and then remove a small amount of the colony using a sterile long-handled inoculating needle. Avoid any stringlike growth that reaches into the oil. This usually results in sterile subcultures.

      (3) Drain as much mineral oil as possible from the inoculum. Recap the tube and return it to storage.

      (4) Transfer the inoculum to a tube of Sabouraud dextrose broth labeled with the accession number.

      (5) Incubate at 30°C until growth appears.

      (6) Subculture to a PDA slant.

      (7) Prepare a tease mount and confirm the identity of the isolate.

## DIFFICULT-TO-REVIVE CULTURES

Cultures that no longer appear to be viable may be occasionally revived. Several techniques can be tried before discarding these cultures as dead.

1. Procedure for attempting to revive cultures with broth
   a. To a culture tube of an apparently nonviable isolate, aseptically pipette 2–3 ml of sterile Sabouraud dextrose broth.
   b. Incubate the culture at 30°C and examine it for the presence of new growth.
   c. Transfer new growth with a long-handled inoculating needle to a PDA slant.
   d. If new growth is not present after 3–4 weeks, discard the culture as nonviable and note this on the culture collection data sheet.
2. Procedure for attempting to revive cultures with agar overlays
   a. To an apparently nonviable isolate, aseptically pipette a few milliliters of molten Sabouraud dextrose agar cooled to 48–50°C. Just cover the top of the colony with the molten agar.
   b. Incubate the culture at 30°C and examine it for new growth emerging through the thin agar overlay.
   c. Transfer the new growth with a long-handled inoculating needle to a PDA slant.
   d. If new growth is not present after 3–4 weeks, discard the isolate as nonviable and note this on the culture collection data sheet.
3. Procedure for attempting to revive cultures by homogenization
   a. Transfer as much as possible of an apparently nonviable isolate to 1 ml of sterile distilled water in a test tube.
   b. With a long-handled inoculating needle, chop up the fungus.
   c. Transfer the entire contents of the test tube to a Petri dish containing PDA. Wrap the edge of the dish with parafilm to retard dehydration.
   d. Incubate the culture plate at 30°C and examine it for the presence of new growth.
   e. If new growth is not present after 3–4 weeks, discard as nonviable and note this on the culture collection data sheet.

## MITES

If one disaster to a culture collection can be singled out as a catastrophe, mites are that disaster. Mites are very minute arachnids that feed upon fungi when given the opportunity. As mites walk from one culture to another, they carry on their bodies bacteria and other fungi. These microorganisms will then rapidly contaminate the culture.

# Mites

Mites enter culture collections primarily as a result of poor laboratory housekeeping. Sources for mites include food in the laboratory, contaminants in clinical specimens (especially hair, nail, and skin), on insects, and in cultures obtained from other laboratories and institutions that have a mite infestation problem. The end product of a mite infestation can be the loss of the entire collection of cultures that are not in storage.

The first step in combating a mite infestation is to clean up the laboratory with a good disinfectant and immediately discard all the contaminated cultures. If a culture is contaminated and must be saved, several steps can be taken. Mite control is simple; the real problem is keeping mites out of the collection in the first place.

1. Cotton-plugged tubes for refrigerator storage
   a. Place 1 or 2 drops of mite poison on the cotton plug of the culture tube to be protected.
   b. Allow the plug to dry overnight.
   c. Mark the plug with a marking pen or with dye so that the culture is labeled as poisoned.
   d. Place the culture in the refrigerator for storage.
2. Contaminated cultures
   a. Transfer the mite-infested fungus to a tube of medium containing hexachlorocyclohexane. This agent will effectively kill mites.
   b. A second technique involves placing the mite-infested cultures into a plastic bag containing crystals of naphthalene or paradichlorobenzene, and then sealing the bag for approximately 1 week. If screw caps are used, they must be loosened. The latter chemical has a tendency to induce mutations in fungi. After treatment with the paradichlorobenzene, subsequent subcultures should be monitored.
3. Incubators or refrigerators
   If mites are present in incubators or refrigerators, they can be eliminated by using either naphthalene or paradichlorobenzene. If yeast assimilation tests are being conducted, *do not* use these chemicals at the same time in the same incubator. Many yeasts will utilize the vapors from these chemicals as a carbon source resulting in false-positive biochemical data.
   a. Clean the incubators or refrigerators with 70% ethanol.
   b. Place a 150-mm Petri dish containing crystals of naphthalene or paradichlorobenzene into the appliance. Approximately 1 week will be necessary to ensure that the mites have been killed.
   c. Discard the chemicals after use.
4. Barrier techniques for mite control

Culture tubes containing fungi can be protected from mites by using parafilm or cigarette paper seals. The use of parafilm is by far the simplest technique. The top of the culture tube is simply sealed with a piece of parafilm. Parafilm allows for good aeration, but prevents mites from walking into the cultures. Cigarette paper seals work equally well, but require more time and supplies for sealing the tubes.
5. Laboratory furniture
Cultures maintained on laboratory furniture with legs can be protected from mite infestation by placing each leg on a Petri dish that has been lightly coated with petroleum jelly. This technique will not prevent the spread of mites via dirty hands and contaminated culture tubes.

## MAILING CULTURES

The importation and transfer of fungi require the use of permits issued either by the United States Public Health Service (USPHS) or the United States Department of Agriculture (USDA), depending upon the nature of the fungus. Permits for the importation and transfer of medically important fungi can be obtained from the Office of Biosafety, Center for Disease Control, 1600 Clifton Road, N.E., Atlanta, GA 30333; and for fungi of agricultural significance must be obtained from the USDA, Animal and Plant Health Inspection Service, Federal Building, Hyattsville, MD 20782. In addition to these permits, if animal pathogens are to be imported or transferred, a permit must be obtained from the Chief Staff Veterinarian, Organisms and Vectors, Veterinary Services, APHIS, USDA, Federal Building, Hyattsville, MD 20782.

When fungi are sent through the mails, they must be in culture tubes, *not* plates. Petri dishes are readily broken and the agar and fungi are usually splashed around in the dish. For short distances, screw-cap tubes work well, but culture tubes with cotton plugs appear to be more suitable for long distances, especially cultures being shipped to foreign countries. Cotton-plugged tubes allow for better aeration. If yeasts that produce gas are to be mailed, they must be sent in cotton-plugged tubes in order to prevent the buildup of gas and possible subsequent breakage of the tube. Whether screw-cap tubes or culture tubes with cotton plugs are being used, the caps and plugs must be secured with tape to ensure that they do not become loose or opened in transit.

Federal regulations as outlined in Interstate Quarantine Regulations 42 CFR, Part 72.25 Etiologic Agents revised July 31, 1972 clearly outline the packaging and labeling requirements for etiologic agents. Basically, each tube is wrapped separately and the mouth of the tube is sealed with waterproof tape. The culture tubes are placed into a container containing an absorbent packing material. This container is then placed into a second container. The outer container must contain the appropriate etiologic agent and biohazard labels as explained in the Federal Register, Vol. 37, No. 127, June 30, 1972 and current item No. 257 from the Center for Disease Control. If the cultures are being mailed out of the country, various customs labels may be required too.

## DEPOSITING UNUSUAL ISOLATES IN MAJOR CULTURE COLLECTIONS

The major culture collections include the American Type Culture Collection (ATCC), 12301 Parklawn Drive, Rockville, MD 20852, U.S.A.; the Centraalbureau voor Schimmelcultures (CBS), Oösterstraat 1, Baarn, Netherlands; the ARS Culture Collection (NRRL), Northern Regional Research Service, U.S.D.A., 1815 N. University Street, Peoria, IL 61604, U.S.A.; and the Commonwealth Mycological Institute (CMI), Ferry Lane, Kew, Surrey, England.

These organizations encourage individuals to deposit free of charge unusual isolates. A primary function of the culture collection is to serve as a clearing house for fungi of interest to other mycologists. Each collection has its own guidelines for receiving new isolates. Prior to sending a culture for deposit, it is important to write the culture collection and obtain directions for deposit of isolates.

## KILLED CULTURES FOR STUDY OR TEACHING

Dangerous fungi, such as *Blastomyces dermatitidis, Coccidioides immitis,* and *Histoplasma capsulatum*, should be killed prior to being used as teaching materials. A satisfactory method for killing these and other fungi utilizes formalin.

1. Using a screw-cap culture tube, remove the cap and replace it with a cotton plug saturated with 40% formalin. Some mycologists prefer to use a small ball of cotton soaked in 40% formalin that is inserted into the cap, which is then screwed down tightly. Both techniques work equally well. Dangerous fungi are worked with *only* in the biological safety cabinet.
2. Incubate the tube at 36°C for 48 hours.

3. Remove the cotton plug and transfer a small amount of the fungus to a growth medium such as Sabouraud dextrose agar. Replace the cap. If the fungus is nonviable, nothing else need be done. If the fungus is viable, replace the cotton plug in the original tube for another 48-hour period and then recheck for viability.

*Selected References*

1. Carmichael, J. W. (1962). Viability of mold cultures stored at $-20°C$. *Mycologia* **54**:432–436.
2. Carmichael, J. W. (1963). Dried mold colonies on cellophane. *Mycologia* **55**:283–288.
3. C. M. I. (1960). "Herb. I. M. I. Handbook. Methods in Use at the Commonwealth Mycological Institute." Commonwealth Mycological Institute, Kew, Surrey, England.
4. C. M. I. (1968). "Plant pathologist's pocketbook." Commonwealth Mycological Institute, Kew, Surrey, England.
5. Hwang, S., W. F. Kwolek, and W. C. Haynes (1976). Investigation of ultralow temperature for fungal cultures. III. Viability and growth rate of mycelial cultures following cryogenic storage. *Mycologia* **68**:377–387.
6. McGinnis, M. R., A. A. Padhye, and L. Ajello (1974). Storage of stock cultures of filamentous fungi, yeasts, and some aerobic actinomycetes in sterile distilled water. *Appl. Microbiol.* **28**:218–222.
7. Pridham, T. G. (1974). "Micro-organism Culture Collections: Acronyms and Abbreviations." USDA, ARS, Peoria, Illinois.
8. Smith, R. S. (1967). Control of tarsonemid mites in fungal cultures. *Mycologia* **59**:600–609.
9. Snyder, W. C., and H. N. Hansen (1946). Control of culture mites by cigarette paper barriers. *Mycologia* **38**:455–462.
10. Stevens, R. B., ed. (1974). "Mycology Guidebook." Univ. of Washington Press, Seattle.
11. Tuite, J. (1969). "Plant Pathological Methods: Fungi and Bacteria." Burgess, Minneapolis, Minnesota.

*Chapter 8*

# Quality Control

During the past several years, mycologists have realized that quality control (QC) must be an integral component of a sound medical mycology program. The ultimate goal of QC is to ensure that the results reported are accurate, reliable, and reproducible. This will significantly enhance the efficiency of the laboratory, strengthen the creditability of the results reported, and improve patient care. The time necessary for QC varies from one laboratory to another and according to the magnitude of the program implemented.

QC is best handled by one individual. This will ensure that all the QC data are recorded and interpreted in a uniform manner. A complete program includes evaluation of all media and reagents, monitoring of equipment, review and reevaluation of test procedures, and evaluation of each person's performance. Each laboratory must design its own QC program that is tailored to meet the specific needs, goals, and expectations of the laboratory.

## GENERAL RECOMMENDATIONS

QC records should be kept for at least 2 years before they are discarded. If the records are numerous, they can be bound as a permanent book on a regular basis. Instructions for every routine procedure that is performed in the laboratory must be readily available. These instructions, or procedural manuals, should be reviewed, dated, and initialed by the reviewer once each year. The reviewer may be either the laboratory supervisor or the laboratory director. Whenever procedures are modified or changed, the new protocol must be dated and initialed by the laboratory director.

All the media, reagents, and stains to be used in the mycology laboratory must have recorded on the container the dates when they were received, first opened, and are to be discarded. Each item should be periodically checked, and if an item appears to be unsatisfactory, it must immediately be removed from the laboratory to prevent its use. Only the smallest amount that is needed in the laboratory should be ordered in order to prevent waste and use of excessive space for storage, and to maintain the freshness of the supplies. A 6-month supply is a reasonable amount to maintain.

The routine procedures used in the laboratory should be those that have been published in reputable mycological publications and evaluated in a competent manner. When new or improved techniques are published, they are compared to the techniques already in use prior to deciding whether or not they should be utilized. The procedures presently being used in the laboratory may be the most ideal for that particular laboratory.

A complete QC program requires that the appropriate fungal cultures be available for monitoring the quality and performance of the media and test procedures. QC cultures can be obtained from the major culture collections or from the clinical laboratory. These cultures must be well characterized and kept in the culture collection. To maintain an efficient work flow in the medical mycology laboratory, supplies, equipment, and the work area must be arranged in an orderly manner. The work areas should be kept clean and must be swabbed daily with a disinfectant, such as 5% phenol.

Each piece of equipment used in the mycology laboratory must meet the manufacturer's specifications and claims. The required monitoring of the laboratory equipment will be discussed later in this chapter. Glassware used in the mycology laboratory must also be monitored.

1. All chipped, damaged, or etched glassware should be discarded to prevent accidents.
2. Sterilized glassware must be checked for sterility on a regular basis and then stored for no more than 3 weeks prior to use.
3. Sterilized glassware as well as all clean glassware should be covered with aluminum foil.
4. All glassware should be free of detergents.

All irregularities must be immediately corrected and brought to the attention of the supervisor. The corrective action taken is documented on the QC forms.

## MEDIA CONTROL

The performance of both commercial and laboratory prepared media must be monitored (Form 8.1). In monitoring the performance of media, a record containing the following information should be prepared for each lot of medium that is tested (Form 8.2).

1. Identification of medium, including name of medium, source, lot number, date received, and expiration date.
2. Preparation of medium (if laboratory prepared) including method of sterilization, special materials added, and final pH value of the medium.
3. Evaluation of packaging and appearance of medium, including condition of packaging, color and clarity of medium, moisture content of medium, microbial or other contamination.
4. Sterility determination, including number of units tested and conditions and length of incubation.
   a. Five percent of the units in each lot of medium should be tested for sterility.
   b. The sampled units should be incubated at 35°C and room temperature for 3 days and inspected daily for indications of contamination.
   c. The sampled units used for testing are discarded at the completion of the evaluation. They are not used in the laboratory.
   d. If microbial growth is detected in 5% of the sampled units, the lot must be resampled. If contamination of 5% or greater is noted again, the entire lot is assumed to be contaminated and is discarded.
5. Performance evaluation including organisms used, incubation conditions, expected results, and observed results.
   a. The performance of 1 unit of each lot of medium is tested with each organism.
   b. The medium is inoculated with the appropriate test organisms that give positive and negative reactions. When the medium has passed the performance and sterility determinations, that particular lot is ready for use.

## EQUIPMENT CONTROL

Performance of each of the following types of equipment found in the medical mycology laboratory must be routinely monitored.

**Form 8.1.** Media Quality Control Summary Sheet

| Media | Expiration time (days from date of manufacture) | Containers | Storage conditions | Sterility | Performance controls Positive | Performance controls Negative | Expected results Positive | Expected results Negative |
|---|---|---|---|---|---|---|---|---|
| Example: caffeic acid agar | 14 days in plates | 15 × 100 mm | 4°C in dark | Yes | *Cryptococcus neoformans* | *Cryptococcus albidus* | Brown to black colony within 3–5 days at 30°C | White to cream colony |

**Form 8.2.** Media Quality Control Worksheet

Medium or reagent _____
QC fungi _____ (positive) _____ (negative)

| Lot No. | Appearance[a] | Performance | | Sterility at 30° and 37°C | | Corrective action or comments | Date and technologist |
|---|---|---|---|---|---|---|---|
| | | Satisfactory | Unsatisfactory | 1, 2, 4 days | 1, 2, 4 days | | |
| | | | | | | | |
| | | | | | | | |

[a] Color, clarity, moisture, agar firmness, agar depth, volume, slant, butt.

## A. Equipment File

An equipment file should be maintained for each piece of equipment and should include the following information (Form 8.3).

1. The first section of each file contains
   a. The identification of the particular piece of equipment in terms of the type of unit, the manufacturer's model and serial numbers, hospital or laboratory serial numbers, and the location of the unit.
   b. Terms of any applicable warranty.
   c. The operating procedures for the unit, both those provided by the manufacturer and any abbreviated versions used in the laboratory.
2. The second section is a maintenance section which
   a. Specifies the terms of any applicable service contracts including contract number, effective dates, and how to obtain the necessary service.
   b. Specifies the routine preventive maintenance required for the particular unit.
   c. Is a record of both the preventive and repair work performed on the unit.
3. The third section is a performance monitoring section which
   a. Contains a statement of the performance standards and monitoring required for the unit.
   b. Is a record of routine monitoring and actions necessary to ensure that the performance standards are met.

## B. Performance Standards

The performance standards for each piece of equipment are established according to the manufacturer's performance specifications and the acceptable range permitted for the procedures for which the piece of equipment is being used.

1. Freezers, incubators, and refrigerators
   A temperature log sheet should be placed on each piece of equipment and the temperature be recorded the first thing in the morning. A temperature variation of $\pm 1°C$ is acceptable for most pieces of equipment. If $37°C$ is desired, then the incubator should be set at $36°C$.
   The concentration of $CO_2$ in $CO_2$ incubators is recorded; this is determined with a Fyrite $CO_2$ instrument. In general, $CO_2$ incubators are adjusted to contain 5% $CO_2$.

|     Form 8.3.   Equipment File Form     |

1. Unit Identification
   Name of Unit  _____
   Manufacturer:
      Serial No.  _____
      Model No.  _____
   Hospital No.  _____
   Laboratory No.  _____
   Location  _____
2. Warranty Information
   Date of Purchase _____
   Date Received _____
   *Manufacturer's Warranty*
      Warranty No. _____
      Covers:  a. _____  From ____ To ____
               b. _____  From ____ To ____
               c. _____  From ____ To ____
               d. _____  From ____ To ____
               e. _____  From ____ To ____
      For Service _____
      Address _____
      Telephone _____
   *Other Warranties*
      Name _____
      Address _____
      Telephone _____
      Covers:  a. _____  From ____ To ____
               b. _____  From ____ To ____
3. Service Contracts
   Name _____
   Address _____
   Telephone _____
   Covers:  a. _____  From ____ To ____
            b. _____  From ____ To ____
            c. _____  From ____ To ____

   Name _____
   Address _____
   Telephone _____
   Covers:  a. _____  From ____ To ____
            b. _____  From ____ To ____
            c. _____  From ____ To ____
4. Routine Preventive Maintenance
   Frequency               Nature of Maintenance
   _____              _____
   _____              _____
   _____              _____

5. Performance Monitoring
   Frequency               Nature of Monitoring
   _____              _____
   _____              _____
   _____              _____

|  | Daily | Monthly | Quarterly | Semiannually |
|---|---|---|---|---|
| Record temperature | + | | | |
| Record $CO_2$ concentration | + | | | |
| Check pilot lights | + | | | |
| Check door seal | | + | | |
| Defrost, clean, or both | | | + | |
| Recalibrate thermometers or temperature recording devices | | | | + |
| Check if instrument is level | | | | + |

2. Water baths

   Water baths should be filled only with distilled or deionized water. This will prevent the accumulation of salts on the walls of the bath. While in use, a temperature variation of $\pm 1°C$ is usually acceptable.

   |  | Daily | Monthly | Semiannually |
   |---|---|---|---|
   | Record temperature | + | | |
   | Check water level | + | | |
   | Replace water | + | | |
   | Clean the bath | | + | |
   | Recalibrate thermometers | | | + |

3. Biological safety cabinets

   Biological safety cabinets must be monitored carefully because of the potentially dangerous nature of the organisms confined. Whenever the cabinet is being used, nothing should be placed on the grid panels, because this could disrupt the air flow pattern. The air velocity across the opening of the cabinet should be at least 75 linear feet per minute (NSF standard for Class II safety cabinets). The cabinets should be set at 90–100 linear feet per minute across the opening of the cabinet. When the output of a UV lamp is 70% or less of its initial rated output, it should be replaced. The output should be at least 253.7 nm (Form 8.4).

   |  | Daily | Bimonthly | Monthly | Semiannually |
   |---|---|---|---|---|
   | Check air pressure gauge | + | | | |
   | Check air flow pattern in front of cabinet with a smoke stick | + | | | |
   | Disinfect the cabinet with disinfectant | + | | | |
   | Check air velocity across cabinet front | | + | | |
   | Clean UV lamps with alcohol gauze | | + | | |
   | Check UV lamp output | | | + | |
   | Recertify cabinet | | | | + |

**Equipment Control**

| | Daily | | Bimonthly | | | | |
|---|---|---|---|---|---|---|---|
| | Pressure Gauge | Smoke Stick | Clean UV Lights | Air Velocity | UV Light Output | CORRECTIVE ACTION | Initials |
| 1 | | | | | | | |
| 2 | | | | | | | |
| 3 | | | | | | | |
| 4 | | | | | | | |
| 5 | | | | | | | |
| 6 | | | | | | | |
| 7 | | | | | | | |
| 8 | | | | | | | |
| 9 | | | | | | | |
| 10 | | | | | | | |
| 11 | | | | | | | |
| 12 | | | | | | | |
| 13 | | | | | | | |
| 14 | | | | | | | |
| 15 | | | | | | | |
| 16 | | | | | | | |
| 17 | | | | | | | |
| 18 | | | | | | | |
| 19 | | | | | | | |
| 20 | | | | | | | |
| 21 | | | | | | | |
| 22 | | | | | | | |
| 23 | | | | | | | |
| 24 | | | | | | | |
| 25 | | | | | | | |
| 26 | | | | | | | |
| 27 | | | | | | | |
| 28 | | | | | | | |
| 29 | | | | | | | |
| 30 | | | | | | | |
| 31 | | | | | | | |

**Form 8.4. Laminar Flow Safety Cabinet**

Cabinet:_____ Serial No.: _____ Month of _____ , 19__

SPECIFICATIONS:  a. UV light output 253.7 nm ($= 5200\ \mu W\ cm^2$ or greater)
b. Minimum Velocity 90 linear ft/min

4. Autoclaves

   Autoclaves should be checked each Friday with commercially available spore strips according to the manufacturer's instructions. This will permit the incubation of the strips over the weekend with a final status report for each autoclave on the following Monday. Whenever materials are being autoclaved in autoclave bags, the bags should not be tightly tied, because steam may not reach the material to be sterilized.

|  | Each load | Weekly | Monthly | Semiannually |
|---|---|---|---|---|
| Check sterilizing cycle | + | | | |
| Check sensitive indicator tape | + | | | |
| Record temperature and pressure | + | | | |
| Spore strip | | + | | |
| Record peak temperature | | + | | |
| Clean the autoclave | | | + | |
| Check door gasket | | | + | |
| Recalibrate and check temperature and pressure gauges, and timer | | | | + |

5. pH meter

|  | Each use | Daily |
|---|---|---|
| Set temperature compensation if not automatic | + | |
| Standardize against certified buffer | + | |
| Check electrodes | + | |
| Insure that the electrodes are immersed in buffer or distilled water | | + |

6. Analytical balances

|  | Each use | Daily | Quarterly | Annually |
|---|---|---|---|---|
| Use weighing paper or boats | + | | | |
| Clean pan and base of balance | + | + | | |
| Insure balance is level | | + | | |
| Adjust zero point | | + | | |
| Lubricate where necessary | | | + | |
| Calibrate with NBC Class S weights | | | + | |
| Recertify balance | | | | + |

7. Spectrophotometers

|  | Daily | Monthly | Annually |
|---|---|---|---|
| Check drift | + | | |
| Check for shorts | + | | |
| Check photocell | + | | |
| Check calibration of wavelength with nickel sulfate and cobalt ammonium sulfate standards | | + | |
| Check monochromator | | + | |
| Check bypass with standards | | + | |
| Clean cuvette well and excitor lamp | | + | |
| Dust and clean the instrument | | + | |
| Recertify | | | + |

# Equipment Control

8. Microscopes

|  | After use | Daily | Weekly | Annually |
|---|---|---|---|---|
| Clean oil immersion objective with lens paper | + | | | |
| Remove slides | + | | | |
| Cover microscope with dust cover | + | | | |
| Adjust optic system if necessary | | + | | |
| Clean optic system and microscope | | | + | |
| Overhaul microscope | | | | + |

9. Centrifuges

When using a centrifuge, the operator must ensure that the heads are symmetrically loaded, tube caps are sealed correctly, tubes are in safety centrifuge cups, and swinging buckets are symmetrically arranged. The chamber should be checked for cleanliness and accidents after each run. The centrifuge is calibrated with a tachometer or strobe light at least semiannually depending upon how frequently the centrifuge is used.

|  | Quarterly |  | Semiannually | Annually |
|---|---|---|---|---|
| Check with tachometer or strobe | + | or | + | |
| Check timer | + | | | |
| Check brushes, bearings, and internal parts | | | + | |
| Check balance of rotors and trunnions | | | + | |
| Recertify | | | | + |

C. *Monitoring of the Parameters Used in Evaluating Equipment Performance*

Monitoring should be performed according to the procedures listed below.

1. Temperature
    a. All thermometers used to monitor temperature must be calibrated against an NBS standard thermometer. Thermometers used to monitor temperatures above 0°C are calibrated at the temperature at which they will be used.
    b. Thermometers used to monitor temperatures above 0°C must have the sensing section (bulb in mercury thermometers) immersed in

water. In heated air incubators, the thermometer is inserted into a small bottle of water that is sealed with a one-hole rubber stopper. In heating units that operate above 100°C (such as heating blocks), the thermometer should be inserted into a small container of mineral oil that is inserted into the heated area.

c. The peak temperature of steam sterilizers should be measured according to the manufacturer's instructions with a peak temperature thermometer.

d. Constant-temperature incubators not equipped with automatic alarms or with continual recording thermometers should be checked at regular intervals (monthly) with a maximum–minimum registering thermometer for a 24–48 hour period.

e. Calibration of thermometers

(1) Calibration of laboratory thermometers used in the range of 20–40°C are calibrated semiannually against a NBS standard thermometer at the actual temperature at which they are used.

(a) Immerse the standard thermometer and thermometer to be calibrated in a water bath.

(b) Adjust the temperature of the water bath until the standard thermometer reads the exact temperature at which the thermometer to be calibrated is used.

(c) Observe and record the temperature readings of the standard thermometer and the laboratory thermometer. Calculate and record the temperature correction that must be applied to the laboratory thermometer for agreement with the reading of the standard thermometer.

Example: desired temperature of use = 37°C; reading of standard thermometer = 37°C; observed temperature reading of laboratory thermometer = 36°C; temperature correction = 37°C − 36°C = +1°C; corrected temperature reading of laboratory thermometer = 36°C + 1°C.

For calibration of laboratory thermometers used in incubators in the range of 20–40°C, carry out the calibration procedure described above in a water bath adjusted to the exact temperature at which the incubator is operated.

(2) Laboratory thermometers used below 20°C are calibrated semiannually at either 0°C or −78.5°C.

(a) Calibration of thermometers used between +20°C and −40°C. (i) Prepare an ice-water solution in a polystyrene container. The solution is prepared by adding crushed ice to the water and then stirring for several minutes to allow the solution to cool and stabilize. (ii) Immerse the thermometers to be calibrated and the standard thermometer in the ice-water solution and allow all temperature readings to stabilize. (iii) Observe and record the temperature readings. Calculate and record the temperature correction for each thermometer being calibrated as described previously.

(b) Calibration at $-78.5°C$. (i) Prepare an isopropanol–Dry Ice solution in a Dewar flask. Prepare the isopropanol–Dry Ice solution by pouring isopropanol into the Dewar flask to a level of about 2 inches below the top of the flask. Slowly add chunks of Dry Ice. When the gas evolution has slowed, begin to add powdered Dry Ice until the solution becomes viscous. Add enough powdered Dry Ice to form a 2-inch layer on the bottom of the flask. (ii) Immerse the thermometers to be calibrated and the standard thermometer in the isopropanol–Dry Ice solution and allow all temperature readings to stabilize. (iii) Observe and record the temperature readings. (iv) Calculate and record the temperature correction factor for each thermometer being calibrated as described previously.

2. $CO_2$ level
   a. A Fyrite $CO_2$ instrument is used to monitor $CO_2$ content.
   b. The instrument is operated according to the manufacturer's instructions.
   c. The test sample should be drawn from a sampling port. When the doors of the incubator are opened to draw the sample, the readings will be invalid.
3. Air flow
   a. Air flow velocity is measured with an air flow meter (thermoanemometer) according to the manufacturer's instructions. The velocity across the front of a laminar flow safety cabinet should never be less than 75 linear ft/minute with a variation of 1 ft/minute from the average face velocity. The recommended velocity is 90–100 linear ft/minute. These are NSF recommended values for Class II safety cabinets.
   b. Air flow patterns are measured with a smoke stick according to the manufacturer's instructions.
4. UV lamp output
   a. The output of UV lamps is always measured after the bulbs have been cleaned with 70% ethanol and allowed to warm up for 5 minutes.

b. The output of the lamp is measured with a UV meter (photoelectric UV intensity meter) according to the manufacturer's instructions. It should be 253.7 nm with a UV irradiation intensity of at least 40 microwatts/cm$^2$ on the work surface.
   c. The UV lamp output meter should be recalibrated once a year.
5. Analytical balance calibration
   a. A set of certified weights must be used to calibrate the analytical balances.
   b. These weights are stored in a cool dry place away from any corrosive fumes.
   c. The weights should never be handled with bare hands. Use either tongs or gloves when handling the weights.
6. Sterility
   a. Sterility checks of sterilizing equipment should be performed with spore strips according to the manufacturer's instructions.
7. Centrifuge speed
   a. Centrifuge speeds are calibrated with a tachometer or a stroboscope according to the manufacturer's instructions.

## PROFICIENCY EVALUATIONS

The proficiency of the laboratory can be monitored by subscribing to any of several proficiency testing programs. These programs in many instances do not accomplish this objective. On numerous occasions, fungi, which should not be sent, are distributed. Many laboratories select only their best people to work on the unknowns because of the pressure to score 100%. Thus, proficiency testing programs become a game between the subscribing laboratory and the testing organization.

Internal unknowns prepared by the supervisory staff are more effective in determining the level of proficiency of each individual and the mycology laboratory overall. These unknowns should be "sneaked in" as "real" clinical specimens or referred cultures for identification assistance. It is important to determine proficiency levels under normal routine conditions. An internal program has the major advantage that each step can be monitored and discussed with the individual working on the unknown. This means that corrections can be made when an error is made.

*Selected References*

1. Blazevic, D. J., C. T. Hall, and M. E. Wilson (1976). Practical quality control procedures

## Selected References

for the clinical microbiology laboratory. Cumitech 3, American Society for Microbiology, Washington, D.C.
2. Center for Disease Control (1977). "Laboratory Safety at the Center for Disease Control," DHEW Publ. No. CDC 77-8118. Center for Disease Control, Atlanta, Georgia.
3. Ellis, R. J. (1974). "Manual of Quality Control Procedures for Microbiological Laboratories." Center for Disease Control, Atlanta, Georgia.
4. Hamlin, W. B., J. K. Duckworth, P. R. Gilmer, and M. V. Stevens (1974). "Laboratory Instrument Maintenance and Function Verification." College of American Pathologists, Chicago, Illinois.

*Chapter 9*

# Synopsis of the Mycoses

## ASPERGILLOSIS

A.  Synonyms
    None

B.  Definition
    Aspergillosis is a spectrum of diseases caused by members of the genus *Aspergillus*. The clinical manifestation and severity of the disease depends upon the physiologic state of the patient and the species of *Aspergillus* involved. Lowered host resistance due to such factors as underlying debilitating disease, chemotherapy, disruption of normal flora, and an inflammatory response due to the use of antimicrobial agents and steroids can predispose the patient to colonization, invasive disease, or both. *Aspergillus* spp. are frequently secondary opportunistic pathogens in patients with bronchiectasis, carcinoma, other mycoses, sarcoid, and tuberculosis.

C.  Forms of the disease
    1.  Colonization
    2.  Infection
    3.  Allergy
    4.  Toxicoses

D.  Prognosis and therapy
    Prognosis depends upon the type and severity of disease as well as the physiological status of the patient. Allergic aspergillosis typically becomes chronic, whereas colonization may remain chronic or become invasive. Allergic aspergillosis has been successfully treated with prednisone, disodium chromoglycate, and inhalation of nystatin. The prolonged use of steroids in cases of chronic aspergillosis should be approached with caution. Aspergillomas may be treated by

surgical resection and amphotericin B. The aspergilli are not extremely sensitive to amphotericin B, but may be more responsive to 5-fluorocytosine. Systemic and meningitic forms are generally fatal, regardless of therapy.

E. Histopathology

The tissue reaction in aspergillosis is acute suppurative inflammation with areas of ischemic necrosis. The fungus proliferates as septate hyphae 2.5–4.5 μm in diameter (Fig. 9.1). The hyphae can be characterized as branching dichotomously (approximately 45° angle) with the overall appearance of an army on the march. The hyphae may branch irregularly and appear similar to hyphae found in zygomycosis. Blood vessel invasion, thrombosis, infarction, and dissemination are extremely frequent.

F. Laboratory
1. Direct examination

    Clinical material, such as fluids, sputa, or tissue, is mounted in 10% KOH. Long, branching, hyaline, septate hyphae approximately 3.0 μm in diameter typify aspergillosis. The demonstra-

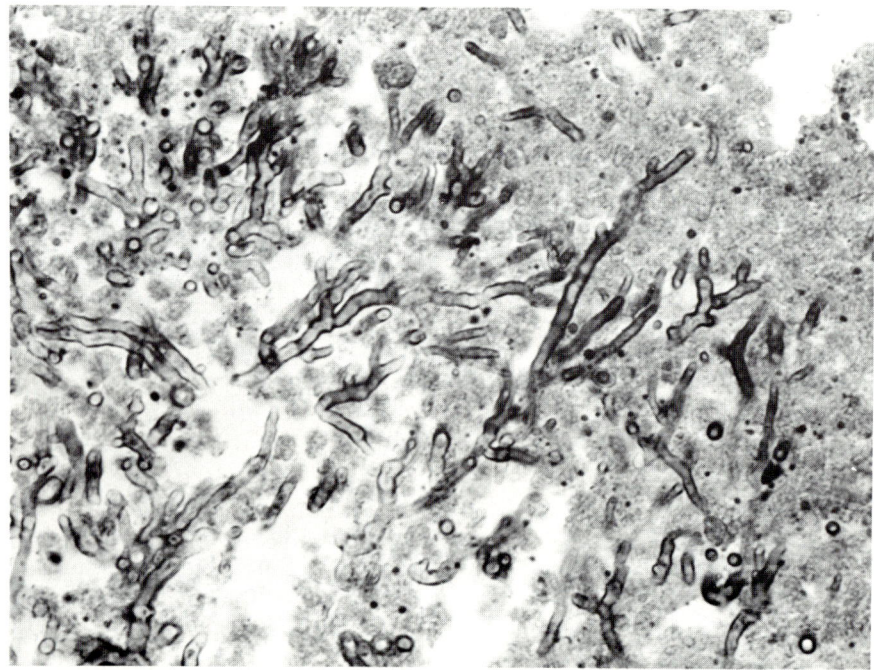

Fig. 9.1 *Aspergillus fumigatus.* The septate hyphae are branching dichotomously, lung tissue, GMS, 400 ×.

tion of hyphae in the clinical specimen and the repeated recovery of the same species of *Aspergillus* in culture is critical in supporting the diagnosis of aspergillosis. It must always be remembered that a number of other fungi can be morphologically identical to *Aspergillus* in tissue. On rare occasions, the hyphae of an *Aspergillus* sp. may have lateral conidia in tissue.
2. Isolation
Inoculate the clinical material onto Sabouraud dextrose agar and incubate at 30°C. The aspergilli are sensitive to cycloheximide, hence they will not grow on media containing this antimicrobial agent. Discard negative cultures after 4 weeks.
G. Mycology (principal fungi)
  1. *Aspergillus flavus*
  2. *Aspergillus fumigatus*
  3. *Aspergillus glaucus* group
  4. *Aspergillus nidulans*
  5. *Aspergillus niger*
  6. *Aspergillus terreus* group
H. Natural habitat
Plant material, soil, ubiquitous

## BLASTOMYCOSIS

A. Synonyms
Chicago disease, Gilchrist's disease, North American Blastomycosis
B. Definition
Blastomycosis may be a benign and self-limiting infection or a chronic granulomatous and suppurative mycosis in which the primary infection is initiated in the lungs with frequent, subsequent dissemination to other body sites, especially the skin and bone. The disease is most prevalent in males 40–60 years of age and in children. Blastomycosis may coexist with bronchogenic carcinoma, histoplasmosis, severe pulmonary disease, or tuberculosis.
C. Forms of the disease
  1. Chronic cutaneous and osseous
  2. Primary pulmonary
  3. Systemic
D. Prognosis and therapy
Therapy is necessary. Amphotericin B is the drug of choice, and at least 1.5 gm must be given to avoid relapse. Hydroxystilbamidine has been used with success in treating the cutaneous form of the disease, but is of limited value in treating other forms of blastomycosis.

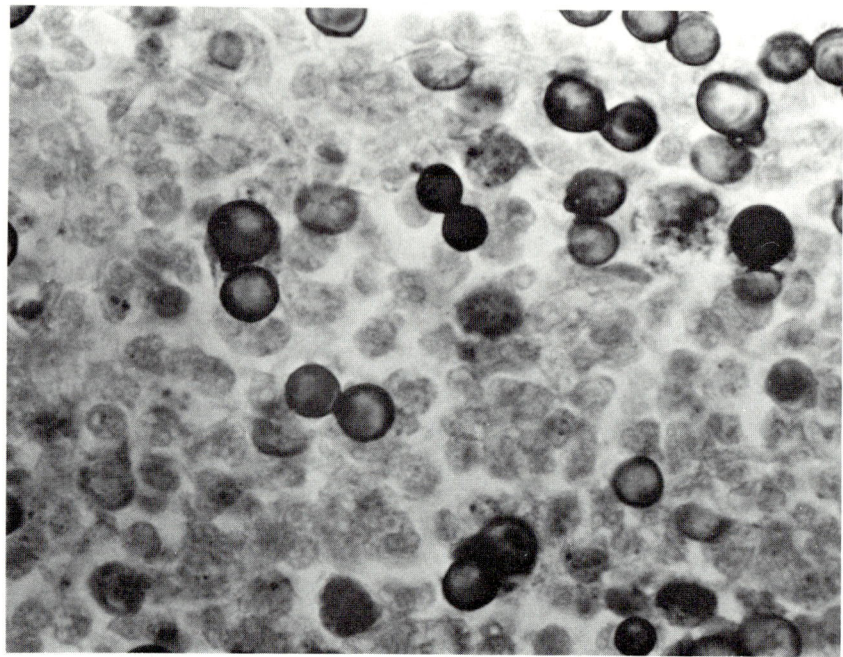

**Fig. 9.2** *Blastomyces dermatitidis.* Note the broad attachment of the blastoconidia to the parent cells of the yeast form of this dimorphic fungus, lung tissue, GMS, 400 ×.

E. Histopathology

The tissue response is a combination of acute suppurative and granulomatous inflammation. These may vary proportionately from one person to another and from one site to another in the same individual. The lung generally has widespread granulomatous inflammation with small areas of abscess formation. Fungi are usually demonstratable at the edge of the abscess. Skin involvement typically shows pseudoepitheliomatous hyperplasia with focal microabscesses in the papillary dermis. The yeast cells are globose to ovoid in shape and approximately 8–15 $\mu$m in diameter. The single blastoconidium is attached by a broad base to the parent cell (Fig. 9.2). In most instances, predominantly single cells without attached blastoconidia are seen. The cell wall of the yeast is thick and appears doubly refractile.

F. Laboratory
  1. Direct examination
     Clinical material, such as fluids, prostate fluid, sputa, or tissue, is examined in 10% KOH (Fig. 9.3). The fungus usually occurs as a

# Blastomycosis

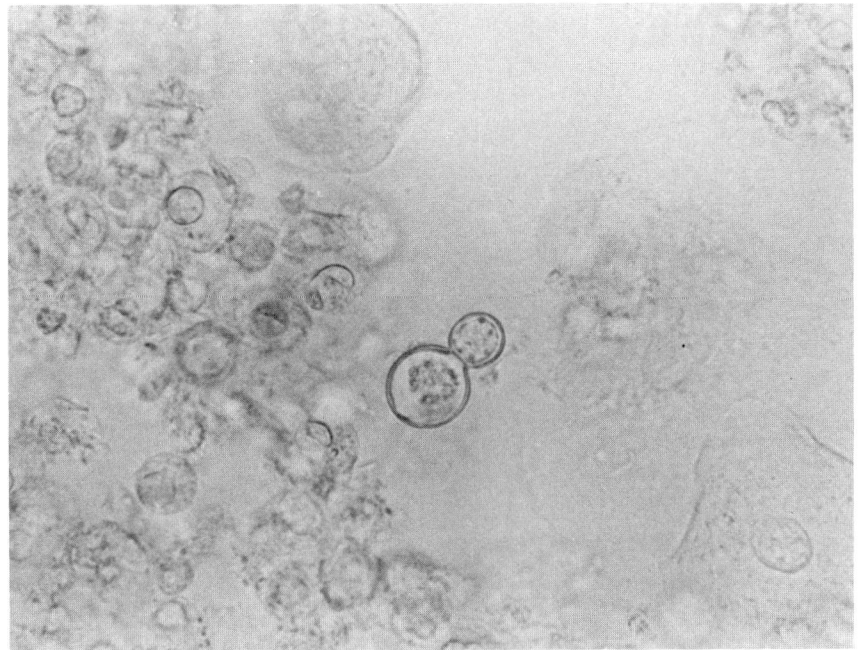

**Fig. 9.3** *Blastomyces dermatitidis*. A yeast cell with a broadly attached blastoconidium can be seen in the center of the field. The cell wall appears thick and refractile, lung tissue, 10% potassium hydroxide, 400 ×.

thick-walled, globose yeast that measures 8–15 μm in diameter. Some yeast cells have been reported to be up to 30 μm in diameter. The fungus may also form yeast cells that are less than 8 μm in diameter. Each blastoconidium is attached to the parent cell by a broad base. Owing to their size, *Blastomyces dermatitidis* could be confused with *Coccidioides immitis* or *Cryptococcus neoformans* under some circumstances.

2. Isolation

   Inoculate the clinical material onto Sabouraud dextrose agar, brain heart infusion agar, yeast extract–phosphate agar, and a medium with cycloheximide, and then incubate at 30°C. The cultures should be kept 4 weeks before discarding as negative. *Blastomyces dermatitidis* grows best on the yeast extract agar.

3. Laboratory confirmation

   The mould form to yeast form conversion is necessary to ensure that the fungus suspected to be *B. dermatitidis* is not a similar fungus, such as a species of *Chrysosporium* or *Sepedonium*. The mould to yeast conversion can be readily accomplished by inoculating Kelley's agar or blood agar supplemented with glutamine and then incubating the inoculated tubes at 37°C. The yeast form will begin to develop within a few days. The entire colony does not have to be converted to the yeast form in order to consider the fungus to be *B. dermatitidis*. An exoantigen technique is available.

G. Mycology
  1. *Blastomyces dermatitidis*
  2. *Ajellomyces dermatitidis* (sexual form)
H. Natural habitat
   Unknown

## CANDIDIASIS

A. Synonyms
   Candidosis, moniliasis, thrush
B. Definition
   Candidiasis is a primary or secondary mycotic infection caused by a member of the genus *Candida*. The clinical manifestations may be acute, subacute, or chronic to episodic. The disease is very difficult to diagnose because members of the genus *Candida* are also commonly recovered from healthy people.
C. Forms of the disease
  1. Allergic
  2. Cutaneous
  3. Mucocutaneous
  4. Systemic
D. Prognosis and therapy
   The prognosis depends almost entirely on the type and severity of the predisposing conditions and the subsequent clinical form of candidiasis. Nystatin is effective in controlling thrush, cutaneous disease, paronychias, chronic esophageal disease, vaginitis, and gastrointestinal infections. Amphotericin B can be used topically and is the drug of choice in treating systemic disease (that is, endocarditis, meningitis, granuloma, chronic mucocutaneous or disseminated disease). Approximately 60% of *Candida albicans* isolates recovered from previously untreated patients are sensitive to 5-fluorocytosine. The drug has been useful in the treatment of systemic disease. Susceptibility testing and monitoring of serum levels for 5-fluorocytosine are mandatory when this antimycotic agent is being utilized.

E. Histopathology

The tissue reaction is initially acute suppurative inflammation followed by granulomatous inflammation. Microabscess formation is fairly common. Blastoconidia and pseudohyphae are both typically seen in tissue sections (Fig. 9.4). These forms are better accentuated by special stains such as in the PAS and GMS techniques for fungi. The blastoconidia are ovoid and usually 3–4 μm in diameter. Under some circumstances, *Candida* species may produce true hyphae either separately or in conjunction with blastoconidia and pseudohyphae.

F. Laboratory
   1. Direct examination
      Ovoid budding yeast cells approximately 3–7 μm in diameter, pseudohyphae, true hyphae, or both are usually seen in clinical specimens mounted in 10% KOH. At times, it can be extremely difficult to differentiate such fungi as *Aspergillus*, *Trichosporon*, and *Geotrichum* sp. from a *Candida* sp. in clinical specimens because they are all able to produce true hyphae.
   2. Isolation
      Inoculate the clinical material onto Sabouraud dextrose agar.

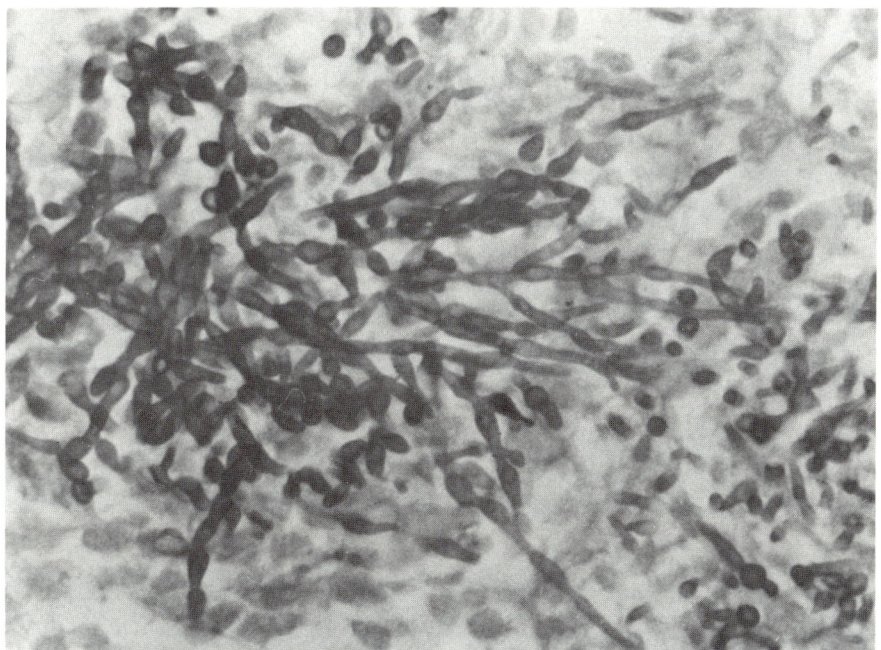

Fig. 9.4  *Candida albicans.* Pseudohyphae and blastoconidia, kidney tissue, PAS, 400 ×.

Many species of *Candida* (that is, *C. krusei, C. parapsilosis*, and *C. tropicalis*—some isolates) are sensitive to cycloheximide. Media with cycloheximide should be used with caution. Incubate the media at 30°C. Growth is usually present within 2–5 days. Blood and spinal fluid should be processed by the filtration technique.
G. Mycology (principal fungi)
   1. *Candida albicans*
   2. *Candida guilliermondii*
   3. *Candida krusei*
   4. *Candida parapsilosis*
   5. *Candida pseudotropicalis*
   6. *Candida stellatoidea*
   7. *Candida tropicalis*
H. Natural habitat
   Man, ubiquitous

## CHROMOBLASTOMYCOSIS

A. Synonyms
   Chromomycosis (in part)
B. Definition
   Chromoblastomycosis is a chronic localized infection of the skin and subcutaneous tissue that follows the traumatic implantation of the etiologic agent. The lesions are verrucoid, ulcerated, and crusted, and may be flat or raised 1–3 cm. Satellite lesions may develop following autoinoculation and by lymphatic spread to adjacent areas. The mycosis usually remains localized with extensive keloid formation. After many years, the lesions may resemble the head of a cauliflower. Some etiologic agents of this disease (*Fonsecaea pedrosoi* and *Phialophora verrucosa*) may disseminate to the brain. Elephantiasis and lymph stasis can occur as a result of secondary infections.
C. Forms of the disease
   1. Verrucous dermatitis
   2. Brain abscess syndrome
   3. Single or multiple cysts
   4. Local or systemic lesions
D. Prognosis and therapy
   The infection usually remains localized, but hematogenous dissemination to the brain may occur with a grave prognosis. Early stages of chromoblastomycosis are treated with surgical excision, electrodesiccation, or cryosurgery. Amphotericin B and 5-fluorocytosine used in combination is the therapy of choice.

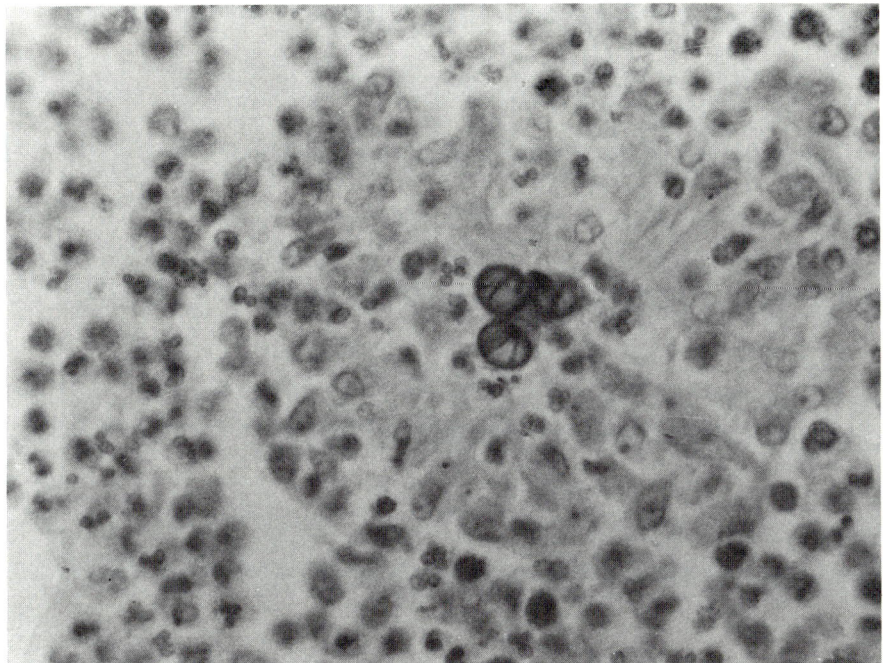

**Fig. 9.5** *Fonsecaea pedrosoi.* The muriform sclerotic bodies are present in a subcutaneous microabscess. The brown color of their cell walls can be seen in this H and E stained section, 400 ×.

E. Histopathology

The skin lesions show a hyperkeratous pseudoepitheliomatous hyperplasia and keratolytic microabscesses in the epidermis. Dematiaceous hyphae and sclerotic bodies are found in the stratum corneum, with essentially only sclerotic bodies in the areas of dermal inflammation. The sclerotic bodies are round, thick-walled, muriform, chestnut brown, and 5–12 μm in diameter (Fig. 9.5). Brain abscesses are typically multilocular and well demarcated with thick walls. Irregular dematiaceous hyphae are in these abscesses.

F. Laboratory
1. Direct examination

Superficial crusts mounted in 10% KOH contain dematiaceous, septate branching hyphae 2–5 μm in diameter. Pus and granulation tissue obtained by curettage, or biopsy specimens of the epidermis and subcutaneous tissues, typically contain dematiaceous round, thick-walled, muriform, sclerotic bodies 5–12 μm in diameter.

2. Isolation
Inoculate the clinical specimens onto Sabouraud dextrose agar and a medium containing cycloheximide. Incubate at 30°C and discard negative cultures in 4 weeks.
G. Mycology (principal fungi)
1. *Cladosporium carrionii*
2. *Fonsecaea compacta*
3. *Fonsecaea pedrosoi*
4. *Phialophora verrucosa*
H. Natural habitat
Soil and woody plant material

## COCCIDIOIDOMYCOSIS

A. Synonyms
San Joaquin Valley fever, Valley fever
B. Definition
Coccidioidomycosis is a respiratory infection that typically resolves rapidly. The mycosis can become acute, chronic, severe, or fatal. The disease may result in a chronic pulmonary condition or disseminate to the meninges, bones, joints, and subcutaneous and cutaneous tissues. The initial tissue response in rapidly disseminating disease is suppuration, whereas chronic and advancing infections are characterized by a granulomatous reaction with some areas being a mixed-type cellular response. It is believed that recovery results in immunity to reinfection. Approximately 60% of patients with primary infections are asymptomatic, 40% have mild to acute pulmonary disease and approximately 0.5% develop serious disease. About 25% of the patients with disseminated disease have meningitis.
C. Forms of the disease
1. Primary
   a. Pulmonary
   b. Cutaneous
2. Secondary
   a. Pulmonary
   b. Disseminated
D. Prognosis and therapy
Primary coccidioidomycosis is treated with bed rest and restricted activity. Steroids may be used to control allergic reactions. Untreated secondary disease has a grave prognosis. The drug of choice is amphotericin B. Meninigitis usually requires intrathecal as well as intravenous administration of amphotericin B. 5-Fluorocytosine has

little value in the treatment of coccidioidomycosis. Some patients treated with miconazole have a high relapse rate.

E. Histopathology

The tissue reaction is acute suppurative and granulomatous inflammation. Acute suppuration is usually present around the arthroconidia and after a spherule ruptures. Granulomatous inflammation usually occurs around developing spherules (Fig. 9.6). Hyphae may be present in pulmonary cavities and meningeal lesions without arthroconidia, which can lead to confusion with the hyphae of an *Aspergillus* sp.

F. Laboratory

1. Direct examination

   Clinical specimens, such as fluids, sputa, and tissue, are examined in 10% KOH. Spherules 30–60 μm in diameter with a thick wall (up to 2 μm) and endospores 2–5 μm in diameter are characteristic of *Coccidioides immitis*. Endospores are released when the wall of the spherule ruptures. Endospores that are no longer in a spherule may remain closely appressed to each other, resulting in a potential confusion with the yeast cells of

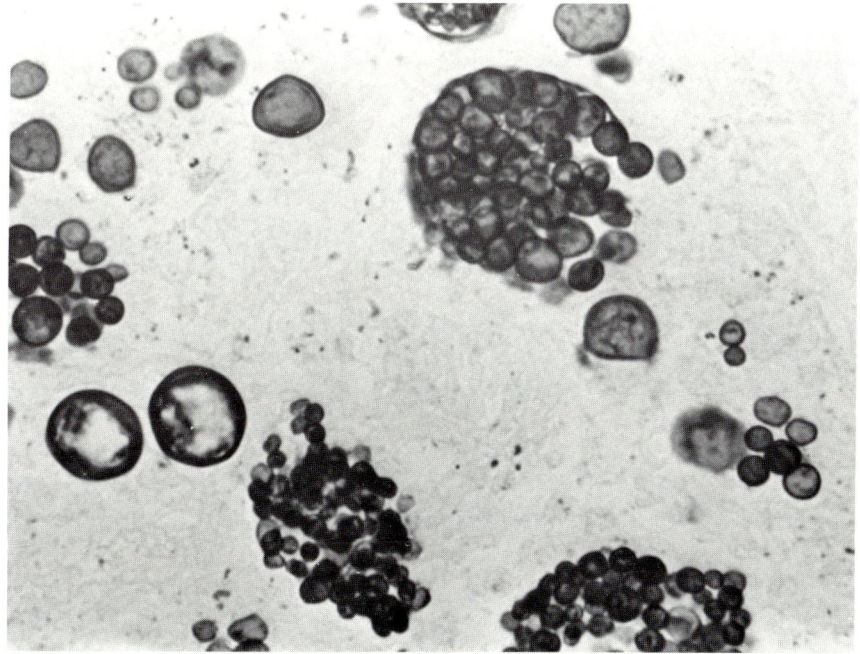

**Fig. 9.6** *Coccidioides immitis.* Several spherules are releasing their endospores. The enlarging cells are young, developing spherules, lung tissue, GMS, 400 ×.

*Blastomyces dermatitidis.* This is especially true if the spherule wall is no longer visible and the clinical specimen has been homogenized.

2. Isolation

   Inoculate the clinical material onto Sabouraud dextrose agar and a medium containing cycloheximide and incubate at 30°C. Cultures should be kept 4 weeks before discarding as negative. The fungus is fast growing and readily produces barrel-shaped arthroconidia 2.5–4 × 3–6 µm with a disjunctor cell between each arthroconidium. *Coccidioides immitis* is a dangerous fungus and should be handled at all times with due respect in a Class II or III biological safety cabinet.

3. Laboratory confirmation

   Confirmation of *C. immitis* is required because other fungi, such as members of the Gymnoascaceae, may develop an anamorph similar to *Coccidioides. In vitro* procedures including special conversion media and an exoantigen procedure are available. Animal studies may be necessary in some instances.

G. Mycology
   1. *Coccidioides immitis*
H. Natural habitat

   Alkaline soil of the Lower Sonoran Life Zone in North, Central, and South America.

## CRYPTOCOCCOSIS

A. Synonyms

   European blastomycosis, torulosis

B. Definition

   Cryptococcosis is a chronic, subacute to acute pulmonary, systemic, or meningitic disease. The primary infection is in the lungs. Following inhalation of the fungus, the primary infection may remain localized or disseminate. On dissemination, the fungus usually shows a predilection for the central nervous system. Primary pulmonary infections have no diagnostic symptoms and usually are asymptomatic. Central nervous system disease is the form most frequently diagnosed.

C. Forms of the disease
   1. Central nervous system
   2. Cutaneous and mucocutaneous
   3. Osseous
   4. Pulmonary
   5. Visceral

D. Prognosis and therapy

Localized pulmonary lesions in noncompromised patients have a good prognosis. They usually heal without treatment. Hematogenous spread to the central nervous system has a grave prognosis unless treated immediately. Systemic infections are usually fatal, especially in debilitated patients, whereas primary cutaneous or mucocutaneous lesions typically resolve spontaneously. Chronic disease is usually characterized by alternating intervals of remission and exacerbation, but eventually is fatal. Amphotericin B is the drug of choice. Chronic pulmonary lesions and osteal lesions may be managed by surgical excision. Many strains rapidly develop resistance to 5-fluorocytosine during chemotherapy, hence susceptibility testing is required. 5-Fluorocytosine and amphotericin B are used concurrently in the treatment of meningitis.

E. Histopathology

The tissue reaction is initially a myxoid degeneration with the area of inflammation assuming a gelatinous appearance. Large numbers of round yeast cells are found in the mucoid matrix. As the lesion progresses, a granulomatous reaction ensues. Organisms decrease

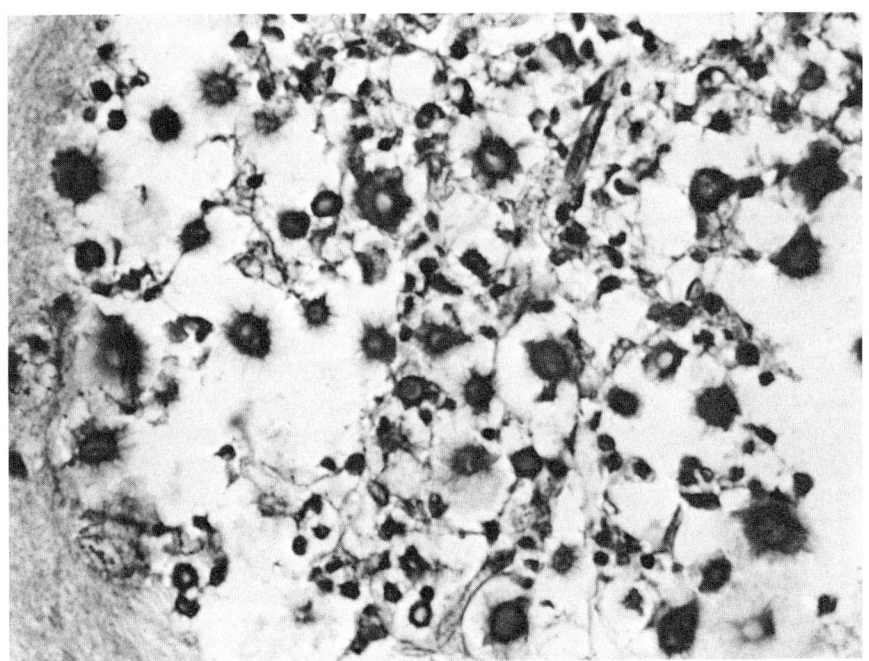

**Fig. 9.7** *Cryptococcus neoformans.* The capsules appear as sun bursts around the yeast cells, brain tissue, mucicarmine stain, 1000 ×.

numerically and are usually found in giant cells and histiocytes. In old healed granulomata, the yeasts are usually dead with disintegrated capsules. They may be difficult to see in H & E stained slides. The yeasts are round, typically encapsulated, and 5–15 μm in diameter (Fig. 9.7). The blastoconidia are attached by a narrow neck. The capsules stain pink by the mucicarmine technique.

F. Laboratory
1. Direct examination
Globose yeast cells are easily seen in most clinical materials, such as cerebrospinal fluid and pulmonary tissue mounted in 10% KOH or India ink. A capsule may or may not be present.
2. Isolation
Inoculate aspirates and tissue (processed in tissue homogenizer) onto Sabouraud dextrose agar and incubate at 30°C. *Cryptococcus neoformans* is sensitive to cycloheximide. Growth is usually present in 2–5 days. Spinal fluid should be processed by the filtration technique.

G. Mycology
1. *Cryptococcus neoformans*
2. *Filobasidiella neoformans* (sexual form)

H. Natural habitat
Fruit, pigeon manure, plants

## EYE INFECTIONS

A. Mycotic keratitis
1. Definition
Following trauma to the cornea by plant material, soil, or surgery, mycotic ulcers develop with an associated severe inflammatory reaction, vascularization, ciliary flush, flare of the anterior chamber, and folding of Descemet's membrane. The initial tissue reaction may be minimal if corticosteroid therapy is being utilized. The ulcer is characterized by a raised epithelium with a white shaggy border. There is frequently a radiating margin from the ulcer which contains hyphae. A sterile hypopyon will eventually develop.
2. Prognosis and therapy
Nystatin has limited value and amphotericin B irritates the infected tissue. Pimaricin appears to be the drug of choice. 5-Fluorocytosine should be considered when yeasts are involved (susceptibility testing will be necessary). Following the resolution of the infection, surgery may be necessary, depending upon the degree of damage to the eye.

3. Histopathology

   The lesions typically advance into the deep stroma of the cornea and contain hyphae that are 3–4 μm in diameter with some swollen cells (Fig. 9.8). The fungus usually develops throughout the entire depth of the cornea. It is not uncommon for hyphae to be only in the middle and deeper layers. Early in the disease, there is an acute suppurative inflammatory process accompanied by coagulative necrosis. Hyphae are typically aligned parallel to the lamellae of the cornea.

4. Laboratory

   a. Direct examination

   The diagnosis of mycotic keratitis must include the demonstration of the fungus in corneal scrapings and the recovery of a compatible fungus. Clinical material can be mounted in 10% KOH or stained by the Gram, PAS, GMS, or Giemsa techniques. Fungi are usually deep within the corneal structure, not on the surface. Extensive debridement may b necessary to obtain satisfactory clinical material. Swabs ar unsatisfactory.

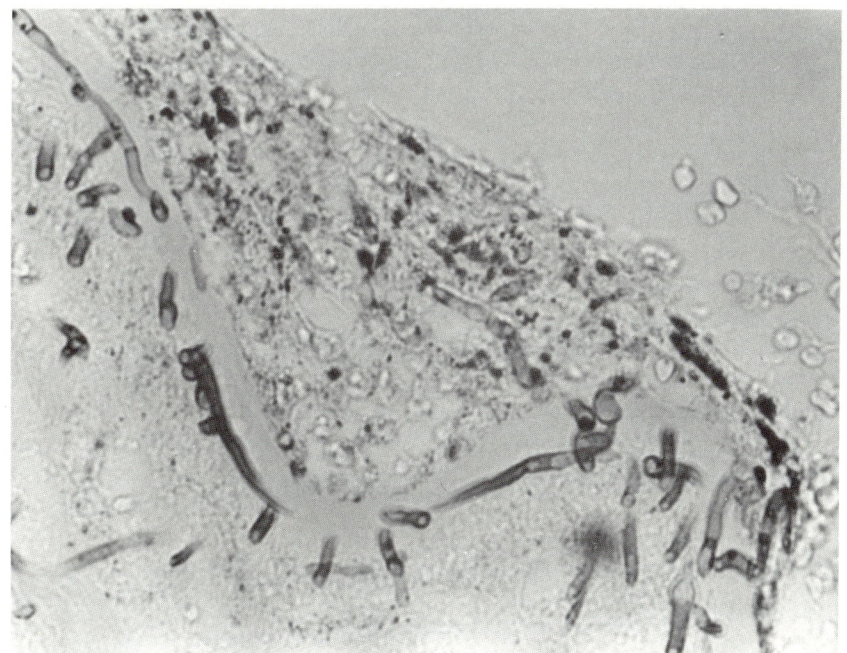

**Fig. 9.8** *Petriellidium boydii.* The hyphae are laying parallel to the eye tissue in this cross section of an eye, GMS, 400 ×.

b. Isolation
     Inoculate the specimens onto Sabouraud dextrose agar and incubate at 30°C. Cycloheximide may inhibit the growth of many of the etiologic agents of mycotic keratitis. A medium containing cycloheximide, if used, cannot be used alone.
  5. Mycology (principal fungi)
     a. *Acremonium* sp.
     b. *Aspergillus flavus*
     c. *Aspergillus fumigatus*
     d. *Aspergillus niger*
     e. *Candida albicans*
     f. *Fusarium oxysporum*
     g. *Fusarium solani*
B. Endogenous oculomycosis
  1. Definition
     This form of eye infection results from fungal dissemination from another body site. Eye involvement is typically a terminal event following widespread dissemination. The mycosis may involve the orbit, retina, optic nerve, sclera, conjunctiva, and adjacent tissue. The diseases in order of frequency are: candidiasis, cryptococcosis, coccidioidomycosis, blastomycosis, sporotrichosis, paracoccidioidomycosis, and histoplasmosis. The most common organism is *Candida albicans*.
  2. Prognosis and therapy
     Amphotericin B, 5-fluorocytosine, or both are typically considered.
C. Extension oculomycosis
  1. Definition
     Extension oculomycosis represents a special form of rhinocerebral zygomycosis in the diabetic patient. The infection starts in the upper portion of the nasal septum and extends into the orbit of the eye, frontal sinuses, major cerebral vessels, and subsequently the central nervous system. *Rhizopus oryzae* and *R. arrhizus* are most commonly involved. Symptoms include orbital pain, ophthalomoplegia, ptosis, localized anesthesia, proptosis, limitation of movement, fixation of pupil and loss of vision.
  2. Prognosis and therapy
     Control of diabetes is the most important factor. Systemic, local amphotericin B, or both and surgery are typically required.
  3. Laboratory
     a. Direct examination
        Clinical material, especially from the tissue surrounding the eye if the eye is not enucleated, is mounted in 10% KOH and

then examined for sparsely septate, irregularly branching hyphae that are 6–15 μm in diameter.
   b. Isolation
      Techniques for Zygomycetes
4. Mycology
   Same as zygomycosis
5. Natural habitat
   Ubiquitous

# HAIR, NAIL, AND SKIN

A. Onychomycosis
   1. Synonyms
      None
   2. Definition
      An infection of the nail caused by a mould (Fig. 9.9) or yeast.
   3. Mycology (principal fungi)
      a. *Acremonium* sp.

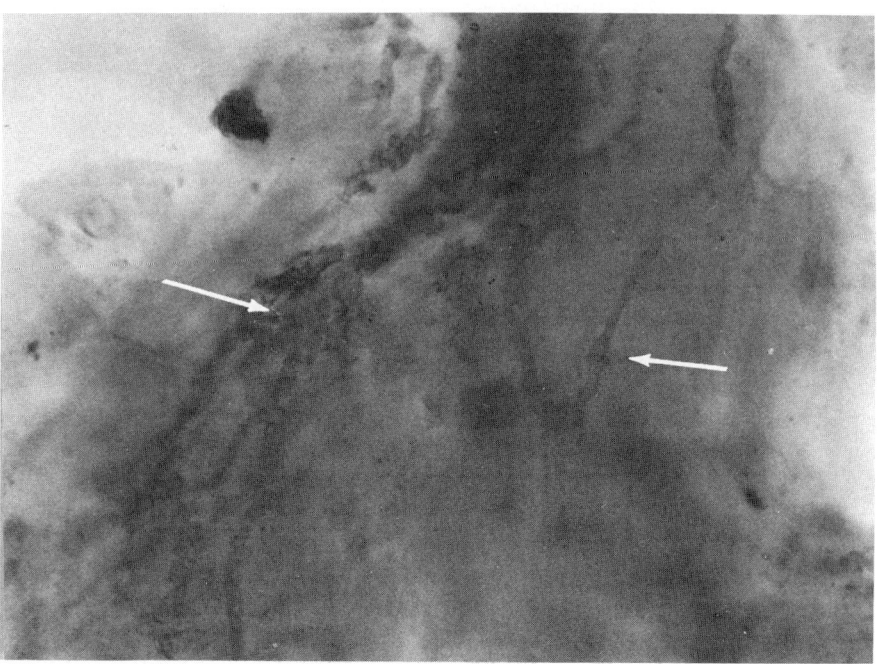

Fig. 9.9 *Scopulariopsis brevicaulis.* The hyphae in the nail tissue are barely visible (arrows), PAS, 400 ×.

b. *Aspergillus* sp.
c. *Aspergillus fumigatus*
d. *Candida albicans*
e. *Fusarium oxysporum*
f. *Scopulariopsis brevicaulis*
4. Natural habitat
   Ubiquitous
B. Piedra
  1. Synonyms
     None
  2. Definition
     Piedra is an infection of the hair shaft characterized by the presence of firm irregular nodules (Fig. 9.10). The nodules are composed of fungal elements cemented together along the hair shaft. Multiple infections of the same strand are common.
  3. Mycology
     a. Black piedra: *Piedraia hortae*

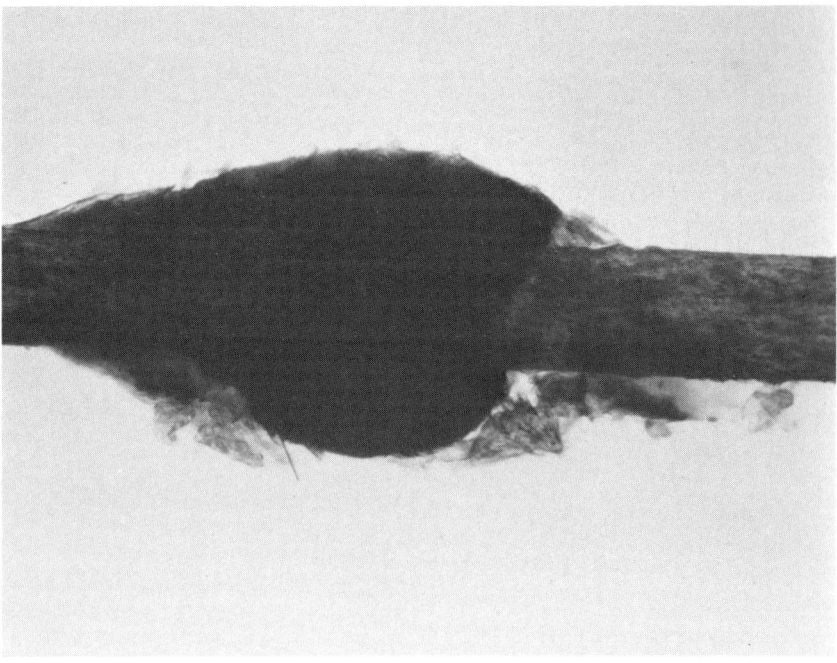

A

**Fig. 9.10** Piedra. A. An ascostroma of *Piedraia hortae* is forming a black nodule around the hair. B. *Trichosporon beigelii* is forming a white nodule that consists of hyphae and arthroconidia (arrow) around the hair, 400 ×.

        b. White piedra: *Trichosporon beigelii*
    4. Natural habitat
       Ubiquitous
C. Pityriasis versicolor
    1. Synonyms
       Tinea alba, tinea versicolor
    2. Definition
       Pityriasis versicolor is a mild to chronic, but usually asymptomatic infection of the stratum corneum. The lesions are characterized by a branny or furfuraceous consistency; they are discrete or concrescent and appear as discolored or depigmented areas of the skin. The affected areas are principally the chest, abdomen, upper limbs, and back. The diagnosis is made on clinical grounds in association with a KOH mount demonstrating the presence of yeast cells in clusters and short hyphal elements (Fig. 9.11).
    3. Mycology
       a. *Malassezia furfur*
       b. This yeast is not usually cultured since it is lipophilic.

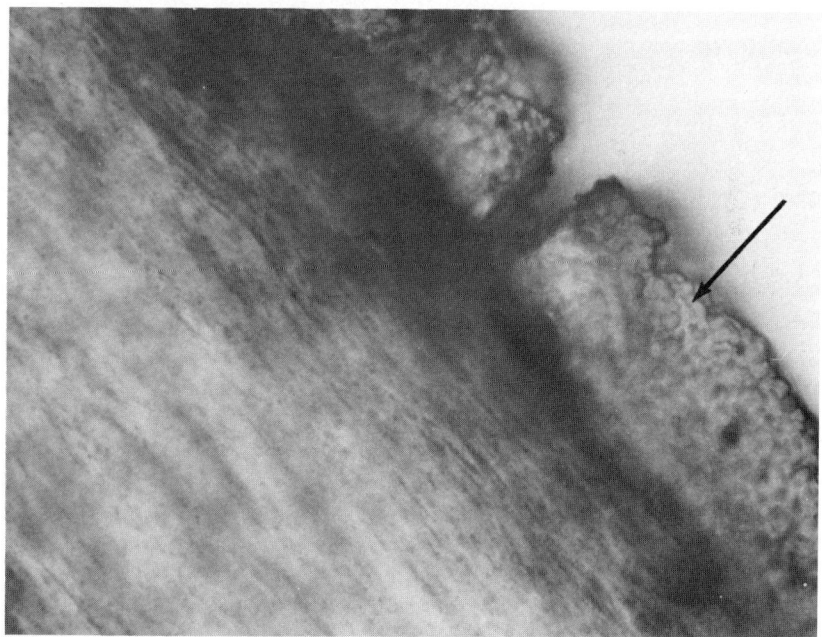

**Fig. 9.10** Continued

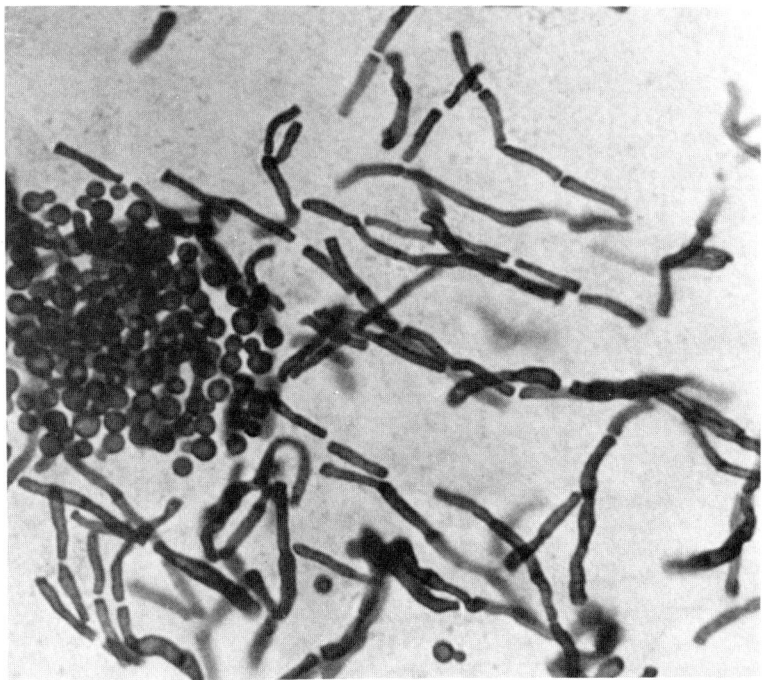

**Fig. 9.11** *Malassezia furfur.* Clusters of bottle-shaped yeast cells and short truncate hyphae are typical of this yeast in the stratum corneum, PAS, 400 ×.

*Malassezia furfur* can be cultured by adding olive oil to the isolation medium.
4. Natural habitat
   Man
D. Tinea barbae
   1. Synonyms
      Ringworm of the beard
   2. Definition
      Tinea barbae is an infection of the bearded areas of the face and neck, hence being restricted to adult males. Lesions are of two types; a mild superficial form that resembles tinea corporis and a form that is a severe, deep, pustular folliculitis.
   3. Mycology (principal dermatophytes)
      a. *Microsporum canis*
      b. *Microsporum gypseum*
      c. *Trichophyton megninii*
      d. *Trichophyton mentagrophytes*

   e. *Trichophyton rubrum*
   f. *Trichophyton schoenleinii*
   g. *Trichophyton verrucosum*
  4. Natural habitat
   Animals, man, soil
 E. Tinea capitis
  1. Synonyms
   Ringworm of the scalp and hair
  2. Definition
   Tinea capitis is an infection of the scalp, eyebrows, and eyelashes caused by species of the genera *Microsporum* and *Trichophyton*. It is characterized by the production of a scaly erythematous lesion and by alopecia that may become severely inflamed with the formation of deep ulcerative kerion eruptions. The latter often results in keloid formation and scarring with permanent alopecia.
  3. Mycology (principal dermatophytes)
   a. *Microsporum audouinii*
   b. *Microsporum canis*
   c. *Microsporum distortum*
   d. *Microsporum gypseum*
   e. *Trichophyton megninii*
   f. *Trichophyton mentagrophytes*
   g. *Trichophyton rubrum*
   h. *Trichophyton schoenleinii*
   i. *Trichophyton tonsurans*
   j. *Trichophyton verrucosum*
  4. Natural habitat
   Animals, man, soil
 F. Tinea corporis
  1. Synonyms
   Ringworm of the body
  2. Definition
   Tinea corporis is an infection of the glabrous skin that is generally restricted to the stratum corneum. The clinical symptoms are mainly due to the host inflammatory response to fungal metabolites acting as toxins and allergens. Lesions vary from simple scaling, scaling with erythema, and vesicles to deep granulomata. Lanugo hair in the involved area may be invaded, the follicle often acting as a reservoir for recrudescence of the disease.
  3. Mycology (principal dermatophytes)
   a. *Epidermophyton floccosum*

  b. *Microsporum audouinii*
  c. *Microsporum canis*
  d. *Microsporum gypseum*
  e. *Trichophyton megninii*
  f. *Trichophyton mentagrophytes*
  g. *Trichophyton rubrum*
  h. *Trichophyton schoenleinii*
  i. *Trichophyton tonsurans*
  j. *Trichophyton verrucosum*
 4. Natural habitat
  Animals, man, soil

G. Tinea cruris
 1. Synonyms
  Jock itch, ringworm of the groin
 2. Definition
  Tinea cruris is an infection of the groin, perineum, and perianal region that is acute or chronic and generally severely pruritic. The lesion is sharply demarcated with a raised erythematous margin and thin dry epidermal scaling.
 3. Mycology (principal dermatophytes)
  a. *Epidermophyton floccosum*
  b. *Microsporum canis*
  c. *Trichophyton mentagrophytes*
  d. *Trichophyton rubrum*
 4. Natural habitat
  Man

H. Tinea favosa
 1. Synonyms
  Favus
 2. Definition
  Tinea favosa is characterized by the occurrence of dense masses of mycelium and epithelial debris forming yellowish cup-shaped crusts called scutula. The scutulum develops at the surface of a hair follicle with the hair shaft in the center of the raised lesion. Removal of these crusts reveals an oozing, moist, red base. After a period of years, atrophy of the skin occurs leaving a cicatricial alopecia and scarring. Scutula may be formed on the scalp or the glabrous skin.
 3. Mycology
  a. *Microsporum gypseum*
  b. *Trichophyton schoenleinii*
 4. Natural habitat
  Man, soil

I. Tinea imbricata
   1. Synonyms
      Tinea circinata
   2. Definition
      Tinea imbricata is a geographically restricted form of tinea corporis caused by *Trichophyton concentricum*. It is characterized by polycyclic, papulosquamous patches of scales scattered over most of the body.
   3. Mycology
      *Trichophyton concentricum*
   4. Natural habitat
      Man
J. Tinea manuum
   1. Synonyms
      None
   2. Definition
      Most dermatophyte infections of the hand, particularly of the dorsal aspect, are similar to tinea corporis. Tinea manuum refers to those infections where the interdigital areas and the palmar surfaces are involved and show characteristic pathologic features similar to tinea pedis.
   3. Mycology (principal dermatophytes)
      a. *Epidermophyton floccosum*
      b. *Microsporum audouinii*
      c. *Microsporum canis*
      d. *Microsporum gypseum*
      e. *Trichophyton megninii*
      f. *Trichophyton mentagrophytes*
      g. *Trichophyton rubrum*
      h. *Trichophyton tonsurans*
      i. *Trichophyton verrucosum*
   4. Natural habitat
      Animals, man, soil
K. Tinea nigra
   1. Synonyms
      Pityriasis nigra, tinea nigra palmaris
   2. Definition
      Tinea nigra is a superficial, asymptomatic fungal infection of the stratum corneum characterized by brown to black nonscaly macules. The palmar surfaces are most often affected, but lesions may occur on the plantar and other surfaces of the skin.
   3. Mycology
      a. *Exophiala werneckii*

            b.  *Stenella araguata*
        4.  Natural habitat
            Plants, soil
    L.  Tinea pedis
        1.  Synonyms
            Athlete's foot, ringworm of the foot
        2.  Definition
            Tinea pedis is an infection of the feet principally involving the toe webs and soles. The lesions are of several types, varying from mild, chronic, and scaling to acute, exfoliative, pustular, and bullous.
        3.  Mycology (principal dermatophytes)
            a.  *Epidermophyton floccosum*
            b.  *Trichophyton mentagrophytes*
            c.  *Trichophyton rubrum*
            d.  *Trichophyton tonsurans*
        4.  Natural habitat
            Man
    M.  Tinea unguium
        1.  Synonyms
            Ringworm of the nail
        2.  Definition
            Tinea unguium is an invasion of the nail plate by a dermatophyte. The disease is of two principal types: (a) leukonychia mycotica (superficial white onychomycosis) in which invasion is restricted to patches or pits on the surface of the nail; and (b) invasive, subungual dermatophytosis (ringworm of the nail) in which the lateral or distal edges of the nail are first involved followed by establishment of the infection beneath the nail plate.
        3.  Mycology (principal dermatophytes)
            a.  *Epidermophyton floccosum*
            b.  *Microsporum audouinii*
            c.  *Microsporum canis*
            d.  *Microsporum gypseum*
            e.  *Trichophyton mentagrophytes*
            f.  *Trichophyton rubrum*
            g.  *Trichophyton schoenleinii*
            h.  *Trichophyton tonsurans*
        4.  Natural habitat
            Animals, man, soil
    N.  Prognosis and therapy
        Most cases of onychomycosis resolve when the conditions causing the abnormal nails are corrected. In chronic infections caused by

**Hair, Nail, and Skin**

filamentous fungi, griseofulvin is usually ineffective. Amphotericin B (topical), gentian violet, resorcin, iodine, nystatin, thiabendazole, and glutaraldehyde have been used with varying degrees of success. Piedra is controlled by shaving or removing the infected hair. With or without therapy, lesions of pityriasis versicolor persist, spread, disappear, reappear, and become chronic. Keratolytic agents (Whitfield's ointment, salicylic acid), mild fungicides (sodium hyposulfite), sulfur-containing ointments, or selium sulfide will control the lesions. Miconazole appears to be helpful. Tinea nigra is controlled with keratolytic agents, iodine, salicylic acid, or sulfur. *Exophiala werneckii* is resistant to griseofulvin. Tinea unguium is most resistant to therapy. Miconazole is the drug of choice. Tinea is controlled primarily with miconazole. Griseofulvin, haloprogin, and sodium tolnaftate are occasionally used.

O. Laboratory
   1. Direct mount
      Skin scrapings (Fig. 9.12), hair (Fig. 9.13) or pulverized nail

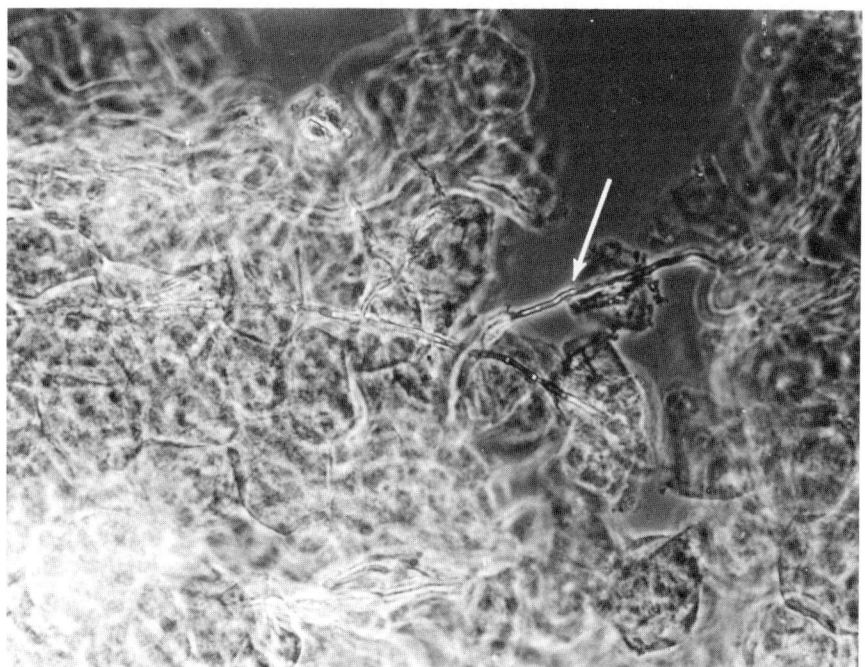

**Fig. 9.12** *Trichophyton mentagrophytes*. The hyphae (arrow) of dermatophytes are often difficult to see in 10% potassium hydroxide preparations of stratum corneum, 430 ×, phase-contrast microscopy.

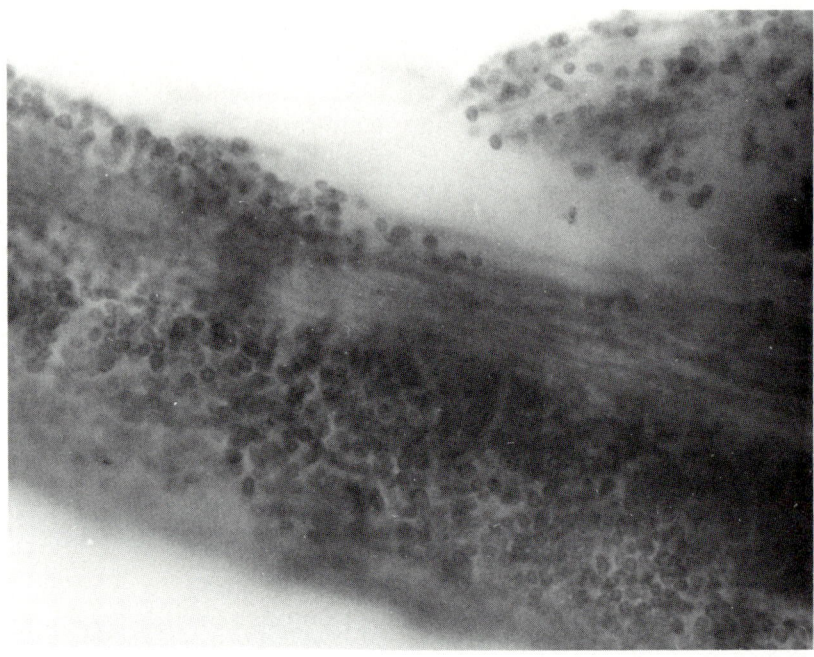

**Fig. 9.13** *Microsporum canis.* Ectothrix hair invasion is characterized by the presence of arthroconidia around the hair. The cuticle of the hair has been destroyed by the fungus, PAS, 400×.

fragments are mounted in 10% KOH. Depending upon the etiologic agent, hyphae, hyphae and arthroconidia, yeasts, yeasts and pseudohyphae, yeasts and hyphae may be seen.

2. Isolation

Inoculate the clinical specimens onto Sabouraud dextrose agar and a medium containing cycloheximide. Incubate at 30°C and discard negative cultures after 2–4 weeks. Dermatophytes and many yeasts are not affected by cycloheximide, whereas opportunistic pathogens, such as species of *Aspergillus* and *Scopulariopsis,* are sensitive to cycloheximide. These fungi will not grow on a medium containing cycloheximide. Dermatophyte test medium (DTM) has little value in isolating these fungi.

## HISTOPLASMOSIS CAPSULATI

A. Synonyms
North American histoplasmosis

B. Definition
Approximately 95% of the cases of histoplasmosis capsulati are inapparent, subclinical, or benign. Five percent of the cases have chronic progressive lung disease, chronic cutaneous or systemic disease, or an acute fulminating fatal systemic disease. All stages of this disease may mimic tuberculosis. Histoplasmosis may coexist with actinomycosis, other mycoses, sarcoidosis, or tuberculosis.

C. Forms of the disease
1. Disseminated
2. Pulmonary

D. Prognosis and therapy
Disseminated, chronic cavitary, mucocutaneous, or systemic disease require therapy. Amphotericin B is the drug of choice and recovery is typically fast with essentially no relapse if adequate drug is given and the patient has no underlying debilitating disease.

E. Histopathology
The histopathological picture in acute disseminated histoplasmosis is different from that seen in the more chronic disease, and in solitary pulmonary nodules ("coin lesion"). In the first entity, *H. capsulatum* is localized in histiocytes and reticuloendothelial cells. The cells enlarge, but with no evidence of inflammation. The intracellular budding yeasts are approximately 3 $\mu$m in diameter (Fig. 9.14), similar to *Leishmania* sp., but do not contain a kinetoplast. In addition, *Leishmania* does not stain with the special stains used for fungi. Older lesions are well-developed granulomata and have a central area of caseation resembling tuberculosis. The solitary pulmonary nodules are well organized and usually have a circumferential rim of calcification accounting for its visibility on chest X-ray. Fungi within these nodules are usually dead. *Histoplasma capsulatum* cells are found in the center of the lesions.

F. Laboratory
1. Direct examination
   The direct detection of fungi in clinical material such as bone marrow, sputum, and tissue is usually difficult. Material stained by the PAS, Giemsa, or GMS methods are superior to KOH preparations.
2. Isolation
   Inoculate the clinical material onto Sabouraud dextrose agar, yeast extract–phosphate agar, a medium containing cycloheximide and Sabhi agar with blood. Incubate cultures at 30°C and do not discard until 12 weeks.
3. Laboratory confirmation

The mould-form-to-yeast-form conversion is necessary to ensure that the fungus is not a species of *Chrysosporium* or *Sepedonium*. Transfer the fungus to a test tube containing brain heart infusion agar with glutamine and incubate at 37°C. As soon as the yeast begins to develop, this is sufficient to consider the fungus *H. capsulatum*. An exoantigen technique is available.

G. Mycology
1. *Histoplasma capsulatum* var. *capsulatum*
2. *Ajellomyces capsulatus* (sexual form)

## HISTOPLASMOSIS DUBOISII

A. Synonyms
   African histoplasmosis
B. Definition

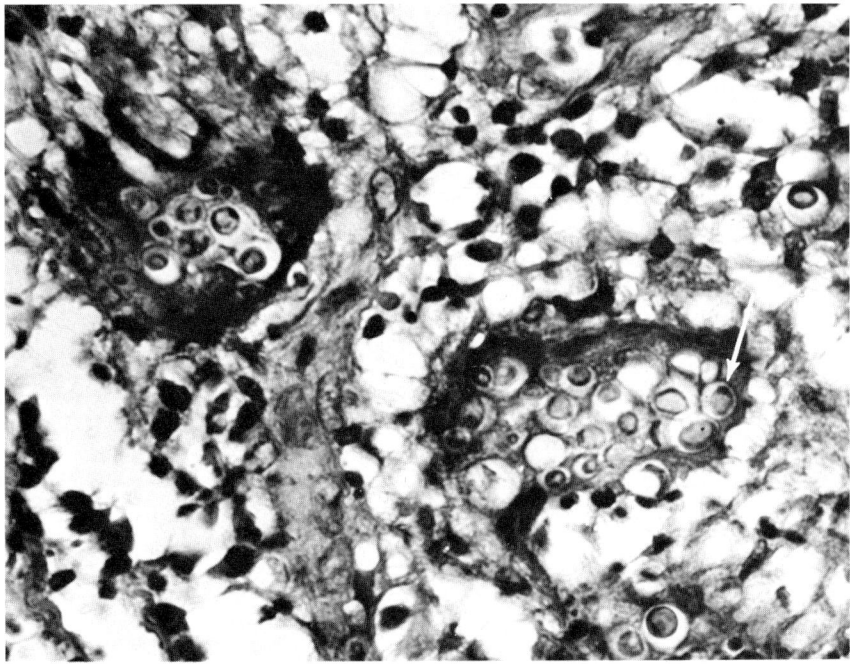

**Fig. 9.14** *Histoplasma capsulatum*. The yeast form of this dimorphic fungus occurs within giant cells. During staining by the H and E procedure, the cytoplasm tends to pull away from the cell wall of the yeasts (arrow), leaving the false impression that the yeast has a capsule, spleen tissue, 1000 ×.

Histoplasmosis duboisii is a mycotic infection primarily involving cutaneous, liver, lung, lymphatic, subcutaneous, and osseous tissues. Skin and bone are the most frequently invaded sites. The etiologic agent grows as a large yeast within the giant cells as well as small cells that are typical of those seen in histoplasmosis capsulati. Nodular and ulcerative cutaneous and osteolytic lesions of bone that disseminate or remain localized are the primary clinical characteristics of histoplasmosis duboisii.
C. Forms of the disease
 1. Disseminated
 2. Localized
D. Prognosis and therapy
 Isolated lesions may heal spontaneously or require surgical management. Disseminated disease has a grave prognosis, especially if the liver and spleen are involved. Amphotericin B is the drug of choice.
E. Histopathology
 Little cellular reaction to the fungi are noted with the exception of large numbers of giant cells (up to 80 μm) and macrophages. Neutrophils are usually present, especially during necrosis. The globose to ovoid, thick-walled yeasts are 7–15 μm (average 10 μm) in diameter and may form rudimentary pseudohyphae consisting of 4 or 5 cells. Large aggregates of yeast cells can be readily seen within giant cells and extracellularly following necrosis of the host tissue. Unlike *Blastomyces dermatitidis*, the blastoconida are not attached to the parent cell by a broad neck.
F. Laboratory
 1. Direct examination
  Clinical specimens such as tissue are examined in 10% KOH. The large yeast cells should be readily visible. Care must be taken to ensure that *B. dermatitidis* is not confused with the etiologic agent of histoplasmosis duboisii since they both occur in Africa.
 2. Isolation
  Inoculate the clinical material onto Sabouraud dextrose agar, yeast extract–phosphate agar, a medium containing cycloheximide, and Sabhi with blood agar. Incubate the cultures at 30°C and discard as negative in 12 weeks.
 3. Laboratory confirmation
  The mould-form-to-yeast-form conversion is required to ensure that the fungus recovered is not a species of *Chrysosporium* or *Sepedonium*. The etiologic agents of histoplasmosis capsulati and histoplasmosis duboisii are morphologically identical at 30°C.

The mould-to-yeast conversion is done on brain heart infusion agar with glutamine incubated at 37°C. Not all cells have to be converted to the yeast form before one may conclude that the fungus is *H. capsulatum*.
G. Mycology
   1. *Histoplasma capsulatum* var. *duboisii*
   2. *Ajellomyces capsulatus* (sexual form)

## LOBOMYCOSIS

A. Synonyms
   Keloidal blastomycosis, Lobo's disease
B. Definition
   Lobomycosis is a chronic cutaneous infection that is localized and manifested as keloids, verrucoid to nodular lesions, crusty plaques, and tumors. The fungus grows as globose cells that are connected to each other by a narrow neck. The cells may form branching chains. Developing lesions are well defined, smooth, painless and easily moved around since they lie free over the deeper tissues. Older lesions typically become verrucoid and ulcerative with satellite lesions resulting from autoinoculation.
C. Clinical forms
   1. Cutaneous
D. Prognosis and therapy
   Lesions are managed by surgical excision. Since frequent relapse occurs, the excision must be wide. Surgery may result in new lesions.
E. Histopathology
   Nodules consist of subepidermal histiocytic granulomas that lie between the overlying skin and subcutaneous tissue. Fibrous tissue is dispersed between large numbers of giant cells and histiocytes. The giant cells are 40–80 $\mu$m in diameter. In older lesions, pyogenic infiltrates, parakeratosis, and acanthosis are present. Pseudoepitheliomatous hyperplasia and intraepidermal abscesses are absent. The fungus occurs as chains of globose cells 7–14 $\mu$m (average 9–10 $\mu$m) in diameter (Fig. 9.15). Each cell is connected to the adjacent cell by a narrow neck. Some yeast cells occur within giant cells and macrophages, but the majority surround these cells.
F. Laboratory
   1. Direct examination
      Clinical material, cutaneous and subcutaneous tissue, is mounted in 10% KOH and examined for the presence of chains of globose cells.

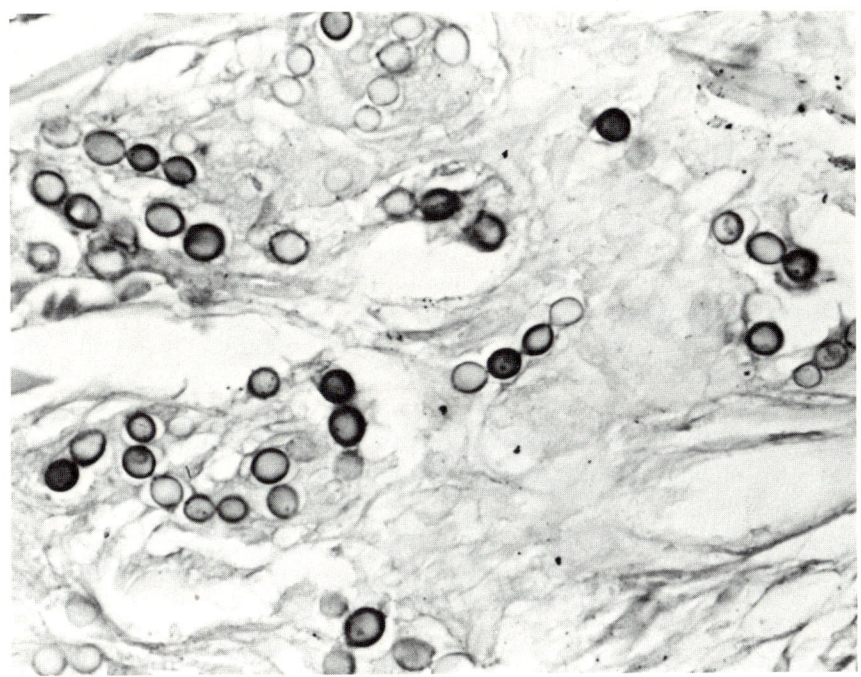

**Fig. 9.15** *Loboa loboi*. The organism forms chains of hyaline cells that are connected to each other by a small neck, subcutaneous tissue, 400 ×.

    2. Isolation
       The fungus has not been cultured.
G. Mycology
    1. *Loboa loboi*
H. Natural habitat
    Unknown

## MYCETOMA

A. Synonyms
    Madura foot, maduromycetoma, maduromycosis
B. Definition
    Mycetoma is a clinical syndrome characterized by tumefaction, draining sinuses, and granules (grains). Mycetomas are localized infections that involve cutaneous and subcutaneous tissue, fascia, and bone. Lesions consist of abscesses, granulomata, and draining sinuses. Following implantation of the etiologic agent, the primary

lesion becomes locally invasive, indolent, tumorlike, or as a small, painless subcutaneous swelling that becomes phlegmonous. The lesions rupture, resulting in sinus tracts, swelling and distortion of the body part infected. Granules are present in pus and in tissue around the draining sinus tracts.
C. Prognosis and therapy
Mycetomas caused by fungi are usually resistant to chemotherapy. Antimycotic drugs have been used with varied degrees of success in conjunction with surgery. Amputation is usually the final action.
D. Histopathology
The ulcer or sinus tract opening is surrounded by raised or flat margins. The abscess is filled with pyogenic materials and granules which are often covered by exudate. The wall of the abscess has granulomatous inflammation, chronic inflammation, and granulation tissue. Granules are present in the tissue (Fig. 9.16).
E. Laboratory
1. Direct examination

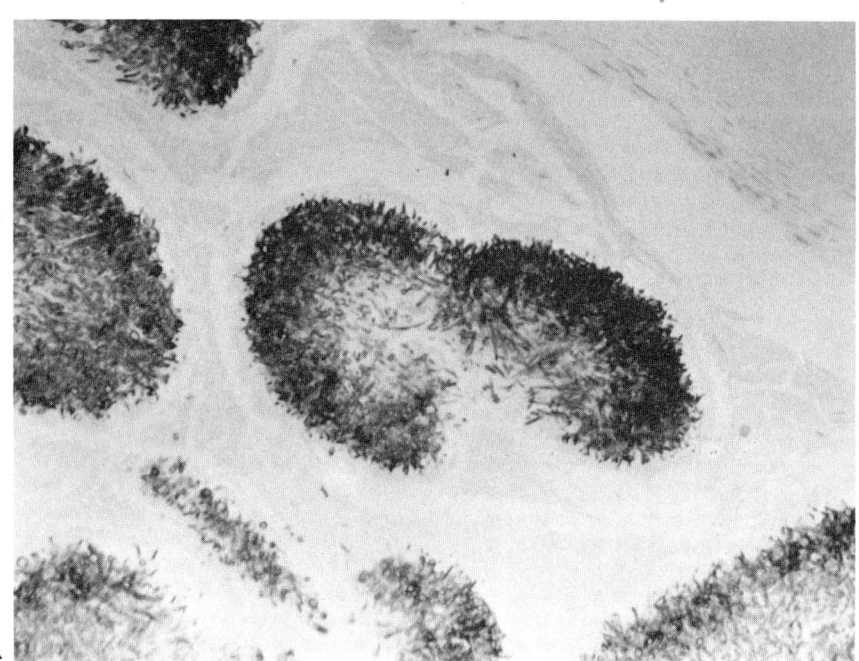

**Fig. 9.16** *Madurella mycetomatis,* subcutaneous tissue, GMS. A. Granules or grains are large fungal structures composed of hyphae, 250 ×. B. The hyphae composing the granule are often swollen and irregular in shape, 400 ×.

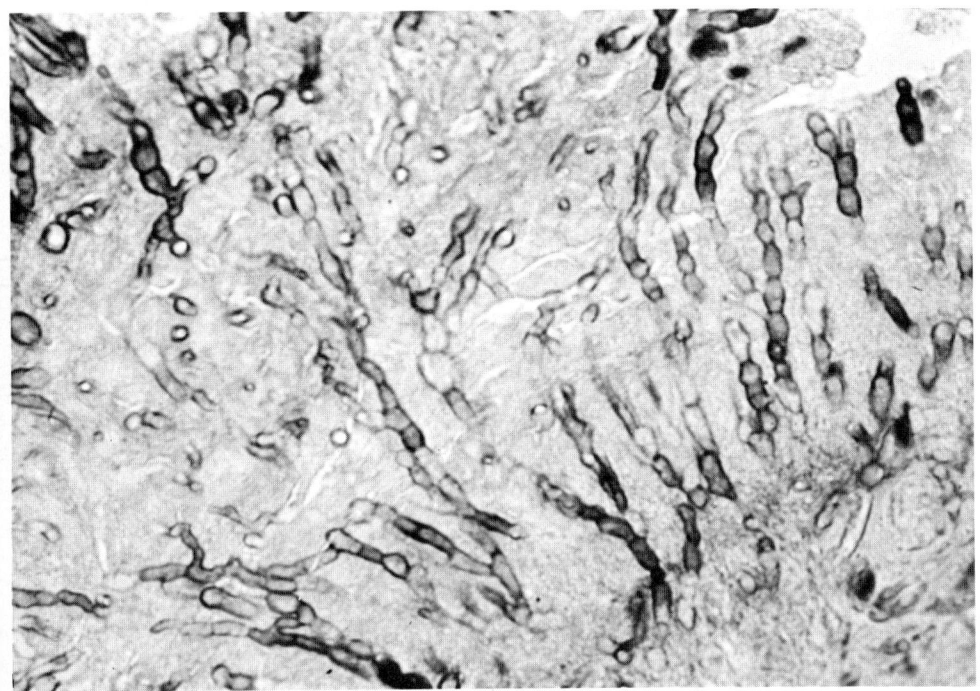

**Fig. 9.16** Continued

Pus, exudate, or tissue should be macroscopically examined for granules. Granules are mounted in sterile saline and then crushed. Actinomycete granules are composed of filaments 0.5–1.0 μm in diameter as well as coccoid and bacillary elements. Fungal hyphae are 2–5 μm in diameter with many intercalary swollen cells.
2. Isolation
Specimens containing fungi are inoculated onto Sabouraud dextrose agar and incubated at 30°C. The granules should be washed in sterile water or in an antibiotic solution prior to inoculation. Some fungi are sensitive to cycloheximide, thus Sabouraud dextrose agar and a medium containing cycloheximide should be used together.
F. Mycology (principal fungi)
  1. Eumycotic mycetoma (granule color)
     a. *Acremonium falciforme* (white)
     b. *Acremonium recifei* (white)
     c. *Aspergillus nidulans* (white)

d. *Exophiala jeanselmei* (black)
e. *Leptosphaeria senegalensis* (black)
f. *Madurella grisea* (black)
g. *Madurella mycetomatis* (black)
h. *Neotestudina rosatii* (white)
i. *Petriellidium boydii* (white to yellow)
j. *Pyrenochaeta romeroi* (black)

G. Natural habitat
Ubiquitous (primarily soil)

## OTOMYCOSIS

A. Synonyms
Fungal ear infection, mycotic otitis externa

B. Definition
Otomycosis is a superficial mycotic infection of the outer ear canal. The infection may be either subacute or acute and is characterized by inflammation, pruritus, scaling, and severe discomfort. The mycosis results in inflammation, superficial epithelium exfoliation, masses of debris containing hyphae, suppuration, and pain. Secondary bacterial infections are common.

C. Prognosis and therapy
Otomycosis is a chronic recurring mycosis. Burrow's solution or 5% aluminum acetate solution should be used to reduce the swelling and remove the debris. An aqueous solution of 0.02–0.1% phenyl mercuric acetate, 1% thymol in metacresyl acetate, or iodochlorohydroxyquin should be considered if drying the ear does not work satisfactorily.

D. Histopathology
Inflammatory response with hyphae in the epithelium and in the exudate

E. Laboratory
1. Direct examination
Epithelial debris placed in 10% KOH should reveal the presence of hyphae and in some instances the fruiting structures of the etiologic agent.
2. Isolation
The clinical material is inoculated onto Sabouraud dextrose agar and incubated at 30°C. Since most of the fungi that cause this infection are sensitive to cycloheximide, a medium with cycloheximide has little value. Additional media containing antibacterial agents may be helpful if there is a heavy bacterial growth in the clinical material.

F. Mycology (principal fungi)
   1. *Aspergillus fumigatus*
   2. *Aspergillus niger*
   3. *Candida albicans*
   4. *Candida tropicalis*
G. Natural habitat
   Ubiquitous

## PARACOCCIDIOIDOMYCOSIS

A. Synonyms
   South American blastomycosis
B. Definition
   Paracoccidioidomycosis is a chronic granulomatous disease that originates as a pulmonary infection. Dissemination occurs resulting in ulcerative granulomata in the nasal, and buccal, occasionally the gastrointestinal mucosa. Lymph nodes are commonly involved. Paracoccidioidomycosis is frequently found associated with other diseases, that is, Chagas' disease, helminth infections, malnutrition, schistosomiasis, or tuberculosis. The infection is commonly seen as lesions on the oropharynx and gingivae. It is less frequently seen in the alimentary tract and anorectal area.
C. Forms of the disease
   1. Disseminated
   2. Mucocutaneous–lymphangitic
   3. Pulmonary
D. Prognosis and therapy
   The prognosis is similar to that for the other systemic mycoses. Amphotericin B is the drug of choice with a course of 1.0 gm. Sulfonamides can be used to treat and control very mild forms of the disease.
E. Histopathology
   Areas of granulomatous inflammation containing focal areas of central caseation mixed with pyogenic abscesses are usually present. Many giant cells are in the granulomata, which contain the organisms. The fungus occurs as a budding yeast with cells 12–14 $\mu$m in diameter. The central cell is surrounded by numerous blastoconidia of various sizes that are attached by narrow necks (Fig. 9.17).
F. Laboratory
   1. Direct examination
      Sputum, biopsy material (base and outer edge of ulcers), crusts or pus (suppurative draining lymph nodes) typically contain the yeast form. Material is mounted in 10% KOH for examination.

510                                                        9  Synopsis of the Mycoses

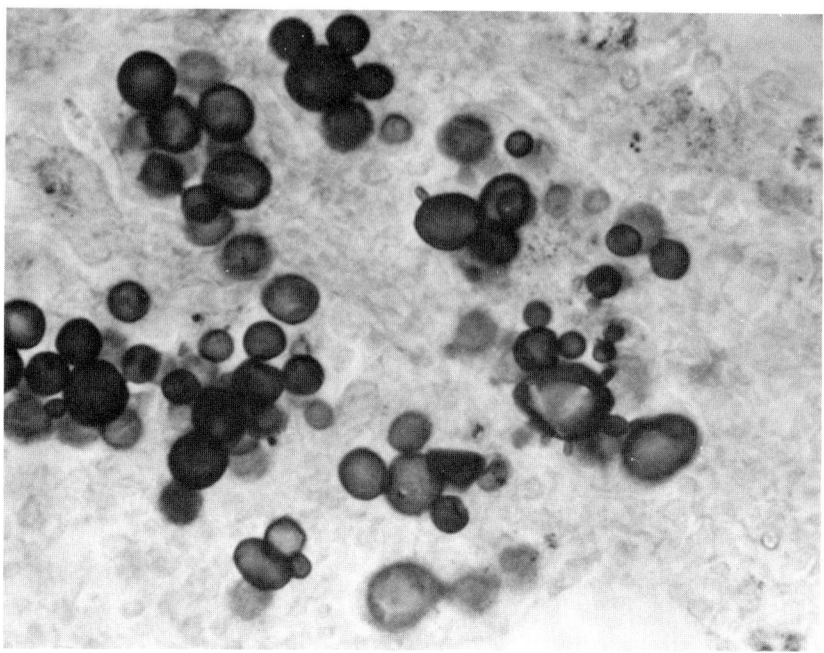

**Fig. 9.17** *Paracoccidioides brasiliensis.* Multiple budding is characteristic of the yeast form of this dimorphic fungus. Many blastoconidia can be seen around each parent cell, oropharynx, GMS, 400 ×.

    The fungus is characterized by multiple budding with globose young cells 2–10 µm in diameter to globose mature cells 30 µm in diameter or greater at the center. Some cells may reach 60 µm in diameter.
  2. Isolation
    Inoculate the clinical material onto Sabouraud dextrose agar and a medium containing cycloheximide. Incubate cultures at 30°C and do not discard as negative until 4 weeks. The colony may require 10 or more days to reach 1 cm in diameter.
  3. Laboratory confirmation
    The mould-form-to-yeast-form conversion is necessary since *Paracoccidioides brasiliensis* is usually sterile. Conidia may be formed which are similar to those produced by the genus *Chrysosporium.* Inoculate the fungus on brain heart infusion agar supplemented with glutamine and incubate at 37°C.
G. Mycology
  1. *Paracoccidioides brasiliensis*
H. Natural habitat
  Soil, wood

# PHAEOHYPHOMYCOSIS

A. Synonyms
   Cerebral chromomycosis, chromoblastomycosis (in part), chromomycosis (in part), cladosporiosis, phaeomycotic cyst, phaeosporotrichosis, subcutaneous mycotic cyst
B. Definition
   Phaeohyphomycosis consists of a group of mycotic infections characterized by the presence of dematiaceous septate hyphae in tissue. The hyphae may be short to elongate, distorted or swollen, regularly shaped, or any combination of the above.
C. Forms of the disease
   1. Abscesses
   2. Localized
D. Prognosis and therapy
   Most cases of phaeohyphomycosis can be controlled by surgical excision and chemotherapy. Amphotericin B and 5-fluorocytosine are the drugs of choice. Miconazole may be helpful in some instances. Invasion of the brain has a grave prognosis.
E. Histopathology
   The histopathology is extremely varied, ranging from tissue reactions associated with walled abscesses to active tissue invasion by hyphae.
F. Laboratory
   1. Direct examination
      Clinical materials such as pus and tissue are mounted in 10% KOH for examination. The dematiaceous nature (Fig. 9.18) of the hyphal elements is a key characteristic for the diagnosis of phaeohyphomycosis. The hyphae may be regular in shape or variable.
   2. Isolation
      The specimens are inoculated onto Sabouraud dextrose agar and a medium containing cycloheximide and then incubated at 30°C. Many of the etiologic agents of phaeohyphomycosis are sensitive to cycloheximide. The cultures are discarded as negative in 4 weeks. The isolated fungus must be compatible with the clinical disease and tissue morphology (that is, dematiaceous) before it can be concluded that it is the etiologic agent involved.
G. Mycology (principal fungi)
   1. *Cladosporium bantianum*
   2. *Curvularia* sp.
   3. *Drechslera* sp.
   4. *Exophiala jeanselmei*

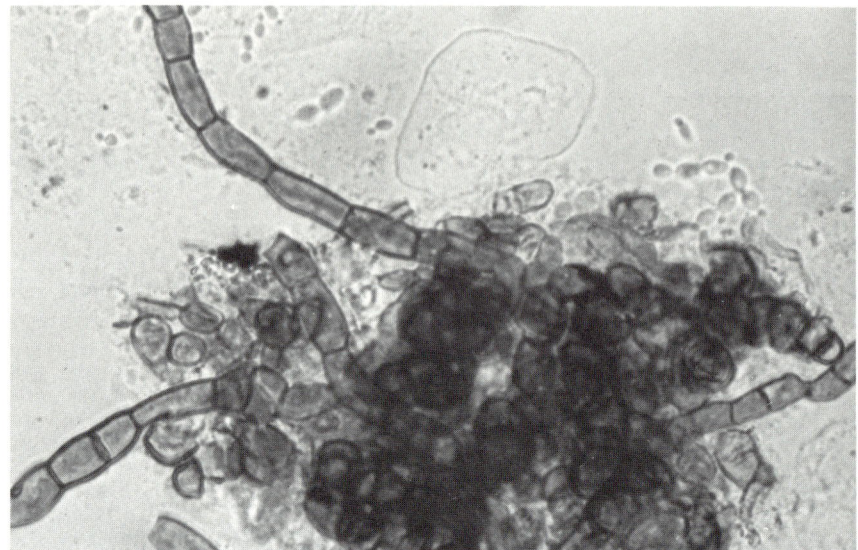

**Fig. 9.18** Dematiaceous hyphae in sputum, 10% potassium hydroxide, 400 ×.

H. Natural Habitat
   Ubiquitous

## RHINOSPORIDIOSIS

A. Synonyms
   None
B. Definition
   Rhinosporidiosis is a mycotic infection of the mucous membranes characterized by the development of polyps. The symptoms vary depending upon the stage of tumor development and site infected. The polyps are usually pink to purple and friable.
C. Forms of the disease
   1. Cutaneous
   2. Dissemination (rare)
   3. Nasal
   4. Ocular
D. Prognosis and therapy
   The polyps are chronic but not painful. Surgical removal of polyps by hot or cold snare techniques are utilized in order to minimize recurrence. Local injection of amphotericin B may be helpful.
E. Histopathology

Large numbers of well defined cysts typically lie just beneath the hyperplastic epithelium. The stroma is dense with chronic inflammation and occasional purulent microabscesses. The spherules reach a size of 300 μm in diameter and contain large numbers of endospores that are 7–9 μm in diameter at maturity (Fig. 9.19). The released endospores incite a polymorphonuclear inflammatory reaction, abscess formation, and some tissue necrosis. Granulation tissue and scarring are usually prominent.

F. Laboratory
  1. Direct examination
     Excised macerated tissue or nasal discharge is mounted in 10% KOH for examination. Spherules and large numbers of free endospores are typically present.
  2. Isolation
     The organism has not been cultured.
G. Mycology
  1. *Rhinosporidium seeberi*
H. Natural habitat
   Unknown

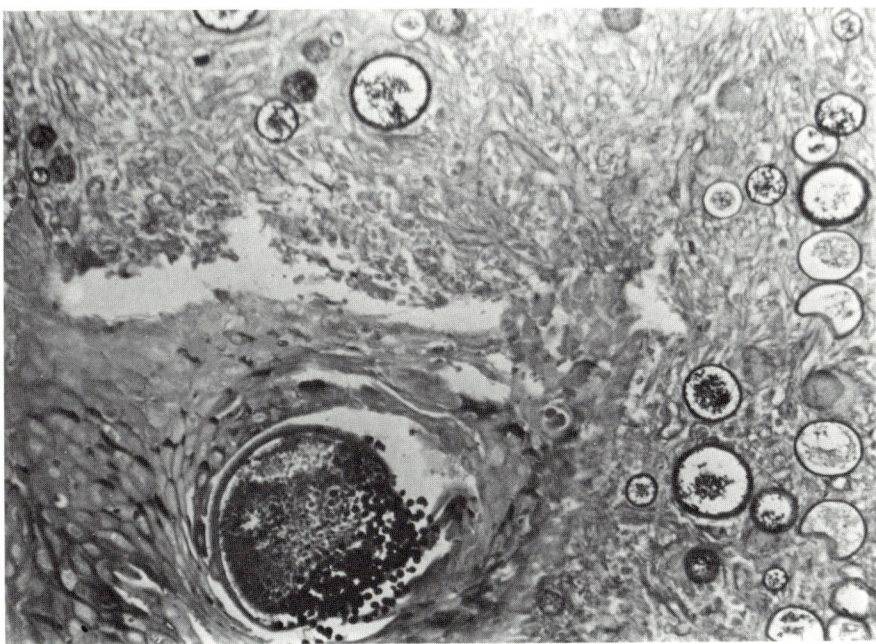

**Fig. 9.19** *Rhinosporidium seeberi.* Extremely large spherules with endospores are characteristic of this organism, nasal polyp, PAS, 250 ×.

## SPOROTRICHOSIS

A. Synonyms
   None
B. Definition
   Sporotrichosis is a chronic infection characterized by nodular lesions of cutaneous or subcutaneous tissues and adjacent lymphatics that suppurate, ulcerate, and drain. Secondary spread to articular surfaces, bone, and muscle may occur. The mycosis may occasionally involve the CNS, lungs, genitourinary system, or all of them. The fungus gains entry via trauma to the skin or by inhalation in the case of pulmonary disease. Symptoms vary depending upon site and method of inoculation.
C. Forms of the disease
   1. Cutaneous
   2. Disseminated
   3. Lymphocutaneous
   4. Pulmonary
D. Prognosis and therapy
   Lymphocutaneous, cutaneous, and mucocutaneous sporotrichosis are chronic infections. Dissemination is rare. Prognosis of disseminated disease is grave as spontaneous cure is unknown. Oral potassium iodide is used in most cases of sporotrichosis. Treatment is continued for at least 4 weeks following clinical cure. Amphotericin B is used to treat relapsed lymphocutaneous disease, pulmonary and disseminated sporotrichosis. Other drugs with varying degrees of success include dihydroxystilbamidine and 5-fluorocytosine. Antibacterial antibiotics are useful when secondary bacterial infections occur.
E. Histopathology
   The pattern of inflammation is characteristically well circumscribed and granulomatous with central areas of acute suppuration. In the skin, this pattern is similar to that seen in blastomycosis and coccidioidomycosis. Demonstration of the organism in tissue is very difficult because the fungi are not numerous. The fungus is yeastlike, subglobose to ovoid, 3–5 $\mu$m in diameter (Fig. 9.20) with multiple blastoconidia. The yeasts are not encapsulated. Asteroid body may be present and consists of a globose to ovoid, basophilic cell, 3–5 $\mu$m in diameter with radiating eosinophilic rays up to 10 $\mu$m in diameter. Asteroid body formation appears to be more common in secondary lesions than in primary ones.
F. Laboratory

# Sporotrichosis

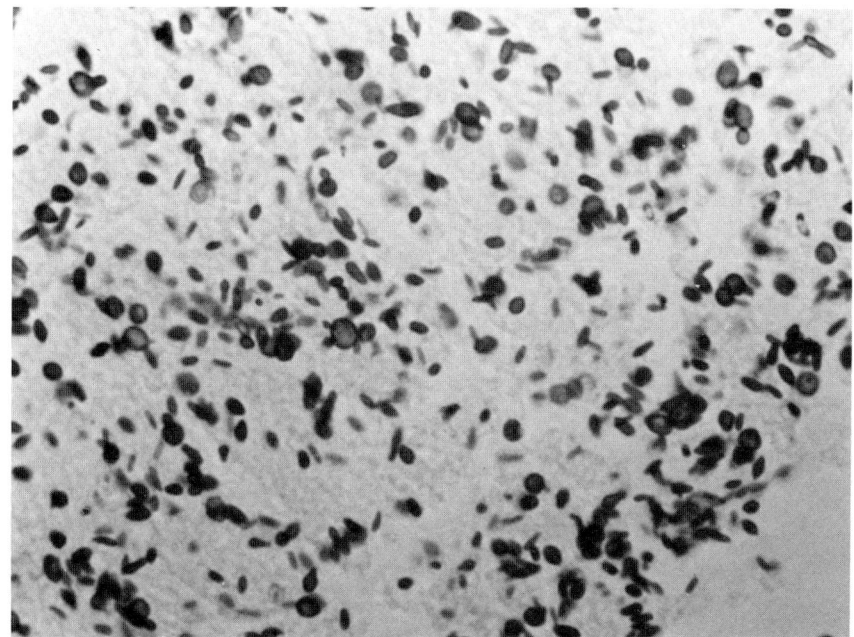

**Fig. 9.20** *Sporothrix schenckii*. The yeast form of this dimorphic fungus is producing blastoconidia in tissue, inoculated mouse, GMS, 400 ×.

1. Direct examination
   Typically unrewarding. Fluorescent antibody staining techniques may be helpful. Diastase digestion prior to staining with H & E or PAS may be helpful.
2. Isolation
   Inoculate the aspirates, material from curettage, or swabbings from open lesions onto Sabouraud dextrose agar and a medium containing cycloheximide. Incubate the media at 30°C. Growth is usually present in 3–5 days.
3. Laboratory confirmation
   The mould-form-to-yeast-form conversion is necessary since other fungi are morphologically similar. Transfer the fungus to brain heart infusion agar and incubate at 37°C in 5–10% $CO_2$.

G. Mycology (principal fungus)
   1. *Sporothrix schenckii*
H. Natural habitat
   Plant material

## ZYGOMYCOSIS

A. Synonyms

Entomophthoromycosis, mucormycosis, phycomycosis, subcutaneous phycomycosis, rhinoentomophthoromycosis, rhinomucormycosis, rhinophycomycosis

1. Zygomycosis caused by *Conidiobolus* sp.
   a. Definition
   
   This infection is a chronic inflammatory or granulomatus disease that is typically restricted to the nasal submucosa and characterized by polyps or palpable restricted subcutaneous masses. Symptoms include nasal swelling beginning in the inferior turbinates, which may extend to the foramina, ostia, paranasal sinuses, submucosa, and sutures. The infections are typically bilateral, but may be unilateral. Masses may be disfiguring, palpable, and anchored to underlying structures. Epidermis may become acanthotic and erythematous. Eyelids may be swollen. X-rays show opaque antrum, obliteration of nasal air spaces, and mucosal thickening. Over 80% of the cases have been in males.
   
   b. Prognosis and treatment
   
   The disease is relatively benign, sometimes clearing spontaneously. Potassium iodide, amphotericin B, or both are the drugs of choice.
   
   c. Histopathology
   
   The hyphae are regularly septate, 4–10 $\mu$m (average 8 $\mu$m) in diameter with an eosinophilic sheath (Splendore–Hoeppli phenomenon) 2–6 $\mu$m in diameter. The eosinophilic material has a fingerlike arrangement similar to that found in sporotrichosis, coccidioidomycosis, blastomycosis, paracoccidioidomycosis, rarely candidiasis and schistosomiasis. Vascular invasion is absent. Cellular reaction may be acute, chronic, or both. Chronic inflammatory reactions are granulomatous with infiltrates containing foreign body giant cells and phagocytized hyphae. The acute reaction consists of eosinophils, lymphocytes, and plasma cells. Eosinophils may result in an eosinophilic abscess.
   
   d. Laboratory: (1) Direct examination. Soft vesicles, scrapings of infected mucosa, or both are mounted in 10% KOH and examined for the presence of broad, septate, doubly refractile hyphae. (2) Isolation. Inoculate the clinical material onto Sabouraud dextrose agar. Do not use a medium containing

cycloheximide, as these fungi are sensitive to this agent. If bacterial contamination is suspected, break tissue apart in sterile water or broth containing 500 mg of streptomycin and 1 mega-unit of penicillin. Incubate at 30°C. Growth is typically present in 48 hours. The technique for forcibly discharged conidia in Chapter 5 can be used to recover the etiologic agent.
    e. Mycology (principal fungus): *Conidiobolus coronatus*
    f. Habitat
       Soil
2. Subcutaneous zygomycosis
    a. Definition
Subcutaneous zygomycosis is a chronic inflammatory or granulomatous disease generally restricted to the limbs, chest, back, or buttocks and characterized by massive palpable, indurated, nonulcerating subcutaneous masses. The disease is primarily in children with a predominance in males. The mycosis begins as a subcutaneous nodule. The swelling is firm, well circumscribed, painless with some pruritis. The mass is palpable and attached to the overlying skin, but not the underlying fascia. The skin is atrophic and discolored or hyperpigmented. The mass increases in size and may involve the entire arm, shoulder, upper body, face, neck, entire leg or buttocks, or both. Internal organs have been reported to be occasionally involved. Leukocytosis (up to 29,000) and eosinophilia (up to 30%) may be present.
    b. Prognosis and treatment
The prognosis is generally good and the gross disfigurement usually resolves. Potassium iodide, amphotericin B, or both are the drugs of choice.
    c. Histopathology
Same as *Conidiobolus coronatus*. Hyphal elements are 10–40 $\mu$m in diameter and the hyphae are usually sparse in the granuloma.
    d. Laboratory: (1) Direct examination. Examination of biopsy material in 10% KOH should reveal broad, septate, doubly refractile hyphae. (2) Isolation. Same as *Conidiobolus coronatus*
    e. Mycology: *Basidiobolus ranarum*
    f. Habitat
       Soil, dung

3. Zygomycosis
   a. Definition
      Mycosis caused by members of the Mucorales are generally acute and rapidly developing in debilitated patients. The disease typically involves the rhino–facial–cranial area, lungs, gastrointestinal tract, skin, or less commonly other organ systems. The disease is associated with the acidotic diabetic, malnourished children, severely burned patients and other diseases such as leukemia and lymphoma, immunosuppressive therapy, or use of cytotoxins and corticosteroids. The fungi show a predilection for vessel (arterial) invasion resulting in embolization and necrosis of surrounding tissue. Suppurative pyogenic reactions develop. Infections are typically acute and fulminant. Rhinocerebral disease in acidotic patients usually results in death, often within a few days.
   b. Forms of the disease: (1) Rhinocerebral. (2) Thoracic. (3)

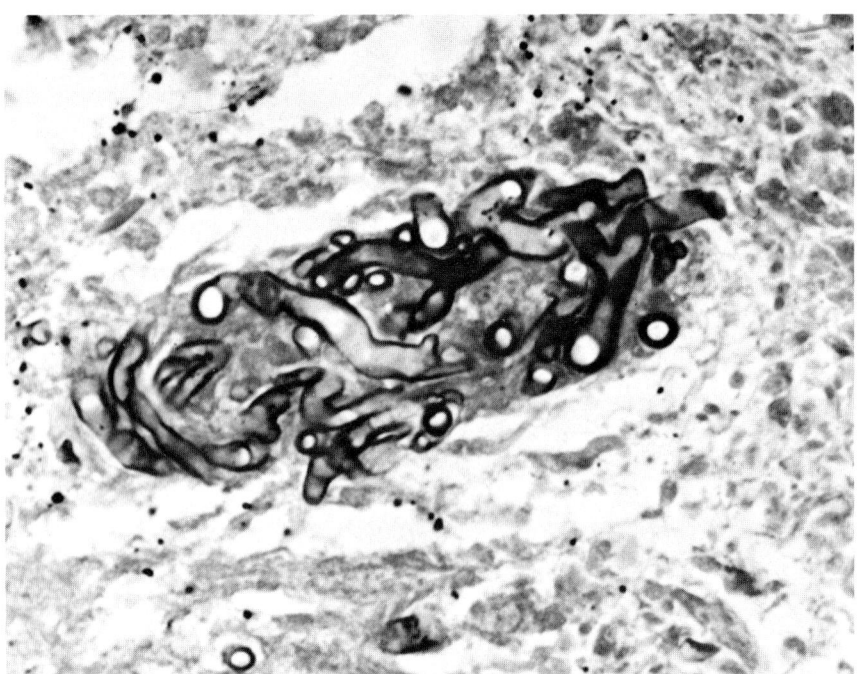

**Fig. 9.21** *Rhizopus arrhizus.* The hyphae in the blood vessel are large, sparsely septate, and irregular in shape and diameter, H and E, 400 ×.

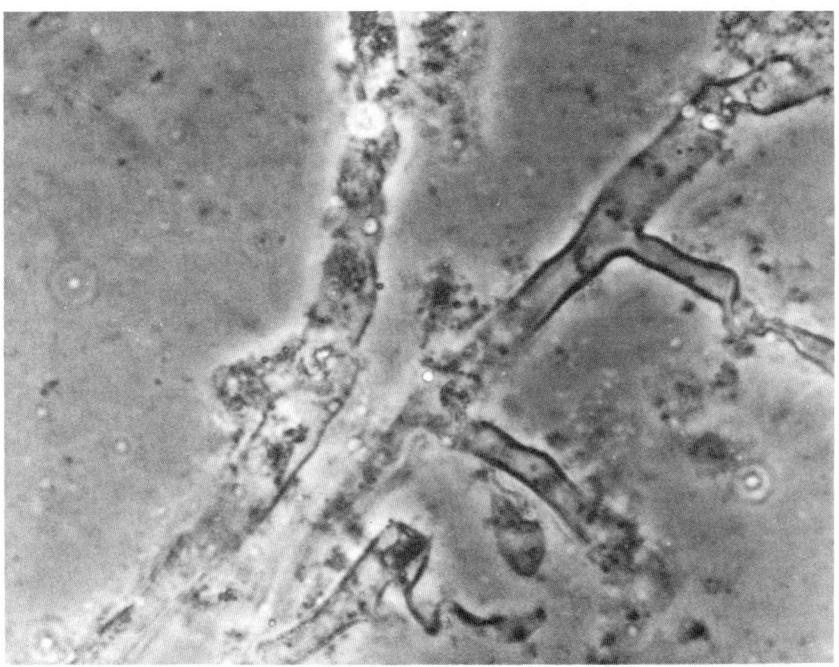

**Fig. 9.22** *Cunninghamella bertholletiae.* The hyphae of this fungus are typical of those seen in zygomycosis, sputum, 10% potassium hydroxide, 400 ×.

        Abdominal–pelvic and gastric. (4) Cutaneous
- c. Prognosis and treatment
   The prognosis is grave, especially when the rhinocerebral area is involved in patients with uncontrolled diabetes. Most cases of gastric and pelvic disease are diagnosed at autopsy. Many cases occur in patients with pulmonary disease, leukemia, or with lymphomas. These are usually fatal. Control of the diabetes, surgical debridement of involved tissue, and amphotericin B are recommended.
- d. Histopathology
   The tissue reaction is usually slight. Acute suppurative inflammation predominates with focal areas of granulomatous inflammation. Hyphae usually vary from 6–50 $\mu$m in diameter, are sparsely septate and irregularly branched (Fig. 9.21). The organism characteristically invades the walls of adjacent blood vessels, producing thrombosis and infarction, but rarely disseminates through the vessels.

Table 9.1. Summary of Selected Mycoserology[a]

| Mycosis | Test | Interpretation | Prognostic value | Limitations |
|---|---|---|---|---|
| Aspergillosis | CF | Titer ≥ 1:8 suggestive of disease | 4-Fold change in titer | Completely specific with lines of identity. Patients with invasive aspergillosis are usually immunologically compromised. False-positive reactions may occur |
| | ID | 1–2 bands = allergic, aspergilloma or aspergillosis<br><br>3 + bands = positive aspergilloma or invasive aspergillosis | Loss of bands or 4-fold change in titer | |
| Blastomycosis | CF | Titer greater than 1:8 to only the homologous antigen is suggestive of disease | 4-Fold change in titer | Less than 50% of patients react. Cross-reactions common. Elevated titer may occur in terminal cancer patients |
| | ID | A or A and B bands associated with active disease | Loss of bands | 20% of patients do not react |
| Candidiasis | CIE, ID, LA | Rising titers in LA and ID suggestive of visceral disease. CIE bands suggestive of systemic disease | 4-Fold change in titer or loss of bands. 4 or more bands in ID indicates disseminated disease | Cross-reactions common. Previous *Candida* infections give false-positive results. False negatives are not uncommon |
| Coccidioidomycosis | CF | Titer ≥ 1:32 suggestive of disease | Parallels severity of disease | 10% of patients do not react |
| | ID | Presence of bands suggestive of disease | Unknown | 10% of patients do not react |

| | | | | |
|---|---|---|---|---|
| Cryptococcosis | TP | Positive 3 weeks to 6 months | None | None |
| | IFA (Ab) | Rising titer | 4-Fold change in titer | Some cross-reactions. |
| | LA (Ag) | Any titer suggests active disease | 4-Fold change in titer | Cross-reactions with rheumatoid arthritis. 8% of patients do not react |
| Histoplasmosis | CF | Titer 1:8 suggestive of disease | 4-Fold change in titer | Cross-reactions with other mycoses. 10–20% of patients do not react |
| | ID | "M" band: past infection, skin test or early disease; "H" band: active disease | Loss of "H" band | Effected by *Histoplasma* skin test |
| Paracoccidioido-mycosis | CF | Titer greater than 1:8 suggestive of disease | 4-Fold change in titer | Some cross-reactivity with other mycoses |
| | ID | Lines of identity | Change in titer | Completely specific, 90% sensitivity |
| Sporotrichosis | SLA | Titer of 4 or greater diagnostic of disease | 4-Fold change in titer | Specific and sensitive |

[a] Abbreviations:
CF, complement fixation; CIE, counterimmunoelectrophoresis; ID, immunodiffusion; Ab, antibody; Ag, antigen; IFA, indirect fluorescent antibody; LA, latex agglutination; TP, tube precipitin; SLA, slide latex agglutination.

e. Laboratory: (1) Direct examination. A rapid diagnosis is critical. Fungal elements are usually not numerous in discharges. Scraping from the upper turbinates, aspirated material from sinuses, sputum in pulmonary disease, and biopsy material mounted in 10% KOH typically contain thick-walled, refractile hyphae 6–15 $\mu$m in diameter (Fig. 9.22). Swollen cells (up to 50 $\mu$m) and distorted hyphae may be present. (2) Isolation. Inoculate the clinical material onto Sabouraud dextrose agar and incubate at 30°C. A medium containing cycloheximide is not used because these fungi are sensitive to cycloheximide. Sterile bread in a test tube may recover Zygomycetes when other media fail. A noninoculated tube of sterile bread is necessary for quality control, since Zygomycetes are commonly associated with bread.
f. Mycology (principal fungi): (1) *Absidia corymbifera*. (2) *Rhizomucor pusillus*. (3) *Rhizopus arrhizus*. (4) *Rhizopus oryzae*
g. Habitat
Soil

*Selected References*

1. Baker, R. D., ed. (1971). "Human Infection with Fungi, Actinomycetes and Algae." Springer-Verlag, Berlin and New York.
2. Emmons, C. W., C. H. Binford, J. P. Utz, and K. J. Kwon-Chung (1977). "Medical Mycology," 3rd ed. Lea & Febiger, Philadephia.
3. Lacaz, C. da Silva (1977). "Micologia Médica Fungos, Actinomicetos e Algas de Interesse Médico," 6th ed. Sarvier, São Paulo, Brazil.
4. Rippon, J. W. (1974). "Medical Mycology: The Pathogenic Fungi and the Pathogenic Actinomycetes." Saunders, Philadephia.

*Chapter 10*

# Media and Reagents

### ALPHACEL AGAR FOR THE GYMNOASCACEAE

1. Formulation

   | | |
   |---|---|
   | Alphacel | 20.0 gm |
   | Magnesium sulfate | 1.0 gm |
   | Potassium phosphate | 1.0 gm |
   | Sodium nitrate | 1.0 gm |
   | Tomato paste (Hunt's) | 10.0 gm |
   | Oatmeal (Beech-Nut for babies) | 10.0 gm |
   | Agar | 15.0 gm |
   | Distilled water | 1 liter |

2. Preparation
   a. Mix reagents.
   b. Bring to a boil.
   c. Cool and adjust pH to 5.6 with sodium hydroxide.
   d. Autoclave for 20 minutes at 15 psi.
   e. Dispense 20.0-ml aliquots into sterile Petri dishes.
   f. Allow to harden.
3. Storage
   a. 4°C
4. Shelf life
   a. 14 days
5. Quality control
   a. Sterility
   b. pH reaction approximately 5.6
   c. Performance; not necessary prior to use
6. Comments
   Alphacel agar is ideal for stimulating the formation of ascocarps in the Gymnoascaceae. Alphacel can be purchased from Nutritional Biochemical Co., Cleveland, Ohio.

## ANTIBIOTIC MEDIUM 3 FOR AMPHOTERICIN B SUSCEPTIBILITY TESTING, 1% AGAR

1. Formulation

   | | |
   |---|---|
   | Beef extract | 1.5 gm |
   | Yeast extract | 1.5 gm |
   | Peptone (Bacto) | 5.0 gm |
   | Glucose | 1.0 gm |
   | Sodium chloride | 3.5 gm |
   | Dipotassium phosphate | 3.68 gm |
   | Monopotassium phosphate | 1.32 gm |
   | Noble agar | 10.0 gm |
   | Distilled water | 1 liter |

2. Preparation
   a. Mix reagents.
   b. Bring to a boil.
   c. Dispense 6.5-ml aliquots into $16 \times 125$ mm test tubes.
   d. Autoclave for 15 minutes at 15 psi.
   e. Stand the test tubes vertically.
3. Storage
   a. 4°C
4. Shelf life
   a. 30 days
5. Quality control
   a. Sterility
   b. Performance; not necessary prior to use
6. Comments

   This medium is commercially available without agar. Prepare according to the manufacturer's instructions and then add the Noble agar.

## ANTIBIOTIC MEDIUM 3 FOR AMPHOTERICIN B SUSCEPTIBILITY TESTING, 2% AGAR

1. Formulation

    | | |
    |---|---|
    | Beef extract | 1.5 gm |
    | Yeast extract | 1.5 gm |
    | Peptone (Bacto) | 5.0 gm |
    | Glucose | 1.0 gm |
    | Sodium chloride | 3.5 gm |
    | Dipotassium phosphate | 3.68 gm |
    | Monopotassium phosphate | 1.32 gm |
    | Noble agar | 20.0 gm |
    | Distilled water | 1 liter |

2. Preparation
    a. Mix reagents.
    b. Bring to a boil.
    c. Dispense 27.5-ml aliquots into 25 × 125 mm screw-cap test tubes.
    d. Autoclave for 15 minutes at 15 psi.
    e. Stand test tubes vertically.
3. Storage
    a. 4°C
4. Shelf life
    a. 30 days
5. Quality control
    a. Sterility
    b. Performance; not necessary prior to use
6. Comments
    This medium is commercially available without agar. It is prepared according to the manufacturer's instructions, after which the Noble agar is added.

## *ASPERGILLUS* DIFFERENTIAL MEDIUM

1. Formulation

    | | |
    |---|---|
    | Tryptone | 15.0 gm |
    | Yeast extract | 10.0 gm |
    | Ferric citrate | 0.5 gm |
    | Agar | 15.0 gm |
    | Distilled water | 1 liter |

2. Preparation
    a. Mix reagents.
    b. Add distilled water to 1 liter.
    c. Bring to a boil.
    d. Dispense 7.0-ml aliquots into 16 × 125 mm test tubes.
    e. Autoclave for 15 minutes at 15 psi.
    f. Slant the tubes.
3. Storage
    a. 4°C
4. Shelf life
    a. 30 days
5. Quality control
    a. Sterility
    b. Performance

    | Fungus | Incubation temperature | Result |
    |---|---|---|
    | *Aspergillus flavus* | 30°C | Bright yellow-orange reverse pigmentation |

6. Comments

    The reverse pigmentation of *A. sulphureus*, *A. sclerotiorum*, and *A. thomii* is indistinguishable from that of *A. flavus* on *Aspergillus* differential medium.

# BRAIN HEART INFUSION (BHI) AGAR

1. Formulation

   | | |
   |---|---|
   | Calf brains, infusion | 200.0 gm |
   | Beef heart, infusion | 250.0 gm |
   | Peptone | 10.0 gm |
   | Glucose | 2.0 gm |
   | Sodium chloride | 5.0 gm |
   | Disodium phosphate | 2.5 gm |
   | Agar | 15.0 gm |
   | Distilled water | 1 liter |

2. Preparation
   a. Mix reagents in a 2-liter flask.
   b. Bring to a boil.
   c. Dispense 7.0-ml aliquots in $16 \times 125$ mm test tubes or 15.0 ml aliquots into $25 \times 125$ mm test tubes.
   d. Autoclave for 15 minutes at 15 psi.
   e. Slant the tubes.
3. Storage
   a. 4°C
4. Shelf life
   a. 30 days in test tubes
   b. 14 days in Petri dishes
5. Quality control
   a. Sterility
   b. Performance

   | Fungus | Incubation temperature | Result |
   |---|---|---|
   | *Aspergillus flavus* | 25°C | Good growth |

6. Comments
   Commercially available media may be substituted; this is prepared according to the manufacturer's instructions. Media in test tubes can be melted and poured into sterile Petri dishes if necessary. The medium can be enriched with 5% sheep blood.

## BUFFERED YEAST NITROGEN BASE FOR SYNERGISM STUDIES

1. Formulation
   a. Yeast nitrogen base

   | | |
   |---|---|
   | Asparagine | 1.5 gm |
   | Glucose | 10.0 gm |
   | Yeast nitrogen base | 6.7 gm |
   | Distilled water | 1 liter |

   b. Buffer

   | | |
   |---|---|
   | Morpholinopropane sulfonic acid | 15.89 gm |
   | Tris-(hydroxymethyl)-aminomethane | 10.08 gm |
   | Distilled water | 100.00 ml |

2. Preparation
   a. Yeast nitrogen base
      (1) Mix reagents.
      (2) Sterilize by filtration.
   b. Buffer
      (1) Mix reagents.
      (2) Autoclave for 15 minutes at 15 psi.
   c. Add 5.0 ml of buffer to 95.0 ml of yeast nitrogen base.
3. Storage
   a. 4°C
4. Shelf life
   a. 30 days
5. Quality control
   a. Sterility
   b. Performance; not necessary prior to use

# CAFFEIC ACID AGAR

1. Formulation

   | | |
   |---|---|
   | Glucose | 5.0 gm |
   | Ammonium sulfate | 5.0 gm |
   | Yeast extract | 2.0 gm |
   | Potassium phosphate | 0.8 gm |
   | Magnesium sulfate | 0.7 gm |
   | Caffeic acid | 0.18 gm |
   | Ferric citrate solution | 4.0 ml |
   | Noble agar | 20.0 gm |
   | Distilled water | 1 liter |

2. Preparation
   a. Add 10.0 mg of ferric citrate to 20.0 ml of distilled water. This is the ferric citrate solution.
   b. Mix reagents.
   c. Add distilled water to 1 liter.
   d. Bring to a boil.
   e. Autoclave for 12 minutes at 15 psi.
   f. Dispense 15.0-ml aliquots into sterile Petri dishes.
   g. Allow to harden.
3. Storage
   a. 4°C in the dark
4. Shelf life
   a. 14 days
5. Quality control
   a. Sterility
   b. Color
      (1) Discard if it becomes dark
   c. Performance

   | Fungus | Incubation temperature | Result |
   |---|---|---|
   | *Cryptococcus neoformans* | 30°C | Black colonies |
   | *Cryptococcus albidus* | 30°C | Cream to tan colonies |

6. Comments
   Caffeic acid agar must be protected from the light. The results appear to be better when the agar is dispensed in Petri dishes instead of test tubes. Chloramphenicol can be added to the caffeic acid agar if necessary.

## CARBON BASAL ASSIMILATION MEDIUM FOR YEASTS (AUXANOGRAPHIC)

1. Formulation

   | | |
   |---|---|
   | Yeast nitrogen base | 6.7 gm |
   | Noble agar | 20.0 gm |
   | Distilled water | 1 liter |

2. Preparation
   a. Mix reagents.
   b. Bring to a boil.
   c. Dispense 25.0-ml aliquots into 25 × 200 mm screw-cap test tubes.
   d. Autoclave for 15 minutes at 15 psi.
   e. Stand the test tubes vertically.
3. Storage
   a. 4°C
4. Shelf life
   a. 30 days
5. Quality control
   a. Sterility
   b. Performance; not necessary prior to use
6. Comments

   The medium is melted and placed in a water bath set at 50–52°C prior to use.

## 10 Media and Reagents

# CARBON DISKS FOR YEASTS

1. Formulation

    | | |
    |---|---|
    | Carbon source (glucose, galactose, etc.) | 3.0 gm |
    | Distilled water | 100.0 ml |

2. Preparation
    a. Mix reagents.
    b. Sterilize by filtration.
    c. Saturate 6-mm sterile sensitivity disks in the solution.
    d. Dry disks in a sterile Petri dish.
3. Storage
    a. 4°C
4. Shelf life
    a. Six months
5. Quality control
    a. Sterility
    b. Performance

| Fungus | Incubation temperature | Result |
|---|---|---|
| *Candida guilliermondii*, *Cryptococcus laurentii*, and *Torulopsis inconspicua* | 30°C | Presence or absence of growth, depending upon the carbon source and yeast |

6. Comments

    Some carbon sources in disks are commercially available. It is important to quality control all carbon sources since they may be contaminated with other sugars.

## CARBON SOURCES, FERMENTATION

1. Formulation

    | | |
    |---|---|
    | Carbon source (glucose, galactose, etc.) | 6.0 gm |
    | Raffinose only | 12.0 gm |
    | Distilled water | 100.0 ml |

2. Preparation
    a. Mix reagents.
    b. Sterilize by filtration.
3. Storage
    a. 4°C
4. Shelf life
    a. 30 days.
5. Quality control
    a. Sterility
    b. Performance

| Fungus | Incubation temperature | Result |
|---|---|---|
| *Candida guilliermondii*, *Cryptococcus laurentii*, and *Torulopsis inconspicua* | 25°C | Presence or absence of fermentation, depending upon the carbon source and the yeast |

6. Comments

    The various carbon sources are tested at a final concentration of 2%, except raffinose, which is tested at 4%. A carbon source may be heated slightly if it will not go into solution.

## CARBON SOURCES, WICKERHAM LIQUID ASSIMILATION

1. Formulation

   | | |
   |---|---|
   | Yeast nitrogen base | 6.7 gm |
   | Carbon source | |
   | (glucose, galactose, etc.) | 5.0 gm |
   | Raffinose only | 10.0 gm |
   | Distilled water | 100.0 ml |

2. Preparation
   a. Mix reagents.
   b. Sterilize by filtration.
   c. Dispense 0.5-ml aliquots into 4.5 ml of sterile distilled water in 16 × 125 mm test tubes.
3. Storage
   a. 4°C
4. Shelf life
   a. 30 days
5. Quality control
   a. Sterility
   b. Performance

   | Fungus | Incubation temperature | Result |
   |---|---|---|
   | *Candida guilliermondii*, *Cryptococcus laurentii*, and *Torulopsis inconspicua* | 25°C | Presence or absence of growth, depending upon the carbon source and the yeast |

6. Comments
   The solutions can be warmed if the carbon source does not go into solution immediately. Raffinose is used as a 1% solution in contrast to the other sugars, which are used in 0.5% solutions. These solutions are used in the Wickerham liquid assimilation test.

## CASITONE MEDIUM FOR MICONAZOLE SUSCEPTIBILITY TESTING, AGAR

1. Formulation

   | | |
   |---|---|
   | Casitone (Bacto) | 5.0 gm |
   | Yeast extract | 5.0 gm |
   | Glucose | 5.0 gm |
   | Noble agar | 20.0 gm |
   | Distilled water | 1 liter |

2. Preparation
   a. Mix reagents.
   b. Bring to a boil.
   c. Dispense 27.5-ml aliquots in 25 × 150 mm screw-cap test tubes.
   d. Autoclave for 15 minutes at 15 psi.
   e. Stand the test tubes vertically.
3. Storage
   a. 4°C
4. Shelf life
   a. 30 days
5. Quality control
   a. Sterility
   b. Performance; not necessary prior to use
6. Comments
   The medium is melted and placed in a water bath set at 50–52°C prior to use.

## CASITONE MEDIUM FOR MICONAZOLE SUSCEPTIBILITY TESTING, BROTH

1. Formulation

    | | |
    |---|---|
    | Casitone (Bacto) | 5.0 gm |
    | Yeast extract | 5.0 gm |
    | Glucose | 5.0 gm |
    | Distilled water | 1 liter |

2. Preparation
    a. Mix reagents.
    b. Dispense 100.0-ml aliquots into 250-ml flasks.
    c. Autoclave for 15 minutes at 15 psi.
3. Storage
    a. 4°C
4. Shelf life
    a. 30 days
5. Quality control
    a. Sterility
    b. Performance; not necessary prior to use

## CEREAL AGAR FOR ASCOCARP PRODUCTION IN THE GYMNOASCACEAE

1. Formulation

   | | |
   |---|---|
   | Precooked mixed cereal | 10.0 gm |
   | Dipotassium phosphate | 1.5 gm |
   | Magnesium sulfate | 1.0 gm |
   | Sodium nitrate | 1.0 gm |
   | Agar | 18.0 gm |
   | Distilled water | 1 liter |

2. Preparation
   a. Mix reagents.
   b. Bring to a boil.
   c. Cool; adjust pH to 5.6.
   d. Autoclave for 15 minutes at 15 psi.
   e. Dispense 15.0-ml aliquots into sterile Petri dishes.
   f. Let the medium harden.
3. Storage
   a. 4°C
4. Shelf life
   a. 14 days
5. Quality control
   a. Sterility
   b. pH reaction approximately 5.6
   c. Performance; not necessary prior to use

## CEREAL AGAR FOR HYPHOMYCETES

1. Formulation

|  |  |
|---|---|
| Precooked mixed cereal | 100.0 gm |
| Agar | 15.0 gm |
| Distilled water | 1 liter |

2. Preparation
    a. Mix reagents.
    b. Bring to a boil.
    c. Dispense 7.0-ml aliquots into 16 × 125 mm test tubes.
    d. Autoclave for 10 minutes at 10 psi.
    e. Slant the test tubes.
3. Storage
    a. 4°C
4. Shelf life
    a. 30 days
5. Quality control
    a. Sterility
    b. Performance

| Fungus | Incubation temperature | Result |
|---|---|---|
| *Trichophyton mentagrophytes* | 25°C | Good production of conidia |

6. Comments
    Cereal agar can be supplemented with 50.0 mg of chloramphenicol per liter if bacterial contamination may be a problem.

## CHRISTENSEN'S UREA AGAR OR BROTH

The medium is commercially available as a dehydrated preparation. The medium is prepared according to the manufacturer's instructions. The medium is dispensed in 7.0-ml aliquots into 16 × 125 mm test tubes. The medium is stored at 4°C for 30 days. The performance is evaluated when it is used.

## CONVERSE LIQUID MEDIUM (LEVINE MODIFICATION) FOR *COCCIDIOIDES*

1. Formulation

    | | |
    |---|---|
    | Ammonium acetate | 1.23 gm |
    | Glucose | 4.0 gm |
    | Dipotassium phosphate | 0.52 gm |
    | Potassium phosphate | 0.4 gm |
    | Magnesium sulfate | 0.4 gm |
    | Zinc sulfate | 0.002 gm |
    | Sodium chloride | 0.014 gm |
    | Sodium carbonate | 0.012 gm |
    | Tamol | 0.5 gm |
    | Calcium chloride | 0.002 gm |
    | Agar (Ionagar No. 2, Agarose, or purified agar) | 10.0 gm |
    | Distilled water | 1 liter |

2. Preparation
    a. Mix reagents.
    b. Bring to a boil.
    c. Autoclave for 15 minutes at 15 psi.
    d. Dispense 15.0-ml aliquots into sterile Petri dishes.
    e. Allow to harden.
3. Storage
    a. 4°C
4. Shelf life
    a. 14 days
5. Quality control
    a. Sterility
    b. Performance

| Fungus | Incubation temperature | Result |
|---|---|---|
| *Coccidioides immitis* | 40°C in a candle jar | Production of spherules and endospores |

## CORNMEAL AGAR

1. Formulation

   | | |
   |---|---|
   | Cornmeal | 50.0 gm |
   | Agar | 15.0 gm |
   | Distilled water | 1 liter |

2. Preparation
   a. Mix cormeal in 500.0 ml of distilled water.
   b. Heat for 1 hour or autoclave for 10 minutes at 15 psi.
   c. Filter the suspension through cheesecloth.
   d. Bring volume up to 1 liter and add agar.
   e. Bring to a boil.
   f. Dispense 7.0-ml aliquots into 16 × 125 mm test tubes.
   g. Autoclave for 15 minutes at 15 psi.
   h. Slant the test tubes.
3. Storage
   a. 4°C
4. Shelf life
   a. 30 days in test tubes
   b. 14 days in Petri dishes
5. Quality control
   a. Sterility
   b. Performance

   | Fungus | Incubation temperature | Result |
   |---|---|---|
   | *Aspergillus flavus* | 25°C | Good growth and conidia production |
   | *Trichophyton rubrum* | 25°C | Red pigment |
   | *Candida albicans* | 25°C | Chlamydospores |

6. Comments

   Depending upon its purpose, the appropriate quality control organism would be selected. If the cornmeal agar is to be used for chlamydospore development in the Dalmau techique, 10.0 ml of Tween 80 is added to the medium prior to sterilization. After sterilization, it is dispensed in 15.0-ml aliquots into sterile Petri dishes.

## COTTONSEED AGAR

1. Formulation

    | | |
    |---|---|
    | Pharmamedia | 20.0 gm |
    | Glucose | 20.0 gm |
    | Agar | 15.0 gm |
    | Distilled water | 1 liter |

2. Preparation
    a. Mix reagents.
    b. Bring to a boil.
    c. Adjust pH to 6.0 with either 1 $N$ HCl or 1 $N$ NaOH.
    d. Dispense in 10.0-ml aliquots into 15 × 125 mm test tubes.
    e. Autoclave for 15 minutes at 15 psi.
    f. Slant the test tubes.
3. Storage
    a. 4°C
4. Shelf life
    a. 30 days
5. Quality control
    a. Sterility
    b. pH reaction of 6.0
    c. Performance

    | Fungus | Incubation temperature | Result |
    |---|---|---|
    | *Blastomyces dermatitidis* | 37°C | Yeast form |

6. Comments

    Cottonseed agar is excellent for the mould-to-yeast conversion of *B. dermatitidis*. This medium is unsatisfactory for the mould-to-yeast conversion of other dimorphic fungi. Pharmamedia can be obtained from Traders Oil Mill Co., Traders Protein Division, Fort Worth, Texas.

# CZAPEK–DOX-SOLUTION AGAR

1. Formulation

    | | |
    |---|---|
    | Magnesium sulfate | 0.5 gm |
    | Potassium chloride | 0.5 gm |
    | Dipotassium phosphate | 1.0 gm |
    | Ferrous sulfate | 0.01 gm |
    | Sodium nitrate | 3.0 gm |
    | Sucrose | 30.0 gm |
    | Agar | 15.0 gm |
    | Distilled water | 1 liter |

2. Preparation
    a. Mix reagents.
    b. Bring to a boil.
    c. Dispense 7.0-ml aliquots into 16 × 125 mm test tubes.
    d. Autoclave for 15 minutes at 15 psi.
    e. Slant the test tubes.
3. Storage
    a. 4°C
4. Shelf life
    a. 30 days in test tubes
    b. 14 days in Petri dishes
5. Quality control
    a. Sterility
    b. Performance

| Fungus | Incubation temperature | Result |
|---|---|---|
| *Aspergillus flavus* | 25°C | Good growth, yellow to green colony |

## CZAPEK–DOX-SOLUTION AGAR FOR *ASPERGILLUS*

1. Formulation

    | | |
    |---|---|
    | Sodium nitrate | 3.0 gm |
    | Dipotassium phosphate | 1.0 gm |
    | Magnesium sulfate | 0.5 gm |
    | Potassium chloride | 0.5 gm |
    | Ferrous sulfate | 0.01 gm |
    | Glucose | 30.0 gm |
    | Agar | 15.0 gm |
    | Distilled water | 1 liter |

2. Preparation
    a. Mix the reagents.
    b. Bring to a boil.
    c. Dispense 7.0-ml aliquots into 16 × 125 mm test tubes.
    d. Autoclave for 15 minutes at 15 psi.
    e. Slant the test tubes.
    f. For plates, autoclave medium in a flask.
        (1) Aseptically dispense 25.0-ml aliquots into sterile Petri dishes.
        (2) Allow medium to harden.
3. Storage
    a. 4°C
4. Shelf life
    a. 30 days in test tubes
    b. 14 days in Petri dishes
5. Quality control
    a. Sterility
    b. Performance

| Fungus | Incubation temperature | Result |
|---|---|---|
| *Aspergillus flavus* | 25°C | Good growth, colonies thin, at first yellow, becoming green |

## FERMENTATION BROTH

1. Formulation

    | | |
    |---|---|
    | Bromothymol blue | 0.04 gm (use analytical balance) |
    | Powdered yeast extract | 4.5 gm |
    | Peptone | 7.5 gm |
    | Distilled water | 1 liter |

2. Preparation
    a. Dissolve bromothymol blue in 3.0 ml of 95% ethanol.
    b. Mix reagents and add bromothymol blue.
    c. Adjust pH to 7.0.
    d. Dispense 2.0-ml aliquots into 16 × 125 mm test tubes with screw caps.
    e. Place 1 Durham tube into each test tube, opening down.
    f. Autoclave for 15 minutes at 15 psi.
    g. Allow medium to cool.
    h. To each tube, aseptically add 1.0 ml of 6.0% aqueous solution of carbon source to be tested, which has been previously filtered through a 0.22-$\mu$m filter.
3. Storage
    a. 4°C
4. Shelf life
    a. 30 days
5. Quality control
    a. Sterility
    b. Color
        (1) Discard if color is not blue-green
    c. Performance; not necessary prior to use

## GERM TUBE TEST MEDIUM

1. Formulation
    Pooled human serum
2. Preparation
    a. Dispense 0.3-ml aliquots into 12 × 75 mm test tubes.
    b. Stopper with cotton plugs.
3. Storage
    a. −70°C
4. Shelf life
    a. One year
5. Quality control
    a. Performance

| Fungus | Incubation temperature | Result |
|---|---|---|
| *Candida albicans* | 37°C in 2.5 hours | Germ tubes present |
| *Candida tropicalis* | 37°C in 2.5 hours | Germ tubes absent |

6. Comments
    Bovine serum works well. Each lot of human sera must be evaluated before it is used.

## GLUCOSE-YEAST EXTRACT MEDIUM FOR *COCCIDIOIDES*

1. Formulation

    | | |
    |---|---|
    | Glucose | 10.0 gm |
    | Yeast extract | 5.0 gm |
    | Agar | 15.0 gm |
    | Distilled water | 1 liter |

2. Preparation
    a. Mix reagents.
    b. Bring to a boil.
    c. Dispense 7.0-ml aliquots into 16 × 125 mm test tubes.
    d. Autoclave for 15 minutes at 15 psi.
    e. Slant the test tubes.
3. Storage
    a. 4°C
4. Shelf life
    a. 30 days
5. Quality control
    a. Sterility
    b. Performance

| Fungus | Incubation temperature | Result |
|---|---|---|
| *Aspergillus flavus* | 25°C | Good growth |

## GORODKOWA'S MEDIUM FOR ASCOSPORES

1. Formulation

    | | |
    |---|---|
    | Glucose | 0.63 gm |
    | Sodium chloride | 1.3 gm |
    | Beef extract | 2.5 gm |
    | Agar | 2.5 gm |
    | Distilled water | 250.0 ml |

2. Preparation
    a. Mix reagents.
    b. Bring to a boil.
    c. Dispense 7.0-ml aliquots into 16 × 125 mm test tubes.
    d. Autoclave for 15 minutes at 15 psi.
    e. Slant the test tubes.
3. Storage
    a. 4°C
4. Shelf life
    a. 30 days in test tubes
    b. 14 days in Petri dishes
5. Quality control
    a. Sterility
    b. Performance

| Fungus | Incubation temperature | Result |
|---|---|---|
| *Saccharomyces cerevisiae* | 25°C | Production of asci and ascospores |

## GRAM STAIN REAGENTS, BURKE'S MODIFICATION

1. Formulation
   a. Crystal violet solution

   | | |
   |---|---|
   | Crystal violet | 1.0 gm |
   | Distilled water | 100.0 ml |

   b. Sodium bicarbonate solution

   | | |
   |---|---|
   | Sodium bicarbonate | 5.0 gm |
   | Distilled water | 100.0 ml |

   c. Iodine solution

   | | |
   |---|---|
   | Iodine | 1.0 gm |
   | Potassium iodide | 2.0 gm |
   | Distilled water | 100.0 ml |

   d. Acetone–alcohol solution

   | | |
   |---|---|
   | Acetone | 50.0 ml |
   | Ethanol, 95% | 50.0 ml |

   e. Safranin solution

   | | |
   |---|---|
   | Safranin | 0.5 gm |
   | Distilled water | 100.0 ml |

2. Preparation
   a. Prepare solutions separately
3. Storage
   a. Brown bottles
4. Shelf life
   a. Six months
5. Quality control
   a. Not necessary

## HAIR TEST, *in Vitro*

1. Formulation

    | | |
    |---|---|
    | Yeast extract | 10.0 gm |
    | Distilled water | 90.0 ml |

2. Preparation
    a. Mix reagents.
    b. Sterilize by filtration.
3. Storage
    a. 4°C
4. Shelf life
    a. Three months
5. Quality control
    a. Sterility
    b. Performance; not necessary prior to use
6. Comments

    Hairs of children are necessary in this test too. They are sterilized for 15 minutes at 15 psi in an autoclave. The hairs can be kept in a Petri dish at room temperature for months.

# HAY INFUSION AGAR

1. Formulation

   | | |
   |---|---|
   | Decomposing hay | 50.0 gm |
   | Dipotassium phosphate | 2.0 gm |
   | Agar | 15.0 gm |
   | Tap water | 1 liter |

2. Preparation
    a. Mix hay and tap water.
    b. Autoclave for 30 minutes at 15 psi.
    c. Filter through cheesecloth.
    d. Add reagents to the hay infusion.
    e. Cool and adjust pH to approximately 6.2.
    f. Bring to a boil.
    g. Dispense 7.0-ml aliquots into $16 \times 125$ mm test tubes.
    h. Autoclave for 15 minutes at 15 psi.
    i. Slant the test tubes.
3. Storage
    a. 4°C
4. Shelf life
    a. 30 days in test tubes
    b. 14 days in Petri dishes
5. Quality control
    a. Sterility
    b. pH reaction approximately 6.2
    c. Performance; not necessary prior to use
6. Comments
    The medium is often used to enhance the development of conidia or spores.

## *HISTOPLASMA* MOULD-TO-YEAST-FORM CONVERSION MEDIUM

1. Formulation

   | | |
   |---|---|
   | Brain heart infusion agar base | 5.2 gm |
   | Glutamine | 1.0 ml |
   | Sheep blood | 5.0 ml |
   | Distilled water | 100.0 ml |

2. Preparation
   a. Prepare brain heart infusion agar base according to the manufacturer's instructions.
   b. Autoclave for 15 minutes at 15 psi.
   c. Add 1.0 ml glutamine (200 mmols/ml).
   d. Add sheep blood.
   e. Dispense 7.0-ml aliquots into sterile 16 × 125 mm test tubes.
   f. Slant the test tubes.
3. Storage
   a. 4°C
4. Shelf life
   a. 30 days
5. Quality control
   a. Sterility
   b. Performance

   | Fungus | Incubation temperature | Result |
   |---|---|---|
   | *Histoplasma capsulatum* | 37°C | Yeast form |

6. Comments
   The stock glutamine solution must be kept frozen prior to use. This medium works well for the mould-to-yeast conversion of *H. capsulatum*.

# HUGH AND LEIFSON AGAR FOR DERMATOPHYTES

1. Formulation

   | | |
   |---|---|
   | Sodium chloride | 5.0 gm |
   | Dipotassium phosphate | 0.3 gm |
   | Peptone | 2.0 gm |
   | Agar | 15.0 gm |
   | Distilled water | 1 liter |

2. Preparation
    a. Mix reagents.
    b. Bring to a boil.
    c. Dispense 7.0-aliquots into $16 \times 125$ mm test tubes.
    d. Autoclave for 15 minutes at 15 psi.
    e. Slant the test tubes.
3. Storage
    a. 4°C
4. Shelf life
    a. 30 days
5. Quality control
    a. Sterility
    b. Performance

    | Fungus | Incubation temperature | Result |
    |---|---|---|
    | *Trichophyton mentagrophytes* | 25°C | Good growth |

6. Comments

    This medium is used for growing inoculum for carbon assimilation studies for the dermatophytes.

## KELLEY'S AGAR

1. Formulation

    | | |
    |---|---|
    | Glucose | 10.0 gm |
    | Bacto peptone | 10.0 gm |
    | Sodium chloride | 5.0 gm |
    | Beef extract | 3.0 gm |
    | Hemoglobin solution | 20.0 ml |
    | Agar | 15.0 gm |
    | Distilled water | 980.0 ml |

2. Preparation
    a. Add 5.0 ml of citrated sheep blood to 15.0 ml of distilled water. This is the hemoglobin solution.
    b. Mix the other reagents.
    c. Bring to a boil.
    d. Add the hemoglobin solution.
    e. Dispense 7.0-ml aliquots into 16 × 125 mm test tubes.
    f. Autoclave for 10 minutes at 15 psi.
    g. Slant the test tubes.
3. Storage
    a. 4°C
4. Shelf life
    a. 30 days
5. Quality control
    a. Sterility
    b. Performance

| Fungus | Incubation temperature | Result |
|---|---|---|
| *Blastomyces dermatitidis* | 37°C | Yeast form |

## KLEYN'S ACETATE AGAR FOR ASCOSPORES

1. Formulation

    | | |
    |---|---|
    | Bacto tryptose | 2.5 gm |
    | Glucose | 0.62 gm |
    | Sodium chloride | 0.62 gm |
    | Sodium acetate trihydrate | 5.0 gm |
    | Agar | 15.0 gm |
    | Distilled water | 1 liter |

2. Preparation
    a. Mix reagents.
    b. Bring to a boil.
    c. Dispense 7.0-ml aliquots into 16 × 125 mm test tubes.
    d. Autoclave for 15 minutes at 15 psi.
    e. Slant the test tubes.
3. Storage
    a. 4°C
4. Shelf life
    a. 30 days
5. Quality control
    a. Sterility
    b. Performance

| Fungus | Incubation temperature | Result |
|---|---|---|
| *Saccharomyces cerevisiae* | 25°C | Production of asci and ascospores |

## LACTOPHENOL AND LACTOPHENOL COTTON BLUE MOUNTING MEDIA

1. Formulation
    a. Lactophenol

    | | |
    |---|---|
    | Phenol, concentrated | 20.0 ml |
    | Lactic acid | 20.0 ml |
    | Glycerol | 40.0 ml |
    | Distilled water | 20.0 ml |

    b. Lactophenol cotton blue

    | | |
    |---|---|
    | Phenol, concentrated | 20.0 ml |
    | Lactic acid | 20.0 ml |
    | Gylcerol | 40.0 ml |
    | Cotton blue | 0.05 gm |
    | Distilled water | 20.0 ml |

2. Preparation
    a. Lactophenol
        (1) Mix reagents.
    b. Lactophenol cotton blue
        (1) Dissolve cotton blue in distilled water.
        (2) Add phenol, lactic acid and glycerol.
3. Storage
    a. Room temperature
4. Shelf life
    a. One year, filter through filter paper if dye precipitates out of solution.
5. Quality control
    a. Not necessary

## MALT EXTRACT AGAR

1. Formulation

    | | |
    |---|---|
    | Malt extract | 20.0 gm |
    | Peptone | 1.0 gm |
    | Glucose | 20.0 gm |
    | Agar | 15.0 gm |
    | Distilled water | 1 liter |

2. Preparation
    a. Mix reagents.
    b. Bring to a boil.
    c. Dispense 7.0-ml aliquots into 16 × 125 mm test tubes.
    d. Autoclave for 15 minutes at 15 psi.
    e. Slant the test tubes.
3. Storage
    a. 4°C
4. Shelf life
    a. 30 days in test tubes
    b. 14 days in Petri dishes
5. Quality control
    a. Sterility
    b. Performance

    | Fungus | Incubation temperature | Result |
    |---|---|---|
    | *Saccharomyces cerevisiae* | 25°C | Good growth |

## MALT EXTRACT (ME) AGAR

1. Formulation

    | | |
    |---|---|
    | Malt extract | 20.0 gm |
    | Agar | 12.0 gm |
    | Distilled water | 400.0 ml |

2. Preparation
    a. Mix agar and distilled water.
    b. Bring to a boil.
    c. Cool, add malt extract and mix.
    d. Dispense 7.5-ml aliquots into $16 \times 125$ mm test tubes.
    e. Autoclave for 15 minutes at 15 psi.
    f. Slant the test tubes.
3. Storage
    a. 4°C
4. Shelf life
    a. 30 days in test tubes
    b. 14 days in Petri dishes
5. Quality control
    a. Sterility
    b. Performance

    | Fungus | Incubation temperature | Result |
    |---|---|---|
    | *Saccharomyces cerevisiae* | 25°C | Good growth |

6. Comments

    The medium can be acidified with hydrochloric acid to a pH reaction of 3.7 if it is to be used for purifying bacterially contaminated yeast cultures.

## MALT EXTRACT AGAR FOR *ASPERGILLUS*

1. Formulation

    | | |
    |---|---|
    | Malt extract | 20.0 gm |
    | Peptone (Difco) | 1.0 gm |
    | Glucose | 20.0 gm |
    | Agar | 20.0 gm |
    | Distilled water | 1 liter |

2. Preparation
    a. Mix reagents.
    b. Bring to a boil.
    c. Dispense 7.0-ml aliquots into 16 × 125 mm test tubes.
    d. Autoclave for 15 minutes at 15 psi.
    e. Slant the test tubes.
    f. For plates, autoclave medium in a flask.
        (1) Aseptically dispense 25.0-ml aliquots into sterile Petri dishes.
        (2) Allow medium to harden.
3. Storage
    a. 4°C
4. Shelf life
    a. 30 days in test tubes
    b. 14 days in Petri dishes
5. Quality control
    a. Sterility
    b. Performance

| Fungus | Incubation temperature | Result |
|---|---|---|
| *Aspergillus flavus* | 25°C | Rapid growth, yellowish-green colonies |

## MARTIN'S MEDIUM (MODIFIED)

1. Formulation

    | | |
    |---|---|
    | Yeast extract | 0.5 gm |
    | Potassium phosphate | 1.0 gm |
    | Magnesium sulfate | 0.5 gm |
    | Peptone | 5.0 gm |
    | Glucose | 10.0 gm |
    | Rose bengal | 0.033 gm |
    | Agar | 15.0 gm |
    | Tap water | 1 liter |

2. Preparation
    a. Mix reagents.
    b. Bring to a boil.
    c. Autoclave for 15 minutes at 15 psi.
    d. Dispense 15.0-ml aliquots into sterile Petri dishes.
    e. Allow to harden.
3. Storage
    a. 4°C in the dark
4. Shelf life
    a. 30 days in test tubes
    b. 14 days in Petri dishes
5. Quality control
    a. Sterility
    b. Performance

    | Fungus | Incubation temperature | Result |
    |---|---|---|
    | *Aspergillus flavus* | 25°C | Restricted colonies |

6. Comments

    Martin's medium must be protected from strong light. The rose bengal can become very fungistatic. This medium is ideal for retarding the growth of fast growing fungi.

## M-3 MEDIUM FOR AMPHOTERICIN B SUSCEPTIBILITY TESTING, BROTH

1. Formulation

    | | |
    |---|---|
    | Beef extract | 1.5 gm |
    | Yeast extract | 1.5 gm |
    | Peptone (Bacto) | 5.0 gm |
    | Glucose | 1.0 gm |
    | Sodium chloride | 3.5 gm |
    | Dispotassium phosphate | 3.68 gm |
    | Monopotassium phosphate | 1.32 gm |
    | Distilled water | 1 liter |

2. Preparation
    a. Mix reagents.
    b. Dispense 100.0-ml aliquots into 250-ml flasks.
    c. Autoclave for 15 minutes at 15 psi.
3. Storage
    a. 4°C
4. Shelf life
    a. 30 days
5. Quality control
    a. Sterility
    b. Performance; not necessary prior to use
6. Comments
    This medium is commerically available. It is prepared according to the manufacturer's instructions.


## MERTHIOLATE FOR SERUM

1. Formulation

    | | |
    |---|---|
    | Sodium borate | 1.4 gm |
    | Merthiolate | 1.0 gm |
    | Distilled water | 100.0 ml |

2. Preparation
    a. Dissolve sodium borate in water.
    b. Add merthiolate.
3. Storage
    a. Room temperature
4. Shelf life
    a. Six months
5. Quality control
    a. Not necessary
6. Comments
    One-tenth milliliter of the 1% merthiolate in 1.4% sodium borate is added to each 10.0 ml of serum.

## MITE CONTROL

1. Formulation

    | | | |
    |---|---|---|
    | Hexachlorocyclohexane | 0.01 | gm |
    | Any mycological medium | 1 | liter |

2. Preparation
    a. Add the hexachlorocyclohexane to 1 liter of any mycological medium.
    b. Sterilize as usual.
3. Storage
    a. Same as for medium
4. Shelf life
    a. Same as for medium
5. Quality control
    a. Same as for medium

## $N$-ACETYL-L-CYSTEINE (NALC) REAGENTS

1. Formulation
    a. 0.1 M sodium citrate solution

    | | | |
    |---|---|---|
    | Sodium citrate | 29.4 | gm |
    | Distilled water | 1 | liter |

    b. NALC powder

    | | |
    |---|---|
    | NALC powder | 0.25 gm |

2. Preparation
    a. Sodium citrate solution
        (1) Mix reagents.
        (2) Autoclave for 15 minutes at 15 psi.
        (3) Place in brown bottle.
3. Storage
    a. Sodium citrate in a brown bottle at 4°C
    b. NALC in a dry screw-cap bottle at 4°C
4. Shelf life
    a. 30 days
5. Quality control
    a. Sterility
    b. Performance; not necessary prior to use
6. Comments
    The NALC and sodium citrate solution are mixed immediately prior to use. The NALC digestant should be no more than 24 hours old.

## NITRATE ASSIMILATION MEDIUM

1. Formulation

   | | |
   |---|---|
   | Yeast carbon base | 11.7 gm |
   | Potassium nitrate | 0.78 gm |
   | Distilled water | 100.0 ml |

2. Preparation
   a. Mix reagents.
   b. Sterilize by filtration.
   c. Dispense 0.5-ml aliquots into $16 \times 125$ mm sterile test tubes containing 4.5 ml of sterile distilled water.
3. Storage
   a. 4°C
4. Shelf life
   a. 30 days
5. Quality control
   a. Sterility
   b. Performance; not necessary prior to use
6. Comments

   The final concentration is $1 \times$. This medium is used for the Wickerham liquid nitrate assimilation test.

## NITRATE REAGENTS

1. Formulation
   a. Reagent A (sulfanilic acid)

      | | | |
      |---|---|---|
      | Sulfanilic acid | 8.0 gm | |
      | Acetic acid, 5 $N$ | 1 | liter |

   b. Reagent B ($\alpha$-naphthylamine)

      | | | |
      |---|---|---|
      | $\alpha$-Naphthylamine | 5.0 gm | |
      | Acetic acid, 5 $N$ | 1 | liter |

2. Preparation
   a. Reagent A
      (1) Add 1 part glacial acetic acid to 2.5 parts distilled water. This is 5 $N$ acetic acid.
      (2) Dissolve sulfanilic acid in 5 $N$ acetic acid.
   b. Reagent B
      (1) Add 1 part glacial acetic acid to 2.5 parts distilled water. This is 5 $N$ acetic acid.
      (2) Dissolve $\alpha$-naphthylamine in 5 $N$ acetic acid.
3. Storage
   a. Room temperature in a brown bottle
4. Shelf life
   a. 30 days
5. Quality control
   a. Not necessary

## NITROGEN ASSIMILATION MEDIUM FOR YEASTS (AUXANOGRAPHIC)

1. Formulation

    | | |
    |---|---|
    | Yeast carbon base | 11.7 gm |
    | Noble agar | 20.0 gm |
    | Distilled water | 1 liter |

2. Preparation
    a. Mix reagents.
    b. Bring to a boil.
    c. Dispense 15.0-ml aliquots into 25 × 125 mm test tubes.
    d. Autoclave for 15 minutes at 15 psi.
    e. Stand the test tubes vertically.
3. Storage
    a. 4°C
4. Shelf life
    a. 30 days
5. Quality control
    a. Sterility
    b. Performance; not necessary prior to use
6. Comments

    The medium is melted and cooled to 50–52°C in a water bath prior to use.

## NUTRIENT AGARS FOR DERMATOPHYTES, CARBON STUDIES

1. Formulation
    a. Basal medium

        | | |
        |---|---|
        | Potassium phosphate | 1.0 gm |
        | Magnesium sulfate | 0.5 gm |
        | Ammonium sulfate | 5.0 gm |
        | Agar (Ion, Noble, or purified) | 15.0 gm |
        | Distilled water | 1 liter |

    b. Growth supplement

        | | |
        |---|---|
        | Thiamine | 1.0 mg |
        | Inositol | 250.0 mg |
        | Nicotinic acid | 10.0 mg |
        | Histidine | 150.0 mg |
        | Distilled water | 100.0 ml |

    c. Carbon sources

        | | |
        |---|---|
        | Carbon source (glucose, mannose, etc.) | 0.5 gm |
        | Distilled water | 100.0 ml |

2. Preparation
    a. Basal medium
        (1) Mix reagents.
        (2) Bring to a boil.
    b. Growth supplement
        (1) Mix reagents.
        (2) Add 20.0 ml to the 1 liter of basal medium.
    c. Dispense 80.0-ml aliquots into 125-ml flasks.
    d. Autoclave for 15 minutes at 15 psi.
    e. Add 20.0 ml of filter-sterilized carbon source to each 80.0 ml of basal medium.
    f. Dispense 7.0-ml aliquots into 16 × 125 mm test tubes.
    g. Slant the test tubes.
3. Storage
    a. 4°C
4. Shelf life
    a. 30 days in test tubes
    b. 14 days in Petri dishes
5. Quality control
    a. Sterility
    b. Performance

| Fungus | Incubation temperature | Result |
|---|---|---|
| *Candida guilliermondii*, *Cryptococcus laurentii*, and *Torulopsis inconspicua* | 25°C | Presence or absence of growth, depending upon the carbon source and the yeast |

6. Comments
    The various carbon sources are tested at a final concentration of 1%. The medium may also be dispensed in 20.0-ml aliquots into sterile Petri dishes. Petri dishes permit the testing of several isolates at once. Yeasts are used for quality control because of their rapid growth rate.

## NUTRITIONAL AGARS FOR *TRICHOPHYTON*

The media are commercially available from Difco Laboratories. The media are prepared according to the manufacturer's instructions. The media are dispensed in 7.0-ml aliquots into 16 × 125 mm test tubes. The media are stored at 4°C for 30 days. Performance is evaluated when a medium is used.

## OATMEAL AGAR FOR THE GYMNOASCACEAE

1. Formulation

   | | |
   |---|---|
   | Tomato paste (Hunt's) | 10.0 gm |
   | Oatmeal (Beech-Nut for babies) | 10.0 gm |
   | Magnesium sulfate | 1.0 gm |
   | Potassium phosphate | 1.0 gm |
   | Sodium nitrate | 1.0 gm |
   | Agar | 15.0 gm |
   | Distilled water | 1 liter |

2. Preparation
   a. Mix reagents.
   b. Bring to a boil.
   c. Cool, adjust pH to 5.6 with sodium hydroxide.
   d. Autoclave for 20 minutes at 15 psi.
   e. Dispense 20.0-ml aliquots into sterile Petri dishes.
   f. Allow to harden.
3. Storage
   a. 4°C
4. Shelf life
   a. 14 days
5. Quality control
   a. Sterility
   b. pH reaction approximately 5.6
   c. Performance; not necessary prior to use
6. Comments

   The medium is excellent for stimulating the formation of gymnothecia by members of the Gymnoascaceae. The medium is commonly used for the genera *Arthroderma* and *Nannizzia*.

## PEPTONE DISKS FOR YEASTS

1. Formulation

    | | |
    |---|---|
    | Peptone | 30.0 gm |
    | Distilled water | 1 liter |

2. Preparation
    a. Mix reagents.
    b. Autoclave for 15 minutes at 15 psi.
    c. Saturate 6-mm sterile sensitivity disks in the solution.
    d. Dry disks in a sterile Petri dish.
3. Storage
    a. 4°C
4. Shelf life
    a. Six months
5. Quality control
    a. Sterility
    b. Performance; not necessary prior to use

## PERIODIC ACID–SCHIFF STAIN REAGENTS

1. Formulation
   a. Periodic acid solution

   | | |
   |---|---|
   | Periodic acid | 5.0 gm |
   | Distilled water | 100.0 ml |

   b. Basic fuchsin solution

   | | |
   |---|---|
   | Basic fuchsin | 0.1 gm |
   | Ethanol, absolute | 5.0 ml |
   | Distilled water | 95.0 ml |

   c. Sodium metabisulfite solution

   | | |
   |---|---|
   | Sodium metabisulfite | 1.0 gm |
   | Hydrochloric acid, 1 $N$ | 10.0 ml |
   | Distilled water | 190.0 ml |

2. Preparation
   a. Periodic acid solution
      (1) Mix reagents in a brown bottle.
      (2) Tighten the cap.
   b. Basic fuchsin
      (1) Mix ethanol and distilled water in a brown bottle.
      (2) Add basic fuchsin, mix by rotating container.
      (3) Tighten the cap.
   c. Sodium metabisulfite
      (1) Add the HCl to the distilled water in a brown bottle.
      (2) Add sodium metabisulfite.
      (3) Tighten the cap.
3. Storage
   a. 4°C in a brown bottle
4. Shelf life
   a. Several days
   b. Discard reagents when the controls are no longer stained properly.
5. Quality control
   a. Not necessary
6. Comments
       The stock periodic acid powder is kept in a desiccator. The reagents are discarded when the controls no longer stain properly. The reagents are not tested prior to their use.

## PHOSPHATE BUFFER, 0.07 $M$ ($M/15$)

1. Formulation
   a. Solution A

   | | | |
   |---|---|---|
   | Disodium phosphate (anhydrous) | 9.47 gm | |
   | Distilled water | 1 | liter |

   b. Solution B

   | | | |
   |---|---|---|
   | Monopotassium phosphate | 9.07 gm | |
   | Distilled Water | 1 | liter |

2. Preparation
   a. Mix reagents separately to prepare solutions A and B. Use volumetric flasks.
   b. Mix 61.1 ml of solution A and 38.9 ml of solution B.
   c. pH should be 7.0, check with a pH meter.
   d. Autoclave for 15 minutes at 15 psi.
3. Storage
   a. 4°C
4. Shelf life
   a. 30 days
5. Quality control
   a. Sterility
   b. pH reaction of 7.0
   c. Performance; not necessary prior to use

## POLYVINYL ALCOHOL MOUNTING MEDIUM

1. Formulation

   | | |
   |---|---|
   | Polyvinyl alcohol granules (PVA) | 10.0 gm |
   | Lactic acid, 85% | 80.0 ml |
   | Distilled water | 20.0 ml |

2. Preparation
   a. Heat the PVA in the distilled water in a 55°C water bath. Stir frequently.
   b. Add lactic acid and transfer to a boiling water bath. Stir occasionally.
   c. Remove PVA when a clear syrup is obtained.
3. Storage
   a. Room temperature
4. Shelf life
   a. One to several years
5. Quality control
   a. Not necessary

## POTASSIUM HYDROXIDE SOLUTIONS

1. Formulation
   a. 10% KOH

   |  |  |
   |---|---|
   | Potassium hydroxide | 10.0 gm |
   | Distilled water | 100.0 ml |

   b. 10% KOH plus glycerol

   |  |  |
   |---|---|
   | Potassium hydroxide | 10.0 gm |
   | Glycerol | 20.0 ml |
   | Distilled water | 80.0 ml |

   c. 10% KOH plus DMSO

   |  |  |
   |---|---|
   | Potassium hydroxide | 10.0 gm |
   | Dimethyl sulfoxide (DMSO) | 40.0 ml |
   | Distilled water | 60.0 ml |

2. Preparation
   a. Mix reagents for solutions A and B.
   b. Mix the DMSO and the distilled water. Use a safety pipetting device and mix in a chemical fume hood.
   c. Add KOH to the DMSO.
3. Storage
   a. Room temperature
4. Shelf life
   a. Six months
5. Quality control
   a. Not necessary

## POTASSIUM NITRATE DISKS FOR YEASTS

1. Formulation

   | | |
   |---|---|
   | Potassium nitrate | 30.0 gm |
   | Distilled water | 1 liter |

2. Preparation
   a. Mix reagents.
   b. Autoclave for 15 minutes at 15 psi.
   c. Saturate 6 mm sterile sensitivity disks in the solution.
   d. Dry disks in a sterile Petri dish.
3. Storage
   a. 4°C
4. Shelf life
   a. Six months
5. Quality control
   a. Sterility
   b. Performance; not necessary prior to use

## POTATO DEXTROSE AGAR

1. Formulation

   | | |
   |---|---|
   | Potato infusion | 500.0 ml |
   | Glucose | 10.0 gm |
   | Agar | 15.0 gm |
   | Tap water | 1 liter |

2. Preparation
   a. Peel and dice 200.0 gm of old-crop potatoes.
   b. Add potatoes to 500.0 ml of tap water.
   c. Boil for 1 hour or cook in autoclave for 10 minutes at 15 psi.
   d. Filter through cheesecloth.
   e. Bring volume up to 500.0 ml with tap water.
   f. Add reagents to infusion.
   g. Bring to a boil.
   h. Dispense 7.0-ml aliquots into $16 \times 125$ mm test tubes.
   i. Autoclave for 15 minutes at 15 psi.
   j. Slant the test tubes.
3. Storage
   a. 4°C
4. Shelf life
   a. 30 days in test tubes
   b. 14 days in Petri dishes
5. Quality control
   a. Sterility
   b. Performance

   | Fungus | Incubation temperature | Result |
   |---|---|---|
   | *Aspergillus flavus* | 25°C | Good growth |

6. Comments

   Potato dextrose agar (PDA) is commercially available. "Homemade" PDA seems to be more ideal.

## POTATO SUCROSE OR DEXTROSE AGAR FOR *FUSARIUM*

1. Formulation

   | | |
   |---|---|
   | Potato infusion | 500.0 ml |
   | Sucrose or glucose | 20.0 gm |
   | Agar | 20.0 gm |
   | Distilled water | 1 liter |

2. Preparation
   a. Peel and dice 200.0 gm of old-crop potatoes.
   b. Add potatoes to 500.0 ml of distilled water.
   c. Boil for 1 hour or cook in autoclave for 10 minutes at 15 psi.
   d. Filter through cheesecloth.
   e. Bring volume up to 500.0 ml with distilled water.
   f. Add reagents to infusion.
   g. Bring to a boil.
   h. Dispense 7.0-ml aliquots into $16 \times 125$ mm test tubes.
   i. Autoclave for 15 minutes at 15 psi.
   j. Slant the test tubes.
3. Storage
   a. 4°C
4. Shelf life
   a. 30 days in test tubes
   b. 14 days in Petri dishes
5. Quality control
   a. Sterility
   b. Performance

   | Fungus | Incubation temperature | Result |
   |---|---|---|
   | *Fusarium solani* | 25°C | Good growth |

6. Comments
   The media can be sterilized and then dispensed in 15.0-ml aliquots into sterile Petri dishes. If additional plates are needed, slants can be melted and repoured into Petri dishes.

## RICE EXTRACT AGAR

This medium is commercially available and is prepared according to the manufacturer's instructions. Rice extract agar and rice extract agar supplemented with 1% Tween 80 are used to stimulate the formation of chlamydospores by *Candida albicans*. The medium is stored at 4°C for up to 14 days in Petri dishes.

## RICE GRAINS

1. Formulation

   | | |
   |---|---|
   | Unfortified white rice grains | 8.0 gm |
   | Distilled water | 25.0 ml |

2. Preparation
   a. Mix reagents in a 125-ml flask.
   b. Autoclave for 15 minutes at 15 psi.
3. Storage
   a. 4°C
4. Shelf life
   a. 30 days
5. Quality control
   a. Sterility
   b. Performance; not necessary prior to use

## SABHI AGAR

1. Formulation

   | | |
   |---|---|
   | Glucose | 21.0 gm |
   | Neopeptone | 5.0 gm |
   | Proteose peptone | 5.0 gm |
   | Calf brains, infusion | 100.0 gm |
   | Beef heart, infusion | 125.0 gm |
   | Sodium chloride | 2.5 gm |
   | Disodium phosphate | 1.25 gm |
   | Chloromycetin | 1.0 gm |
   | Agar | 15.0 gm |
   | Whole blood (human bank blood, outdated; sheep or fresh human) | approx. 100.0 ml |
   | Distilled water | 900.0 liter |

2. Preparation
   a. Mix reagents except chloromycetin and blood.
   b. Bring to a boil.
   c. Autoclave for 15 minutes at 15 psi.
   d. Cool to 50–52°C.
   e. Add chloromycetin to 10.0 ml of sterile distilled water.
   f. Add 0.4 ml of chloromycetin to the medium.
   g. Add whole blood to the medium.
   h. Dispense 15.0-ml aliquots into 25 × 125 mm test tubes.
   i. Slant the test tubes.
3. Storage
   a. 4°C
4. Shelf life
   a. 14 days
5. Quality control
   a. Sterility
   b. Performance

   | Fungus | Incubation temperature | Result |
   |---|---|---|
   | *Aspergillus flavus* | 25°C | Good growth |

6. Comments
   Sabhi can be manufactured without blood.

## SABOURAUD DEXTROSE AGAR

1. Formulation

   | | |
   |---|---|
   | Neopeptone | 10.0 gm |
   | Glucose | 20.0 gm |
   | Agar | 15.0 gm |
   | Distilled water | 1 liter |

2. Preparation
    a. Mix reagents.
    b. Bring to a boil.
    c. Dispense 7.0-ml aliquots into 16 × 125 mm test tubes.
    d. Autoclave for 10 minutes at 15 psi.
    e. Slant the test tubes.
3. Storage
    a. 4°C
4. Shelf life
    a. 30 days in test tubes
    b. 14 days in Petri dishes
5. Quality control
    a. Sterility
    b. Color
    c. Performance

    | Fungus | Incubation temperature | Result |
    |---|---|---|
    | *Aspergillus flavus* | 25°C | Good growth |

6. Comments
    The medium can also be dispensed in 15.0-ml aliquots into sterile Petri dishes. The glucose concentration can be increased to 40.0 gm per liter. This medium is recommended for studying the colonial morphology of dermatophytes. Sabouraud dextrose agar is commercially available and should be prepared according to the manufacturer's instructions.

## SABOURAUD DEXTROSE AGAR FOR DERMATOPHYTE MAINTENANCE

1. Formulation

    | | |
    |---|---|
    | Neopeptone | 10.0 gm |
    | Glucose | 20.0 gm |
    | Yeast extract | 5.0 gm |
    | Agar | 15.0 gm |
    | Distilled water | 1 liter |

2. Preparation
    a. Mix reagents.
    b. Bring to a boil.
    c. Dispense 7.0-ml aliquots into 16 × 125 mm test tubes.
    d. Autoclave for 10 minutes at 15 psi.
    e. Slant the test tubes.
3. Storage
    a. 4°C
4. Shelf life
    a. 30 days
5. Quality control
    a. Sterility
    b. Color
    c. Performance

| Fungus | Incubation temperature | Result |
|---|---|---|
| *Trichophyton mentagrophytes* | 25°C | Good growth |

## SABOURAUD DEXTROSE AGAR FOR DERMATOPHYTE SPORULATION

1. Formulation

   | | |
   |---|---|
   | Neopeptone | 2.5 gm |
   | Glucose | 5.0 gm |
   | Yeast extract | 1.25 gm |
   | Sodium chloride | 20.0 gm |
   | Agar | 20.0 gm |
   | Distilled water | 1 liter |

2. Preparation
   a. Mix reagents.
   b. Bring to a boil.
   c. Dispense 7.0-ml aliquots into 16 × 125 mm test tubes.
   d. Autoclave for 10 minutes at 15 psi.
   e. Slant the test tubes.
3. Storage
   a. 4°C
4. Shelf life
   a. 30 days in test tubes
   b. 14 days in Petri dishes
5. Quality control
   a. Sterility
   b. Color
   c. Performance

| Fungus | Incubation temperature | Result |
|---|---|---|
| *Trichophyton mentagrophytes* | 25°C | Good sporulation |

# SABOURAUD DEXTROSE AGAR WITH CYCLOHEXIMIDE AND CHLORAMPHENICOL, OR CHLORAMPHENICOL ALONE

1. Formulation

    | | |
    |---|---|
    | Peptone | 10.0 gm |
    | Glucose | 10.0 gm |
    | Cycloheximide | 0.5 gm |
    | Chloramphenicol | 0.05 gm |
    | Agar | 15.0 gm |
    | Distilled water | 1 liter |

2. Preparation
    a. Dissolve cycloheximide in 10.0 ml of acetone.
    b. Dissolve chloramphenicol in 10.0 ml of 95% ethanol.
    c. Mix reagents, cycloheximide, and chloramphenicol.
    d. Bring to a boil.
    e. Dispense in 7.0-ml aliquots into 16 × 125 mm test tubes.
    f. Autoclave for 10 minutes at 15 psi.
    g. Slant the test tubes.
3. Storage
    a. 4°C
4. Shelf life
    a. 30 days in test tubes
    b. 14 days in Petri dishes
5. Quality control
    a. Sterility
    b. Color
    c. Performance

    | Fungus | Incubation temperature | Result |
    |---|---|---|
    | *Trichophyton mentagrophytes* | 25°C | Good growth |
    | *Aspergillus flavus* | 25°C | No growth |

6. Comments
    Mycosel and Mycobiotic Agar are two commerically available media. They should be prepared according to the manufacturer's instructions. From a practical point, only the positive quality control organism is probably necessary. Sabouraud dextrose agar with chloramphenicol is prepared as above except that the cycloheximide is omitted.

## SABOURAUD DEXTROSE BROTH

1. Formulation

    | | |
    |---|---|
    | Neopeptone | 10.0 gm |
    | Glucose | 20.0 gm |
    | Distilled water | 1 liter |

2. Preparation
    a. Mix reagents.
    b. Dispense 7.0-ml aliquots into 16 × 125 mm test tubes.
    c. Autoclave for 10 minutes at 15 psi.
3. Storage
    a. 4°C
4. Shelf life
    a. 30 days
5. Quality control
    a. Sterility
    b. Color
    c. Performance

| Fungus | Incubation temperature | Result |
|---|---|---|
| *Candida albicans* | 25°C | Good growth |

## SODIUM CARBONATE FOR BLOOD CULTURES

1. Formulation

    | | |
    |---|---|
    | Sodium carbonate | 0.4 gm |
    | Distilled water | 500.0 ml |

2. Preparation
    a. Mix reagents.
    b. Dispense 50.0-ml aliquots into 125-ml flasks.
    c. Autoclave for 15 minutes at 15 psi.
3. Storage
    a. Room temperature
4. Shelf life
    a. 30 days
5. Quality control
    a. Sterility
    b. Performance; not necessary prior to use

## SOIL EXTRACT AGAR

1. Formulation

    | | |
    |---|---|
    | Soil | 500.0 gm |
    | Glucose | 2.0 gm |
    | Yeast extract | 1.0 gm |
    | Potassium phosphate | 0.5 gm |
    | Agar | 15.0 gm |
    | Tap water | 1 liter |

2. Preparation
    a. Mix 500.0 gm of garden soil and 1 liter of tap water.
    b. Autoclave for 3 hours at 15 psi.
    c. Filter through Whatman No. 2 filter paper. This is the soil infusion.
    d. Add reagents and bring volume up to 1 liter.
    e. Bring to a boil.
    f. Dispense 7.0-ml aliquots into 16 × 125 mm test tubes.
    g. Autoclave for 15 minutes at 15 psi.
    h. Slant the test tubes.
3. Storage
    a. 4°C
4. Shelf life
    a. 30 days in test tubes
    b. 14 days in Petri dishes
5. Quality control
    a. Sterility
    b. Performance

    | Fungus | Incubation temperature | Result |
    |---|---|---|
    | *Chrysosporium* sp. | 25°C | Good growth and production of conidia |

6. Comments

    Soil extract agar is excellent for maintaining *Histoplasma capsulatum* and *Blastomyces dermatitidis*. It is also excellent for stimulating the production of conidia. It can also be used to stimulate ascocarp development in *B. dermatitidis*.

## STARVATION MEDIUM FOR YEASTS

1. Formulation

    | | |
    |---|---|
    | Yeast nitrogen base | 0.67 gm |
    | Glucose | 0.1 gm |
    | Distilled water | 100.0 ml |

2. Preparation
    a. Mix reagents.
    b. Filter sterilize.
    c. Dispense 10.0-ml aliquots into 16 × 125 mm test tubes.
3. Storage
    a. 4°C
4. Shelf life
    a. 30 days
5. Quality control
    a. Sterility
    b. Performance; not necessary prior to use
6. Comments

    The above formulation results in a 1 × strength solution. This medium is used to starve yeasts for the Wickerham carbon assimilation tests.

## TRITON X-100 FOR BLOOD CULTURES

1. Formulation

    | | |
    |---|---|
    | Triton X-100 | 1.0 ml |
    | Distilled water | 500.0 ml |

2. Preparation
    a. Mix reagents.
    b. Dispense 50.0-ml aliquots into 125-ml flasks.
    c. Autoclave for 15 minutes at 15 psi.
3. Storage
    a. Room temperature
4. Shelf life
    a. 30 days
5. Quality control
    a. Sterility
    b. Performance; not necessary prior to use.

## VARIDASE FOR BLOOD CULTURES

Varidase is a commercially available enzyme preparation. It consists of streptokinase (5000 units)–streptodornase (1250 units). The preparation is prepared fresh with each use in a 1.5% concentration. The commercial preparation is maintained at 4°C.

## V-8 JUICE AGAR, 18%

1. Formulation

    | | |
    |---|---|
    | V-8 Juice | 180.0 ml |
    | Calcium carbonate | 2.0 gm |
    | Agar | 15.0 gm |
    | Distilled water | 805.0 ml |

2. Preparation
    a. Mix reagents.
    b. Bring to a boil.
    c. Dispense in 7.0-ml aliquots into 16 × 125 mm test tubes.
    d. Autoclave for 15 minutes at 15 psi.
    e. Slant the test tubes.
3. Storage
    a. 4°C
4. Shelf life
    a. 30 days
5. Quality control
    a. Sterility
    b. Performance

    | Fungus | Incubation temperature | Result |
    |---|---|---|
    | *Aspergillus fumigatus* | 25°C | Good growth |

6. Comments
    V-8 juice agar, 18%, is excellent for the stimulation of conidium production in the hyphomycetes. Colonies develop well without starvation. The medium is not recommended for pycnidium-forming fungi.

## V-8 JUICE FOR ASCOSPORES

1. Formulation

   | | |
   |---|---:|
   | V-8 Juice | 350.0 ml |
   | Compressed yeast | 5.0 gm |
   | Agar | 14.0 gm |
   | Distilled water | 340.0 ml |

2. Preparation
   a. Mix agar and distilled water.
   b. Bring to a boil.
   c. Mix V-8 juice and compressed yeast in a second flask.
   d. Adjust V-8 juice-yeast solution to pH 6.8.
   e. Heat for 10 minutes in flowing steam.
   f. Readjust pH to 6.8 when the solution is cool.
   g. Mix the agar and V-8 juice–yeast solutions.
   h. Dispense 7.0-ml aliquots into $16 \times 125$ mm test tubes.
   i. Autoclave for 15 minutes at 15 psi.
3. Storage
   a. 4°C
4. Shelf life
   a. 30 days
5. Quality control
   a. Sterility
   b. Performance

| Fungus | Incubation temperature | Result |
|---|:---:|---|
| *Saccharomyces cerevisiae* | 25°C | Production of asci and ascospores |

## WATER AGAR, 2%

1. Formulation

    | | | |
    |---|---|---|
    | Agar | 20.0 | gm |
    | Distilled water | 1 | liter |

2. Preparation
    a. Mix reagents.
    b. Bring to a boil.
    c. Dispense 15.0-ml aliquots into 25 × 125 mm test tubes.
    d. Autoclave for 15 minutes at 15 psi.
3. Storage
    a. 4°C
4. Shelf life
    a. 30 days in test tubes
    b. 14 days in Petri dishes
5. Quality control
    a. Sterility
    b. Performance; not necessary prior to use
6. Comments
    The water agar is melted and poured into sterile Petri dishes prior to use.

## WATER AGAR FOR SUSCEPTIBILITY TESTING, 2%

1. Formulation

    | | | |
    |---|---|---|
    | Noble agar | 20.0 | gm |
    | Distilled water | 1 | liter |

2. Preparation
    a. Mix the reagents.
    b. Bring to a boil.
    c. Dispense 27.5-ml aliquots into 25 × 150 mm screw-cap test tubes.
    d. Autoclave for 15 minutes at 15 psi.
    e. Stand test tubes upright.
3. Storage
    a. 4°C
4. Shelf life
    a. 30 days
5. Quality control
    a. Sterility
    b. Performance; not necessary prior to use
6. Comments
    The agar is melted and placed in a water bath at 50–52°C prior to use.

## YEAST EXTRACT–MALT EXTRACT (YM) AGAR

1. Formulation

   | | | |
   |---|---|---|
   | | Yeast extract | 3.0 gm |
   | | Malt extract | 3.0 gm |
   | | Peptone | 5.0 gm |
   | | Glucose | 10.0 gm |
   | | Agar | 15.0 gm |
   | | Distilled water | 1 liter |

2. Preparation
   a. Mix reagents.
   b. Bring to a boil.
   c. Dispense 7.0-ml aliquots into $16 \times 125$ mm test tubes.
   d. Autoclave for 15 minutes at 15 psi.
   e. Slant the test tubes.
3. Storage
   a. 4°C
4. Shelf life
   a. 30 days in test tubes
   b. 14 days in Petri dishes
5. Quality control
   a. Sterility
   b. Performance

   | Fungus | Incubation temperature | Result |
   |---|---|---|
   | *Saccharomyces cerevisiae* | 25°C | Good growth |

6. Comments
   The pH can be adjusted to 3.7 with dilute hydrochloric acid. Acidified YM agar or broth can be used to purify yeast cultures that have a bacterial contaminant.

## YEAST EXTRACT-PHOSPHATE AGAR

1. Formulation
   a. Solution A

   | | | |
   |---|---|---|
   | Yeast extract | 1.0 gm | |
   | Agar | 15.0 gm | |
   | Distilled water | 1 liter | |

   b. Solution B

   | | |
   |---|---|
   | Disodium phosphate, anhydrous | 4.0 gm |
   | Monopotassium phosphate | 6.0 gm |
   | Distilled water | 30.0 ml |

   c. Solution C

   | | |
   |---|---|
   | Ammonium hydroxide, concentrated | 1.0 ml |

2. Preparation
   a. Solution A
      (1) Mix reagents.
      (2) Bring solution to a boil.
   b. Solution B
      (1) Mix reagents.
      (2) Adjust pH to 6.0 with either 1 $N$ HCl or 1 $N$ NaOH.
   c. Add 2.0 ml of solution B to solution A.
   d. Autoclave for 15 minutes at 15 psi.
   e. Dispense into sterile Petri dishes (35 ml per dish).
3. Storage
   a. 4°C
4. Shelf life
   a. 14 days
5. Quality control
   a. Sterility
   b. pH reaction of 6.0
   c. Performance

   | Fungus | Incubation temperature | Result |
   |---|---|---|
   | *Blastomyces dermatitidis* | 25°C | Good growth |

6. Comments
   Approximately 0.1–0.5 ml of the contaminated specimen that has been concentrated is placed onto the medium. One drop (0.05 ml) of solution C is placed onto the medium surface away from the sediment. The ammonium hydroxide will diffuse throughout the medium. Cycloheximide cannot be incorporated into the medium because the ammonium hydroxide will inactivate it. Antibacterial agents such as chloramphenicol can be added to the medium.

## YEAST MORPHOLOGY AGAR

Yeast morphology agar is commercially available and is prepared according to the manufacturer's instructions. The prepared medium is stored at 4°C for 30 days in test tubes and 14 days in Petri dishes. Yeast morphology agar is used to study yeast morphology, to stimulate the production of asci and ascospores, and in susceptibility testing with 5-fluorocytosine. In the latter use, the medium is dispensed in 100.0-ml aliquots into 250-ml flasks.

| Fungus | Incubation temperature | Result |
|---|---|---|
| *Saccharomyces cerevisiae* | 30°C | Good growth |

## YEAST NITROGEN BASE, BUFFERED FOR SYNERGISM STUDIES

1. Formulation
   a. Yeast nitrogen base

   | | |
   |---|---|
   | Yeast nitrogen base | 6.7 gm |
   | L-Asparagine | 1.5 gm |
   | Glucose | 10.0 gm |
   | Distilled water | 100.0 ml |

   b. Buffer

   | | |
   |---|---|
   | Morpholinopropane sulfonic acid | 15.89 gm |
   | Tris-(hydroxymethyl)-aminomethane | 10.08 gm |
   | Distilled water | 100.0 ml |

2. Preparation
   a. Yeast nitrogen base
      (1) Mix reagents.
      (2) Sterilize by filtration.
   b. Buffer
      (1) Mix reagents.
      (2) Autoclave for 15 minutes at 15 psi.
      (3) Cool.
   c. Add 5.0 ml of buffer to the yeast nitrogen base.
3. Storage
   a. 4°C
4. Shelf life
   a. 30 days
5. Quality control
   a. Sterility
   b. Performance; not necessary prior to use

## YEAST NITROGEN BASE MEDIUM FOR 5-FLUOROCYTOSINE SUSCEPTIBILITY TESTING, BROTH

1. Formulation

    | | |
    |---|---|
    | L-Asparagine | 1.5 gm |
    | Glucose | 10.0 gm |
    | Yeast nitrogen base | 6.7 gm |
    | Distilled water | 100.0 ml |

2. Preparation
    a. Mix reagents.
    b. Sterilize by filtration.
3. Storage
    a. 4°C
4. Shelf life
    a. 30 days
5. Quality control
    a. Sterility
    b. Performance; not necessary prior to use
6. Comments

    The above formulation results in a 10 × strength solution. The solution can be heated slightly if all the reagents do not go into solution immediately.

# Glossary

A, an, apo: Used as a prefix to mean without.
Abscess: A localized accumulation of pus in a cavity resulting from the disintegration of tissue.
Abscission: Detachment of conidia from their conidiophores.
Abstriction: The cutting off of a portion of a hypha by fission through a double septum to form a conidium.
Acerose: Needle-shaped.
Acervulus (pl. acervuli): A tightly bound mat of hyphae giving rise to short, closely packed conidiophores. Fungi that produce acervuli are generally plant pathogens. The acervulus forms under the epidermis or cuticle of the plant, and is usually circular and of a constant size.
Achlorophyllous: Lacking chlorophyll.
Acicular: Needle-shaped.
Acid-fast: A cell wall property in which basic dyes are not removed from the cell wall by mineral acids during a staining reaction.
Acroauxic: Restricted in growth to the apical region.
Acrogenous: Developing at the apex of the conidiophore.
Acropetal: Produced toward the apex; with reference to a chain of conidia, the youngest conidium is at the tip and the oldest is at the base.
Acropleurogenous: Developing at the apex and along the sides.
Actinomycete: A filamentous Gram-positive bacterium.
Actinomycotic granule: A granule formed by an actinomycete.
Actinomycotic mycetoma: A mycetoma caused by an actinomycete.
Actinomycosis: An opportunistic bacterial infection caused by an actinomycete. The most frequent etiologic agent is *Actinomyces israelii*.
Aculeate: Spiny, pointed.
Acuminate: Gradually tapering to a point.
Acute: Sharp; in medicine, a short and severe course.
Acute suppurative inflammation: A pattern of inflammation characterized by vascular congestion, exudation of plasma proteins, and accumulations of polymorphonuclear leukocytes. Implies a short temporal course.
Additive: Having a combined effect equal to the sum of the individual effects.
Adenopathy: Enlargement of glands, especially lymphatic glands.
Adiaspore: A large, globose, thick-walled cell in the lungs of animals and man that resulted from the inhalation and subsequent enlargement of a conidium produced by *Chrysosporium parvum*. These structures are produced *in vitro* under the appropriate conditions.

Adnate: Broadly attached.
Aerial hyphae: Hyphae above the nutrient agar surface.
Aerobic: Being able to grow in the presence of molecular oxygen.
Aleurioconidium (pl. aleurioconidia): A thallic conidium that develops as an expanded end of an undifferentiated hypha or on a short pedicel and is released by rupture of the supporting cell. The term has been applied to a number of different structures and is therefore not recommended for describing conidia.
Aleuriospore: *See* Aleurioconidium.
Aliquot: A portion.
Allantoid: Slightly curved and rounded at the ends, sausage-shaped.
Allele: One of two or more genes that occupy corresponding loci on homologous chromosomes.
Allergen: A substance capable of inducing a specific hypersensitivity.
Allergic: Possessing hypersensitivity to a particular allergen.
Alopecia: Loss of hair.
Alternate: Made up of a succession of arthroconidia and vegetative cells. Approximately one half of the cells of the parent hypha become arthroconidia while the remaining vegetative cells degenerate, resulting in an alternation of arthoconidia and disjunctor cells.
Alternate arthroconidium: An arthroconidium separated by disjunctor cells and released by their rupture.
Alveolate: Pitted, honeycomb-like.
Ameroconidium (pl. ameroconidia): One-celled conidium.
Amerospore: One-celled spore.
Amphigenous: Developing on all sides.
Amphipathic: Having both hydrophilic and hydrophobic properties.
Ampulla (pl. ampullae): A swollen conidiogenous cell with a number of points or areas from which conidia will develop. In most instances, conidium development is synchronized.
Ampulliform: Flask-shaped.
Anaerobic: Being able to grow in the absence of molecular oxygen.
Anamorph: An asexual or somatic reproductive structure, specialized or generalized, but neither morphologically nor karyologically sexual.
Anastomosis (pl. anastomoses): Fusion between two hyphae, like a bridge.
Angular: Not rounded, with abrupt angles.
Annellate: Having annellations.
Annellation: A ring of outer cell wall material remaining at the apex of an annellide that resulted from the release of an annelloconidium.
Annellide: A percurrent, indeterminate conidiogenous cell in which the first conidium is holoblastic and each successive conidium is enteroblastic. As each basipetally formed conidium is released, a ring of outer cell wall material remains at the tip of the annellide forming an annellation.
Annellidic: Pertaining to an annellide, a type of conidium development.
Annelloconidium (pl. annelloconidia): A conidium produced from an annellide.
Annellophore: A specialized hypha upon which an annellide develops.
Annular frill: Skirtlike remanent of cell wall material at the base of a conidium.
Annulate: With a ring.
Antagonism: An increase, twofold or greater, in the MIC of one drug in the presence of an otherwise subinhibitory concentration of a second drug.
Anterior: At the front.
Antheridium (pl. antheridia): A male gametangium.
Anthropophilic: Preferring man.

# Glossary

Antibody: An immunoglobulin that interacts only with the antigen that induced its formation.
Antigen: Any substance that is capable of inducing the synthesis of antibodies.
Antimicrobic: An agent that suppresses the growth of, or kills, a microorganism.
Apedicellate: Without a pedicel.
Apex (pl. apices): The tip.
Apical: Pertaining to the apex.
Apiculate: Having a short projection at one or both ends.
Apiculus: A short projection at the end of a conidium or spore.
Apophysis: A swelling. The term is primarily applied to the swelling of a sporangiophore immediately below the columella.
Apothecium (pl. apothecia): A flat to cup-shaped open ascocarp. The asci are in a hymenium.
Appendage: An outgrowth.
Appendiculate: Having one or more appendages.
Appressed: Lying flat.
Appressorium (pl. appressoria): A flattened hyphal organ from which a small peg (infection peg) develops and subsequently penetrates a host's epidermal cell.
Arachnoid: Cobweb-like.
Arcuate: Moderately curved.
Area: A space or spot.
Arthric: Developing by the conversion and subsequent disarticulation of a determinate conidiogenous hypha. *See* Thallic-arthric.
Arthroaleurie: *See* Alternate arthroconidium.
Arthroconidium (pl. arthroconidia): A thallic conidium that is released by fission through a double septum or fragmentation/lysis of a disjunctor cell.
Arthrospore: *See* Arthroconidium.
Articulate: Jointed.
Ascocarp: A complex fruiting body containing asci. The sterile tissue of the ascocarp is haploid.
Ascogenous hypha: A specialized hypha from which one or more asci are produced.
Ascogonium (pl. ascogonia): A female gametangium produced by an ascomycete.
Ascoma (pl. ascomata): *See* Ascocarp.
Ascomycetes: A group of fungi that produce asci.
Ascospore: A haploid spore produced within an ascus following karyogamy and meiosis.
Ascostroma (pl. ascostromata): An ascocarp characterized by cavities or locules resulting from compression of surrounding tissue or lysis in the fruiting body prior to ascus formation. Bitunicate asci typically occur individually or in clusters.
Ascus (pl. asci): A saclike structure containing ascospores that were formed as a result of karyogamy and meiosis. Asci are characteristic of the Ascomycetes.
Ascus mother cell: The hook cell (or other dikaryotic cell) at the tip of an ascogenous hypha in which karyogamy occurs.
Aseptate: Lacking septa.
Asexual reproduction: Development by mitosis.
Aspergillosis: An infection of man or lower animals caused by a member of the genus *Aspergillus*.
Asperulate: Slightly roughened
Assimilation: The ability to use a carbon or nitrogen source for growth with oxygen serving as the final electron acceptor. Assimilation is read as the presence or the absence of growth.

Asteroid: Starlike, radiant.
Asteroid body: A globose to oval basophilic staining yeast cell in tissue surrounded by a eosinophilic covering approximately 10 $\mu$m thick consisting of a precipitated antibody–antigen complex.
Asymmetrical: With reference to conidia or spores, flattened on one side; not symmetrical.
Atypical: Abnormal.
Author: In nomenclature, the person to whom the publication or name is credited.
Autotroph: A microorganism that can grow without utilizing organic substrates as an energy source.
Auxanographic technique: A method for determining the ability of yeasts to utilize various carbon and nitrogen sources for growth. The technique consists of placing the carbon or nitrogen source directly onto the surface of a solid medium seeded with the yeast to be evaluated.
Azygospore: A body resembling a zygospore that was formed without the fusion of gametangia.
Bacillate: Rod-shaped.
Ballistoconidium (pl. ballistoconidia): A conidium that is forcibly discharged.
Ballistospore: A spore that is forcibly discharged.
Balloon form: An enlarged, globose conidium that resembles a balloon in shape.
Basal tuft: A cluster of asci or conidiophores in the bottom of a fruiting body.
Basauxic: Restricted in growth to the base.
Basidiocarp: A fruiting body that produces basidia.
Basidioma (pl. basidiomata): See Basidiocarp.
Basidiomycetes: A group of fungi that produce basidia.
Basidiospore: A haploid spore produced on a basidium following karyogamy and meiosis.
Basidium: A cell upon which basidiospores form as a result of karyogamy and meiosis. Basidia are characteristic of the Basidiomycetes.
Basipetal: Produced toward the base; with reference to a chain of conidia, the oldest conidium is at the apex and the youngest is at the base.
Beak: An elongated tip.
Biconic: With reference to conidia, shaped like two cones attached to each other at their bases.
Biflagellate: Having two flagella.
Bifurcate: Forking in twos.
Binomial: The scientific name of an organism consisting of a genus name and a species epithet.
Biopsy: The removal and examination of tissue in order to make a precise diagnosis.
Bipolar budding: Developing at the opposite poles of the parent cell.
Bipolar heterothallism: A genetic incompatiblity system involving a single locus.
Biseriate: With reference to the genus *Aspergillus*, phialides arising from metulae; in two series or rows.
Bitunicate: Having two walls.
Bivalvate: With reference to conidia, lens-shaped with a hyaline rim.
Biverticillate: With reference to the genus *Penicillium*, with two or rarely three levels of branching directly below the phialides.
Biverticillate asymmetrical: With reference to the genus *Penicillium*, having biverticillate branching not regularly and evenly spaced about the central axis of the conidiophore; one-sided.
Biverticillate symmetrical: With reference to the genus *Penicillium*, having biverticillate branching regularly and evenly spaced about the central axis of the conidiophore; symmetrical.

# Glossary

Black yeast: A dematiaceous fungus that produces a conspicuous unicellular budding form resulting in a black pasty colony.
Blastic: Involving a conidium in which the conidium initial enlarges as *de novo* growth and then becomes differentiated from its parent cell by a septum. The conidium results from part of the parent cell.
Blastoconidia (sing. blastoconidium): Holoblastic conidia that are produced solitarily, synchronously, or in acrogenous chains. Blastoconidia are typically released by fission through double septa.
Blastomycosis: An infection of man and lower animals caused by *Blastomyces dermatitidis*. The term has been misapplied by some mycologists to describe any infection caused by a yeast.
Blastospore: *See* Blastoconidia.
Botryoaleuriospore: *See* Botryoconidium.
Botryoblastoconidia (sing. botryoblastoconidium): Blastoconidia that developed synchronously from an ampulla.
Botryoblastospore: *See* Botryoblastoconidia.
Botryoconidium (pl. botryoconidia): A conidium in an apical cluster that developed successively and basipetally from a conidiogenous cell.
Botryose: In a cluster, like grapes.
Branch: A specialized hypha upon which metulae arise in the penicillia. The branches originate at the apex of an erect conidiophore.
Bud: A young conidium. Usually used to denote the young blastoconidia of yeasts.
Budding: Asexual multiplication by the production of a small outgrowth or bud from a parent cell.
Byssoid: Composed of delicate hyphae.
Caducous: Deciduous.
Caespitose: In dense groups or tufts.
Calyciform: Cup-shaped.
Candidiasis: An infection of man and lower animals caused by a member of the genus *Candida*. Both the terms candidiasis and candidosis are etymologically correct. Owing to common usage, candidiasis is the preferred term.
Candidosis: *See* Candidiasis.
Capitate: In heads.
Capsule: A hyaline gelatinous sheath surrounding a cell.
Carotenoid: An orange, red, or yellow pigmented polyisoprenoid lipid.
Carry-over: A condition in which stored nutrients in yeast cell, carried-over carbon and nitrogen compounds from the original culture medium, or both result in background growth during assimilation tests.
Catenate: *See* Catenulate.
Catenulate: In chains.
Caudate: Having a tail at the base.
Cell: Any unit, conidium, or spore that is separated from its neighbors, usually by a wall or septum.
Cell wall: The wall enclosing a cell. In fungi it consists of a complex network of fibrils with the spaces filled by polymers.
Cellulose: A carbohydrate with the formula $(C_6H_{10}O_5)_n$.
Centrum: The central area of a fruiting body.
Cerebriform: Having brainlike folds.
Cespitose: *See* Caespitose.
Chancre: A primary papular lesion.
Channel: A secondarily induced pore in the outer wall of a conidiogenous cell that is usually thick and darkly pigmented.

Chemotherapy: The treatment of a disease with chemical agents.
Chitin: A linear molecule consisting of $\beta$-1, 4 linked $N$-acetylglucosamine residues; a major component of most fungal cell walls.
Chlamydospore: A thallic conidium that becomes rounded and enlarged with an increase in cell wall thickness and protoplasm density. Chlamydospores are released by the disintegration of the surrounding cells. In essence, they are survival or resting conidia. This term has been misapplied to the enlarged cells produced by *Candida albicans* and some similar yeasts. The "chlamydospore" of *C. albicans* is a thick-walled vesicle, since it neither germinates nor produces conidia when mature.
Chromoblastomycosis: A mycotic infection of the cutaneous and subcutaneous tissues characterized by the development in tissue of dematiaceous sclerotic bodies.
Chromomycosis: An ambiguous term that encompasses two different diseases. See Chromoblastomycosis and Phaeohyphomycosis.
Chronic: Lasting a long period of time.
Chronic inflammation: A pattern of inflammation marked by fibrous tissue proliferation (scarring) and accumulations of mononuclear cells (lymphocytes, histiocytes, and plasma cells). It implies a long temporal course.
Cicatrized: Having scars.
Circinate: Coiled.
Cirrhus (pl. cirrhi): A ribbonlike mass of conidia or spores held together by mucus flowing from an ostiole.
Clamp connection: A specialized hyphal-bridge found in some Basidiomycetes that permits the simultaneous mitosis of two nuclei to occur in such a position that dikaryons ($n + n$) of compatible nuclei are duplicated.
Clavate: Club-shaped; swollen at the distal end.
Clavulate: Somewhat club-shaped.
Cleistothecium (pl. cleistothecia): A completely enclosed ascocarp characterized by a distinct peridium and usually with randomly dispersed asci. Cleistothecia are typically round and nonostiolate. A cleistothecium may also be defined as containing randomly dispersed asci, a hymenium, or a basal bush of asci.
Coccidioidomycosis: An infection of man and lower animals caused by *Coccidioides immitis*.
Coenocytic: Having a cell, an individual hypha, or other structural unit containing numerous nuclei.
Coil: *See* Spiral.
Coin lesion: A small, globose, calcified pulmonary lesion.
Collapsed: Sunken.
Collarette: A small collar. A collar of cell wall remnants at the tip of a phialide, which resulted from the rupture of the tip during the release of the first phialoconidium.
Colony: A fungus growing from a single point and forming a thallus.
Columella (pl. columellae): A sterile domelike structure at the tip of a sporangiophore or within a sporocarp or sporangium.
Columnar: Forming a column.
Concave: Hollowed.
Concrescent: Growing together.
Conic: Cone-shaped.
Conidial: Referring to conidia.
Conidial state: An anamorph or asexual stage in the development of a fungus characterized by the formation of conidia.
Conidiogenous: Giving rise to conidia.
Conidiogenous cell: A cell that produces conidia.

# Glossary

Conidiogenous locus (pl. conidiogenous loci): Any point, area, or zone where conidia arise from a conidiogenous cell.
Conidioma (pl. conidiomata): A specialized, multihyphal, conidium-bearing structure. Conidiomata is a general term that includes acervuli, pycnidia, sporodochia, and synnemata.
Conidiophore: A specialized hypha upon which conidia develop.
Conidiospore (in part): See Conidium.
Conidium (pl. conidia): An asexual, usually deciduous, nonmotile propagule that forms in any manner other than by cytoplasmic cleavage, free-cell formation, or conjugation. Ascospores, basidiospores, sporangiospores, zoospores, and zygospores are not considered to be conidia.
Conidium initial: The cell or portion of a cell from which the conidium will originate.
Conjugation: Copulation or fusion of sexual elements.
Connective: The trace of cell wall material between conidia.
Conspicuous: Prominent, obvious.
Copulation: Fusion of two sex cells.
Convolute: Folded, coiled.
Coremium (pl. coremia): See Synnema. Sometimes used for a loosely bound synnema.
Coriaceous: Leathery.
Cottony: See Floccose. Having aerial hyphae that are loose and coarse.
Crateriform: Hollowed out.
Crosswall: A septum, partition.
Crozier: The hook at the tip of an ascogenous hypha.
Cryptococcosis: An infection of man and lower animals caused by *Cryptococcus neoformans*.
Cutaneous: Pertaining to the skin.
Cylindrical: Cylindric, having parallel walls and circular cross-section.
Deciduous: Separating at maturity.
Deliquescent: Dissolving or becoming fluid at maturity.
Dematiaceous: Having conidia, spores, or hyphae that are brown to black.
Denticle: A small projection or peg.
Denticulate: Bearing denticles.
Dendritic: Treelike with irregular branching.
Dermatophyte: A fungus belonging to the genera *Epidermophyton, Microsporum,* or *Trichophyton* with the ability to infect hair, nail, skin.
Dermatitis: Inflammation of the skin.
Determinate: Involving conidiophores or conidiogenous cells in which growth permanently ceases at or just before the occurrence of conidiogenesis.
Deuteromycetes: See Fungi Imperfecti.
Diagnosis: In nomenclature, a statement by an author which in his or her opinion distinguishes the taxonomic group from all others.
Dichotomous: Branching into two more or less equal branches.
Dictyoconidium (pl. dictyoconidia): A conidium with vertical and horizontal septa; a muriform conidium.
Dictyospore: A spore with vertical and horizontal septa; a muriform spore.
Didymoconidium (pl. didymoconidia): A two-celled conidium.
Didymospore: A two-celled spore.
Diffluent: Readily dissolving.
Dikaryon: Two closely associated nuclei that were probably derived from different parent cells and which divide simultaneously.

Dikaryotic: Having two closely associated nuclei behaving as one but not fused, $n + n$ number of chromosomes.

Dimorphic: Having two morphological forms. The term is commonly used to describe those fungi that grow as a mould at room temperature and either a yeast or spherule in tissue, depending upon the species of fungus.

Diploid: Containing the $2n$ number of chromosomes.

Diplophase: That part of the life cycle in which the cells are diploid.

Discrete: Separate, distinct.

Discrete conidiogenous cell: With a distinct shape, different from the vegetative cells.

Disjunctor cell: An empty cell that fragments, undergoes lysis, or both thereby releasing a conidium.

Dissemination: Distribution in a wide area.

Distorted: Twisted out of shape.

Divaricate: Branching at a 90° angle.

Divergent: Separating, going apart.

Dolioform: Barrel-shaped.

Dolipore septum (pl. dolipore septa): A septum found in the Basidiomycetes that expands or flares out in the middle of the septum.

Double septum: A septum that consists of two layers of wall material with a very thin zone between them where separation by lytic enzyme activity will eventually occur.

Downy: Having a short and dense mycelial texture.

Dubious: Doubtful.

Dysgonic: Slowly growing variant.

Eccentric: Away from the center.

Echinulate: Delicately spiny.

Ectothrix: Natural hair invasion by a dermatophyte characterized by arthroconidia on the outside and mycelium within the hair shaft. The cuticle of the hair is destroyed.

Effuse: Spread out, radiate.

Ellipsoid: With reference to conidia and spores, more or less elliptical when viewing the conidium or spore through its longer axis.

Elliptical: Oval, with symmetric curve.

Elongate: Lengthened.

Encapsulated: Having a capsule.

Endemic: Peculiar to a particular geographic area or locality.

Endoarthroconidium (pl. endoarthroconidia): *See* Alternate arthroconidium.

Endoconidiophore: *See* Phialide.

Endoconidium (pl. endoconidia): A phialoconidium produced within an elongated tubular phialide. Endoconidium may also refer to a conidium produced within a hypha.

Endogenous: Originating from within.

Endogenous oculomycosis: An infection of the eye resulting from dissemination of the etiologic agent from another body site.

Endospore: A spore produced within a spherule. In reality, endospores are sporangiospores. The term is maintained for a specific reproductive propagule in tissue.

Endothrix: Natural hair invasion by a dermatophyte characterized by the development of arthroconidia within the hair shaft only. The cuticle of the hair remains intact.

Enteroarthric: Involving only the inner cell wall layer(s) in thallic-arthric conidium development. The outer wall usually separates from the newly formed wall of the endogenous conidium.

Enteroblastic: Involving only the inner cell wall layer(s) of the conidiogenous cell in blastic conidium development.

Epigean: On the ground.

Erect: Upright.
Etiologic: Pertaining to the cause(s) of the disease.
Eukaryotic: Having a highly organized nucleus bounded by a nuclear membrane.
Eumycotic granule: A granule produced by a fungus.
Eumycotic mycetoma: A mycetoma caused by a true fungus.
Evanescent: Disappearing.
Exoconidium (pl. exoconidia): A conidium formed on the surface of a hypha.
Exogenous: With reference to conidiogenous cells, a condition in which the contents of the conidiogenous cell protrude beyond an opening, from which the conidium develops.
Extension oculomycosis: A special form of rhinocerebral zygomycosis with the etiologic agent usually extending from the nasal area to the orbit of the eye.
Exudate: With reference to colonies, droplets of fluids that may be of various colors formed at the surface of the colony.
Falcate: Curved like a sickle.
Fascicle: A bundle of hyphae.
Fasciculate: Having a mealy, rough, or granular margin; having a cluster of elongate ascospores in an ascus.
Favic chandelier: A swollen and rapidly branching hyphal apex that looks like a chandelier or the horns of an elk. Produced by many of the dermatophytes, especially *Trichophyton schoenleinii*.
Favus: A form of tinea capitis characterized by the development of scutula.
Fixed: Having sites on a hypha that give rise to conidia that remain in one place. Each site may give rise to more than one conidium.
Fermentation: The ability of a fungus to use a carbon source for growth with organic compounds serving as the electron donor and acceptor. Fermentation is read as the production of gas.
Fertile: Bearing or producing conidia, spores, or both.
Filament: Thread, a hypha.
Filamentous: Having filaments.
Filiform: Threadlike.
Fission: With reference to conidium release, the breakdown of the thin layer between the two thickened cell-wall layers of a double septum, resulting in the separation of the two cells; to split one cell into two cells.
Fistula: An abnormal tubular connection between two points.
Flagellum (pl. flagella): A whiplike structure used for motility.
Flexuous: Wavy.
Floccose: Having a cottony mass of hyphae over the surface of a nutrient agar with the conidiophores appearing as branches from these aerial hyphae; cottony.
Foot cell: The basal area of the conidiophore of *Aspergillus* where it merges with the hypha giving the impression of a foot (heel and toes). The base of the phialoconidium of *Fusarium* is also referred to as a foot cell.
Form–genus (pl. form–genera): A genus formed on the basis of asexual morphological, physiological characteristics, or both, to accommodate a group of similar fungi (i.e., form–species). Form–genera do not imply phylogenetic relationships. The term was originally coined for fossils, but it is used for the Fungi Imperfecti too.
Form–species: An artificial species formed on the basis of asexual morphological, physiological characteristics, or both, to accommodate a group of similar individuals. Form–species do not imply phylogenetic relationships. The term was originally coined for fossils, but it is used for the Fungi Imperfecti too.
Formae speciales: A group of physiological strains within a species that are morphologically indistinguishable; abbrev. f. sp.

Fracture: The rupture or breakage of the cell wall at some point other than at a septum.
Fragmentation: The separation of a hypha into a number of conidia.
Free-cell formation: The process in an ascus by which a portion of the cytoplasm in the ascus surrounds each haploid nucleus and then becomes enveloped by a cell wall resulting in an ascospore.
Fruiting body: A large and complex fungal structure that gives rise to conidia or spores.
Fungi Imperfecti: Those fungi that apparently lack the ability to reproduce by sexual means. In some instances, teleomorphs are discovered and the fungus is then classified in the Ascomycetes or Basidiomycetes. The term Fungi Imperfecti is preferred over the division name Deuteromycota, as the latter name implies equal taxonomic status to the divisions based upon sexual reproduction.
Fungus (pl. fungi): An achlorophyllous, eukaryotic, unicellular to filamentous organism that usually reproduces by both sexual and asexual means. Fungi are susceptible to antimycotic agents, but not generally to antibacterial agents.
Fuseaux: A French term for macroconidia.
Fusiform: Spindle-shaped, tapering toward the end.
Gametangial contact: Sexual reproduction involving two gametangia coming into contact with each other without fusion. The male gamete migrates through a pore or tube into the female gametangium.
Gametangial copulation: Sexual reproduction by fusion of two gametangia giving rise to a zygote or dikaryon.
Gametangium (pl. gametangia): A cell that contains gametes or functions in place of a gamete.
Gamete: A sex cell or sex nucleus that will fuse with a compatible sex cell or sex nucleus during sexual reproduction.
Gangliospore: An older term for a holoblastic conidium.
Gemma (pl. gemmae): Chlamydospore-like cell produced by some of the Zygomycetes.
Geniculate: Bent like a knee.
Genus (pl. genera): A taxonomic grouping usually consisting of several species.
Geophilic: Growing in the soil.
Germ pore: A thin circular area in the conidium or spore wall through which germination occurs.
Germ slit: A thin area in the wall of the conidium or spore that transgresses the length of the conidium or spore, through which germination occurs.
Germ tube: The initial hypha that develops from a conidium or spore.
Giant cell: *See* Gemma.
Glabrous: Smooth.
Globose: Round.
Gloeoid ball: A mass of conidia held together by a mucuslike material resulting in a ball-like cluster of conidia.
Granular: Coarse.
Granule: An organized mass of hyphae or actinomycetous filaments with or without a crystalline matrix in a mycetoma.
Granuloma: A mass or nodule of granulation tissue.
Granulomatous inflammation: A distinctive pattern of tissue reaction manifested by collections of modified histiocytes (epithelioid cells) surrounded by or mixed with mononuclear cells, primarily lymphocytes and plasma cells. Often the area of inflammation contains Langhan's or foreign body-type giant cells.
Gregarious: Densely aggregated.
Gummatous: Having a soft, gummy tumor.
Guttulate: Containing one or more oil droplets.

Gymnothecium (pl. gymnothecia): A cleistothecium-like ascocarp in which the peridial hyphae are extremely loosely organized and the asci are randomly distributed within the ascocarp. Gymnothecia are usually round and nonostiolate and are associated with the Gymnoascaceae.
Habitat: Ecological niche where a fungus normally lives and grows.
Haploid: Having the reduced, or $n$ number of chromosomes.
Haplophase: That part of the life cycle of a fungus in which the cells are haploid.
Haustorium (pl. haustoria): A modified intracellular hypha which absorbs nutrients from a host cell.
Helicoconidium (pl. helicoconidia): A curved or spiral-shaped conidium.
Helicospore: A curved or spiral-shaped spore.
Hemispheric: Half of a sphere.
Heterogametangium (pl. heterogametangia): A gametangium of one "sex" that is morphologically distinguishable from a gametangium of the opposite "sex."
Heterogeneous: Different from each other.
Heterokaryotic: Involving the association of genetically different nuclei within the same cell.
Heterothallic: Self-sterile and requiring two compatible thalli for sexual reproduction to occur.
Heterotrophic: Requiring organic compounds as an energy source.
Heterozygous: Having different alleles at a particular locus.
Hilum: A scar at the base of a conidium.
Hirsute: Hairy.
Histoplasmosis capsulati: An infection of man and lower animals caused by *Histoplasma capsulatum* var. *capsulatum*, characterized by pulmonary involvement and the presence of small yeast cells in macrophages.
Histoplasmosis duboisii: An infection of man and lower animals caused by *Histoplasma capsulatum* var. *duboisii*, characterized by cutaneous and subcutaneous tissue involvement and the development of large yeast cells in macrophages.
Holoarthric: Involving all the cell wall layers in thallic-arthric conidium development.
Holoblastic: Involving all the cell wall layers of the conidiogenous cell in blastic conidium development.
Holomorph: The whole fungus.
Holothallic: Involving all the cell wall layers of the conidiogenous or sporogenous cell in thallic development.
Holotype: In nomenclature, the one specimen or element used by the author or designated by him as the nomenclatural type.
Homogeneous: Having parts of one kind, uniform.
Homogenous: Having the same origin.
Homonym: In nomenclature, an identical name.
Homothallic: Being self-compatible; sexual reproduction can take place with one thallus.
Hülle (also spelled Hüllen) cells: Extremely thickened large sterile cells with a small lumen that are usually associated with cleistothecia produced by members of the Eurotiaceae.
Hyaline: Colorless.
Hyalo-: A prefix meaning hyaline to lightly colored.
Hymenium (pl. hymenia): A layer or zone of asci, basidia, or conidiophores.
Hyperplasia: Abnormal multiplication of cells.
Hypha (pl. hyphae): A single filament of a fungus.
Hyphal body: A hyphal fragment found in the Entomophthorales.
Hyphopodium (pl. hyphopodia): An appressorium of constant size and shape.

Hypogean: Under the ground.
Imbricate: Having an overlapping regular pattern.
Immature: Lacking complete growth.
Immersed: Growing within, such as within the nutrient agar.
Immunity: Protection against a particular disease.
Imperfect state: An anamorph or asexual stage of development characterized by a specific form(s) of conidia or spores.
Incompatible: Not combining.
Indeterminate: Involving conidiophores or conidiogenous cells in which growth continues to occur during or between the development of successive conidia. *See also* Proliferous.
Inflammation: Following injury or tissue destruction, a local protective response of the body (mainly leukocytes) to destroy, dilute, or wall off the etiologic agent and injured tissue.
Inoperculate: Without a cap or lid.
Inordinate: Random.
Integrated: With reference to conidiogenous cells, incorporated into the main axis of the conidiophore.
Integrated conidiogenous cell: A conidiogenous cell that is incorporated within the main axis or branch of a conidiophore, either in a terminal or intercalary position.
Intercalary: Within a hyphal element.
Intercellular: Between cells.
Internode: Between nodes.
Interstitial: Between spaces in a tissue.
Intertriginous: Occurring on apposed skin surfaces.
Intracellular: Within cells.
Intrahyphal hypha: A hypha that is within the walls of a preexisting hypha.
Ischemic: Pertaining to a deficiency of blood, in part due obstruction of a blood vessel.
Isogametangium (pl. isogametangia): A gametangium of one "sex" that is morphologically indistinguishable from a gametangium of the opposite "sex."
Isthmus: A connection or short neck.
Karyogamy: The fusion of two nuclei.
Keratin: A scleroprotein containing large amounts of sulfur, such as cystine.
Keratinophilic: Preferring keratin.
Keratitis: Inflammation of the cornea.
Kerion: A severe pustular inflammation involving the hair follicles.
Lageniform: Flask-shaped.
Lanceolate: Lance-shaped.
Lanose: With reference to colony texture, woolly. A tufted appearance with conidiophores arising from the aerial hyphae.
Lateral: Along a side.
Lectotype: In nomenclature, a type selected from the original material upon which the taxonomic group was based. A lectotype is selected when a holotype was not designated, or when the holotype has been lost or destroyed.
Lenticular: Double convex.
Lentiform: Lens-shaped.
Lignicolous: Wood inhabiting.
Limoniform: Lemon-shaped.
Lobomycosis: A chronic cutaneous infection of man and lower animals caused by *Loboa loboi*.
Lobulate: Having lobes.
Localized: Within a small area.

# Glossary

Locule: A cavity within an ascostroma.
Loose: Loosely bound together.
Lunate: Crescent-shaped.
Lysis: Dissolution of a cell wall.
Macro-: A prefix meaning large.
Macroconidium (pl. macroconidia): The larger of two different sizes of conidia produced by a fungus in the same manner.
Macronematous: Having a conidiophore that is morphologically different from the vegetative hyphae.
Macula (pl. maculae): An area distinguished by color from its surrounding area.
Megaspore: A term used by Sabouraud for large-spored ectothrix hair invasion.
Meiosis: The process of nuclear reduction division resulting in haploid nuclei.
Membranous: Membranelike, thin.
Meristem: The site where growth occurs.
Meristematic: Having growth.
Merosporangium (pl. merosporangia): A cylindrical sporangium with the sporangiospores aligned in a row.
Metula (pl. metulae): A sterile branch below the phialides of *Aspergillus* (biseriate only) and *Penicillium* (bi- and polyverticillate only) species.
Micro-: A prefix meaning small.
Microconidium (pl. microconidia): The smaller of two different sizes of conidia produced by a fungus in the same manner.
Microides: A term Sabouraud used for small-spored ectothrix hair invasion.
Micrometer: A unit of linear measurement being $10^{-3}$ mm; abbrev. µm.
Micron: *See* Micrometer.
Micronematous: Having a conidiophore that is morphologically similar to the vegetative hyphae.
Minimal fungicidal concentration: The smallest concentration of an antifungal agent that will kill a fungus under standard conditions; abbrev. MFC.
Minimal inhibitory concentration: The smallest concentration of an antifungal agent that will inhibit the growth of the fungus under standard conditions, abbrev. MIC.
Mitosis: The process of nuclear division by which the two daughter nuclei receive a complement of chromosomes identical with that of the parent.
Moniliaceous: Refers to those fungi that produce free conidiophores and are hyaline to brightly colored.
Moniliasis: *See* Candidiasis.
Moniliform: Beadlike, having swellings.
Monilioid: *See* Moniliform.
Monoblastic: With reference to blastic conidiogenous cells, having one blown-out area at a single point.
Monokaryotic: Having one nucleus.
Mononematous: Having solitary free conidiophores.
Monophialide: *See* Phialide.
Monophialidic: With reference to phialides, having one opening (meristematic site).
Monopodial: Restricted in growth to the same apex.
Monoporogenous: With reference to porogenous conidiogenous cells, having one channel or pore.
Monoverticillate: With reference to the genus *Penicillium*, phialides arising from the apex of the conidiophore.
Mold, mould: A filamentous fungus.
Mucedinaceous: *See* Moniliaceous.

Mucilaginous: Sticky or slimy.

Mucormycosis: *See* Zygomycosis. The term is unacceptable as it implies mycoses caused only by *Mucor* species, even though it was originally proposed for any infection in man and lower animals caused by a member of the order Mucorales.

Multiperforate septum: Having many pores (micropores) in the septum.

Multiple budding: Developing successive crops of conidia that remain attached to the parent cells. There may be several layers of conidia, each layer decreasing in size toward the periphery. Commonly seen in *Paracoccidioides brasiliensis*.

Multipolar budding: Developing at different sites on the surface of the parent cell.

Multiseptate: Having several septa.

Muriform: Having horizontal and vertical septa.

Mutation: A permanent genetic change that cannot be traced to genetic recombination during meiosis.

Mycelia Sterilia: An order of the Fungi Imperfecti consisting of fungi that do not produce conidia or spores.

Mycelium: The mass of hyphae making up the thallus of a fungus.

Mycetoma: An infection of man and lower animals caused by a number of different fungi and actinomycetes classically characterized by draining sinuses, granules, and tumefaction.

Mycology: The branch of science that studies fungi and their biology.

Mycoserology: The study of mycological antigen–antibody reactions *in vitro*.

Mycosis (pl. mycoses): A disease caused by a fungus.

Mycotic: Pertaining to a fungal disease.

Mycotic keratitis: A mycotic ulcer of the eye usually following trauma to the cornea.

Name: In nomenclature, a name that has been validly published.

Necrosis: Death of cells, groups of cells, or localized tissue.

Nematophagous: Trapping nematodes.

Neotype: In nomenclature, a specimen designated to replace the holotype when all the original material is believed to be lost or destroyed.

Niger: Black.

Nocardiosis: A chronic suppurative infection of man and lower animals caused by a member of the genus *Nocardia*. Species of *Nocardia* are aerobic actinomycetes.

Node: With reference to the Zygomycetes, the point where a stolon (runner) contacts a surface. The term node is also used for a center from which hyphae arise or a swelling develops.

Nodosus: Having a number of joints.

Nodular organ: A knot of hyphae, especially prevalent in some dermatophytes.

Nodulate: Having intermittent nodes or swellings.

*Nomen*: A Latin word meaning name.

Nomenclatural type: The original specimen or element upon which the name is based.

Nomenclature: The system governing the naming of organisms and their groupings.

Nonseptate: Without septa.

Obclavate: Club-shaped in reverse; the distal region is smaller.

Oblong: Rectangle-like with rounded ends.

Obovate: Egg-shaped in reverse; the distal region is larger.

Obpyriform: Pear-shaped in reverse; the distal region is larger.

Oculomycosis: An infection of the eye caused by a fungus.

Oidium (pl. oidia): *See* Arthroconidium.

Olivaceous: Olive-gray color.

Ontogeny: With reference to conidia, the development of a conidium; development of the individual fungus.

Onychia: Inflammation of the nail matrix.

# Glossary

Onychomycosis:   An infection of the nail by yeasts, moulds, or both.

Oospore:   A thick-walled spore that developed from a large, naked, nonmotile female gamete (oosphere) following fertilization or parthenogenesis. Oospores are characteristic of the Oomycetes.

Operculum (pl. opercula):   A lid.

Orthophialide:   *See* Phialide.

Osmophilic:   Having the ability to grow under conditions of high osmotic pressure.

Ostiolate:   Having an ostiole or mouth.

Ostiole:   A mouth or opening. The term is also used to describe the necklike structure arising from ascocarps, which terminates in an opening or mouth. The ostiole is usually lined with periphyses.

Otomycosis:   A superficial fungal infection of the outer ear canal.

Oval:   Egg-shaped, with asymmetric curve.

Pallescent:   Turning pale.

Paniculate:   Branched.

Papilla (pl. papillae):   A nipple, small elevation.

Paracoccidioidomycosis:   A chronic granulomatous infection caused by *Paracoccidioides brasiliensis*.

Paraphysis (pl. paraphyses):   A sterile hypha found in a hymenium that arose as part of the fruiting body.

Parasexual cycle:   A mechanism, in the filamentous fungi, by which the recombination of genetic material occurs through mitosis rather than meiosis. The process involves the formation of diploid nuclei in heterokaryotic haploid hyphae; multiplication of the diploid nuclei along with the haploid nuclei; sorting of the diploid homokaryon; segregation and recombination via crossing-over during mitosis; and haplodization of the diploid nuclei.

Parasite:   An organism that obtains its food by living on or in another living organism.

Paronychia:   Inflammation of the tissue folds surrounding finger or toe nails.

Parthenogenesis:   A modification of sexual reproduction in which the female gamete alone gives rise to a normal offspring.

Pathogen:   An organism that produces disease.

Pathogenesis:   The developmental sequence of events resulting in a disease.

Pectinate:   Comb-shaped.

Pectinate hypha:   A comblike hypha typically produced by some dermatophytes.

Pedicel:   A slender stalk.

Pedicellate:   Having a pedicel.

Pellicle:   A filmlike or skinlike surface growth.

Pelliculate:   Forming a pellicle.

Pendulous:   Hanging down.

Penicillus (pl. penicilli):   The brushlike conidiophore of *Penicillium*.

Percurrent:   Developing new apices through the previous ones.

Perfect state:   That portion of the life cycle characterized by sexual reproduction. The teleomorph.

Perforating organ:   An organized mass of hyphae produced by a dermatophyte or other keratinophilic fungus in the process of perforating hair *in vitro*.

Peridial hyphae:   The hyphae making up the outside covering wall of a fruiting body.

Peridium (pl. peridia):   The outside wall covering of some fruiting bodies, such as a gymnothecium, perithecium, or sporangium.

Periphery:   The outer boundary.

Periphysis (pl. periphyses):   The short hairlike hyphae lining the inside of an ostiole or port of perithecia, pycnidia, and pycnia.

Perithecium (pl. perithecia):   A tightly enclosed ascocarp characterized by asci in a basal tuft or hymenium layer. Perithecia are usually flask-shaped and ostiolate.

Persistent:   Remaining intact.
Petri dish:   A round plastic or glass dish with vertical walls and flat bottom and a slightly larger corresponding lid that fits over the bottom portion of the dish.
Phaeo-:   A prefix meaning dark.
Phaeohyphomycosis:   An infection of man and lower animals caused by a number of dematiaceous fungi, characterized by the development of dematiaceous hyphae in the tissue that are short to elongate, distorted or swollen, regular, or irregular in form.
Phialide:   A determinate conidiogenous cell in which the first conidium is holoblastic and each successive conidium is enteroblastic. Each new basipetally formed conidium's wall arises *de novo* from a fixed conidiogenous locus. A collarette may be present at the tip of the phialide.
Phialidic:   Refers to conidium ontogeny involving a phialide.
Phialoconidium (pl. phialoconidia):   A conidium produced from a phialide.
Phialospore:   *See* Phialoconidium.
Phragmoconidium (pl. phragmoconidia):   A conidium having two or more transverse septa.
Phragmospore:   A spore having two or more transverse septa.
Phycomycetes:   An old mycological class name that originally contained the two subclasses Oomycetidae and Zygomycetidae. The archaic class Phycomycetes has been replaced by the classes Chytridiomycetes, Hyphochytridiomycetes, Oomycetes, Plasmodiophoromycetes, Trichomycetes, and Zygomycetes. The term is now only of historical interest. These organisms are no longer considered to be fungi (except Chytridiomycetes, Trichomycetes and Zygomycetes) by some.
Phycomycosis:   *See* Zygomycosis.
Piedra:   An infection of the hair shaft characterized by the presence of irregular nodules. Black piedra is caused by *Piedraia hortae* and white piedra by *Trichosporon beigelii*.
Pionnotes:   A mass of conidia having a fatty or greasy appearance. Pionnotes are formed by various species of *Fusarium*.
Pionnotes sporodochium (pl. pionnotes sporodochia):   A small sporodochium that is close to the surface of the medium without a stroma. The conidia formed from such a sporodochium develop as a continuous slimy layer. Pionnotes sporodochia are formed by various species of *Fusarium*.
Pityriasis:   Having fine to branny scales. The term pityriasis is used as a modifier.
Pityriasis versicolor:   A mild to chronic, but usually asymptomatic infection of the stratum corneum caused by *Malassezia furfur*.
Plagiophialide:   *See* Phialide.
Plasmodium (pl. plasmodia):   A multinucleate motile feeding mass of naked protoplasm.
Plasmogamy:   Fusion of two protoplasts, but not their nuclei.
Pleomorphic:   Having more than one form. The term pleomorphic has also been used to describe the changes a dermatophyte colony can go through in which it becomes irreversibly sterile.
Pleuracrogenous:   Borne at the tip and along the sides of a conidiophore or conidiogenous cell.
Pleurophialide:   *See* Phialide.
Ploidy:   Refers to the number of basic sets of chromosomes, $1n$, $2n$, etc.
Polar:   At the ends or poles of a cell.
Poly-:   A prefix meaning many.
Polyblastic:   With reference to a blastic conidiogenous cell, having several points where conidia are produced.
Polymorphic:   Having more than one form. Polymorphic is often used to denote hyphomycetes having more than one anamorph or mode of conidiogenesis.

Polyp: A protruding growth from the mucous membrane.
Polyphialide: *See* Sympodial phialide.
Polyphialidic: With reference to a phialide, having more than one meristematic site or opening.
Polyploid: Having more than two sets of homologous chromosomes.
Polyporogenous: With reference to a porogenous conidiogenous cell, having several pores or channels.
Polyverticillate: With reference to the genus *Penicillium*, having a complex penicillus consisting of several whorls of branches below the phialides.
Poroconidium (pl. poroconidia): A holoblastic conidium produced through a minute pore or channel in the cell wall of the conidiophore or conidiogenous cell.
Porogenous: With reference to conidiogenesis, having a pore formed at the junction of the conidiogenous cell and conidium.
Porospore: *See* Poroconidium.
Posterior: At the rear.
Potentiation: Having a twofold reduction in the MIC of one drug in the presence of an otherwise subinhibitory concentration of a second drug.
Progametangium (pl. progametangia): A cell that gives rise to a gametangium.
Progressive: A condition in which an area giving rise to conidia moves forward sympodially, percurrently, or into successive conidia that are developing in an acropetal manner.
Prokaryote: An organism that does not have a true nucleus, a bacterium. The nuclear material is spread throughout the cytoplasm.
Proliferate: To grow, reproduce, spread.
Proliferous: Reproducing by vegetative means, as in sympodia or percurrent proliferation.
Promycelium: A hypha originating from a teliospore upon which basidiospores will develop.
Propagule: An individual unit that can give rise to another organism.
Prophialide: *See* Metula.
Prostrate: Lying flat.
Pruinose: Powdery.
Pseudo-: A prefix meaning false.
Pseudoconidium (pl. pseudoconidia): *See* Sporangiolum.
Pseudo-germ-tube: *See* Germ tube. The term coined for germ-tube-like growths from conidia and spores in which the conidium or spore does not swell prior to germination. Pseudo-germ-tube was introduced for the "germ tubes" of *Candida albicans*. There is little reason to maintain this term.
Pseudohypha (pl. pseudohyphae): In essence, a series of blastoconidia that remain attached to each other forming a hyphalike filament.
Pseudomycelium: A large quantity of pseudohyphae.
Pseudoparenchyma (pl. pseudoparenchymata): A tissue consisting of oval to round cells in which the hyphae have lost their individuality.
Pseudopionnotes: *See* Pionnotes sporodochium.
Pseudoperithecium (pl. pseudoperithecia): Uniloculate ascostroma.
Pseudoplasmodium (pl. pseudoplasmodia): An aggregate of amoeboid cells of the Acrasiales.
Pseudoseptum (pl. pseudosepta): A partial cross-wall that resembles a septum but does not entirely reach across the conidium from one wall to the other.
Pubescent: Hairy.
Pulvinate: Cushionlike.
Punctate: Dotted; marked by narrow pores or perforations.
Punctiform: Very small.

**Pusillus:** Tiny.
**Pycnidioconidium (pl. pycnidioconidia):** A conidium formed within a pycnidium.
**Pycnidiospore:** *See* Pycnidioconidium.
**Pycnidium (pl. pyncidia):** An asexual fruiting body in which conidia are produced. The wall may be of various thicknesses and textures; the pyncidium may be a dissolved hole in a stroma; several fruiting bodies can be lumped together; it may contain a layer of distinct conidiophores; the wall cells may give rise directly to the conidia; and the conidia and conidiophores may be renewed. Pycnidia are usually round to flasked-shaped and ostiolate.
**Pycnosclerotium (pl. pycnosclerotia):** A hard-walled structure without conidia that resembles a pycnidium.
**Pyreniform:** Nut-shaped.
**Pyriform:** Pear-shaped; smaller at the distal end.
**Raceme:** A series of individual conidiophores, sporangiophores, or branches arising along a central hypha or stolon.
**Racemose:** Having a cluster of conidiophores or sporangiophores with each conidium or sporangium on a pedicel.
**Rachis:** An extension of a sympodial proliferating conidiogenous cell bearing conidia.
**Racket cell:** A hyphal cell that is swollen at one end.
**Racket hypha:** A series of racket cells in a single hypha.
**Racquet cell:** *See* Racket cell.
**Racquet hypha:** *See* Racket hypha.
**Radiate:** Radiating from a common center.
**Radulaspore:** A term used by Mason to describe the conidia of *Botrytis*.
**Ramoconidium (pl. ramoconidia):** An apical cell of a branched conidiophore that secedes and functions as a conidium, as in the shield cells of *Cladosporium* species.
**Ramose:** Abundantly branching.
**Random:** Lacking a pattern.
**Recurved:** Bent backward.
**Reniform:** Kidney-shaped.
**Retrogressive:** Developing by the conversion of a conidiogenous cell or hypha into conidia. The conidiogenous cell becomes shorter during the successive development of the conidia.
**Rhexolytic:** With reference to conidium secession, the circumscissile rupture of the wall of the cell below the basal septum of the conidium. The rupture may result from mechanical stress, lytic enzyme activity, or both.
**Rhinoentomophthoromycosis:** *See* Zygomycosis. The term was originally proposed for a chronic inflammatory to granulomatous infection usually restricted to the nasal submucosa characterized by polyps or palpable restricted subcutaneous masses. The infection is commonly caused by *Conidiobolus coronatus*, not by species of *Entomophthora*.
**Rhinosporidiosis:** An infection of the mucous membranes characterized by the development of polyps. The infection is caused by *Rhinosporidium seeberi*.
**Rhizoid:** A short branching hypha that resembles a root.
**Rhizomorph:** A thick organized cordlike structure consisting of a mass of hyphae in which the hyphae have lost their individuality. The structure resembles the tip of a root.
**Ringworm:** A term used to denote superficial fungus infections caused by dermatophytes.
**Rostrate:** Beaked.
**Rudimentary:** Primitive, poorly developed.
**Rugose:** Coarsely wrinkled.
**Saprobe:** An organism that uses dead organic matter as a source of food.
**Saprophyte:** *See* Saprobe.
**Sarciniform:** Packetlike.

# Glossary

Schizogenous: Arising from splitting or separating.
Schizolytic: With reference to conidium secession, fission through a double septum separating a conidium and conidiogenous cell, or between two adjacent conidia. The separation is centripetal due to lytic enzyme activity.
Schizophialide: *See* Phialide.
Sclerotium (pl. sclerotia): A hard mass of cells that remain dormant for long periods of time during unfavorable environmental conditions. Sclerotia germinate when favorable environmental conditions return.
Sclerotic body: A cluster of thick-walled, dematiaceous, rounded cells, some of which are muriform. Sclerotic bodies are diagnostic of chromoblastomycosis.
Scolecoconidium (pl. scolecoconidia): A conidium with a length to width ratio of 20:1 or greater.
Scolecospore: A spore with a length to width ratio of 20:1 or better.
Scutulum (pl. scutula): A yellow cup-shaped crust consisting of dense masses of mycelium and epithelial debris.
Secession: Release of mature conidia from their conidiogenous cells.
Self-compatible: Self-fertile, being able to reproduce sexually with itself.
Self-incompatible: Self-sterile, not being able to reproduce sexually with itself.
Semi-: A prefix meaning half.
Semiendogenous: Having conidia formed partly within the opening of a phialide or similar conidiogenous cell.
Semimacronematous: Having a conidiophore that is only slightly morphologically different from the vegetative hyphae.
Septal pore: An opening through a septum in a hypha or conidium.
Septate: Having cross-walls or septa.
Septum (pl. septa): A cross-wall in a conidium, hypha, or spore.
Serial: Restricted conidium differentiation and delimination in sequence prior to the initiation of the next new conidium.
Serum (pl. sera): Clear portion of blood separated from its solid components.
Sessile: Not on a stalk, but attached directly by its base.
Seta (pl. setae): A spine or bristlelike appendage usually occurring as a projection from a fruiting body.
Setula (pl. setulae): A delicate appendage arising from the surface of a conidium.
Sexual reproduction: Involving the fusion of two compatible haploid nuclei.
Shield cell: A conidium of *Cladosporium* that has the general shape of a shield.
Simple: Nonbranched.
Single: A conidium by itself that does not contribute to the formation of additional conidia.
Sinuous: Wavy.
Sinus: An abnormal channel.
Smut: A disease of plants caused by members of the Ustilaginales.
Solitary: Alone, by one's self.
Sparsely septate: Having rare septa.
Species: A closely related group of individuals that resemble each other to some degree. A species is the basic unit of classification and shows phylogenetic relationships.
Spherule: A sporangiumlike structure with a thick wall that is produced within tissue and *in vitro* by *Coccidioides immitis*.
Spicule: *See* Denticle.
Spine: A sharply pointed process.
Spinose: Having spines.
Spinulose: Having small spines.

Spiral hypha: A hypha that spirals.
Sporangiolum (pl. sporangiola): A small sporangium producing a small number of sporangiospores.
Sporangiophore: A specialized hypha upon which a sporangium develops.
Sporangiospore: An asexual spore produced within a sporangium.
Sporangium (pl. sporangia): A saclike structure in which the entire internal contents are cleaved into asexual spores.
Spore: A propagule derived by sexual or asexual means. If by asexual means, a cleavage process is usually involved.
Sporidium (pl. sporidia): *See* Basidiospore.
Sporodochium (pl. sporodochia): A cushion-shaped stroma or mat of hyphae that is covered with conidiophores.
Sporogenous: Giving rise to spores.
Sporogenous cell: A cell that gives rise to spores.
Sporogenous cell (in part): *See* Conidiogenous cell.
Sporophore: A specialized hypha that gives rise to spores.
Sporotrichosis: An infection of man and lower animals caused by *Sporothrix schenckii*.
Sputum (pl. sputa): Material collected from the bronchi, lungs, and trachea that is discharged through the mouth.
Squamulose: Scaly.
Stable: Having a determinate conidiogenous cell that is not converted into conidia retrogressively.
State: A phase or condition in the life cycle of a fungus, i.e. conidial state, etc.
Stauroconidium (pl. stauroconidia): A forked or stellate conidium.
Staurospore: A forked or stellate spore.
Stellate: Star-shaped.
Sterigma (pl. sterigmata): A supporting pedicel or denticlelike structure originating from a basidium upon which a basidiospore will develop.
Sterile: Not producing conidia or spores.
Stilbaceous: Producing synnemata.
Stolon: A runner, a horizontal hypha from which new hyphae, rhizoids, sporangiophores, or any combination of these structures arise.
Strain: A group of individuals within a species or variety with one or more characteristics that are unique to them.
Stratum corneum: The outer layer of the epidermis consisting of dead desquamating cells.
Striate: Having lines or minute furrows.
Stroma: A compact vegetative structure on which or within which fruiting bodies develop.
Stylospore: An obsolete term for an elongated pycnidioconidium or any conidium or spore on a pedicel or hypha.
Sub-: A prefix meaning below, under, somewhat, slightly, or approximately.
Subacute: Somewhat acute, a condition between acute and chronic.
Subcutaneous: Below the skin.
Subcutaneous zygomycosis: A zygomycete infection involving the subcutaneous tissue.
Subiculum (pl. subicula): A loose to crustlike mat of hyphae upon which fruiting bodies are formed.
Subglobose: Not quite round or spherical.
Subjacent: Just below.
Sublanose: Slightly woolly.
Submerged: Growing into the nutrient agar.
Substrate: A substance used for growth.

Subulate: Tapering to a slender point.
Superficial: Near the surface.
Suppurative: Producing pus.
Suspensor: A supporting hypha for a gamete or gametangium.
Symbiosis: Two unlike organisms living together.
Symmetrical: *See* Biverticillate symmetrical.
Sympodial: Pertaining to indeterminate vegetative proliferation of a conidiophore or conidiogenous cell that is characterized by the successive development of new subterminal-lateral apices associated with successive areas of conidium development. The conidiophore or conidiogenous cell becomes swollen or increases in length, often taking on a geniculate appearance.
Sympodial phialide: A phialide that undergoes intermittent sympodial growth.
Sympodioconidium (pl. sympodioconidia): A conidium produced from a sympodial conidiophore or conidiogenous cell. The term is not recommended because it defines a conidium on the basis of its conidiogenous cell.
Sympodiospore: *See* Sympodioconidium.
Sympodula: A sympodial conidiogenous cell.
Synchronized: Occurring together at one time; the simultaneous differentiation of conidia.
Synergy: Having a fourfold or greater reduction in the MIC of one drug in the presence of an otherwise subinhibitory concentration of a second drug.
Synnema (pl. synnemata): A compact elongated group of erect conidiophores that are cemented together, their conidia being produced at the apex, along the sides of the upper portion of the synnema, or both.
Synonym: Another name for a species or group of fungi. A synonym is usually a later or illegitimate name under the rules of botanical nomenclature. An obligate (i.e., nomenclatural) synonym is one of two or more names based upon the same type, and a facultative (i.e., taxonomic) synonym is one of two or more names based upon different types, but judged to apply to the same taxonomic group.
Systemic: Affecting the body as a whole.
Taxon (pl. taxa): In nomenclature, any taxonomic group.
Taxonomy: The systematic classification of organisms.
Teleomorph: A reproductive organ that is either morphologically, karyologically, or both, specialized for generating meiospores or their homologs, whether by normal sexual or parthenogenetic means.
Teliospore (also spelled teleutospore): A usually thick-walled resting spore in which karyogamy occurs. It functions as a component of the basidium. Teliospores are produced by members of the Uredinales and Ustilaginales.
Tenuous: Delicate.
Terminal: At the end.
Thallic: Involving a conidium in which the young conidium initial does not begin to develop until after it has been delimited by a septum. The conidium originates from the entire parent cell.
Thallic–arthric: With reference to thallic conidium development, fragmentation and disarticulation of fertile, determinate hyphae into chains of conidia.
Thallospore: An old term for conidium that was produced directly from a hypha without a distinct conidiophore.
Thallus (pl. thalli): The vegetative growth of a fungus.
Thermophile: Being able to grow and sporulate at 45°C and above.
Tinea: A superficial fungus infection of the skin.
Tinea barbae: A superficial fungus infection of the bearded areas of the face and neck.

Tinea capitis: A superficial fungus infection of the scalp.
Tinea corporis: A superficial fungus infection of the glabrous skin that is usually restricted to the stratum corneum.
Tinea cruris: A superficial fungus infection of the groin, perineum, and perianal region.
Tinea favosa: A superficial fungus infection of the scalp characterized by the development of scutula.
Tinea imbricata: A superficial fungus infection of the body characterized by concentrically arranged rings of papulosquamous patches of scales.
Tinea manuum: A superficial fungus infection of the hand, especially the interdigital areas and palmar surface.
Tinea nigra: An asymptomatic superficial fungus infection of the stratum corneum characterized by brown to black nonscaly macules.
Tinea pedis: A superficial fungus infection of the feet that involves the toe webs and soles.
Tinea unguium: A superficial fungus infection of the nail plate by a dermatophyte.
Tinsel: With reference to flagella, a flagellum with brushlike appendages.
Toruloid: Having swellings at intervals.
Translucent: Transmitting light.
Tretic: Originating through a narrow channel or pore in the cell wall of the conidiophore or conidiogenous cell. *See* Porogenous.
Tretoconidium (pl. tretoconidia): A blastic conidium produced through a minute channel in the cell wall of the conidiophore or conidiogenous cell. The term poroconidium is more widely used.
Trichogyne: Extension of an ascogonium that fuses with a fertilizing cell.
Truncate: Ending abruptly, cut-off sharply.
Tubercle: Wartlike protuberance.
Tuberculate: Having tubercles or small wartlike processes.
Tumefaction: A swelling; edema.
Turbinate: Top-shaped.
Type: *See* Nomenclatural type.
Ubiquitous: Everywhere.
Ulcer: A surface excavation of the skin due to the sloughing of inflammatory necrotic tissue.
Umbilicate: Having a small hollowed area.
Umbo: A raised mound.
Umbonate: Having an umbo.
Uncinate: Hooked.
Undulate: Wavy.
Uniflagellate: Having one flagellum.
Uniloculate: Having one locule. An uniloculate ascostroma has been referred to in the past as a pseudoperithecium.
Uniperforate septum: Having one pore through the septum.
Uniseriate: With reference to the genus *Aspergillus*, phialides arising directly from the vesicle; having one series or row.
Unitunicate: Having one wall.
Vacuole: In a cell, a minute cavity devoid of protoplasm.
Valid: In nomenclature, the first publication of a name in accordance with the applicable rules.
Vegetative: Assimilative.
Velutinous: Velvety in texture.

# Glossary

Velvety: With reference to colony texture, conidiophores forming a fairly dense, even stand, arising from the vegetative hyphae that are submerged in the nutrient agar.
Venter: That portion of a phialide that lies between the base of the phialide and the conidiogenous locus.
Verrucose: Having many warts.
Verruculose: Having many small warts or verrucae.
Versicolor: Having different colors.
Verticil: A whorl of conidiophores or conidiogenous cells from a common point or node.
Verticillate: In whorls or verticils.
Vesicle: A swollen cell; the swollen apex of the conidiophore of an *Aspergillus* sp.; the swollen apex of a sporangiophore as in species of *Syncephalastrum*.
Vesiculose: Composed of vesicles.
Virulence: The degree of pathogenicity of an organism.
Whiplash: With reference to flagella, a flagellum without brushlike appendages.
Whorl: A cluster radiating from a common point.
Wild type: An initial isolate from nature.
Wood's lamp: A lamp that emits ultraviolet radiation at approximately 365 nm. The lamp is used to help diagnose tinea capitis and erythrasma (a superficial bacterial infection).
Woronin body: A rounded or oval, cytoplasmic organelle bound by a single membrane that is highly refractive formed within the cells of Ascomycetes and Fungi Imperfecti.
Yeast: In a strict sense, a unicellular budding fungus that reproduces by both sexual and asexual means. In this handbook, yeast and yeastlike will be used interchangeably. Some mycologists restrict the term yeasts to Ascomycetes that do not produce ascocarps, whether or not budding cells are present. This latter concept is not generally accepted.
Yeastlike: Having a unicellular budding form that reproduces by asexual means only. In this handbook, yeastlike and yeast will be used interchangeably.
Zonate: Having concentric bands or rings.
Zoophilic: Preferring animals.
Zoospore: A motile asexual spore.
Zygomycosis: An infection of man and lower animals caused by any member of the class Zygomycetes.
Zygospore: A resting spore that resulted from the fusion of two similar gametangia. Zygospores are characteristic of the Zygomycetes.
Zygote: A diploid cell that results from the fusion of two haploid cells.

*Appendix A*

# Some Simple Symmetrical Shapes*

In medical mycology, it is important to use a standardized descriptive terminology for shapes. Standardized terms permit medical mycologists to communicate effectively with each other as well as to help eliminate much of the confusion associated with shapes and their numerous names.

Figures 1–23 illustrate the terminology recommended by the Systematics Association Committee for Descriptive Biological Terminology for some of the simple symmetrical plane shapes. More commonly used names have been placed in parentheses following the standardized terms where appropriate. The paired figures 3–4, 5–6, 7–8, 9–10, 11–12, 14–15, 16–17, 18–19, and 20–21 represent the extremes for each shape. Figures 24–32 consist of nonstandardized shapes, with their common names, that are of special interest to medical mycologists.

*Adapted by permission from *Taxon* 11:145–156, 1962.

## Appendix A

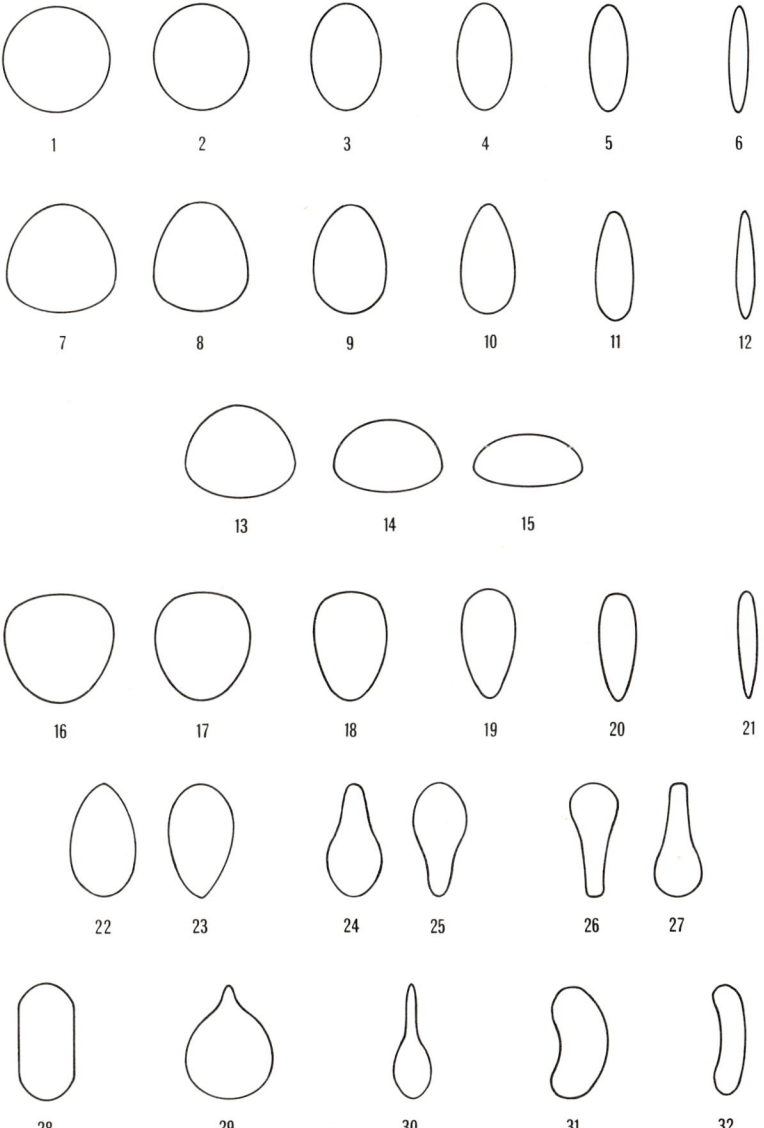

**Figs. 1–32.** Terminology. 1, circular (globose, spherical); 2, broadly elliptic (subglobose); 3, elliptic (broadly ellipsoidal); 4, elliptic (ellipsoidal, elongate); 5, narrowly elliptic (oval); 6, narrowly elliptic (fusiform); 7, broadly ovate; 8, broadly ovate; 9, ovate (ovoid); 10, ovate (ovoid); 11, narrowly ovate; 12, narrowly ovate; 13, very broadly ovate; 14, depressed ovate; 15, depressed ovate; 16, broadly obovate; 17, broadly obovate; 18, obovate (obovoid); 19, obovate (obovoid); 20, narrowly obovate; 21, narrowly obovate; 22, ovate; 23, obovate; 24, obpyriform; 25, pyriform; 26, clavate; 27, obclavate; 28, oblong; 29, ampulliform; 30, lageniform; 31, reniform; 32, allantoid.

*Appendix B*

# Commonly Encountered Synonyms and Other Obsolete Names

Many physicians and medical mycologists in the past have published and used names for fungi in complete ignorance, or even disregard, of the principles of nomenclature and taxonomy. Important isolates, often including type cultures, were not maintained for future medical mycologists to study. Even today, descriptions of the etiologic agents causing unusual mycoses are not always included in the case reports. As in the past, cultures are rarely saved. Thus, it is often difficult, if not impossible, to determine the true identity of many of the the reported etiologic agents causing disease in man and lower animals. With these thoughts in mind, a limited listing of major synonyms and obsolete names are tabulated below. The list has been deliberately kept short in order to avoid mentioning many of these old names once again in print.

| Synonym | Currently accepted name |
| --- | --- |
| *Absidia ramosa* (Lindt) Lendner, 1908 | *Absidia corymbifera* (Cohn) Saccardo et Trotter, 1912 |
| *Achorion* Remak, 1845 | *Trichophyton* Malmsten, 1845 |
| *Acrotheca* Fuckel, 1860 | *Ramularia* Unger, 1833 |
| *Acrotheca aquaspersa* Borelli, 1972 | *Rhinocladiella* Nannfeldt, 1934 |
| *Aleurisma* Link, 1809 | *Trichoderma* Persoon ex Gray, 1821 |
| *Allescheria boydii* Shear, 1922 | *Petriellidium boydii* (Shear) Malloch, 1970 |
| *Alternaria tenuis* Nees, 1816–1817 | *Alternaria alternata* (Fr.) Keissler, 1912 |

Appendix B

| Synonym | Currently accepted name |
|---|---|
| *Arachniotus trisporus* Hotson, 1936 | *Byssochlamys nivea* Westling, 1909 |
| *Aspergillus glaucus* Link, 1909 | *Aspergillis glaucus* group, which contains several species |
| *Basidiobolus haptosporus* Drechsler, 1947 | *Basidiobolus ranarum* Eidam, 1886 |
| *Basidiobolus meristosporus* Drechsler, 1955 | *Basidiobolus ranarum* Eidam, 1886 |
| *Bipolaris* Shoemaker, 1959 | *Drechslera* Ito, 1930 |
| *Botryodiplodia theobromae* Patouillard, 1892 | *Lasiodiplodia theobromae* (Patouillard) Griffon et Maublanc, 1909 |
| *Cephalosporium* Corda, 1839 | *Acremonium* Link ex. Fries, 1821 |
| *Cephalosporium acremonium* Corda, 1839 | Several species of *Acremonium* Link ex. Fris, 1821 |
| *Cephalosporium cinnabarinum* | Uncertain |
| *Cephalosporium falciforme* Carrión, 1951 | *Acremonium falciforme* (Carrión) Gams, 1971 |
| *Cephalosporium granulomatis* Weidm. et Kligm., 1945 | *Acremonium kiliense* Grütz, 1925 |
| *Cephalosporium infestans* Gaind et Thirum., 1962 | *Acremonium kiliense* Grütz, 1925 |
| *Cephalosporium kiliense* (Grütz) Hartmann, 1926 | *Acremonium kiliense* Grütz, 1925 |
| *Cephalosporium madurae* Padhye, et al., 1962 | *Acremonium kiliense* Grütz, 1925 |
| *Cephalosporium niveolanosum* Benedek, 1928 | *Acremonium kiliense* Grütz, 1925 |
| *Cephalosporium potronii* (Vuill.) Oomen, 1957 | *Acremonium potronii* Vuill., 1910 |
| *Cephalosporium recifei* Leão et Lôbo, 1934 | *Acremonium recifei* (Leão et Lôbo) Gams, 1971 |
| *Cephalosporium roseo-griseum* Saksena, 1955 | *Acremonium roseo-griseum* (Saksena) Gams, 1971 |
| *Cephalosporium serrae* Maffei, 1930 | *Verticillium serrae* (Maffei) v. Beyma, 1939 |
| *Cercospora apii* Fres., 1863 in the sense of Emmons | *Mycocentrospora acerina* (Hartig) Deighton, 1972 |
| *Chmelia slovaca* (Svobodová, Chmel et Bojanovská) Svobodová, 1966 | Uncertain |
| *Chrysosporium pannorum* (Link) Hughes, 1958 | *Geomyces pannorus* (Link) Sigler et Carmichael, 1976 |
| *Cladosporium castellanii* Borelli et Marcano, 1973 | *Stenella araguata* Sydow, 1930 |
| *Cladosporium mansonii* (Castellani), Castellani, 1913 | *Malassezia furfur* (Robin) Baillon, 1889 |
| *Cladosporium trichoides* Emmons, 1952 | *Cladosporium bantianum* (Saccardo) Borelli, 1960 |

| Synonym | Currently accepted name |
|---|---|
| *Cladosporium werneckii* Horta, 1921 | *Exophiala werneckii* (Horta) v. Arx, 1970 |
| *Cryptococcus bacillisporus* Kwon-Chung et Bennett, 1978 | *Cryptococcus neoformans* (Sanfelice) Vuillemin, 1901 |
| *Cryptococcus nigricans* Rich et Stern, 1958 | *Phaeococcus nigricans* (Rich et Stern) de Hoog, 1977 |
| *Dematium* Persoon, 1801 | Confused name |
| *Dematium pullulans* deBary, 1866 | *Aureobasidium pullulans* (deBary) Arn., 1910 |
| *Emmonsia* Ciferri et Montemartini, 1959 | *Chrysosporium* Corda, 1833 |
| *Emmonsia crescens* Emmons et Jellison, 1960 | *Chrysosporium parvum* (Emmons et Ashburn) Carmichael, 1962 |
| *Emmonsia parva* (Emmons et Ashburn) Ciferri et Montemartini, 1959 | *Chrysosporium parvum* (Emmons et Jellison) Carmichael, 1962 |
| *Emmonsiella* Kwon-Chung, 1972 | *Ajellomyces* McDonough et Lewis emend. McGinnis et Katz, 1979 |
| *Emmonsiella capsulata* Kwon-Chung, 1972 | *Ajellomyces capsulatus* (Kwon-Chung) McGinnis et Katz, 1979 (as "*capsulata*") |
| *Entomophthora coronata* (Cost.) Kevork. 1937 | *Conidiobolus coronatus* (Cost.) Batko, 1964 |
| *Exophiala dermatitidis* (Kano) De Hoog, 1977 | *Wangiella dermatitidis* (Kano) McGinnis, 1977 |
| *Filobasidiella bacillispora* Kwon-Chung, 1976 | *Filobasidiella neoformans* Kwon-Chung, 1975 |
| *Fonsecaea dermatitidis* (Kano) Carrión, 1950 | *Wangiella dermatitidis* (Kano) McGinnis, 1977 |
| *Fusarium episphaeria* (Tode) Synder et Hansen, 1945 | *Fusarium dimerum* Penzig, 1882 (in part); *Fusarium merismoides* Corda, 1838 (in part) |
| *Fusarium roseum* Link emend. Snyder et Hansen, 1945 | Several species of *Fusarium* Link ex Gray, 1821 |
| *Fusidium terricola* Miller *et al.*, 1957 | *Sagrahamala terricola* (Miller *et al.*) Subramanian et Pushkaran, 1975 |
| *Heterosporium* Klotzsch, 1877 | *Cladosporium* Link ex Gray, 1821 |
| *Histoplasma duboisii* Vanbreuseghem, 1952 | *Histoplasma capsulatum* var. *duboisii* (Vanbreuseghem) Ciferri, 1960 |
| *Hormiscium* Kunze, 1817 | *Torula* (Persoon) Link ex Gray, 1821 |
| *Hormiscium dermatitidis* Kano, 1934 | *Wangiella dermatitidis* (Kano) McGinnis, 1977 |
| *Hormodendrum* Bonorden, 1853 | *Cladosporium* Link ex Gray, 1821 |
| *Hormonema* Lagerberg et Melin, 1927 | *Aureobasidium* Viala et Boyer, 1891 |
| *Keratinomyces* Vanbreuseghem, 1952 | *Trichophyton* Malmsten, 1845 |
| *Macrosporium* Fries, 1832 | *Alternaria* Nees ex Persoon, 1822 |
| *Madurella mycetomi* (Laveran) Brumpt, 1905 | Correct spelling is *Madurella mycetomatis* |
| *Microides* de Vroey, 1970 | Invalid name, no Latin diagnosis |
| *Monilia albicans* (Robin) Zopf, 1890 | *Candida albicans* (Robin) Berkhout, 1923 |
| *Monilia parakrusei* Castellani et Chalmers, 1919 | *Candida krusei* (Castellani) Berkhout, 1923 |

## Appendix B

| Synonym | Currently accepted name |
|---|---|
| *Monosporium* Bonorden, 1851 | Illegitimate name |
| *Monosporium apiospermum* Saccardo, 1911 | *Scedosporium apiospermum* (Saccardo) Castellani et Chalmers, 1919 |
| *Mortierella mycetomatis* (as "*mycetomi*") | Uncertain |
| *Mucor pusillus* Lindt, 1886 | *Rhizomucor pusillus* (Lindt) Schipper, 1978 |
| *Oospora* Wallroth, 1833 | Illegitimate name |
| *Penicillium crustaceum* Fries, 1829 | Several species of *Penicillium* Link emend. Thom, 1910 |
| *Penicillium glaucum* Link, 1809 | Several species of *Penicillium* Link emend. Thom, 1910 |
| *Penicillium lilacinum* Thom, 1910 | *Paecilomyces lilacinus* (Thom) Samson, 1974 |
| *Peyronellaea* Goidànich, 1946 | *Phoma* Saccardo, 1880 *nom. cons.* |
| *Phialophora compacta* (Carrión) Red. et Cif., 1942 | *Fonsecaea compacta* (Carrión) Carrión, 1940 |
| *Phialophora dermatitidis* (Kano) Emmons, 1963 | *Wangiella dermatitidis* (Kano) McGinnis, 1977 |
| *Phialophora gougerotii* (Matruchot) Borelli, 1955 in the sense of Borelli | *Exophiala jeanselmei* (Langeron) McGinnis et Padhye, 1977 |
| *Phialophora jeanselmei* (Langeron) Emmons, 1945 | *Exophiala jeanselmei* (Langeron) McGinnis et Padhye, 1977 |
| *Phialophora mutabilis* (v. Beyma) Schol-Schwarz, 1970 | *Phialophora hoffmannii* (v. Beyma) Schol-Schwarz, 1970 |
| *Phialophora pedrosoi* (Brumpt) Red. et Cif., 1942 | *Fonsecaea pedrosoi* (Brumpt) Negroni, 1936 |
| *Phialophora spinifera* Nielsen et Conant, 1968 | *Exophiala spinifera* (Nielsen et Conant) McGinnis, 1977 |
| *Pityrosporum* Sabouraud, 1904 | *Malassezia* Baillon, 1889 |
| *Pityrosporum orbiculare* Gordon, 1951 | *Malassezia furfur* (Robin) Baillon, 1889 |
| *Pityrosporum ovale* (Bizzozero) Castellani et Chalmers, 1913 | *Malassezia furfur* (Robin) Baillon, 1889 |
| *Pityrosporum pachydermatis* Weidman, 1925 | *Malassezia pachydermatis* (Weidman) Dodge, 1935 |
| *Prototheca filamenta* Arnold et Ahearn, 1972 | *Fissuricella filamenta* (Arnold et Ahearn) Pore, D'Amato et Ajello, 1977 |
| *Pullularia* Berkhout, 1923 | *Aureobasidium* Viala et Boyer, 1891 |
| *Pullularia pullulans* (deBary) Berkhout, 1923 | *Aureobasidium pullulans* (deBary) Arn., 1910 |
| *Rhinocladiella compacta* (Carrión) Schol-Schwarz, 1968 | *Fonsecaea compacta* (Carrión) Carrión, 1940 |
| *Rhinocladiella pedrosoi* (Brumpt) Schol-Schwarz, 1968 | *Fonsecaea pedrosoi* (Brumpt) Negroni, 1936 |
| *Rhinocladiella spinifera* (Nielsen et Conant) de Hoog, 1977 | *Exophiala spinifera* (Nielsen et Conant) McGinnis, 1977 |
| *Rhizopus nigricans* Ehrenb., 1820 | *Rhizopus stolonifer* (Ehrenb. ex Fr.) Lind., 1913 |

| Synonym | Currently accepted name |
|---|---|
| *Rhodotorula mucilaginosa* (Jörg.) Harrison, 1928 | *Rhodotorula rubra* (Demme) Lodder, 1934 |
| *Sarcinomyces crustaceus* Lindner, 1898 in the sense of Hermanides-Nijhof | *Exophiala werneckii* (Horta) v. Arx, 1970 |
| *Sporotrichum schenckii* (Hektoen et Perkins) de Beurmann et Gougerot, 1906 | *Sporothrix schenckii* Hektoen et Perkins, 1900 |
| *Torulopsis famata* (Harrison) Lodder et Kreger-van Rij, 1952 | *Torulopsis candida* (Saito) Lodder, 1934 |
| *Trichophyton gallinae* (Mégnin) Silva et Benham, 1952 | *Microsporum gallinae* (Mégnin) Grigorakis, 1929 |
| *Trichophyton gypseum* Bodin, 1902 | *Trichophyton mentagrophytes* (Robin) Blanchard, 1896 |
| *Trichophyton interdigitale* Priestley, 1917 | *Trichophyton mentagrophytes* (Robin) Blanchard, 1896 |
| *Trichophyton persicolor* Sabouraud, 1910 | *Microsporum persicolor* (Sabouraud) Guiart et Grigorakis, 1928 |
| *Trichosporon cutaneum* (deBeurmann, Gougerot et Vaucher) Ota, 1926 | *Trichosporon beigelii* (Küch. et Rabenh.) Vuillemin, 1902 |
| *Trichosporon penicillatum* do Carmo-Sousa, 1965 | *Geotrichum penicillatum* (do Carmo-Sousa) v. Arx, 1977 |
| *Zopfia rosatii* (Segretain et Destombes) Hawksw. et Booth, 1974 | *Neotestudina rosatii* Segretain et Destombes, 1961 |

*Appendix C*

# Reported Fungal Pathogens of Man

Over 275 species of fungi have been reported to cause disease in man. Appendix C lists these reported pathogens and separates many of the valid reports from the questionable ones. It is beyond the scope of the appendix to include all the literature pertaining to each fungus. In those instances where only a few case reports have been published, all have been included. Even though a limited number of studies are cited, an attempt was made to review and evaluate a large number of reports. Each reference cited in this appendix has been reviewed and evaluated for its credibility. The proportion of acceptable to questionable reports cited is based upon this author's impression of all the reports evaluated with reference to the particular fungus being reviewed.

The fungi are listed alphabetically by their currently accepted scientific names, which in some instances is not the name used by the original author. This was done in order to avoid obsolete names. The appendix is primarily restricted to the reported pathogenic fungi from the late 1940s to the beginning of 1979. This time frame was selected because the descriptions of the clinical diseases and the taxonomy of the reported etiologic agents in the majority of the reported cases prior to the 1940s are extremely questionable.

The criteria employed to distinguish acceptable from questionable reports and reviews are fourfold. A report was considered to be acceptable when an adequate clinical history was presented that suggested a mycotic infection; the fungus was seen in the clinical specimens; the morphology of the fungus in the clinical specimens was compatible with the reported etiologic agent; and there was adequate evidence that the fungus was identified properly. All the criteria had to be met before the report was considered acceptable. If the criteria were not met, the report was listed as questionable. Since the final decision relied upon the judgment of this author, other mycologists may not necessarily agree with the final disposition of all the cases included in the appendix.

For the most part, the case reports and reviews contain satisfactory clinical summaries, indicating that a particular patient had a fungal infection. A few reports did not contain appropriate evidence that the reported fungus was seen in the clinical specimens. In a few instances, the tissue morphology of the supposed etiologic agent was not compatible with the isolated fungus. As an example, a photomicrograph of a yeast producing blastoconidia in tissue was not considered to be compatible with the etiologic agent being reported as *Geotrichum candidum.*

The majority of the questionable cases were considered as such because the identification of the etiologic agent may have been in error. The mere mention of the name of the fungus without either photographic evidence, or a discussion of the identification, or acknowledgment that a respected mycologist performed the identification, was considered to be unacceptable. It is only necessary to see a photomicrograph of *Cunninghamella* sp. labeled as *Mucor* sp. to realize how important identification data are, especially when unusual and rare fungi are involved. Without doubt, the majority of the questionable reports may have described valid fungal infections, but the authors failed to adequately and convincingly document their reports.

Other factors that were taken into consideration included the repeated recovery of the suspected pathogen and its involvement in more than one body site. This also resulted in some problems. For example, the repeated recovery of *G. candidum* from sputum specimens resulted in the diagnosis of pulmonary geotrichosis in several case reports. We know that the individual's diet can result in the repeated recovery of *G. candidum* from sputa. The dilemma is, should these cases be accepted as pulmonary geotrichosis? In this particular example, the case reports were considered questionable because other data were not available. It should be obvious that all the criteria cannot be applied equally to all case reports and summaries. Thus, individual judgment becomes the single most important factor in rating reports and summaries as either acceptable or questionable. Of the 278 fungi reviewed, only 174 (63%) met the rigid criteria set for considering them to be the etiologic agents of disease.

| Fungi | Representative case reports and summaries | |
|---|---|---|
| | Accepted | Questionable |
| 1. *Absidia corymbifera* | 63 | |
| 2. *Acremonium* sp. | 9, 76 | 17, 170, 175, 255 |

# Appendix C

| Fungi | Representative case reports and summaries | |
|---|---|---|
| | Accepted | Questionable |
| 3. *Acremonium falciforme* | 130 | |
| 4. *Acremonium kiliense* | 234, 253 | 376 |
| 5. *Acremonium potronii* | 98, 99 | |
| 6. *Acremonium recifei* | 8 | |
| 7. *Acremonium roseo-griseum* | 357, 375 | |
| 8. *Alternaria* sp. | 135 | 19, 39, 188 |
| 9. *Alternaria alternata* | 93 | 38, 100, 250, 257, 308 |
| 10. *Alternaria* anamorph of *Pleospora infectoria* | | 100, 107 |
| 11. *Aphanoascus fulvescens* | 292 | |
| 12. *Arthrographis kalrai* | | 54 |
| 13. *Aspergillus amstelodami* | 65 | 97, 140 |
| 14. *Aspergillus awamori* | | 254 |
| 15. *Aspergillus bouffardi*[a] | | 41 |
| 16. *Aspergillus caesiellus* | 252 | |
| 17. *Aspergillus candidus* group | | 28 |
| 18. *Aspergillus candidus* | 15, 185, 355 | 87, 213 |
| 19. *Aspergillus carneus* | 270 | 230 |
| 20. *Aspergillus chevalieri* | | 237 |
| 21. *Aspergillus clavato-nanica* | | 25 |
| 22. *Aspergillus fischeri* | | 112 |
| 23. *Aspergillus flavipes* | | 145, 333 |
| 24. *Aspergillus flavus* group | | 28, 328 |
| 25. *Aspergillus flavus* | 7, 154 | 333 |
| 26. *Aspergillus fumigatus* | 84, 174, 290 | |
| 27. *Aspergillus glaucus* group | 126 | 28, 306 |
| 28. *Aspergillus janus* | | 239 |
| 29. *Aspergillus nidulans* | 166, 199, 200 | 40, 333, 362, 376 |
| 30. *Aspergillus niger* group | | 28, 328 |
| 31. *Aspergillus niger* | 1, 84, 86, 174, 290 | 228 |
| 32. *Aspergillus niveus* | | 313 |
| 33. *Aspergillus ochraceus* | | 249 |
| 34. *Aspergillus oryzae* | 120, 226, 381 | |
| 35. *Aspergillus penicilloides* | 103 | 218 |
| 36. *Aspergillus phialiseptus* | | 171 |
| 37. *Aspergillus restrictus* group | | 209 |
| 38. *Aspergillus restrictus* | 310 | 92 |
| 39. *Aspergillus sclerotiorum* | | 224 |
| 40. *Aspergillus sulphureus* | | 80 |
| 41. *Aspergillus sydowi* | 355 | 12, 53 |
| 42. *Aspergillus terreus* group | | 328 |
| 43. *Aspergillus terreus* | 49, 157, 319, 355, 375 | 3, 87, 219, 291, 376 |
| 44. *Aspergillus terricola* | | 376 |
| 45. *Aspergillus unguis* | 310 | |
| 46. *Aspergillus ustus* | 46, 181 | |
| 47. *Aspergillus versicolor* | 13, 355 | 66, 87 |
| 48. *Aspergillus wentii* | | 145 |

|  | Representative case reports and summaries | |
|---|---|---|
| Fungi | Accepted | Questionable |
| 49. *Aureobasidium pullulans* |  | 147, 305, 346, 349 |
| 50. *Basidiobolus ranarum* | 81, 150, 164, 204 |  |
| 51. Basidiomycete |  | 24 |
| 52. *Beauveria bassiana* | 105 |  |
| 53. *Blastomyces dermatitidis* | 84, 174, 290, 312 |  |
| 54. *Byssochlamys nivea* |  | 298 |
| 55. *Candida albicans* | 84, 174, 290 |  |
| 56. *Candida brumptii* |  | 96 |
| 57. *Candida claussenii* |  | 187 |
| 58. *Candida guilliermondii* | 84, 174, 290 |  |
| 59. *Candida humicola* |  | 247, 324 |
| 60. *Candida ingens* |  | 288 |
| 61. *Candida intermedia* |  | 102, 279 |
| 62. *Candida krusei* | 84, 174, 290 |  |
| 63. *Candida lipolytica* |  | 248, 288 |
| 64. *Candida melinii* |  | 59 |
| 65. *Candida mogii* |  | 87 |
| 66. *Candida parapsilosis* | 68, 84, 174, 264, 290 |  |
| 67. *Candida pseudotropicalis* | 84, 174, 290 |  |
| 68. *Candida pulcherrima* | 227 | 275 |
| 69. *Candida ravautii* | 60 |  |
| 70. *Candida reukaufii* |  | 279, 323 |
| 71. *Candida scottii* |  | 323 |
| 72. *Candida solani* |  | 288, 326 |
| 73. *Candida stellatoidea* | 84, 174, 210, 290 |  |
| 74. *Candida tropicalis* | 84, 174, 290 |  |
| 75. *Candida utilis* |  | 102, 347 |
| 76. *Candida viswanathii* | 304 | 352 |
| 77. *Candida zeylanoides* |  | 75, 102, 168 |
| 78. *Chaetoconidium* sp. | 189 |  |
| 79. *Chaetomium funicolum* |  | 162 |
| 80. *Chaetosphaeronema larense* | 37 |  |
| 81. *Chmelia slovaca* |  | 334 |
| 82. *Chrysosporium evolceanui* |  | 113 |
| 83. *Chrysosporium keratinophilum* |  | 167 |
| 84. *Chrysosporium parvum* | 278, 345 |  |
| 85. *Cladorrhinum* sp. |  | 377 |
| 86. *Cladosporium* sp. |  | 34, 104 |
| 87. *Cladosporium bantianum* | 84, 174, 223, 290 |  |
| 88. *Cladosporium carrionii* | 84, 174, 290 |  |
| 89. *Cladosporium cladosporioides* | 172 | 251, 265, 375 |
| 90. *Cladosporium nigrescens* |  | 376 |
| 91. *Cladosporium oxysporum* |  | 100 |
| 92. *Cladosporium sphaerospermum* |  | 203 |
| 93. *Coccidioides immitis* | 77, 78, 84, 174, 290 |  |
| 94. *Conidiobolus coronatus* | 84, 151, 174, 290 |  |
| 95. *Conidiobolus incongruus* | 82 |  |

## Appendix C

|  | Representative case reports and summaries | |
|---|---|---|
| Fungi | Accepted | Questionable |
| 96. *Coprinus cinereus* | 329, 354 | |
| 97. *Corynespora cassiicola* | 198 | |
| 98. *Cryptococcus albidus* | | 23, 62, 169, 323, 363 |
| 99. *Cryptococcus laurentii* | | 152, 323 |
| 100. *Cryptococcus luteolus* | | 32 |
| 101. *Cryptococcus neoformans* | 84, 174, 290 | |
| 102. *Cunninghamella bertholletiae* | 139, 173 | |
| 103. *Curvularia geniculata* | 156, 246, 358 | |
| 104. *Curvularia lunata* | 200, 245 | 233, 365, 376 |
| 105. *Curvularia pallescens* | 176 | |
| 106. *Curvularia senegalensis* | 100 | |
| 107. *Curvularia verruculosa* | | 100 |
| 108. *Cylindrocarpon tonkinense* | 180 | |
| 109. *Debaryomyces hansenii* | | 22, 158, 339 |
| 110. *Drechslera* sp. | 71, 165 | |
| 111. *Drechslera hawaiiensis* | 106, 371 | |
| 112. *Drechslera rostrata* | 145 | |
| 113. *Drechslera spicifera* | 91, 378 | |
| 114. *Endomycopsis* sp. | | 302 |
| 115. *Epidermophyton floccosum* | 84, 174, 281, 290 | |
| 116. *Exophiala jeanselmei* | 180, 214 | |
| 117. *Exophiala moniliae* | 216 | |
| 118. *Exophiala spinifera* | 243 | |
| 119. *Exophiala werneckii* | 84, 174, 214, 290 | |
| 120. *Fissuricella filamenta* | | 269 |
| 121. *Fonsecaea compacta* | 84, 174, 290 | |
| 122. *Fonsecaea pedrosoi* | 84, 174, 190, 290 | |
| 123. *Fusarium* sp. | 2, 30, 259 | |
| 124. *Fusarium dimerum* | 121, 379, 380 | |
| 125. *Fusarium moniliforme* | 14, 57, 266, 373 | |
| 126. *Fusarium nivale* | 258 | |
| 127. *Fusarium otomycosis* | | 374 |
| 128. *Fusarium oxysporum* | 86, 127, 225, 301 | 194, 376 |
| 129. *Fusarium solani* | 50, 86, 124, 136, 340 | |
| 130. *Geomyces pannorus* | | 167 |
| 131. *Geotrichum* sp. | | 29, 48, 149 |
| 132. *Geotrichum candidum* | 299, 320 | 73, 118, 241, 321, 361 |
| 133. *Graphium* sp. | | 16 |
| 134. *Hansenula anomala* | | 61, 356 |
| 135. *Hansenula polymorpha* | 217 | |
| 136. *Hendersonula toruloidea* | 44, 111, 206 | |
| 137. *Histoplasma capsulatum* var. *capsulatum* | 84, 119, 174, 290 | |
| 138. *Histoplasma capsulatum* var. *duboisii* | 55, 74, 79, 193 | |
| 139. *Kloeckera* sp. | | 202 |
| 140. *Kluyveromyces lactis* | | 96 |

| Fungi | Representative case reports and summaries | |
|---|---|---|
| | Accepted | Questionable |
| 141. *Kluyveromyces marxianus* | | 307 |
| 142. *Lasiodiplodia theobromae* | 280, 283 | |
| 143. *Leptosphaeria senegalensis* | 27 | |
| 144. *Leptosphaeria tompkinsii* | 263, 315 | |
| 145. *Loboa loboi* | 31, 143 | |
| 146. *Lycoperdon* sp. | | 332 |
| 147. *Madurella grisea* | 43, 84, 117, 174, 290 | |
| 148. *Madurella mycetomatis* | 27, 125, 195 | |
| 149. *Malassezia furfur* | 84, 174, 290 | |
| 150. *Malbranchea pulchella* | | 351 |
| 151. *Microascus desmosporus* | 309 | |
| 152. *Microsporum audouinii* | 281, 290 | |
| 153. *Microsporum canis* | 281, 290 | |
| 154. *Microsporum distortum* | 281, 290 | |
| 155. *Microsporum equinun* | 281, 290 | |
| 156. *Microsporum ferrugineum* | 281, 290 | |
| 157. *Microsporum fulvum* | 281, 290 | |
| 158. *Microsporum gallinae* | 341 | |
| 159. *Microsporum gypseum* | 281, 290 | |
| 160. *Microsporum nanum* | 281, 290 | |
| 161. *Microsporum persicolor* | 281, 290 | |
| 162. *Microsporum racemosum* | 10 | 64 |
| 163. *Mortierella* sp. | | 83 |
| 164. *Mortierella mycetomatis*[a] | | 242 |
| 165. *Mortierella niveo-velutina* | | 52 |
| 166. *Mucor hiemalis* | | 360 |
| 167. *Mucor mycetomatis*[a] | | 109 |
| 168. *Mucor ramosissimus* | 42, 350 | |
| 169. *Mucor rouxianus* | 72 | |
| 170. Mycelia Sterilia | 215 | |
| 171. *Mycocentrospora acerina* | 184 | |
| 172. *Neotestudina rosatii* | 316 | |
| 173. *Neurospora sitophila* | | 338 |
| 174. *Oidiodendron cerealis* | 33 | |
| 175. *Paecilomyces* sp. | 128 | 134 |
| 176. *Paecilomyces lilacinus* | 95, 129, 201, 231, 335 | 376 |
| 177. *Paecilomyces variotii* | 212, 325 | |
| 178. *Paecilomyces viridis* | 295 | |
| 179. *Paracoccidioides brasiliensis* | 84, 174, 286, 290 | |
| 180. *Penicillium* sp. | 131 | 51, 94, 183, 196, 232, 244 |
| 181. *Penicillium bacillosporum* | | 148 |
| 182. *Penicillium bertai*[a] | | 336 |
| 183. *Penicillium chrysogenum* | 342 | 376 |
| 184. *Penicillium citrinum* | 115, 124, 146 | 376 |
| 185. *Penicillium commune* | 138 | |
| 186. *Penicillium expansum* | 124 | |
| 187. *Penicillium marneffei* | 70 | |

# Appendix C

| Fungi | Representative case reports and summaries | |
|---|---|---|
| | Accepted | Questionable |
| 188. *Penicillium mycetomagenum*[a] | | 205 |
| 189. *Penicillium oxalicum* | | 376 |
| 190. *Penicillium rubrum* | | 303 |
| 191. *Penicillium rugulosum* | | 239 |
| 192. *Penicillium spinulosum* | 69 | 122 |
| 193. *Petriellidium boydii* | 84, 86, 89, 174, 290 | |
| 194. *Phialophora bubakii* | | 271 |
| 195. *Phialophora hoffmannii* | 261, 327 | |
| 196. *Phialophora parasitica* | 6 | |
| 197. *Phialophora repens* | 222 | |
| 198. *Phialophora richardsiae* | 186, 311 | |
| 199. *Phialophora verrucosa* | 84, 174, 290, 364 | 265 |
| 200. *Phoma* sp. | 372 | 140, 141 |
| 201. *Phoma glomerata* | | 4 |
| 202. *Phoma hibernica* | 21 | |
| 203. *Phoma oculo-hominis* | | 276 |
| 204. *Phyllosticta* sp. | 116 | |
| 205. *Piedraia hortae* | 84, 174, 290, 296 | |
| 206. *Polypaecilum insolitum* | | 369, 370 |
| 207. *Prototheca wickerhamii* | 155, 160, 211 | |
| 208. *Prototheca zopfii* | 67, 155 | |
| 209. *Pseudoarachniotus* sp. | | 300 |
| 210. *Pseudoarachniotus roseus* | 26 | |
| 211. *Pseudoeurotium ovalis* | 88 | |
| 212. *Pyrenochaeta* sp. | | 11 |
| 213. *Pyrenochaeta mackinnonii* | 36 | |
| 214. *Pyrenochaeta unguis-hominis* | 277 | 87 |
| 215. *Rhinocladiella* sp. | 35 | |
| 216. *Rhinosporidium seeberi* | 18, 153, 178 | |
| 217. *Rhizoctonia* sp. | 330 | |
| 218. *Rhizomucor pusillus* | 221 | |
| 219. *Rhizopus arrhizus* | 132, 290 | 267 |
| 220. *Rhizopus microsporus* | 236 | 360 |
| 221. *Rhizopus oryzae* | 179, 353 | |
| 222. *Rhizopus rhizopodiformis* | 20, 108 | |
| 223. *Rhizopus stolonifer* | | 47, 56, 360 |
| 224. *Rhodotorula* sp. | | 133, 182, 191, 192 |
| 225. *Rhodotorula glutinis* | | 323 |
| 226. *Rhodotorula pilimanae* | 235 | |
| 227. *Rhodotorula rubra* | 161, 268 | 58, 87, 289, 297, 314, 323 |
| 228. *Saccharomyces* sp. | | 114, 331 |
| 229. *Saccharomyces cerevisiae* | | 144, 347 |
| 230. *Saccharomyces uvarum* | | 282 |
| 231. *Sagrahamala terricola* | | 14 |
| 232. *Saksenaea vasiformis* | 5 | |
| 233. *Sarcinosporon inkin* | | 220 |
| 234. *Scedosporium apiospermum* | 84, 174, 290 | |
| 235. *Schizophyllum commune* | 159, 285 | |

| Fungi | Representative case reports and summaries | |
|---|---|---|
| | Accepted | Questionable |
| 236. *Scopulariopsis acremonium* | 310 | |
| 237. *Scopulariopsis brevicaulis* | 84, 174, 238, 290, 310, 318, 355 | 87, 208 |
| 238. *Scopulariopsis brumptii* | 123 | |
| 239. *Scopulariopsis candida* | | 102 |
| 240. *Scopulariopsis koningii* | | 142, 310 |
| 241. *Scytalidium hyalinum* | 45 | |
| 242. *Sporobolomyces salmonicolor* | | 163, 260 |
| 243. *Sporormia articulata* | | 348 |
| 244. *Sporothrix cyanescens* | | 137 |
| 245. *Sporothrix schenckii* | 84, 174, 290 | |
| 246. *Stenella araguata* | 207, 274, 287 | |
| 247. *Syncephalastrum racemosum* | | 367 |
| 248. *Taeniolella stilbospora* | 262 | |
| 249. *Tetraploa* sp. | 240 | |
| 250. *Thailandia candida* | | 344 |
| 251. *Torulopsis candida* | | 239 |
| 252. *Torulopsis glabrata* | 84, 174, 290, 317 | |
| 253. *Torulopsis haemulonii* | | 87 |
| 254. *Torulopsis inconspicua* | | 337, 347 |
| 255. *Trichoderma viride* | | 90 |
| 256. *Trichophyton ajelloi* | | 273 |
| 257. *Trichophyton concentricum* | 281, 290 | |
| 258. *Trichophyton equinum* | 281, 290 | |
| 259. *Trichophyton gourvilii* | 281, 290 | |
| 260. *Trichophyton megninii* | 281, 290 | |
| 261. *Trichophyton mentagrophytes* | 281, 290 | |
| 262. *Trichophyton rubrum* | 281, 290 | |
| 263. *Trichophyton schoenleinii* | 281, 290 | |
| 264. *Trichophyton simii* | 281, 290 | |
| 265. *Trichophyton soudanense* | 281, 290 | |
| 266. *Trichophyton terrestre* | 281, 290 | |
| 267. *Trichophyton tonsurans* | 281, 290 | |
| 268. *Trichophyton verrucosum* | 281, 290 | |
| 269. *Trichophyton violaceum* | 281, 290 | |
| 270. *Trichophyton yaoundei* | 281, 290 | |
| 271. *Trichosporon beigelii* | 256, 293, 322 | 197, 343, 359 |
| 272. *Trichosporon capitatum* | 366 | 110, 284 |
| 273. *Trigonopsis variabilis* | | 202 |
| 274. *Tritirachium oryzae* | 177, 294 | |
| 275. *Ustilago maydis* | | 229, 272 |
| 276. *Verticillium graphii* | | 368 |
| 277. *Volutella cinerescens* | 101 | |
| 278. *Wangiella dermatitidis* | 84, 174, 290 | 85 |

[a] This species is not identifiable.

# Appendix C

## References Cited

1. Abboud, I. A., and L. S. Hanna (1970). Ocular fungus. Report of two cases. *Br. J. Ophthalmol.* **54**:477-483.
2. Abramowsky, C. R., D. Quinn, W. D. Bradford, and N. F. Conant (1974). Systemic infection by *Fusarium* in a burned child. The emergence of a saprophytic strain. *J. Pediatr.* **84**:561-564.
3. Agarwal, L. P., S. R. K. Malik, M. Mohan, and L. N. Mahopatra (1962). Orbital aspergillosis. *Br. J. Ophthalmol.* **46**:559-562.
4. Agostini, A., and V. Tredici (1937). Sopra una nuova specie di micete commensale (*Phoma hominis* Agostini et Tredici) isolato da forme cliniche del derma. *Atti Ist. Bot. Univ. Pavia* [*Ser. 4*] **9**:179-189.
5. Ajello, L., D. F. Dean, and R. S. Irwin (1976). The zygomycete *Saksenaea vasiformis* as a pathogen of humans with a critical review of the etiology of zygomycosis. *Mycologia* **68**:52-62.
6. Ajello, L., L. K. Georg, R. T. Steigbigel, and C. J. K. Wang (1974). A case of phaeohyphomycosis caused by a new species of *Phialophora*. *Mycologia* **66**:490-498.
7. Albesi, E. J., and R. C. Zapater (1975). Queratitis por *Aspergillus flavus*. *Arch. Oftalmol. Buenos Aires* **50**:163-168.
8. Albornoz, M. C. Bastardo de (1963-1964). Micetoma (Pie de Madura) debido a *Cephalosporium recifei*. *Dermatol. Venez.* **4**:56-64.
9. Albornoz, M. B. de (1974). *Cephalosporium serrae*, agente etiologico de micetomas. *Mycopathol. Mycol. Appl.* **54**:485-498.
10. Albornoz, M. B. de, C. A. Lopez, and N. Alfonzo (1972). Primer caso de tinea corporis por el *Microsporum racemosum* (Dante Borelli, 1965). *Dermatol. Venez.* **11**:310-318.
11. Albornoz, M. B. de, G. Rodriguez-Garcilazo, and D. Urdaneta-González (1977). Micetomas de localizacion podal de etiologia doble. *Sabouraudia* **15**:187-193.
12. Alecrim, I. C. da, and A. F. Vital (1955). O *Aspergillus sydowi* (Bain. and Sart.) Thom e Church numa lesão ungueal. *An. Fac. Med. Univ. Recife* **15**:229-240.
13. Amicis, E. de (1950). Osservazioni cliniche, micologiche e patogenetiche su tre casi di otomicosi da *Aspergillus versicolor*. *Boll. Mal. Orecchio. Gola Naso* **68**:278-325.
14. Anderson, B., S. S. Roberts, C. Gonzalez, and E. W. Chick (1959). Mycotic ulcerative keratitis. *Arch. Ophthalmol.* **62**:169-179.
15. Anzmlt, B. M. C., and M. Eastman (1975). Onychomycosis due to *Aspergillus candidus*: case report. *N. Z. Med. J.* **82**:13-15.
16. Apostol, J. G., and S. L. Meyer (1972). *Graphium* endophthalmitis. *Am. J. Ophthamol.* **73**:556-569.

17. Arievitch, A. M., Z. G. Stepanisheva, O. V. Tjufilina, Z. I. Kukoleva, A. J. Malkina, and V. V. Teplitz (1966). Gummato-ulcerative cephalosporiosis of the skin. *Mycopathol. Mycol. Appl.* **28**:113–121.
18. Ashworth, J. H. (1923). XVI. On *Rhinosporidium seeberi* (Wernicke, 1903), with special reference to its sporulation and affinities. *Trans. R. Soc. Edinburgh* **53**:301–342.
19. Azar, P., J. V. Aquavella, and R. S. Smith (1975). Keratomycosis due to an *Alternaria* species. *Am. J. Ophthalmol.* **79**:881–883.
20. Baker, R. D., J. H. Seabury, and J. D. Schneidau (1962). Subcutaneous and cutaneous mucormycosis and subcutaneous phycomycosis. *Lab. Invest.* **11**:1091–1102.
21. Bakerspigel, A. (1970). The isolation of *Phoma hibernica* from a lesion on a leg. *Sabouraudia* **7**:261–264.
22. Barney, M., C. W. Dodge, and R. Simmers (1963). *Debaryomyces* infection in Vermont. *Mycopathol. Mycol. Appl.* **19**:246–254.
23. Batista, A. C., and S. T. C. Campos (1962). Criptococose lingual e genital. *Inst. Micol. Univ. Recife, Publ.* **202**, pp. 1–27.
24. Batista, A. C., J. A. Maia, and R. Singer (1955). Basidioneuromycosis on man. *Inst. Micol. Univ. Recife, Publ.* **42**, pp. 53–60.
25. Batista, A. C., H. da Silva Maia, and I. C. Alecrim (1955). Onicomicose produzida por *Aspergillus clavato-nanica* n. sp. *An. Fac. Med. Univ. Recife* **15**:197–203.
26. Batista, A. C., H. da Silva Maia, and W. Cavalcanti (1960). Otomicose produzida por *Waldemaria pernambucensis* n. gen. n. sp. *Inst. Micol. Univ. Recife* **1**:5–12.
27. Baylet, J., R. Camain, and G. Segretain (1959). Identification des agents des maduromycoses du Sénégal et de la Mauritanie. Description d'une espèce nouvelle. *Bull. Soc. Pathol. Exot.* **52**:448–477.
28. Beaney, G. P. E., and A. Broughton (1967). Tropical otomycosis. *J. Laryngol. Otol.* **81**:987–997.
29. Bendove, R. A., and B. I. Ashe (1952). *Geotrichum* septicemia. *Arch. Intern. Med.* **89**:107–110.
30. Benjamin, R. P., J. L. Callaway, and N. F. Conant (1970). Facial granuloma associated with *Fusarium* infection. *Arch. Dermatol.* **101**:598–600.
31. Bhawan, J., R. W. Bain, D. T. Purtilo, N. Gomez, C. Dewan, C. F. Whelan, M. Dolorum, and L. Edelstein (1976). Lobomycosis. An electronmicroscopic, histochemical and immunologic study. *J. Cutan. Pathol.* **3**:5–16.
32. Binder, L., A. Csillag, and G. Tóth (1956). Diffuse infiltration of the lungs associated with *Cryptococcus luteolus*. *Lancet* **270**:1043–1045.
33. Blomqvist, K., and A. Salonen (1969). *Oidiodendron cerealis* isolated from neurodermitis nuchae. *Dermatologica* **139**:158–160.
34. Bojanovsky, A., and G. Lischka (1976). Kutane granulömatose Cladosporiose. *Z. Hautkr.* **51**:658–662.
35. Borelli, D. (1972). *Acrotheca aquaspersa* nova species agente de cromomicosis. *Acta Cient. Venez.* **23**:193–196.
36. Borelli, D. (1976). *Pyrenochaeta mackinnonii* nova species agente de micetoma. *Castellania* **4**:227–234.
37. Borelli, D., R. Zamora, and G. Senabre (1976). *Chaetosphaeronema larense* nova specie agente de micetoma. *Gac. Med. Caracas* **84**:307–318.
38. Borsook, M. E. (1933). Skin infection due to *Alternaria tenuis* with the report of a case. *Can. Med. Assoc. J.* **29**:479–482.
39. Bourlond, A., J. Decroix, F. Dobbelaere, and A. Lissoir (1974). Alternariose dermique. *Ann. Dermatol. Syphiligr.* **101**:413–415.
40. Braf, Z. F., G. Altmann, and E. Ostfeld (1976). Fungal infections after renal transplantation. *Isr. J. Med. Sci.* **12**:674–677.

41. Brumpt, E. (1906). Mycétome noir de Bouffard à *Aspergillus Bouffardi*, n. sp. Brumpt, 1906. "Les Mycétomes," pp. 38–46. Asselin et Houzeau, Paris.
42. Bullock, J. D., L. M. Jampol, and A. J. Fezza (1974). Two cases of orbital phycomycosis with recovery. *Am. J. Ophthalmol.* **78**:811–815.
43. Butz, W. C., and L. Ajello (1971). Black grain mycetoma. A case due to *Madurella grisea*. *Arch. Dermatol.* **104**:197–201.
44. Campbell, C. K., A. Kurwa, A.-H. M. Abdel-Aziz, and C. Hodgson (1973). Fungal infection of skin and nails by *Hendersonula toruloidea*. *Br. J. Dermatol.* **89**:45–52.
45. Campbell, C. K., and J. L. Mulder (1977). Skin and nail infection by *Scytalidium hyalinum* sp. nov. *Sabouraudia* **15**:161–166.
46. Carrizosa, J., M. E. Levison, T. Lawrence, and D. Kaye (1974). Cure of *Aspergillus ustus* endocarditis on a prosthetic valve. *Arch. Intern. Med.* **133**:486–490.
47. Champion, C. K., and T. M. Johnson (1969). Rhino-orbital-cerebral phycomycosis. *Mich. Med.* **68**:807–810.
48. Chang, W. W. L., and L. Buerger (1964). Disseminated geotrichosis. Case report. *Arch. Intern. Med.* 113:356–360.
49. Cheetham, H. D. (1964). Subcutaneous infection due to *Aspergillus terreus*. *J. Clin. Pathol.* **17**:251–253.
50. Cho, C. T., T. S. Vats, J. T. Lowman, J. W. Brandsberg, and F. E. Tosh (1973). *Fusarium solani* infection during treatment for acute leukemia. *J. Pediatr.* **83**:1028–1031.
51. Chute, A. L. (1911). An infection of the bladder with *Penicillium glaucum*. *Boston Med. Surg. J.* **164**:420–422.
52. Ciferri, R., and B. K. Ashford (1929). A new species of *Mortierella* isolated from the human skin. *P. R. J. Publ. Health Trop. Med.* **5**:134–143.
53. Clinicopathological Conference (1969). A case of fungal endocarditis. *Br. Med. J.* **3**:765–770.
54. Cochet, G. (1942–1943). Propriétés physiologiques d'*Arthrographis langeroni* Cochet 1939 agent pathogène d'une onychomycose humaine. *Ann. Parasitol. Hum. Comp.* **19**:157–159.
55. Cockshott, W. P., and A. O. Lucas (1964). Histoplasmosis duboisii. *Quart. J. Med.* **33**:223–238.
56. Coetzee, A. S., and G. F. de Bruin (1974). Mucormycosis case report and review. *S. Afr. Med. J.* **48**:2486–2488.
57. Collins, M. S. and M. G. Rinaldi (1977). Cutaneous infection in man caused by *Fusarium moniliforme*. *Sabouraudia* **15**:151–160.
58. Cramer, H. J., and H. A. Koch (1963). Über die Bedeutung der *Rhodotorula*-Hefen als Krankheitserreger in der Dermatologie. *Dermatol. Wochenschr.* **147**:563–568.
59. Cramer, H. J., H. Liedloff, and H. A. Koch (1968). Singuläres *Candida*-Granulom der Haut mit Hornhaut-Candidose durch eine seltene Hefeart. *Dtsch. Gesundheitswes.* **23**:1554–1558.
60. Crozier, W. J., and H. Coats (1977). A case of onychomycosis due to *Candida ravautii*. *Australas. J. Dermatol.* **18**:139–140.
61. Csillag, A., and L. Brandstein (1954). The role of a blastomyces species in the genesis of interstitial pneumonia of the premature infant. A preliminary report. *Acta Microbiol. Hung.* **1**:525–529.
62. Cunha, T. da, and J. Lusins (1973). *Cryptococcus albidus* meningitis. *South. Med. J.* **66**:1230 and 1243.
63. Darja, M., and M. I. Davy (1963). Pulmonary mucormycosis with cultural identification. *Can. Med. Assoc. J.* **89**:1235–1238.

64. Daum, V., and D. J. McCloud (1976). *Microsporum racemosum*: first isolation in the United States. *Mycopathologia* **59**:183–185.
65. David, M., Charlin, Morice, and Naudascher (1951). Infiltration mycosique à *Aspergillus amstelodami* du lobe temporal simulant un abcès encapsulé. Ablation en masse. Guérison opératoire. *Rev. Neurol. (Paris)* **85**:121–124.
66. Davies, D. (1963). Pulmonary aspergillosis. *Can. Med. Assoc. J.* **89**:392–395.
67. Davies, R. R., H. Spencer, and P. O. Wakelin (1964). A case of human protothecosis. *Trans. R. Soc. Trop. Med. Hyg.* **58**:448–451.
68. Dehghanian, J., J. Partin, and W. K. Schubert (1976). *Candida parapsilosis* infection. *South. Med. J.* **69**:68–69.
69. Delore, P., J. Coudert, R. Lambert, and J. Fayolle (1955). Un cas de mycose bronchique avec localisations musculaires septicémiques. *Presse Med.* **63**:1580–1582.
70. DiSalvo, A. F., A. M. Fickling, and L. Ajello (1973). Infection caused by *Penicillium marneffei*: description of first natural infection in man. *Am. J. Clin. Pathol.* **60**:259–263.
71. Dolan, C. T., L. A. Weed, and D. E. Dines (1970). Bronchopulmonary helminthosporiosis. *Am. J. Clin. Pathol.* **53**:235–242.
72. Douvin, D., Y. Lefichoux, and C. Huguet (1975). Phycomycose gastrique diagnostic anatomo-pathologique et mycologique précoce évolution favorable sous traitement médical puis chirurgical. *Arch. Anat. Pathol.* **23**:133–138.
73. Drach, G. W., C. E. Carlton, O. W. Chenault, and R. F. Dykhuizen (1968). Fungal superinfection: geotrichosis of the urinary tract in association with parathyroid adenoma. *J. Urol.* **100**:82–84.
74. Drouhet, E. (1957). Quelques aspects biologiques et mycologiques de l'histoplasmose. *Arch. Biol. Med.* **33**:439–461.
75. Drouhet, E. (1973). Mycoses du coeur. Encyclopédie Médico-Chirurgicale No. 7, 10 pp.
76. Drouhet, E., L. Martin, G. Segretain, and P. Destombes (1965). Mycose méningo-cérébrale a *Cephalosporium*. *Presse Med.* **73**:1809–1814.
77. Drutz, D. J., and A. Catanzaro (1978). Coccidioidomycosis. Part 1. *Am. Rev. Respir. Dis.* **117**:559–585.
78. Drutz, D. J., and A. Catanzaro (1978). Coccidioidomycosis. Part II. *Am. Rev. Respir. Dis.* **117**:727–771.
79. Dubois, A., P. G. Janssens, P. Brutsaert, and R. Vanbreuseghem (1952). Un cas d'histoplasmose africaine, avec une note mycologique sur *Histoplasma duboisii* n. sp. *Ann. Soc. Belg. Med. Trop.* **32**:569–583.
80. Durie, E. B., and S. Brown (1953). Fungous infections in hospital practice. *Med. J. Aust.* **2**:813–814.
81. Dworzack, D. L., A. S. Pollock, G. R. Hodges, W. G. Barnes, L. Ajello, and A. Padhye (1978). Zygomycosis of the maxillary sinus and palate caused by *Basidiobolus haptosporus*. *Arch. Intern. Med.* **138**:1274–1276.
82. Eckert, H. L, G. H. Khoury, R. S. Pore, E. F. Gilbert, and J. R. Gaskell (1972). Deep *Entomophthora* phycomycotic infection reported for the first time in the United States. *Chest* **61**:392–394.
83. Emmons, C. W. (1964). Phycomycosis in man and animals. *Riv. Patol. Veg. (Pavia)* [*Ser. 3, part 4*] **4**:329–337.
84. Emmons, C. W., C. H. Binford, J. P. Utz, and K. J. Kwon-Chung (1977). "Medical Mycology," 3rd ed. Lea & Febiger, Philadelphia.
85. Engelman, R. M., R. M. Chase, F. C. Spencer, M. V. Benjamin, and S. A. Rosenthal (1971). Mycotic infections on prosthetic and homograft heart valves: report of the first case of endocarditis caused by *Hormodendrum dermatitidis*. *Ann. Surg.* **173**:455–461.
86. English, M. P. (1968). Invasion of the skin by filamentous nondermatophyte fungi. *Br. J. Dermatol.* **80**:282–286.

87. English, M. P., and R. Atkinson (1974). Onychomycosis in elderly chiropody patients. *Br. J. Dermatol.* **91**:67-72.
88. English, M. P., R. R. M. Harman, and J. W. J. Turvey (1967). *Pseudoeurotium ovalis* in toenails. Some problems of mycological diagnosis of nail infections. *Br. J. Dermatol.* **79**:553-556.
89. Ernest, J. T., and J. W. Rippon (1966). Keratitis due to *Allescheria boydii* (*Monosporium apiospermum*). *Am. J. Ophthalmol.* **62**:1202-1204.
90. Escudero Gil, M. R., E. Pino Corral, and R. Muñoz Muñoz (1976). Micoma pulmonar causado por *Trichoderma viride*. *Actas Dermo-Sifiliogr.* **67**:673-680.
91. Estes, S. A., W. G. Merz, and L. G. Maxwell (1977). Primary cutaneous phaeohyphomycosis caused by *Drechslera spicifera*. *Arch. Dermatol.* **113**:813-815.
92. Estrader, F., H. Longefait, G. Lalevée, C. Coury, and P. Constans (1972). *Aspergillus restrictus* forme rare d'aspergillome intracavitaire associée à une tuberculose active. *J. Fr. Med.* **26**:241-249.
93. Farmer, S. G., and R. A. Komorowski (1976). Cutaneous microabscess formation from *Alternaria alternata*. *Am. J. Clin. Pathol.* **66**:565-569.
94. Fazakas, S. (1959). Zusammenfassender Bericht über die sekundären Mykosen bei Erkrankungen des Augenlidrandes, der Bindehaut und der Hornhaut. *Ophthalmologica* **138**:108-118.
95. Fenech, F. F., and C. P. Mallia (1972). Pleural effusion caused by *Penicillium lilacinum*. *Br. J. Dis. Chest* **66**:284-290.
96. Földvári, F., and E. Flórián (1965). Blastomycosis profunda glutealis. *Trans. St. John's Hosp. Dermatol. Soc.* **51**:60-61.
97. Fonseca Filho, O. da (1930). Mycetoma por *Aspergillus amstelodami*. *Rev. Med. Cirurg. Brasil* **38**:415-423.
98. Forster, R. K., and G. Rebell (1975). Therapeutic surgery in failures of medical treatment of fungal keratitis. *Br. J. Ophthalmol.* **59**:366-371.
99. Forster, R. K., G. Rebell, and W. Stiles (1975). Recurrent keratitis due to *Acremonium potronii*. *Am. J. Ophthalmol.* **79**:126-128.
100. Forster, R. K., G. Rebell, and L. A. Wilson (1975). Dematiaceous fungal keratitis. Clinical isolates and management. *Br. J. Ophthalmol.* **59**:372-376.
101. Foster, J. B. T., E. Almeda, M. L. Littman, and M. E. Wilson (1958). Some intraocular and conjunctival effects of amphotericin B in man and in the rabbit. *Arch. Ophthalmol.* **60**:555-564.
102. Fragner, P. (1966). Mykoflora der Onychomykosen. *Mykosen* **9**:29-34.
103. Fragner, P., J. Vitovec, P. Vladik, and Z. Záhoř (1973). *Aspergillus penicilloides* v solitárnim plicnim aspergilomu u srny. *Ceska Mykol.* **27**:151-155.
104. Francois, J., and M. Ryselaere (1972). "Oculomycoses," pp. 66-67. Thomas, Springfield, Illinois.
105. Fréour, P., M. Lahourcade, and P. Chomy (1966). Les champignons *Beauveria* en pathologie humaine à propos d'un cas à localisation pulmonaire. *Presse Med.* **74**:2317-2320.
106. Fuste, F. J., L. Ajello, R. Threlkeld, and J. E. Henry (1973). *Drechslera hawaiiensis*: causative agent of a fatal fungal meningo-encephalitis. *Sabouraudia* **11**:59-63.
107. Garau, J., R. D. Diamond, L. B. Lagrotteria, and S. A. Kabins (1977). *Alternaria* osteomyelitis. *Ann. Intern. Med.* **86**:747-748.
108. Gartenberg, G., E. J. Bottone, G. T. Keusch, and I. Weitzman (1978). Hospitalacquired mucormycosis (*Rhizopus rhizopodiformis*) of skin and subcutaneous tissue. *N. Engl. J. Med.* **299**:1115-1118.
109. Gelonesi, G. (1927). Due nuovi parassiti del "piede di madura." Studio sui micetomi della Somalia Meridionale. *Ann. Med. Nav. Colon.* **33**:283-308.

110. Gemeinhardt, H. (1965). Zur Frage der Pathogenität des Sprobpilzes *Trichosporon capitatum* im Respirationstrakt des Menschen. Ein Beitrag zur Diagnostik der Lungenmykosen. *Z. Tuberk. Erkr. Thoraxorgane* **124**: 190–197.
111. Gentles, J. C., and E. G. V. Evans (1970). Infection of the feet and nails with *Hendersonula toruloidea*. *Sabouraudia* **8**:72–75.
112. Gerber, J., J. Chomicki, J. W. Brandsberg, R. Jones, , and K. J. Hammerman (1973). Pulmonary aspergillosis caused by *Aspergillus fischeri* var. *spinosus:* report of a case and value of serologic studies. *Am. J. Clin. Pathol.* **60**:861–866.
113. Ghosh, G. R., B. Sur, and K. Roy (1976). Dermatomycoses in Cuttack, Orissa and report on pseudocleistothecia formation by strains of *Trichophyton rubrum* Castellani. *Kavaka* **4**:25–30.
114. Giese, W. (1952). Pathogenese und Ätiologie der interstitiellen plasmazellulären Säuglingspneumonie. *Verh. Dtsch. Ges. Pathol.* **36**:284–289.
115. Gilliam, J. S., and S. A. Vest (1951). *Penicillium* infection of the urinary tract. *J. Urol.* **65**:484–489.
116. Gip, L., and H. Paldrok (1967). Onychomycosis caused by *Phyllostictina* Sydow. *Acta Dermatol. Venereol.* **47**:186–189.
117. Gokhalay, B. B., A. A. Padhye, and M. J. Thirumalachar (1968). Madura foot in India caused by *Madurella grisea*. *Sabouraudia* **6**:305–306.
118. Goldman, S., P. R. Lipscomb, and J. A. Ulrich (1969). *Geotrichum* tumefaction of the hand. Report of a case. *J. Bone Jt. Surg.* **51**:587–590.
119. Goodwin, R. A., F. T. Owens, J. D. Snell, W. W. Hubbard, R. D. Buchanan, R. T. Terry, and R. M. Des Prez (1976). Chronic pulmonary histoplasmosis. *Medicine* **55**:413–452.
120. Gordon, M. A., R. S. Holzman, H. Senter, E. W. Lapa, and M. J. Kupersmith (1976). *Aspergillus oryzae* meningitis. *J. Am. Med. Assoc.* **235**:2122–2123.
121. Greer, D. L., C. Brahim, and L. A. González (1973). Queratitis micotica en Colombia. *Trib. Med.* **74**:A15–A20.
122. Grégoire, P. E., R. Linz, and O. Van Damme (1953). Apparitions successives d'un *Penicillium* et d'un *Aspergillus* dans un liquide pleural. *Acta Clin. Belg.* **8**:483–485.
123. Grieble, H. G., J. W. Rippon, N. Maliwan, and V. Daun (1975). Scopulariopsosis and hypersensitivity pneumonitis in an addict. *Ann. Intern. Med.* **83**:326–329.
124. Gugnani, H. C., R. S. Talwar, A. N. U. Njoku-Obi, and H. C. Kodilinye (1976). Mycotic keratitis in Nigeria. A study of 21 cases. *Br. J. Ophthalmol.* **60**:607–613.
125. Gumaa, S. A., A. A. Satir, A. H. Shehata, and E. S. Mahgoub (1975). Tumor of the mandible caused by *Madurella mycetomii*. *Am. J. Trop. Med. Hyg.* **24**:471–474.
126. Gupta, K. R., B. Udhayakumar, P. B. Rao, M. Madhavan, and L. R. Das Gupta (1973). Aspergilloma of the frontal bone. *J. Laryngol. Otol.* **87**:1007–1011.
127. Gutmann, L., S. M. Chou, and R. S. Pore (1975). Fusariosis, myasthenic syndrome, and aplastic anemia. *Neurology* **24**:922–926.
128. Haldane, E. V., J. L. MacDonald, W. O. Gittens, K. Yuce, and C. E. van Rooyen (1974). Prosthetic valvular endocarditis due to the fungus *Paecilomyces*. *Can. Med. Assoc. J.* **111**:963–968.
129. Halde, C., and M. Okumoto (1966). Ocular mycoses: a study of 82 cases. *Proc. Int. Congr. Ophthalmol.*, 20th, Excerpta Med., Int. Congr. Ser. No. 146, part 2, pp. 705–712.
130. Halde, C., A. A. Padhye, L. D. Haley, M. G. Rinaldi, D. Kay, and R. Leeper (1976). *Acremonium falciforme* as a cause of mycetoma in California. *Sabouraudia* **14**:319–326.
131. Hall, W. J. (1974). *Penicillium* endocarditis following open heart surgery and prosthetic valve insertion. *Am. Heart J.* **87**:501–506.

132. Hammer, G. S., E. J. Bottone, and S. Z. Hirschman (1975). Mucormycosis in a transplant recipient. *Am. J. Clin. Pathol.* **64**:389–398.
133. Henig, E. (1973). Ocular mycoses due to *Rhodotorula*. *Harefuah* **84**:142–144
134. Henig, F. E., N. Lehrer, A. Gabbay, and O. Kurz (1973). Paecilomycosis of the lacrimal sac. *Mykosen* **16**:25–28.
135. Higashi, N., and Y. Asada (1973). Cutaneous alternariosis with mixed infection of *Candida albicans*. Report of a patient responding to natamycin. *Arch. Dermatol.* **108**:558–560.
136. Holzegel, K., and H. J. Kempf (1964). Fusariummykose auf der Haut eines Verbrannten. *Dermatol. Wochenschr.* **51**:651–658.
137. Hoog, G. S. de, and G. A. de Vries, (1973). Two new species of *Sporothrix* and their relation to *Blastobotrys nivea*. *Antonie van Leeuwenhoek J. Microbiol. Serol.* **39**:515–520.
138. Huang, S., and L. S. Harris (1963). Acute disseminated penicilliosis: report of a case and review of pertinent literature. *Am. J. Clin. Pathol.* **39**:167–174.
139. Hutter, R. V. P. (1959). Phycomycetous infection (mucormycosis) in cancer patients: a complication of therapy. *Cancer* **12**:330–350.
140. Janke, D. (1950). Bericht mit Bilddemonstrationen klinischer, mykologischer, histologischer und tierexperimenteller Untersuchungen über seltene Mykosen. *Arch. Dermatol. Syph.* **191**:479–482.
141. Janke, D. (1956). Über eine menschenpathogene, aus Lungenveränderungen gezüchtete neue Spezies von *Peyronellaea*. *Mycopathol. Mycol. Appl.* **7**:229–240.
142. Jannin, L. (1912). Mycoses gommeuses a *Scopulariopsis koningi*. *Arch. Parasitol.* **15**:478–489.
143. Jaramillo, D., A. Cortés, A. Restrepo, M. Builes, and M. Robledo (1976). Lobomycosis. Report of the eighth Colombian case and review of the literature. *J. Cutan. Pathol.* **3**:180–189.
144. Jensen, D. P., and D. L. Smith (1976). Fever of unknown origin secondary to Brewer's yeast ingestion. *Arch. Intern. Med.* **136**:332–333.
145. Jones, B. R. (1975). Principles in the management of oculomycosis. *Trans. Am. Acad. Ophthalmol. Otolaryngol.* **79**:OP15–53.
146. Jones, D. B., L. Wilson, R. Sexton, and G. Rebell (1969). Early diagnosis of mycotic keratitis. *Trans. Ophthalmol. Soc. U. K.* **69**:805–813.
147. Jones, F. R., and G. R. Christensen (1974). *Pullularia* corneal ulcer. *Arch. Ophthalmol.* **92**:529–530.
148. Jong, M. A. de (1954). Twee gevallen van schimmelaandoening van de long. *Ned. Tijdschr. Geneeskd.* **98**:2928–2929.
149. Kaliski, S. R., M. L. Beene, and L. Mattman (1952). *Geotrichum* in blood stream of an infant. *J. Am. Med. Assoc.* **148**:1207–1209.
150. Kamalam, A., and A. S. Thambiah (1975). Basidiobolomycosis with lymph node involvement. *Sabouraudia* **13**:44–48.
151. Kamalam, A., and A. S. Thambiah (1978). Lymph node invasion by *Conidiobolus coronatus* and its spore formation *in vivo*. *Sabouraudia* **16**:175–184.
152. Kamalam, A., P. Yesudian, and A. S. Thambiah (1977). Cutaneous infection by *Cryptococcus laurentii*. *Br. J. Dermatol.* **97**:221–223.
153. Kameswaran, S. (1966). Surgery in rhinosporidiosis. Experience with 293 cases. *Int. Surg.* **46**:602–605.
154. Kammer, R. B., and J. P. Utz (1974). *Aspergillus* species endocarditis. The new face of a not so rare disease. *Am. J. Med.* **56**:506–521.
155. Kaplan, W. (1978). Protothecosis and infections caused by morphologically similar green algae. *Proc. Int. Conf. Mycoses*, 4th, *PAHO Sci. Publ.* 356, pp. 218–232.

156. Kaufman, S. M. (1971). *Curvularia* endocarditis following cardiac surgery. *Am. J. Clin. Pathol.* **56**:466–470.
157. Kennedy, W. P. U., L. J. R. Milne, W. Blyth, and G. K. Crompton (1972). Two unusual organisms, *Aspergillus terreus* and *Metschnikowia pulcherrima*, associated with the lung disease of ankylosing spondylitis. *Thorax* **27**:604–610.
158. Kliewe, H., and J. Hofer (1952). Über die Systematik eines pathogenen Sprospilzes. *Frankf. Z. Pathol.* **63**:88–94.
159. Kligman, A. M. (1950). A basidiomycete probably causing onychomycosis. *J. Invest. Dermatol.* **14**:67–70.
160. Klintworth, G. K., B. F. Fetter, and H. S. Nielsen (1968). Protothecosis, an algal infection: report of a case in man. *J. Med. Microbiol.* **1**:211–216.
161. Knoth, W., S. Krause, and K. H. Knoll (1955). Tumorförmige Pilzerkrankung durch eine anaskosporogene Hefe. *Dermatologica* **3**:357–366.
162. Koch, H. A. von, and H. Haneke (1966). *Chaetomium funicolum* Cooke als möglicher Erreger einer tiefen Mykose. *Mykosen* **9**:23–28.
163. Köhlmeier, W., and H. Kreitner (1951). Ein Fall von Mycetoma pedis (Madurafuss) in Wien. *Klin. Med.* **6**:337–342.
164. Koshi, G., T. Kurien, D. Sudarsanam, A. J. Selvapandian, and K. E. Mammen (1972). Subcutaneous phycomycosis caused by *Basidiobolus*. A report of three cases. *Sabouraudia* **10**:237–243.
165. Krachmer, J. H., R. L. Anderson, P. S. Binder, G. O. Waring, J. J. Rowsey, and E. S. Meek (1978). *Helminthosporium* corneal ulcers. *Am. J. Ophthalmol.* **85**:666–670.
166. Krakówka, P., H. Halweg, M. Chimial, and H. Kozaków (1968). Kropidalkowy grzybniak pluc wywolany przez *Aspergillus nidulans* (Eidam) Wint. *Gruźlica Choroby Pluc* **36**:487–491.
167. Krempl-Lamprecht, L. (1965). Über das Vorkommen von Pilzen aus der Gattung *Chrysosporium* auf der Haut und Diskussion ihrer systematischen Stellung. In "Krankheiten durch Schimmelpilze bei Mensch und Tier" (H. Grimmer and H. Rieth, eds.), pp. 136–141. Springer-Verlag, Berlin and New York.
168. Krudysz, J., and W. Kapuscinski (1971). Przypadek iritis tumorosa haemorrhagica mycotica endogenes u piecioletniego dziecka. *Klin. Oczna* **41**:701–704.
169. Krumholz, R. A. (1972). Pulmonary cryptococcosis. A case due to *Cryptococcus albidus*. *Am. Rev. Respir. Dis.* **105**:421–424.
170. Kukoleva, L. I., and A. Ya. Malkina (1967). Sluchai rasprostranennogo gummoznoyazvennogo tsefalosporioza. *Vestn. Dermatol. Venerol.* **41**:76–79.
171. Kwon-Chung, K. J. (1975). A new pathogenic species of *Aspergillus* in the *Aspergillus fumigatus* series. *Mycologia* **67**:770–779.
172. Kwon-Chung, K. J., I. S. Schwartz, and B. J. Rybak (1975). A pulmonary fungus ball produced by *Cladosporium cladosporioides*. *Am. J. Clin. Pathol.* **64**:564–568.
173. Kwon-Chung, K. J., R. C. Young, and M. Orlando (1975). Pulmonary mucormycosis caused by *Cunninghamella elegans* in a patient with chronic myelogenous leukemia. *Am. J. Clin. Pathol.* **64**:544–548.
174. Lacaz, C. da Silva (1977). "Micologia Médica Fungos, Actinomycetos e Algas de Interesse Médico," 6th ed. Sarvier, São Paulo.
175. Lahourcade, M., and L. Texier (1976). A propos d'un cas original de céphalosporiose cutanée superficielle provoquée par *Cephalosporium acremonium*, Corda 1839. *Bull. Soc. Fr. Mycol. Med.* **5**:127–132.
176. Lampert, R. P., J. H. Hutto, W. H. Donnelly, and S. T. Shulman (1977). Pulmonary and cerebral mycetoma caused by *Curvularia pallescens*. *J. Pediatr.* **91**:603–605.
177. Langeron, M. (1947). *Tritirachium brumpti* (Langeron et Lichaa 1934) Langeron 1947 et le genre *Tritirachium* Limber 1940. *Ann. Parasitol. Hum. Comp.* **22**:94–99.

178. Lasser, A., and H. W. Smith (1976). Rhinosporidiosis. *Arch. Otolaryngol.* **102**:308-310.
179. La Touche, C. J., T. W. Sutherland, and M. Telling (1964). Histopathological and mycological features of a case of rhinocerebral mucormycosis (phycomycosis) in Britain. *Sabouraudia* **3**:148-150.
180. Laverde, S., L. H. Moncada, A. Restrepo, and C. L. Vera (1973). Mycotic keratitis; 5 cases caused by unusual fungi. *Sabouraudia* **11**:119-123.
181. Lawrence, T., A. T. Shockman, and H. MacVaugh (1971). *Aspergillus* infection of prosthetic aortic valves. *Chest* **60**:406-414.
182. Leeber, D. A., and I. Scher (1969). *Rhodotorula* fungemia presenting as "endotoxic" shock. *Arch. Intern. Med.* **123**:78-81.
183. Liebler, G. A., G. J. Magovern, P. Sadighi, S. B. Park, and W. J. Cushing (1977). *Penicillium* granuloma of the lung presenting as a solitary pulmonary nodule. *J. Am. Med. Assoc.* **237**:671.
184. Lie-Kian-Joe, N. T. Eng, S. Kertopati, and C. W. Emmons (1957). A new verrucous mycosis caused by *Cercospora apii*. *Arch. Dermatol.* **75**:864-870.
185. Linares, G., P. A. McGarry, and R. D. Baker (1971). Solid solitary aspergillotic granuloma of the brain. Report of a case due to *Aspergillus candidus* and review of the literature. *Neurology* **21**:177-184.
186. Listemann, H. (1975). Die kulturelle Untersuchung eines Tränensteines mit Isolierung des Pilzes *Phialophora richardsiae*. *E. Rodenwaldt-Arch.* **2**:45-52.
187. Littlewood, J. M. (1968). *Candida* infection of the urinary tract. Case report, with a review of the literature and a study of frequency of yeast isolations from the urine of children with bacterial urinary infections. *Br. J. Urol.* **40**:293-305.
188. Lobritz, R. W., T. H. Roberts, R. V. Marraro, P. K. Carlton, and D. J. Thorp (1979). Granulomatous pulmonary disease secondary to *Alternaria*. *J. Am. Med. Assoc.* **241**:596-597.
189. Lomvardias, S., and G. E. Madge (1972). *Chaetoconidium* and atypical acid-fast bacilli in skin ulcers. *Arch. Dermatol.* **106**:875-876.
190. Londero, A. T., and C. D. Ramos (1976). Chromomycosis: a clinical and mycologic study of thirty-five cases observed in the Hinterland of Rio Grande do Sul, Brazil. *Am. J. Trop. Med. Hyg.* **25**:132-135.
191. Louria, D. B., A. Blevins, D. Armstrong, R. Burdick, and P. Lieberman (1967). Fungemia caused by "nonpathogenic" yeasts. *Arch. Intern. Med.* **119**:247-252.
192. Louria, D. B., S. M. Greenberg, and D. W. Molander (1960). Fungemia caused by certain nonpathogenic strains of the family Cryptococcaceae. Report of two cases due to *Rhodotorula* and *Torulopsis glabrata*. *N. Engl. J. Med.* **263**:1281-1284.
193. Lucas, A. O. (1970). Cutaneous manifestations of African histoplasmosis. *Br. J. Dermatol.* **82**:435-447.
194. Lynn, J. R (1964). *Fusarium* keratitis treated with cycloheximide. *Am. J. Opthamol.* **58**:637-641.
195. Mackinnon, J. E. (1954). A contribution to the study of the causal organisms of maduromycosis. *Trans. R. Soc. Trop. Med. Hyg.* **48**:470-480.
196. Maddoux, G. L., J. A. Mohr, and H. G. Muchmore (1972). Pulmonary penicilliosis: a case presentation and a review of the literature. *J. Okla. State Med. Assoc.* **65**:418-421.
197. Madhavan, T., J. Eisses, and E. L. Quinn (1976). Infections due to *Trichosporon cutaneum*, an uncommon systemic pathogen. *Henry Ford Hosp. Med. J.* **24**:27-30.
198. Mahgoub, E. (1969). *Corynespora cassiicola*, a new agent of maduromycetoma. *J. Trop. Med. Hyg.* **72**:218-221.
199. Mahgoub, E. S. (1971). Maduromycetoma caused by *Aspergillus nidulans*. *J. Trop. Med. Hyg.* **74**:60-61.

200. Mahgoub, E. S. (1973). Mycetomas caused by *Curvularia lunata, Madurella grisea, Aspergillus nidulans,* and *Nocardia brasiliensis* in Sudan. *Sabouraudia* **11**:179–182.
201. Malbran, E., E. J. Albesi, H. Daro, and R. C. Zapater (1973). Endoftalmitis por *Penicillium lilacinum. Arch. Oftalmol. Buenos Aires* **48**:253–294.
202. Male, O. (1977). Zur Ätiopathogenese und Epidemiologie der Candidose und verwandter Hefemykosen. *Hautarzt* **28**:286–294.
203. Male, O., and J. Tappeiner (1965). Nagelveränderungen durch Schimmelpilze. *Dermatol. Wochenschr.* **151**:212–221.
204. Mankodi, R. C., L. N. Mohapatra, and R. M. Parekh (1976). Subcutaneous phycomycosis in India. *Indian J. Med. Sci.* **30**:102–105.
205. Mantelli, C., and G. Negri (1915). Ricerche sperimentali sull'agente eziologico di un micetoma a grani neri (*Penicillium mycetogenum* n.f.). *G. Accad. Med. Torino* **21**:161–167.
206. Mariat, F., B. Liautaud, M. Liautaud, and F. G. Marill (1978). *Hendersonula toruloidea,* agent d'une dermatite verruqueuse mycosique observée en Algérie. *Sabouraudia* **16**:133–140.
207. Marcano, C., and B. Hutton (1973). Tinea nigra plantaris por *Cladosporium* sp., segundo caso. *Castellania* **1**:129–131.
208. Markley, A. J., O. S. Philpott, and F. D. Weidman (1936). Deep scopulariopsosis of ulcerating granuloma type confirmed by culture and animal inoculation. *Arch. Dermatol. Syph.* **33**:627–641.
209. Maršálek, E., Z. Zižka, V. Riha, J. Dušek, and C. Dvořáček (1960). Plicni aspergilóza s generalizaci vyvolaná druhem *Aspergillus restrictus. Cas. Lek. Cesk.* **99**:1285–1292.
210. Marsten, J. J., J. L. Greenberg, J. C. Piccinini, and A. M. Rywlin (1969). Aortitis due to *Candida stellatoidea* developing in a supravalvular suture line. *Ann. Thorac. Surg.* **7**:134–138.
211. Mayhall, C. G., C. W. Miller, A. Z. Eisen, G. S. Kobayashi, and G. Medoff (1976). Cutaneous protothecosis. *Arch. Dermatol.* **112**:1749–1752.
212. McClellan, J. R., J. D. Hamilton, G. A. Alexander, W. G. Wolfe, and J. B. Reed (1976). *Paecilomyces varioti* endocarditis on a prosthetic aortic valve. *J. Thorac. Cardiovasc. Surg.* **71**:472–475.
213. McCormick, W. F., S. S. Schochet, P. R. Weaver, and J. A. McCrary (1975). Disseminated aspergillosis. *Aspergillus* endophthalmitis, optic nerve infarction, and carotid artery thrombosis. *Arch. Pathol.* **99**:353–359.
214. McGinnis, M. R. (1977). Human pathogenic species of *Exophiala, Phialophora,* and *Wangiella. Proc. Int. Conf. Mycoses, 4th, PAHO Sci. Publ.* 356, pp. 37–59.
215. McGinnis, M. R., S. Lemon, W. Lamar, and S. Shadomy. Cerebral phaeohyphomycosis due to a member of the Mycelia Sterilia. (In preparation.)
216. McGinnis, M. R., D. F. Sorrell, R. M. Miller, and G. W. Kaminski (1980). Subcutaneous phaeohyphomycosis caused by *Exophiala moniliae. Mycopathologica.* (In press.)
217. McGinnis, M. R., D. Walker, and J. D. Folds (1980). *Hansenula polymorpha* infection in a child with chronic granulomatous disease. *Arch. Pathol. Lab. Med..* (In press.)
218. McMillen, M., and W. I. Metzger (1967). *Aspergillus penicilloides:* human pathogen. *Bacteriol. Proc.* citation M70.
219. Mershon, J. C., D. R. Samuelson, and T. E. Layman (1968). Left ventricular "Fibrous Body" aneurysm caused by *Aspergillus* endocarditis. *Am. J. Cardiol.* **22**:281–285.
220. Mesones, H. A., and C. W. Dodge (1960). *Sarcinomyces inkin* in Brasil. *Mycologia* **52**:800–804.
221. Meyer, R. D., M. H. Kaplan, M. Ong, and D. Armstrong (1973). Cutaneous lesions in disseminated mucormycosis. *J. Am. Med. Assoc.* **225**:737–738.

## Appendix C

222. Meyers, W. M., J. R. Dooley, and K. J. Kwon-Chung (1975). Mycotic granuloma caused by *Phialophora repens. Am. J. Clin. Pathol.* **64**:549–555.
223. Middleton, F. G., P. F. Jurgenson, J. P. Utz, S. Shadomy, and H. J. Shadomy (1976). Brain abscess caused by *Cladosporium trichoides. Arch. Intern. Med.* **136**:444–448.
224. Miguères, J., H. Paczuszynski, and R. Estève (1965). Aspergillome pulmonaire en apparence primitif, traité avec succès par injections trans-thoraciques d'amphotéricine B. *J. Fr. Med. Chir. Thorac.* **19**:59–71.
225. Mikami, R., and G. N. Stemmermann (1958). Keratomycosis caused by *Fusarium oxysporum. Am. J. Clin. Pathol.* **29**:257–262.
226. Miloshev, B., C. M. Davidson, J. C. Gentles, and A. T. Sandison (1966). Aspergilloma of paranasal sinuses and orbit in Northern Sudanese. *Lancet* **1**:746–747.
227. Mizuta, M., W. Mizuta, and K. Tōjyō (1955). A case of acute diffuse moniliasis presumably caused by *Candida pulcherrima. Bull. Yamaguchi Med. Sch.* **3**:11–16.
228. Mofty, A. M. E., and M. M. Nada (1970). Skin granuloma in the Nile Valley. *Int. J. Dermatol.* **9**:33–40.
229. Moore, M., W. O. Russell, and E. Sachs (1946). Chronic leptomeningitis and ependymitis caused by *Ustilago*, probably *U. zeae* (corn smut). Ustilagomycosis, the second reported instance of human infection. *Am. J. Pathol.* **22**:761–777.
230. Morquer, R., and L. Enjalbert (1957). Étude morphologique et physiologique d'un *Aspergillus* nouvellement isolé au cours d'une affection pulmonaire de l'homme. *C. R. Acad. Sci. (Paris)* **244**:1405–1408.
231. Mosier, M. A., B. Lusk, T. H. Pettit, D. H. Howard, and J. Rhodes (1977). Fungal endophthalmitis following intraocular lens implantation. *Am. J. Ophthalmol.* **83**:1–8.
232. Motta, R. (1929). I miceti delle cavità nasali e della gola negli ozenatosi. *Valsalva* **5**:525–557.
233. Mukerji, S., J. R. Patwardhan, and R. K. Gadgil (1971). Bacterial and mycotic infection of the brain. *Indian J. Med. Sci.* **25**:791–794.
234. Murray, I. G., and H. D. Holt (1964). Is *Cephalosporium acremonium* capable of producing maduromycosis? *Mycopathol. Mycol. Appl.* **22**:335–338.
235. Naveh, Y., A. Friedman, D. Merzback, and N. Hashman (1975). Endocarditis caused by *Rhodotorula* successfully treated with 5-fluorocytosine. *Br. Heart J.* **37**:101–104.
236. Neame, P., and D. Rayner (1960). Mucormycosis. A report of twenty-two cases. *Arch. Pathol.* **70**:261–268.
237. Negroni, P., and J. A. Tey (1939). Estudio micologico del primer caso Argentino de micetoma maduromicosico con granos negros. *Rev. Argent. Dermatosifilol.* **23**:584–595.
238. Negroni, R., S. Avervach, R. Russo, and E. Frigerio (1969). Granuloma por *Scopulariopsis brevicaulis. Rev. Derm. Ibero Latin. Am.* **11**:249–254.
239. Neuhann, T. (1976). Clotrimazol in der Behandlung von Keratomykosen. *Klin. Monatsbl. Augenheilkd.* **169**:459–462.
240. Newmark, E., and F. M. Polack (1970). *Tetraploa* keratomycosis. *Am. J. Ophthalmol.* **70**:1013–1015.
241. Nicolau, St.-G., A. Avram, N. Dobrovici, and D. Hatmanu (1959). Aspects clinico-radiologiques des mycétomes du pied contributions à l'étude de l'ostéite mycétomique. *Presse Med.* **67**:1863–1866.
242. Nicolau, S., and R. Evolceanu (1947). Recherches mycologiques dans un cas de "mycétome" du pied a grains noirs (*Mortierella mycetomi*). *Ann. Dermatol. Syphililgr.* **7**:330–343.
243. Nielsen, H. S., and N. F. Conant (1968). A new human pathogenic *Phialophora. Sabouraudia* **6**:228–231.
244. Niño, F. L (1932). Broncomicosis penicilliar. *Sem. Med.* **2**:1015–1020.

245. Nityananda, K., P. Sivasubramaniam, and L. Ajello (1962). Mycotic keratitis caused by *Curvularia lunata* case report. *Sabouraudia* **2**:35-39.
246. Nityananda, K., P. Sivasubramaniam, and L. Ajello (1964). A case of mycotic keratitis caused by *Curvularia geniculata*. *Arch. Ophthalmol.* **71**:456-458.
247. Nitzulescu, V., and M. Niculescu (1975). Ophtalmopathie déterminée par *Candida humicola*. *Arch. Roum. Pathol. Exp. Microbiol.* **34**:357-361.
248. Nitzulescu, V., and M. Niculescu (1976). Considérations sur trois cas de candidose oculaire à *Candida lipolytica*. *Arch. Roum. Pathol. Exp. Microbiol.* **35**:269-272.
249. Novey, H. S., and I. D. Wells (1978). Allergic bronchopulmonary aspergillosis caused by *Aspergillus ochraceus*. *Am. J. Clin. Pathol.* **70**:840-843.
250. Ohashi, Y. (1960). On a rare disease due to *Alternaria tenuis* Nees (Alternariasis). *Tohoku J. Exp. Med.* **72**:78-82.
251. Otčenášek, M., Z. Hubálek, J. Dvořak, and M. Šabatová (1968). Ein weiterer Chromomykose-Fall in der Tschechoslowakei? *Mykosen* **11**:719-724.
252. Otčenášek, M., V. Janečková, R. Kaupa, B. Medek, and D. Nevludová (1976). K etiologii plicnich aspergilomu. *Cesk. Epidemiol. Microbiol. Immunol.* **25**:263-268.
253. Paiva, C., A. C. Batista, and A. Gomes (1960). Endoftalmite micótica pós-operatória por *Hyalopus bogolepofii*. *Rev. Bras. Oftalmol* **19**:193-202.
254. Paldrok, H (1965). Report on a case of subcutaneous dissemination of *Aspergillus niger*, type *awamori*. *Acta Dermatol. Venereol.* **45**:275-282.
255. Papadatos, C., M. Pavlatou, and D. Alexiou (1969). *Cephalosporium* meningitis. *Pediatrics* **44**:749-751.
256. Patterson, J. C., S. L. Laine, and W. B. Taylor (1962). White piedra occurring on the pubic hair of a native caucasian North American. *Arch. Dermatol.* **85**:534-536.
257. Pedersen, N. B., P. A. Mårdh, T. Hallberg, and N. Jonsson (1976). Cutaneous alternariosis. *Br. J. Dermatol.* **94**:201-209.
258. Perz, M. (1966). *Fusarium nivale* jako przyczyna grzybicy rogówki. *Klin. Oczna* **36**:609-612.
259. Peterson, J. E., and T. J. Baker (1959). An isolate of *Fusarium roseum* from human burns. *Mycologia* **51**:453-456.
260. Pfleger, L., and H. Tirschek (1957). Zur Problematik der Hautblastomykose. *Dermatologica* **114**:1-17.
261. Pierach, C. A., G. Gülmen, G. J. Dhar, and J. C. Kiser (1973). *Phialophora mutabilis* endocarditis. *Ann. Intern. Med.* **79**:900-901.
262. Pietrini, P., and W. M. Stewart (1977). Granulome peri-narinaire dû à *Taeniolella stilbospora* (Corda) Hughes. *Bull. Soc. Fr. Mycol. Med.* **6**:97-100.
263. Pietrini, P., W. M. Stewart, G. Segretain, and G. Badillet (1974). Mycétome de la main à *Leptosphaeria tompkinsii* (El-Ani). *Bull. Soc. Fr. Mycol. Med.* **3**:117-120.
264. Plouffe, J. F., D. G. Brown, J. Silva, T. Eck, R. L. Stricof, and F. R. Fekety (1977). Nosocomial outbreak of *Candida parapsilosis* fungemia related to intravenous infusions. *Arch. Intern. Med.* **137**:1686-1689.
265. Polack, F. M., C. Siverio, and R. H. Bresky (1976). Corneal chromomycosis: double infection by *Phialophora verrucosa* (Medlar) and *Cladosporium cladosporioides* (Frescenius). *Ann. Ophthalmol.* **8**:139-144.
266. Polenghi, F., and A. Lasagni (1976). Observations on a case of mycokeratitis and its treatment with BAY b 5097 (Canesten). *Mykosen* **19**:223-226.
267. Pollock, R. A., R. C. Pratt, J. A. Shulman, and J. S. Turner (1975). Nasal mucormycosis: early detection and treatment without radical surgery or amphotericin B. *South. Med. J.* **68**:1279-1282.
268. Pore, R. S., and J. Chen (1976). Meningitis caused by *Rhodotorula*. *Sabouraudia* **14**:331-335.

269. Pore, R. S., R. F. D'Amato, and L. Ajello (1977). *Fissuricella* gen. nov.: a new taxon for *Prototheca filamenta*. *Sabouraudia* **15**:69–78.
270. Pore, R. S., and H. W. Larsh (1968). Experimental pathology of *Aspergillus terreus-flavipes* group species. *Sabouraudia* **6**:89–93.
271. Porto, E., C. Lacaz, E. Sabbaga, P. Chocair, J. A. da Fonseca, E. A. Rivitte, and A. Salebian (1979). *Phialophora bubakii*. Isolamento de abscesso subcutâneo, em transplantado renal. *Rev. Inst. Med. Trop. Sao Paulo* **21**:106–109.
272. Preininger, T. (1937). Durch Maisbrand (*Ustilago maydis*) bedingte Dermatomykose. *Arch. Dermatol. Syph.* **176**:109–113.
273. Presbury, D. G. C., and C. N. Young (1978). *Trichophyton ajelloi* isolated from a child. *Sabouraudia* **16**:233–235.
274. Prisco, J. di, and D. Borelli (1973). Tinea nigra por *Cladosporium* species. *Castellania* **1**:97–100.
275. Proost, J. M., F. M. Maes-Dockx, M. O. Nelis, and J. M. van Cutsem (1972). Miconazole in the treatment of mycotic vulvovaginitis. *Am. J. Obstet. Gynecol.* **112**:688–692.
276. Punithalingam, E. (1976). *Phoma oculo-hominis* sp. nov. from corneal ulcer. *Trans. Br. Mycol. Soc.* **67**:142–143.
277. Punithalingam, E., and M. P. English (1975). *Pyrenochaeta unguis-hominis* sp. nov. on human toe-nails. *Trans. Br. Mycol. Soc.* **64**:539–541.
278. Quilici, M., A. Orsini, D. Basbous, C. Scheiner, A. Dor, and G. Lebreuil (1977). Adiasporomycose pulmonaire disséminée (à propos d'une observation). *Arch. Anat. Cytol. Pathol.* **25**:227–234.
279. Raab, W. (1964). Die gegenseitige Beeinflussung von Tuberkulose und systematisierter Moniliasis. *Dermatol. Wochenschr.* **149**:401–410.
280. Rebell, G., and R. K. Forster (1976). *Lasiodiplodia theobromae* as a case of keratomycoses. *Sabouraudia* **14**:155–170.
281. Rebell, G., and D. Taplin (1970). "Dermatophytes, Their Recognition and Identification," 2nd. ed. Univ. of Miami Press, Miami, Florida.
282. Reiersöl, S., and J. Hoel (1958). *Saccharomyces carlsbergensis*, possibly a pathogenic. *Acta Pathol. Microbiol. Scand.* **44**:313–318.
283. Restrepo, A., M. Arango, H. Velez, and L. Uribe (1976). The isolation of *Botryodiplodia theobromae* from a nail lesion. *Sabouraudia* **14**:1–4.
284. Restrepo, A., and L. de Uribe (1976). Isolation of fungi belonging to the genera *Geotrichum* and *Trichosporum* from human dermal lesions. *Mycopathologia.* **59**:3–9.
285. Restrepo, A., D. L. Greer, M. Robledo, O. Osorio, and H. Mondragón (1971). Ulceration of the palate caused by a basidiomycete *Schizophyllum commune*. *Sabouraudia* **9**:201–204.
286. Restrepo, A., M. Robledo, R. Giraldo, H. Hernández, F. Sierra, F. Gutiérrez, F. Londoño, R. López, and G. Calle (1976). The gamut of paracoccidioidomycosis. *Am. J. Med.* **61**:33–42.
287. Reyes, O., and D. Borelli (1974). Caso de tina por cepa peculiar de *Cladosporium castellanii*. *Dermatol. Venez.* **13**:21–28.
288. Ribet, M., R. Callafe, J. P. Delaby, F. Liber, and A. Hassoun (1975). Septicémies à *Candida* dans un service de chirurgie générale. *Chirurgie* **101**:441–446.
289. Riopedre, R. N., L. de Cesarc, E. Miatello, M. A. Caria, and R. C. Zapater (1960). Aislamiento de *Rhodotorula mucilagnosa* del L.C.R., heces, orina, exudado faringeo y piel de un lactante de 3 meses. *Rev. Assoc. Med. Argent.* **74**:431–434.
290. Rippon, J. W (1974). "Medical Mycology: The Pathogenic Fungi and the Pathogenic Actinomycetes." Saunders, Philadelphia.

291. Rippon, J. W., D. N. Anderson, and M. Soo Hoo (1971). Aspergillosis: comparative virulence, metabolic rate, growth rate and ubiquinone content of soil and human isolates of *Aspergillus terreus. Sabouraudia* **12**:157–161.
292. Rippon, J. W., F. C. Lee, and S. McMillen (1970). Dermatophyte infection caused by *Aphanoascus fulvescens. Arch. Dermatol.* **102**:552–555.
293. Rivera, R., and A. Cangir (1975). *Trichosporon* sepsis and leukemia. *Cancer* **36**:1106–1110.
294. Rodrigues, M. M., P. Laibson, and W. Kaplan (1975). Exogenous corneal ulcer caused by *Tritirachium roseum. Am. J. Ophthalmol.* **80**:804–806.
295. Rodrigues, M. M., and D. MacLeod (1975). Exogenous fungal endophthalmitis caused by *Paecilomyces. Am. J. Ophthalmol.* **79**:687–690.
296. Rodriguez, J. D. (1961). Piedra en Ecuador. *Mycopathol. Mycol. Appl.* **14**:31–38.
297. Romano, A., E. Segal, and T. Ben-Tovim (1973). Epithelial keratitis due to *Rhodotorula. Ophthalmologica* **166**:353–359.
298. Rosenbaum, E. H. (1944). The development and systematic position of *Arachniotus trisporus. Ann. Mo. Bot. Gard.* **31**:184–200.
299. Ross, J. D., K. D. G. Reid, and C. F. Speirs (1966). Bronchopulmonary geotrichosis with severe asthma. *Br. Med. J.* **1**:1400–1402.
300. Roy, A., and M. Chunder (1963). *Pseudoarachniotus* sp. as the aetiological agent of a case of human mycosis. *Bull. Calcutta Sch. Trop. Med.* **11**:108–109.
301. Rush-Munro, F. M., H. Black, and J. M. Dingley (1971). Onychomycosis caused by *Fusarium oxysporum. Australas. J. Dermatol.* **12**:18–29.
302. Sachsenweger, R. (1955). Klinische Befunde und experimentelle Untersuchungen über Augenerkrankungen durch saprophytär wachsende Pilze. *Klin. Monatsbl. Augenheilkd.* **127**:721–730.
303. Sahn, S. A., and S. Lakshminarayan (1973). Allergic bronchopulmonary penicilliosis. *Chest* **63**:286–288.
304. Sandhu, D. K., R. S. Sandhu, and V. C. Misra (1976). Isolation of *Candida viswanathii* from cerebrospinal fluid. *Sabouraudia* **14**:251–254.
305. Sarrat, H., H. Mathe, J. P. Marchand, and I. Faye (1973). Agents étiologiques rares de mycoses sous-cutanées. *Bull. Soc. Pathol. Exot.* **66**:615–620.
306. Schelbert, H. R., and O. F. Muller (1972). Detection of fungal vegetations involving a Starr–Edwards mitral prosthesis by means of ultrasound. *Vasc. Surg.* **6**:20–25.
307. Schmid, K. O. (1955). Zur Ätiologie der interstitiellen plasmocellulären Pneumonie (Saccharomykose) im Säuglingsalter. *Frankf. Z. Pathol.* **66**:426–448.
308. Schnapka, O. (1955). Onychomycosis nigricans. Beitrag zum Krankheitsbild der ' 'schwarzen Nägel." *Arch. Klin. Exp. Dermatol.* **202**:45–50.
309. Schönborn, C., and H. Jahn (1970). *Microascus desmosporus* (Lechmere) Curzi 1931 als Erreger einer Zehennagel-Mykose. *Dermatol. Monatsschr.* **156**:615–626.
310. Schönborn, C., and H. Schmoranzer (1970). Untersuchungen über Schimmelpilzinfektionen der Zehennägel. *Mykosen* **13**:253–272.
311. Schwartz, I. S., and C. W. Emmons (1968). Subcutaneous cystic granuloma caused by a fungus of wood pulp (*Phialophora richardsiae*). *Am. J. Clin. Pathol.* **49**:500–505.
312. Schwarz, J., and K. Salfelder (1977). Blastomycosis. A review of 152 cases. *Curr. Top. Pathol.* **65**:165–200.
313. Seabury, J. H., and M. Samuels (1963). The pathogenetic spectrum of aspergillosis. *Am. J. Clin. Pathol.* **40**:21–33.
314. Segal, E., A. Romano, E. Eylan, R. Stein, and T. Ben-Tovim (1975). *Rhodotorula rubra* —cause of eye infection. *Mykosen* **18**:107–111.
315. Segretain, G., M. André, H. Sarrat, and P. Destombes (1974). *Leptosphaeria tompkinsii,* agent de mycétomes au Sénégal. *Bull. Soc. Fr. Mycol. Med.* **3**:71–74.

316. Segretain, G., and P. Destombes (1961). Description d'un nouvel agent de maduromycose, *Neotestudina rosatii*, n. gen., n. sp. isolé en Afrique. *C. R. Acad. Sci. (Paris)* **253**:2577-2579.
317. Sekhon, A. S. (1978). *Bacteroides fragilis* and *Torulopsis glabrata* septicemia in a patient with gastrointestinal ulcers and chronic renal failure, with review of literature on torulopsosis. *Proc. Int. Conf. Mycoses, 4th, PAHO Sci. Publ.* 356, pp. 167-175.
318. Sekhon, A. S., D. J. Willans, and J. H. Harvey (1974). Deep scopulariopsosis: a case report and sensitivity studies. *J. Clin. Pathol.* **27**:837-843.
319. Seligsohn, R., J. W. Rippon, and S. A. Lerner (1977). *Aspergillus terreus* osteomyelitis. *Arch. Intern. Med.* **137**:918-920.
320. Serban, P., and C. Tascá (1964). Studium über 2 Fälle von Allgemeinmykose mit tödlicher Entwicklung während der Behandlung mit Antibiotika. *Zentralbl. Allg. Pathol.* **105**:185-193.
321. Sheehy, T. W., B. K. Honeycutt, and J. T. Spencer (1976). *Geotrichum* septicemia. *J. Am. Med. Assoc.* **235**:1035-1037.
322. Sheikh, H. A., S. Mahgoub, and K. Badi (1974). Postoperative endophthalmitis due to *Trichosporon cutaneum*. *Br. J. Ophthalmol.* **58**:591-594.
323. Silveira, J. S. (1959). Ensaios clinico-experimentais com tricomicina (cabimicina) em ginecomicopatologia. *Rev. Ginecol. Obstet. (Rio de Janeiro)* **105**:439-464.
324. Silveira, J. S. (1963). Ocorrencia de *Candida humicola* (Daszewska) Diddens & Lodder em uretra de gestante. *Inst. Micol. Univ. Recife, Publ.* 150, pp. 1-9.
325. Silver, M. D., P. G. Tuffnell, and W. G. Bigelow (1971). Endocarditis caused by *Paecilomyces varioti* affecting an aortic valve allograft. *J. Thorac. Cardiovasc. Surg.* **61**:278-281.
326. Simonart, J. (1965). L'ongle et le *Candida albicans*. *Arch. Belg. Dermatol. Syphiligr.* **21**:64-72.
327. Slifkin, M., and H. M. Bowers (1975). *Phialophora mutabilis* endocarditis. *Am. J. Clin. Pathol.* **63**:120-130.
328. Smyth, G. D. L. (1962). Fungal infection of the post-operative mastoid cavity. *J. Laryngol. Otol.* **76**:797-821.
329. Speller, D. C. E., and A. G. MacIver (1971). Endocarditis caused by a *Coprinus* species: a fungus of the toadstool group. *J. Med. Microbiol.* **4**:370-374.
330. Srivastava, O. P., B. Lal, P. K. Agrawal, S. C. Agarwal, B. Chandra, and I. S. Mathur (1977). Mycotic keratitis due to *Rhizoctonia* sp. *Sabouraudia* **15**:125-131.
331. Stein, P. D., A. T. Folkens, and K. A. Hruska (1970). *Saccharomyces* fungemia. *Chest* **58**:173-175.
332. Strand, R. D., E. B. D. Neuhauser, and C. F. Sornberger (1967). Lycoperdonosis. *N. Engl. J. Med.* **277**:89-91.
333. Stuart, E. A., and F. Blank (1955). Aspergillosis of the ear. A report of twenty-nine cases. *Can. Med. Assoc. J.* **72**:334-337.
334. Svobodová, Y. (1966). *Chmelia slovaca* gen. nov. a dematiaceous fungus, pathogenic for man and animals. *Biologia (Bratislava)* **21**:81-88.
335. Takayasu, S., M. Akagi, and Y. Shimizu (1977). Cutaneous mycosis caused by *Paecilomyces lilacinus*. *Arch. Dermatol.* **113**:1687-1690.
336. Talice, R. V., and J. E. Mackinnon (1929). *Penicillium bertai* n. sp. agent d'une mycose broncho-pulmonaire de l'homme. *Ann. Parasitol. Hum. Comp.* **7**:97-106.
337. Tchange, F. K. M., and C. L. Gilardi (1973). Osteomyelitis due to *Torulopsis inconspicua*. *Am. J. Bone Jt. Surg.* **55-A**:1739-1743.
338. Theodore, F. H., M. L. Littman, and E. Almeda (1962). Endophthalmitis following cataract extraction due to *Neurospora sitophila*, a so-called nonpathogenic fungus. *Am. J. Ophthalmol.* **53**:35-39.

339. Thiers, H., J. Coudert, D. Colomb, J. Fayolle, and G. Moulin (1960). État septicémique avec gommes cutanées et musculaires dû à *Debaryomyces kloeckeri* et très amélioré par l'auto-vaccin. *Bull. Soc. Fr. Dermatol. Syphiligr.* **67**:711–714.
340. Thygeson, P., and M. Okumoto (1974). Keratomycosis: a preventable disease. *Trans. Am. Acad. Ophthalmol. Otolaryngol.* **78**:OP433–439.
341. Torres, G., and L. K. Georg (1956). A human case of *Trichophyton gallinae* infection. *Arch. Dermatol.* **74**:191–197.
342. Upshaw, C. B. (1974). *Penicillium* endocarditis of aortic valve prosthesis. *J. Thorac. Cardiovasc. Surg.* **68**:428–431.
343. Vanderdonckt, J., W. Lauwers, and J. Bockaert (1976). Miconazole alcoholic solution in the treatment of mycotic nail infections. *Mykosen* **19**:251–256.
344. Vardhanabhuti, S. (1959). Cultural characteristics and life history of a new human pathogen, *Thailandia candida*, nov. gen. et nov. spec. *Sydowia* [*Ser. 2*] **13**:98–104.
345. Vermeil, C., A. Gordeeff, and M. Geffriaud (1975). Adiaspiromycose pulmonaire humaine: observation d'un nouveau cas en Bretagne. *Mycopathologia* **56**:109–111.
346. Vermeil, C., A. Gordeff, M.-J. Leroux, O. Morin, and M. Bouc (1971). Blastomycose cheloidienne à *Aureobasidium pullulans* (de Bary) Arnaud en Bretagne. *Mycopathol. Mycol. Appl.* **43**:35–39.
347. Veselý, K., M. Petrů, and S. Hontela (1968). Mykologische und klinische Diagnostik der Hefepilze in der weiblichen und Kindergynäkologie. *Zentralbl. Gynaekol.* **90**:1767–1774.
348. Viégas, A. P. (1943). Notas sôbre uma nova espécie de *Sporormia*. *Bragantia* **3**:155–164.
349. Vieira, J. R. (1959). Onicomicose por *Aureobasidium pullulans* (de Bary) Arnaud. *Proc. Int. Congr. Trop. Med. Malar.*, 6th, Vol. 4, pp. 768–777.
350. Vignale, R., J. E. Mackinnon, E. Casella de Vilaboa, and F. Burgoa (1964). Chronic, destructive, mucocutaneous phycomycosis in man. *Sabouraudia* **3**:143–147.
351. Vilanova, X., J. Esteller, and M. Casanovas (1951). Gomme mycosique du cou par *Malbranchea pulchella*. *Ann. Dermatol. Syphiligr.* **78**:566–569.
352. Viswanathan, R., and H. S. Randhawa (1959). *Candida viswanathii* sp. novo isolated from a case of meningitis. *Sci. Cult.* **25**:86–87.
353. Vonlanthen, M., G. Thiel, F. Brunner, F. Harder, M. Keller, M. Stoecklin, H. Ohnacker, W. Jacques, and M. Podvinec (1977). Mucormycose craniale chez un transplanté rénal. *Schweiz. Med. Wochenschr.* **107**:1784–1786.
354. Vries, G. A. de, R. F. O. Kemp, and D. C. E. Speller (1971). Endocarditis caused by *Coprinus delicatulus*. *C. R. Comm. V. Congr. l'ISHAM*, pp. 185–186.
355. Walshe, M. M., and M. P. English (1966). Fungi in nails. *Br. J. Dermatol.* **78**:198–207.
356. Wang, C. J. K., and J. Schwarz (1958). The etiology of interstitial pneumonia. Identification as *Hansenula anomala* of a yeast isolated from lungs of infants. *Mycopathol. Mycol. Appl.* **9**:299–306.
357. Ward, H. P., W. J. Martin, J. C. Ivins, and L. A. Weed (1961). *Cephalosporium* arthritis. *Proc. Mayo Clin.* **36**:337–343.
358. Warren, C. M. (1964). Dangers of steroids in ophthalmology with report of a case of mycotic perforating corneal ulcer. *J. Med. Assoc. Ala.* **33**:229–233.
359. Watson, K. C., and S. Kallichurum (1970). Brain abscess due to *Trichosporon cutaneum*. *J. Med. Microbiol.* **3**:191–193.
360. Watson, K. C., and P. B. Neame (1960). *In vitro* activity of amphotericin B on strains of Mucoraceae pathogenic to man. *J. Lab. Clin. Med.* **56**:251–257.
361. Webster, B. H. (1959). Bronchopulmonary geotrichosis: a review with report of four cases. *Dis. Chest.* **35**:273–281.
362. White, J. H. (1969). Fungal contamination of donor eyes. *Br. J. Ophthalmol.* **53**:30–33.

363. Wieser, H. G. (1973). Zur Frage der Pathogenität des *Cryptococcus albidus*. *Schweiz. Med. Wochenschr.* **103**:475–481.
364. Wilson, L. A., R. R. Sexton, and D. Ahearn (1966). Keratochromomycosis. *Arch. Ophthalmol.* **76**:811–816.
365. Wind, C. A., and F. M. Polack (1970). Keratomycosis due to *Curvularia lunata*. *Arch. Ophthalmol.* **84**:694–696.
366. Winston, D. J., G. E. Balsley, J. Rhodes, and S. R. Linné (1977). Disseminated *Trichosporon capitatum* infection in an immunosuppressed host. *Arch. Intern. Med.* **137**:1192–1195.
367. Wolf, F. T. (1947). Relation of various fungi to otomycosis. *Arch. Otolaryngol.* **46**:361–374.
368. Wright, R. E. (1929). Hypopyon ulcer of the cornea due to *Glenospora graphii*. *Br. J. Ophthalmol.* **13**:496–498.
369. Yamashita, K. (1956). Fungus problems in otolaryngology. *J. Otolaryngol. Jpn.* **59**:129–149.
370. Yamashita, K., and T. Yamashita (1972). *Polypaecilum insolitum* (= *Scopulariopsis divaricata*) isolated from cases of otomycosis. *Sabouraudia* **10**:128–131.
371. Young, C. N., J. G. Swart, D. Ackermann, and K. Davidge-Pitts (1978). Nasal obstruction and bone erosion caused by *Drechslera hawaiiensis*. *J. Laryngol. Otol.* **92**:137–143.
372. Young, N. A., K. J. Kwon-Chung, and J. Freeman (1973). Subcutaneous abscess caused by *Phoma* sp. resembling *Pyrenochaeta romeroi*: unique fungal infection occurring in immunosuppressed recipient of renal allograft. *Am. J. Clin. Pathol.* **59**:810–816.
373. Young, N. A., K. J. Kwon-Chung, T. T. Kubota, A. E. Jennings, and R. I. Fisher (1978). Disseminated infection by *Fusarium moniliforme* during treatment for malignant lymphoma. *J. Clin. Microbiol.* **7**:589–594.
374. Yow-nung, M., and Y. Ta-fuh (1966). A new *Fusarium*, the causal agent of otomycosis. *Acta Microbiol. Sinica* **12**:176–179. (In Chinese.)
375. Zaias, N. (1966). Superficial white onychomycosis. *Sabouraudia* **5**:99–103.
376. Zaias, N., I. Oertel, and D. F. Elliott (1969). Fungi in toe nails. *J. Invest. Dermatol.* **53**:140–142.
377. Zapater, R. C. (1977). Ocular mycology in Argentina. *In* "Recent Advances in Medical and Veterinary Mycology" (K. Iwata, ed.), pp. 245–252. University Park Press, Baltimore, Maryland.
378. Zapater, R. C., E. J. Albesi, and G. H. Garcia (1975). Mycotic keratitis by *Drechslera spicifera*. *Sabouraudia* **13**:295–298.
379. Zapater, R. C., A. de Arrechea, and V. H. Guevara (1972). Queratomicosis por *Fusarium dimerum*. *Sabouraudia* **10**:274–275.
380. Zapater, R. C., M. A. Brunzini, E. J. Albesi, and C. A. Silicaro Arturi (1976). El genero *Fusarium* como agente etiologico de micosis oculares (presentación de 7 casos). *Arch. Oftalmol. Buenos Aires* **51**:279–286.
381. Ziskind, J., P. Pizzolato, and E. E. Buff (1958). Aspergillosis of the brain. Report of a case. *Am. J. Clin. Pathol.* **29**:554–559.

# Taxonomic Index

Numbers in italics denote pages with figures.

## A

*Absidia* van Tieghem, 1876, *18*, 78, 85, 113, 124, 162, 304–306, *312*, *313*, 318, 322, 323
   *corymbifera*, 305, 306, 522
   *ramosa*, 305, 306
   *spinosa*, 115
*Aciculoconidium*, 223, 399
*Acremonium* Link ex Fries, 1821, 12, 54, 78, 85, 110, 156, 175, 179, *180*, 181, 205, 220, 226, 239, 247, 263, 268, 287, 288, 296, 346, 490, 491
   *falciforme*, 507
   *kiliense*, 20
   *recifei*, 507
*Acrodontium*, 187
*Acrotheca*, 217
   *aquaspera*, 267
Actinomycetes, 3, 85
*Aessosporon salmonicolor*, 398
*Ajellomyces* McDonough et Lewis emend. McGinnis et Katz, 1979, 145, 162–164
   *capsulatus*, 120, 163, 231, 502, 504
   *dermatitidis*, *44*, 53, *163*, *164*, 192, 480
Aleuriosporae, 109
*Alleschria*, 172
   *boydii*, 172, 270
*Alternaria* Nees ex Wallroth, 1833 *nom. cons.*, 105, 148, *151*, 156, *181*, 182, 296
   *alternata*, 182
   *tenuis*, 182
Amerosporae, 104, 105
*Angiopoma*, 206
*Arthrinium*, 108, 110

*Arthrobotrys* Corda emend. Schenck, Kendrick et Pramer, 1977, *105*, 147, *160*, 182, *183*
   *amerospora*, 182
*Arthroderma* Currey ex Berkeley, 1860, 145, 164, *165*, 168, 198, 293, 564
   *benhamiae*, 166, 303
   *ciferrii*, 166, 303
   *cuniculi*, 166
   *curreyi*, 166
   *flavescens*, 166, 303
   *gertleri*, 166, 303
   *gloriae*, 166, 303
   *insingulare*, 166, 303
   *lenticularum*, 166, 303
   *multifidum*, 166
   *quadrifidum*, 166, 303
   *simii*, 166, 303
   *tuberculatum*, 166
   *uncinatum*, 166, 303
   *vanbreuseghemii*, 166, 303
*Arthrographis*, 223, 224, 244
Arthrosporae, 109
Ascomycetes, 1, 2, 4, 35, 42–43, 49, 117, 144, 162–175
Ascomycota, 50, 51, 337
*Aspergillus* Micheli ex Link, 1821, 6, 12, 78, 79, 85, 86, 94, 124, 129, 138, 140, 145, *153*, 154, 166, 182–185, *185*, 187–188, 189–190, 326, 413, 420, 425, 475–477, 481, 485, 492, 500, 526
   *candidus*, 188, 189
   *cervinus*, 188, 189
   *clavatus*, 187, 189

*Aspergillus* Micheli ex Link *(cont.)*
  *cremeus*, 188, 190
  *fischeri*, 189
  *flavipes*, 188, 190
  *flavus*, 6, 183, 185, 187, 189, 477, 490, 526, 527, 539, 541, 542, 544, 556, 557, 570, 573, 574, 577
  *fumigatus*, 21, 82, 140, *184*, 185, 187, 189, *476*, 477, 490, 492, 509, 581
  *glaucus*, 185, 187, 189, 477
  *janus*, 190
  *nidulans*, 187, 190, 477, 507
  *niger*, 105, 185, 188, 189, 477, 490, 509
  *ochraceus*, 188, 189
  *ornatus*, 187, 189
  *restrictus*, 187, 189
  *sclerotiorum*, 526
  *sulphureus*, 526
  *sparsus*, 188, 190
  *terreus*, 188, 190, 477
  *thomii*, 526
  *ustus*, 188, 190
  *versicolor*, 188, 190
  *wentii*, 188, 189
*Aureobasidium* Viala et Boyer, 1891, 31, 161, 186, 191, 260
  *pullulans*, 186, 260, 276, 346
*Auxarthron*, 235

**B**

*Basidiobolus* Eidam, 1886, 113, 125, 162, 306–309
  *haptosporus*, 308, 309
  *heterosporus*, 309
  *lacertae*, 309
  *magnus*, 309
  *meristosporus*, 308, 309
  *microsporus*, 309
  *myxophilus*, 309
  *philippinensis*, 309
  *ranarum*, 307, 308, 309, *314*, *315*, 517
Basidiomycetes, 1, 2, 35, 43, 45–46, 115, 118, 161
Basidiomycota, 50, 51, 338
*Basipetospora rubra*, 30
*Beauveria* Vuillemin, 1912, 110, 148, 186–187, 280, 296
  *bassiana*, 187, *192–193*
*Bipolaris*, 206, 208

*Bispora*, 286
Blastocladiomycetes, 50
*Blastomyces* Costantin et Rolland, 1888, 188
*Blastomyces* Gilchrist et Stokes, 1898, 78, 85, 109, 159, 187–188, 191–192
  *dermatitidis*, 3, *8*, *25*, 53, 60, 63, 79, 81, 96, 121, 124, 163, 187, 191–192, *194*, *195*, 230, 457, *478*, *479*, 480, 486, 503, 540, 551, 579, 585
Blastomycetes, 51, 104, 338
Blastosporae, 109
Botryoblastosporae, 109
*Botryodiplodia theobromae*, 178
*Botryotinia*, 193
*Botryotrichum*, 145
*Botrytis* Micheli ex Saint-Amans, 1821, 107, 110, 147, 159, 192–193
  *cinerea*, *8*, *10*, *38*, *149*, *195*
*Bullera*, 398
*Byssoascus*, 244
*Byssochlamys*, 248

**C**

*Calonectria*, 205, 220
*Candida* Berkhout, 1923 nom. cons., 17, 78, 79, 83, 85, 86, 91, 94, 238, 340, 359, 373, 377, 378, 379, 385, 387–389, 390, 402, 520
  *albicans*, *10*, 31, 346, 357, *358*, 359, 364, 365, 366, 373, 389, 390, 402, 414, 480, *481*, 482, 490, 492, 509, 539, 544, 578
  *australis*, 357
  *brumptii*, 364
  *catenulata*, 390, 402
  *claussenii*, 357, 389, 402
  *curvata*, 390, 402
  *guilliermondii*, 389, 390, 402, 482, 531, 532, 533, 563
  *humicola*, 358, 390, 402
  *ingens*, 402
  *kefyr*, 402
  *krusei*, 342, 389, 390, 402, 482
  *lambica*, 389, 390, 402
  *lipolytica*, 390, 402
  *lusitaniae*, 402
  *macedoniensis*, 389, 402
  *membranifaciens*, 389, 402
  *norvegensis*, 402

# Taxonomic Index

*parapsilosis*, 342, 390, 402, 482
*pseudotropicalis*, 364, 389, 390, 402, 482
*rugosa*, 402
*sake*, 402
*sorbosa*, *388*, *402*
*stellatoidea*, 346, 357, 359, 364, 366, 389, 390, 402, 426, 439, 482
*tropicalis*, 342, 357, 364, 366, 390, 402, 414, 482, 509, 544
*utilis*, 390, 402
*valida*, 402
*veronae*, 402
*vini*, 390, 402
*viswanathii*, 402
*zeylanoides*, 402
Carpenteles series, 257
*Cephalosporium*, 179
 *boydii*, 172
*Cephalotheca*, 248
*Cephalotrichum* Link ex Gray, 1821, 147, 152, 193, *196*, 295
*Ceratocystis*, 122, 197, 228, 278
 *minor*, 122
 *montia*, 122
 *multiannulata*, 122
 *narcissi*, 122
 *nigrocarpa*, 122
 *perparvispora*, 122
 *pilifera*, 122
 *stenoceras*, 122, 279
*Cercospora*, *105*, 241, 285
 *apii*, 241
*Chaetomium* Kunze ex Fries, 1829, 145, 165–166, 274
 *globosum*, *167*
*Chalara* (Corda) Rabenh. emend. Nag Raj et Kendrick, 1975, 154, 197, *198*
*Chlamydoabsidia padeni*, 6, 7
*Chrysosporium* Corda, 1833, 85, *105*, 122, 145, 159, 164, 166, 175, 191, 197–198, 230, 234, 249, 250, 280, 479, 502, 503, 510, 579
 *dermatitidis*, 191
 *merdarium*, 188
 *parvum*, 197, 230
 *pruinosum*, *199*, 434
Chytridiomycota, 50
Chytridiomycetes, 1, 2, 50
Chytrids, *see* Chytridiomycetes

*Circinella* v. Tieghem et Le Monnier, 1873, 9, *17*, 162, 309–310, *316*
*Cladosporium* Link ex Gray, 1821, 53, 78, 85, 107, 109, 140, 149, 161, 198–201, *203*, 214, 216, 217, 266, 285
 *bantianum*, 132, 140, *160*, 199, *200*, 201, 511
 *carrionii*, 132, 140, 200, *201*, *202*, 484
 *castellanii*, 285
 *mansonii*, 211, 266
 *trichoides*, 199–200
 *werneckii*, 211
*Clathrospora*, 182
*Coccidioides* Rixford et Gilchrist, 1896, 30, 78, 85, 109, 158, 201–203, 224
 *immitis*, 3, 18, 60, 63, 79, 121, 122, 123, 124, 138, 201–203, *204*, *205*, 235, 457, 479, 484–486, *485*, 538
*Cochliobolus*, 204, 208
Coelomycetes, 51, 103, 104, 144, 145, 175–179
*Conidiobolus* Brefeld, 1884, 113, 125, 162, 310–313, *317*, 516
 *coronatus*, 113, 311–312, *317*, 517
 *incongruus*, 312, 317
*Coniosporium*, 286
*Coremiella*, 223, 235
*Corynascus*, 278
*Cryptococcus* Kützing emend. Phaff et Spencer, 1969, 78, 85, 342, 359, 361, 373, 385, 387, 389, 391–392, 396, 398, 404
 *albidus*, 370, 371, 372, 373, 391, 392, 404, 529
 *bacillisporus*, 391
 *gastricus*, 392, 404
 *infirmo-miniatus*, 391
 *laurentii*, 358, 372, *391*, 392, 404, 531, 532, 533, 563
 *luteolus*, 372, 392, 404
 *neoformans*, 60, 79, 80, 83, 87, 91, 359, 360, 368, 370, 371–372, 389, 391, 392, 404, 420, 479, *487*, 488, 529
 *terreus*, 372, 392, 404
 *uniguttulatus*, 391, 392, 404
*Ctenomyces serratus*, *116*
*Cunninghamella* Matruchot, 1903, 9, 162, 313, 315
 *bertholletiae*, *16*, 315, 318, *519*
 *elegans*, 315

*Curvularia* Boedijn, 1933, 23, *105, 150,*
    151, 157, 203-204, *206,* 208, 511
    *inaequalis, 31*
*Cuspidosporium,* 208
*Cylindrocarpon* Wollenweber, 1913 *nom.
    cons.,* 155, 181, 204-205, *207*
*Cylindrocladium,* 205

**D**

*Dactylaria,* 182, 272
*Debaryomyces* Klöcker, 1909, 375-376,
    399
    *hansenii,* 369, *376,* 383 408
Dematiaceae, 104, 105
*Dendrostilbella boydii,* 172
Deuteromycetes, *see* Fungi Imperfecti
Deuteromycota, 50, 51, 52-53
Dictyosporae, 104, 105
*Dictyotrichiella mansonii,* 267
Didymosporae, 104, 105
*Diheterospora,* 300
*Dipodascus,* 222, 223
Discomycetes, 51
*Dolichoascus,* 279
*Doratomyces,* 196, 295
*Dothichiza,* 186
*Dothidea,* 186
*Drechslera* Ito, 1930, *4,* 5, 17, 23, *27,* 151,
    157, 206, *208,* 228, 511

**E**

*Echinobotryum,* 196
*Emericella,* 43, 185
*Emericellopsis,* 181
*Emmonsia,* 84, 197
    *crescens,* 197
    *parva,* 197
*Emmonsiella, see Ajellomyces*
*Endomyces,* 223
    Endomycetales, 337
*Entelexis,* 399
*Entomophthora coronata,* 311, 312
Entomophthorales, 112, 113
*Epicoccum* Link ex Steudel, 1824, 158, 209
    *nigrum, 209*
*Epidermidophyton* Lang, 1879, 210
*Epidermophyton* Mégnin, 1881, 210
*Epidermophyton* Sabouraud, 1907, 78, 86,
    158, 209-210, 290, 291

*floccosum,* 124, *210,* 495, 496, 497, 498
*stockdaleae,* 210
*Erysiphe,* 108, 222
*Eupenicillium,* 256
*Eurotiopsis gayoni,* 172
*Eurotium* Link ex Fries, 1829, 145, 166,
    *168,* 185
*Eversia,* 286, 287
*Exophiala* Carmichael, 1966, 25, 78, 85,
    86, 152, 186, 211-213, 260, 261, 280,
    287, 300, 346
    *jeanselmei,* 132, 186, 211, *212,* 213, 260,
        262, 266, 508, 511
    *moniliae,* 213
    *spinifera, 34, 152,* 211, *213,* 267
    *werneckii,* 211, 213, *215,* 497, 499

**F**

*Filobasidiella* Kwon-Chung, 1975, 381, 384
    *arachnophila,* 384
    *bacillispora,* 381
    *neoformans,* 381, *384,* 391, 488
*Filobasidium* Olive, 1968, 381, 384, 385
    *floriforme, 385,* 391
    *uniguttulatus,* 391
*Fissuricella,* 341
*Fonsecaea* Negroni, 1936, 53, 54, 78, 85,
    149, 213-214, 216-218, 262, 267
    *compacta,* 214, 217, *221, 222,* 262, 266,
        267, 484
    *pedrosoi,* 120, 132, 140, 214, *217, 218,
        219, 220,* 262, 266, 267, 482, *483,* 484
Fungi Imperfecti, 1, 2, 4, 49, 50, 52, 103,
    110-111, 338
*Fusarium* Link ex Gray, 1821, 6, 54, 78,
    106, 155, 181, 184, 205, 218-220, 342
    *dimerum,* 219
    *epishaeria,* 219
    *moniliforme,* 220
    *oxysporum,* 220, 490, 492
    *roseum,* 219
    *solani, 6, 223,* 490, 571
*Fusidium* Link ex Gray, 1821, 3, 5, 161,
    220-221, *224*

**G**

*Gaeumannomyces,* 264
Gasteromycetes, 51
*Geomyces,* 197, 224

*Geotrichum* Link ex Persoon, 1822, 30, 78, 108, 109, 158, 221–224, 244, 276, 346, 364, 387, 400, 481
  *candidum*, 16, 17, *26*, *157*, 222, 223, 225
  *capitatum*, 400
  *fermentans*, 400
  *penicillatum*, 400
*Gibberella*, 220
  *fujikuroi*, 219
*Gilmaniella*, 232
*Gliocladium* Corda, 1840, 155, 224, *226*
*Gliomastix* Guéguen, 1905, 155, 179, 226–227, 268, 286
  *murorum*, 227
*Graphium* Corda, 1837, *22*, 145, 147, *148*, 152, 172, 227, *228*, *229*, 270
  *fructicola*, 271
*Guignardia*, 186
*Gymnascella aurantiaca*, *116*, *117*
Gymnoascaceae, 43, 115, 198, 202, 523, 564

**H**

*Hanseniaspora* Zikes, 1911, 340, 351, 375, 376–377, 393
  *uvarum*, 377
*Hansenula* H. Sydow et P. Sydow, 1919, 375, 377, 402
  *anomala*, 383, 402
  *californica*, 383, 402
  *polymorpha*, *378*, 383, 402
*Haplosporangium parvum*, 197
Harpochytridiomycetes, 50
Helicosporae, 104, 105
*Helicosporium*, *105*
*Helminthosporium* Link ex Fries, 1821 nom. cons., 108, 156, 208, 228–229
  *solani*, 28, *231*
Hemiascomycetes, 51, 337
*Hendersonula* Spegazzini, 1880, 86, 145, 175, 177, 276
  *toruloidea*, *175*, 177
*Heterosporium*, 199, 272
*Histoplasma* Darling, 1906, 78, 85, 145, 159, 229–231
  *capsulatum*, 3, 60, 63, 78, 79, 81, 82, 83, 91, 96, 98, 100, 120, 121, 122, 124, 163, 230–231, *233*, *234*, 278, 413, 457, 501, *502*, 504, 549, 579

  *capsulatum* var. *capsulatum*, 230, 502
  *capsulatum* var. *duboisii*, 230, 504
  *farciminosum*, 230
*Hormiscium*, 286
  *dermatitidis*, 300
*Hormodendrum*, 199
*Hormonema*, 186
*Humicola* Traaen, 1914, 159, 231–232
  *grisea*, 235
*Hyalodendron*, 201
Hymenomycetes, 51, 338
*Hypocrea*, 224, 289
*Hypomyces*, 278, 294
Hyphomycetes, 51, 103, 104, 106, 109, 144, 147–161, 179–304, 337, 346

**I**

*Isaria*, 187

**K**

*Keratinomyces*, 290
*Kernia*, 274
*Khuskia*, 242
*Kloeckera* Janke, 1923, 340, 376, 387, 393
  *apiculata*, *340*, 383, *393*, 408
*Kluyveromyces* van der Walt emend. van der Walt, 1965, 375, 377–378, 399
  *marxianus*, *379*, 389

**L**

Laboulbeniomycetes, 51
*Lasiodiplodia* Ellis et Everhart apud Clendenin, 1896, 145, 177–178
  *theobromae*, 178
*Leishmania*, 501
*Leptosphaeria* Cesati et de Notaris, 1861, 145, 166–167, 182
  *senegalensis*, 167, *170*, 508
  *tompkinsii*, *47*, *48*, 167, *169*
*Leucosporidium* Fell, Statzell, Hunter et Phaff, 1969, 381, 385–386
*Lipomyces*, 351
*Loboa*, 78, 85
  *loboi*, 505
Loculoascomycetes, 51
*Lomentospora*, 187

## M

*Madurella* Brumpt, 1905, 85, 155, 161, 232–234
  *grisea*, 233, 508
  *mycetomatis*, 233, *236, 237, 506, 507,* 508
*Malassezia* Baillon, 1889, 78, 86, 340, 387, 393–394
  *furfur*, 211, 394, 493, *494*
  *pachydermatis*, *341*, 383, *394*, 408
*Malbranchea* Saccardo, 1882, 30, 122, 158, 197, 203, 222, 224, 234–235, 244
  *albolutea*, *39*, 238
*Margarinomyces*, 263
Melanconiaceae, 104
Melanconiales, 103, 104
*Melanopsamma pomiformis*, 283
*Memnoniella*, 282
Meristem Arthrosporae, 110
Meristem Blastosporae, 110
Microascaceae, 172, 173
*Microascus*, 196, 274
*Microsporum* Gruby, 1843, 78, 86, 109, 124, 131, 145, 158, 159, 165, 168, 235–238, 243–246, 290
  *amazonicum*, 172, 246
  *audouinii*, 6, *9*, 133, 236, 237, 243, 245, *246*, 495, 496, 497, 498
  *boullardii*, 246
  *canis*, 133, 172, 236, 237, *239*, 240, 243, 245, 246, 494, 495, 496, 497, 498, *500*
  *cookei*, *39*, 172, 245, 246
  *distortum*, 237, 243, 246, 495
  *equinum*, 245, 246
  *ferrugineum*,132, 243, 245, 246, 300
  *fulvum*, 172, 245, 246
  *gallinae*, 246, 299
  *gypseum*, 18, 53, 172, 236, 237, *241, 242,* 244, 245, 246, 494, 495, 496, 497, 498
  *magellanicum*, 246
  *nanum*, 172, 244, 245, 246
  *persicolor*, 172, 245, 246
  *praecox*, 246
  *racemosum*, 172, 246
  *ripariae*, 246
  *vanbreuseghemii*, 172, 244, 246
*Micronectriella*, 220
*Mollisia*, 264
*Monascus*, 172

*Monilia* Bonorden, 1851, *nom. cons.*, 109, 138, 161, 238–239, 388
  *sitophila*, *247, 248*
Moniliaceae, 104, 105
Moniliales, 103, 104
*Moniliella*, 157, 223, 388
*Monilinia*, 239
Monoblepharidiomycetes, 50
*Monocillium* Saksena, 1955, 156, 181, 239–240, 287, 288
  *indicum*, 249
*Mortierella* Coemans, 1863, 162, 315–316, *319*
  *mycetomatis*, 316
  *ramanniana*, 315
*Monosporium*, 270
  *apiospermum*, 269, 270
Mucedinaceae, see Moniliaceae
*Mucor* Micheli ex Saint-Amans, 1821, 78, 85, 113, 124, 162, 305, 316, 318, *320,* 321, 322, 323, 413
  *bainieri*, *41, 114*
  *hiemalis*, 320
  *mycetomatis*, *318*
  *pusillus*, 318, 322
Mucorales, 112, 337
*Muellerites*, 186
Mycelia Sterilia, 103, 104, 117, 346
*Myceliophthora*, 197
*Mycocentrospora* Deighton, 1972, 151, 240–241
  *acerina*, 241
*Mycospherella*, 201
*Mycotypha*, 337
*Myxotrichum*, 235, 244
  *chartarum*, *116*

## N

*Nadsonia*, 340
*Nannizzia* Stockdale, 1961, 53, 145, 164, 165, 167–168, 238, 564
  *borellii*, 172
  *cajetani*, 172
  *fulva*, 172
  *gypsea*, 172
  *grubyia*, *171*, 172
  *incurvata*, 172
  *obtusa*, 172
  *otae*, 172

*persicolor*, 172
*racemosa*, 172
*Nectria*, 181, 205, 220, 224, 300
*Nematospora* Peglion, 1897, 375, 378
  *coryli*, *380*
*Neocosmospora*, 181
*Neotestudina* Segretain et Destombes, 1961, 145, 168–170
  *rosatii*, 168, 169, 170, 508
*Neurospora*, 239, 388
*Niesslia*, 240
*Nigrospora* Zimmerman, 1902, 159, 241–242
  *oryzae*, 251

O

*Ochroconis*, 272
*Oidiodendron* Robak, 1932, 109, 158, 223, 224, 242–244, *252*
*Oidium*, 188, 222
Oomycetes, 2
*Oospora*, 222
*Ophiostoma*, 279
*Ovadendron*, 224, 235, 244

P

*Paecilomyces* Bainier, 1907, 155, 179, 181, 244, 247–248, 268, 273
  *variotii*, *253*, 432
*Papulaspora*, 161, 287
*Paracoccidioides* de Almeida, 1930, 78, 85, 161, 248–251
  *brasiliensis*, 3, *38*, 60, 121, 122, 124, 248–251, *254*, *255*, *510*
*Peckiella*, 278
*Penicilliopsis*, 256
*Penicillium* Link ex Gray, 1821, 110, 129, 184, 247, 251–255, *256*, 257–259, *260*, *261*, 273
  *adametzi*, 257
  *bertai*, 255
  *brevi-compactum*, 258
  *camemberti*, 258
  *canescens*, 258
  *chrysogenum*, 258
  *citreo-viride*, 255
  *citrinum*, 258
  *claviforme*, 259
  *commune*, 258
  *corylophilum*, *37*
  *crustaceum*, 255
  *cyclopium*, 259
  *decumbens*, 257
  *digitatum*, 258
  *duclauxi*, 259
  *expansum*, 259
  *frequentans*, 257
  *funiculosum*, 259
  *gladioli*, 258
  *glaucum*, 255
  *granulatum*, 259
  *herquei*, 259
  *implicatum*, 257
  *italicum*, 259
  *janthinellum*, 25
  *javanicum*, 257
  *lilacinum*, 257
  *lividum*, 257
  *luteum*, 259
  *mycetomagenum*, 255
  *nigricans*, 258
  *novae-zeelandiae*, 259
  *ochraceum*, 259
  *oxalicum*, 258
  *pallidum*, 258
  *purpurogenum*, 259
  *raistrickii*, 257
  *restrictum*, 257
  *rogueforti*, 258
  *rugulosum*, 259
  *terrestre*, 258
  *thomii*, 257
  *urticae*, 259
  *viridicatum*, 259
*Petriella*, *45*, 173, 228, *230*, 270, 271, 274
*Petriellidium* Malloch, 1970, 145, 152, 172–173, 228, 270, 271
  *boydii*, *148*, 172, *173*, 270, *489*, 508
*Peziza*, 46
*Phaeococcus* de Hoog, 1977, 152, 156, 161, 186, 211, 256, 260, 262, 346
  *catenatus*, 261
  *exophialae*, 261
  *nigricans*, 261
*Phialophora* Medlar, 1915, 25, 53, 54, 78, 85, 107, 110, 149, 150, 155, 211, 214, 216, 217, 261–265
  *aurantiaca*, 262

*Phialophora* Medlar *(cont.)*
  *dermatitidis*, 263
  *heteromorpha*, 262, 266
  *hoffmannii*, 181, 262, 263, *264*, 346
  *lagerbergii*, *36*
  *luteo-viridis*, 262
  *mutabilis*, 262
  *parasitica*, 265, *267*
  *repens*, *265*
  *richardsiae*, 264, 265, 266
  *spinifera*, 211
  *verrucosa*, 132, 261, *263*, 264, 482, 484
Phialosporae, 110
*Phoma* Saccardo, 1880 *nom. cons.*, 147, 176, 178–179
Phragmosporae, 104, 105
*Pichia* Hansen, 1904, 378–379
  *farinosa*, 379, *381*, 383, 408
  *fermentans*, 389
  *guilliermondii*, 389
  *kudriavzevii*, 389
*Piedraia* Fonseca et Arêa Leão, 1928, 78, 86, 145, 173–174
  *hortae*, *174*, *492*
Pilobolaceae, 113
*Pilobolus*, 113
*Pityrosporum*, 394
Plectomycetes, 51, 115
*Pleospora*, 182, 284
*Podosporiella*, 208
*Podostroma*, 289
Porosporae, 110
*Potebniamyces*, 186
*Pringsheimia*, 186
*Prototheca* Krüger, 1894, 341, 387, 394–395
  *wickerhamii*, *343*, *395*
  *zopfii*, 395
*Pyrenochaeta* de Notaris, 1849, 145, 179
  *romeroi*, 508
  *unguis-hominis*, 23, *177*, *178*
Pyrenomycetes, 51
*Pyrenophora*, 208

**R**

*Ramichloridium*, 267
  *cerophilum*, 267
Ramigena series, 257
*Ramularia*, 217
*Renispora flavissima*, 230

*Rhinocladiella* Nannfeldt, 1934, 53, 110, 150, 211, 214, 216, 265–267, 268, *269*, 270
  *anceps*, 268
  *atrovirens*, 266
  *compacta*, 267
  *mansonii*, 262, 266, 267
  *pedrosoi*, 267
*Rhinosporidium*, 78, 85
  *seeberi*, *513*
*Rhizoctonia*, 6, 117, 161
  *solani*, *119*
*Rhizomucor* (Lucet et Costantin) Wehmer ex Vuillemin, 1931, 162, 305, 318, 320, 322, 323
  *pusillus*, 140, *321*, *322*, 522
*Rhizopus* Ehrenberg ex Corda, 1838, 78, 82, 85, 113, 124, 162, 305, 318, 321, 322, 323–325, 413
  *arrhizus*, 324, 490, *518*, 522
  *hiemalis*, 320
  *microsporus*, 324
  *nigricans*, 324
  *oryzae*,324, 490, 522
  *rhizopodiformis*, 324
  *stolonifer*, *19*, 323, 324
*Rhodosporidium* Banno, 1967, 381, 385, 386, 396
  *dacryoidum*, 396
  *diobovatum*, 396
  *infirmo-miniatum*, 391
  *malvinellum*, 396
  *toruloides*, 396
  *sphaerocarpum*, 396
*Rhodotorula* Harrison, 1927, 346, 359, 373, 386, 387, 391, 395–397, 406
  *aurantiaca*, 397, 406
  *glutinis*, *396*, 397, 406
  *graminis*, 396, 397, 406
  *marina*, 397, 406
  *minuta*, 396, 397, 406
  *pallida*, 396
  *pilimanae*, 397, 406
  *rubra*, 406
*Rutola*, 287

**S**

*Saccharomyces* Meyen ex Hansen, 1883, 338, 342, 375, 379, 399

# Taxonomic Index

*cerevisiae*, 35, *340*, 351, *352*, 379, *382*, 383, 414, 421, 436, 545, 552, 554, 555, 582, 584, 586
*hansenii*, 408
**Saccharomycodes**, 340
**Sagenomella**, 248
**Sagrahamala** Subramanian, 1972, 156, 159, 179, 181, 226, 232, 239, 248, 268, *271*, 287, 288
**Saksenaea vasiformis**, *13*
**Sarcinomyces crustaceus**, 211, *216*
**Sarcinosporon**, 341
*inkin*, *344*
**Sarcophoma**, 186
**Sartorya**, 185
**Scedosporium** Saccardo ex Castellani et Chalmers, 1919, 78, 85, 124, 145, 147, 152, 173, 268–271
*apiospermum*, 172, 173, 270, 271, *272*
**Schizosaccharomyces** Lindner, 1893, 339, 375, 380
*octosporus*, *339*, 383
**Sclerotinia**, 193
**Sclerotium**, 117, 161
**Scolecobasidium** Abbott, 1927, 150, 199, 271–272
*constrictum*, 271
*humicola*, *274*
*terreum*, 271
Scolecosporae, 104, 105
**Scopulariopsis** Bainier, 1907, 25, 78, 79, 86, 94, 107, 147, 152, 196, 272–274, 295, 500
*brevicaulis*, *33*, *35*, 273, 274, *275*, *491*, 492
*koningii*, 273
**Scytalidium** Pesante, 1957, 145, 158, 161, *175*, 177, 186, 223, 235, 274, 276
*lignicola*, 276
**Sepedonium** Link ex Greville, 1824, 109, 145, 159, 175, 230, 276, 277, 278, 300, 479, 502, 503
Sphaerosidales, 103, 104
**Sporendonema**, 203, 224, 235
**Sporobolomyces** Kluyver et van Niel, 1924, 312, 341, 346, 364, 387, 397–398
*salmonicolor*, 342, *397*, 398
**Sporothrix** Hektoen et Perkins, 1900, 78, 85, 110, 122, 150, 182, 278–279, 280
*cyanescens*, 278
*schenckii*, 3, 60, 121, 122, 124, 211, 278, 279, 280, *515*

**Sporotrichum** Link ex Gray, 1821, 159, 278–280, *281*
*aureum*, 29, *113*, 278, 280, *281*
*gougerotii*, 211
**Stachybotrys** Corda, 1837, 155, *282*, *283*
Staurosporae, 104, 105
**Stemphylium** Wallroth, 1833, 110, 156, 283–284, 296
*sarcinaeforme*, *284*
**Stenella** Sydow, 1930, 149, 161, 285
*araguata*, *285*, 498
Stilbaceae, *see* Stilbellaceae
Stilbellaceae, 104
**Streptothrix mycetomatis**, 233
**Stysanus**, 196
**Sydowia**, 186
Sympodulosporae, 110
**Syncephalastrum** Schröter, 1886, 9, 162, 325–326
*racemosum*, *14*, *15*, *324*, *325*, *326*
**Syringospora** Quinq., 1868, 389

# T

**Talaromyces**, 256
Teliomycetes, 51, 338
**Thermoascus**, 248
**Thermomyces**, 232
**Thielavia** Zopf, 1876, *44*, *118*, 145, 174–175, 278
**Torula** Persoon ex Gray, 1821, 156, 161, 286–287
*herbarum*, 286
**Torulaspora**, 376
**Torulomyces** Delitsch, 1943, 156, 181, 239, 287–288
*lagena*, *287*, *288*
**Torulopsis** Berlese, 1894, 78, 85, 340, 342, 359, 373, 375, 377, 378, 379, 385, 387, 388, 389, 391, 396, 398–399, 406
*candida*, 406
*magnoliae*, 406
*maris*, 406
*pintolopesii*, 406
*glabrata*, *398*, 406
*inconspicua*, 406, 531, 532, 533, 563
**Trichoderma** Persoon ex Gray, 1821, 156, 288–289
*viride*, *153*, *154*, 289
Trichomycetes, 50, 112

*Trichophyton* Malmsten, 1845, 78, 86, 124, 131, 132, 140, 145, 158, 159, 164, 289–293, 297–303, 563
  *ajelloi*, 166, *290*, 297, 303
  *concentricum*, 132, 299, 303, 497
  *equinum*, 132, 297, 298, 300, 301, 303
  *fischeri*, 303
  *flavescens*, 166, 303
  *georgiae*, 166, 303
  *gloriae*, 166, 303
  *gourvillii*, 303
  *longifusus*, 303
  *megninii*, 132, 297, 298, 299, 303, 494, 495, 496, 497
  *mentagrophytes*, 125, *126*, *127*, 132, 140, 141, 142, 166, *291*, *292*, *293*, 297, 298, 299, 300, 301, 303, 494, 495, 496, 497, 498, *499*, 537, 550, 575, 576, 577
  *phaseoliforme*, 303
  *rubrum*, 125, 126, 132, 141, 142, 291–292, *294*, 297, 298, 299, 301, 303, 495, 496, 497, 498, 539
  *schoenleinii*, 6, 93, 132, 297, 298, 299, 301, 303, 495, 496, 498
  *simii*, 166, 298, 303
  *soudanense*, 297, 298, 303
  *terrestre*, 140, 166, 297, 298, 303
  *tonsurans*, 132, 236, 292, *295*, 297, 298, 299, 302, 303, 495, 496, 497, 498
  *vanbreuseghemii*, 166, 303
  *verrucosum*, 132, 140, 297, 298, 299, 302, 303, 495, 496, 497
  *violaceum*, 132, 297, 298, 300, 302, 303
*Trichosporon* Behrend, 1890, 78, 86, 157, 223, 359, 364, 387, 399–401, 408, 481
  *beigelii*, 357, *399*, 400, 401, 408, *493*
  *capitatum*, 400, 401, 408
  *cutaneum*, 400
  *fermentans*, 400, 401, 408
  *penicillatum*, 400
  *pullulans*, 401, 408
*Trichothecium* Link ex Gray, 1821, 154, 157, 161, 293–294
  *roseum*, 303, *304*
*Trichurus* Clements et Shear, 1896, 147, 152, 196, 273, 295
  *spiralis*, 305, *306*

*Trimmatostroma*, 110
*Tripospermum*, *105*
*Tritirachium* Limber, 1940, 23, 107, 148, 187, 295–296
  *album*, 32
  *oryzae*, *307*, *308*
Tuberculariaceae, 104

## U

*Ulocladium* Preuss, 1851, 23, 110, 148, 284, 296
  *atrum*, 29, *111*, *309*
*Uncinocarpus*, 235
Uredinales, 53
*Ustilago* (Persoon) Roussel, 1806, 338, 346, 386–387
  *violaceum*, 386

## V

*Venturia*, 201
*Verticillium* Nees ex Steudel, 1824, 155, 159, 181, 247, 276, 296, 300, *310*

## W

*Wangiella* McGinnis, 1977, 156, 186, 211, *214*, 260, 287, 300, 304, 346
  *dermatitidis*, 140, 211, 261, 263, 266, 300, 304, *311*
*Wickerhamiella*, 399

## X

*Xylohypha*, 217, 287
  *curta*, 217

## Z

*Zopfia*, 169, 170
Zygomycetes, 1, 2, 4, 5, 9–11, 40, 49, 50, 53, 80, 112, 113, 114, 129, 139, 144, 304–326
Zygomycota, 50, 53, 112, 113
*Zygorhynchus*, *41*
*Zymonema brasiliense*, 250

# Subject Index

## A

Abscesses
 as clinical specimen, 74, 88–89
 common fungi in, 78
Accidents
 biological hazards of, 60–64
 handling of, 62–64
 in laboratory, 57–59
Aleuriospores, 28
Alphacel agar, composition of, 523
Amphotericin B
 in body fluids, bioassay, 432–435
 fungi susceptible tests for, 412–419
  media, 524, 525, 558
 synergism studies on, 442–444
Ancobon, see 5-Fluorocystine
Antibiotic medium 3, composition of, 524
Apothecium, description of, 43
Arthroconidia, fungi producing, 223–224
Asci
 formation of, 42
 in yeast identification, 350–352
Ascocarps
 medium for tests on, 536
 types of, 42–43
Ascomycetes
 key to, 144–146
 taxonomy of, 162–175
Ascomycetous yeasts
 key to, 375
 taxonomy of, 375–380
Ascospores, media for tests on, 545, 552, 582
Ascostroma, description of, 43
Asexual reproduction, of fungi, 7–34

Aspergilli
 classification of, 187–190
 Czapek-Dox-solution agar for, 542
 malt extract agar for, 556
Aspergillosis
 serology of, 520
 synopsis of, 475–477
*Aspergillus* differential medium, composition of, 526
Assimilation studies
 of moulds, 131
 of yeasts, 352–357
Auxanographic technique
 for assimilation studies, 356–357
 medium, 530
Autoclaves, performance standards for, 467–468

## B

Balances, performance standards for, 468
Barron's classification system, for moulds, 109–120
Basidiomycetous yeasts
 key to, 380–381
 taxonomy of, 381–401
Bioassay procedures, for fungi, 411–446
Biological hazards, of accidents, 60–64
Biopsy, as clinical specimen, 74, 77, 96–98
Blastoconidia, 28
Blastomycosis
 serology of, 520
 synopsis of, 477–480
Blood
 as clinical specimen, 74, 89–90
 common fungi in, 78

655

Blood agar medium, 80
Blood cultures
　sodium carbonate for, 578
　Triton-X for, 580
Blood heart infusion agar (BHIA), 80
Body fluids, drug-level assays of, 432–442
Bone marrow
　as clinical specimen, 74, 91
　common fungi in, 78
Brain heart infusion (BHI) agar, composition of, 527
Brain heart infusion biphasic blood culture medium, 80
Bread medium, 80
Bronchial brush
　as clinical specimen, 74
Bronchial washings, common fungi in, 78

## C

Cabinets, safety type, classes of, 62
Caffeic acid agar, 80
　composition of, 529
*Candida*
　key to, 390
　physiology, 402–403
Candidiasis
　serology of, 520
　synopsis of, 480–482
Candidosis, *see* Candidiasis
Capsules, yeast formation of, 359–361
Carbon basal assimilation medium, composition of, 530
Carbon disks, preparation of, 531
Carbon sources
　for fermentation, 532
　for Wickerham liquid assimilation, 533
Casitone medium, composition of, 534–535
Cell wall, of fungi, 2
Centrifuges, performance standards for, 469
Cereal agar media
　for ascocarp production, 536
　for Hyphomycetes, 537
Cerebrospinal fluid
　as clinical specimen, 75, 91–92
　common fungi in, 78
Chemical hazards, in laboratory, 66–67
Chemical waste, disposal of, 68

Chest X-ray, recommendations for, 58
Chicago disease, *see* Blastomycosis
Chlamydospores, use in yeast identification, 357–359
Chromoblastomycosis, synopsis of, 482–484
Cleistothecium, description of, 43
Clinical specimens, 73–102
　care in handling of, 79–80
　collection of, 73
　fungi in, list, 78
　list of, 74–77
*Coccidioides,* Converse liquid medium for, 538
Coccidioidomycosis
　serology of, 520
　synopsis of, 484–486
Coelomycetes
　key to, 145
　taxonomy of, 175–179
Conidia
　description of, 9
　forcibly discharged
　of moulds, 125–126
　of yeasts, 364
Contact lenses, rules against use of, 59
Converse liquid medium, composition of, 538
Corneal scrapings, common fungi in, 78
Cornmeal agar, composition of, 539
Cottonseed agar, composition of, 540
Cryptococcosis
　serology of, 521
　synopsis of, 486–488
*Cryptococcus*
　key to, 392
　physiology, 404–405
*Cryptococcus neoformans,* pigment formation by, 371–372
Culture collections, of fungi, 447–458
　difficult-to-revive, 454
　killed, for study, 457–458
　mailing, 456–457
　major, 457
　mites in, 454–456
　new isolates, 448
　reconstitution, 450–451
　records, 447–448
　storage, 451–453

# Subject Index

Cycloheximide
  media containing, 81
  resistance to, use in mould identification, 124–125
Cylinders, of gas, storage and use of, 70–71
Czapek-Dox-solution agar, composition of, 541, 542

## D

Dalmau plate
  morphology seen on, 347
  use in yeast identification, 357–359
Dermatophytes
  Hugh and Leifson agar for, 550
  nutrient agars for, 562–563
  test media for, 80, 575, 576
Dimorphic fungi, confirmation of, 121–124
Disinfection, safety rules for, 59–60
Drugs, bioassay of levels of, 432–442

## E

Ear
  common fungi in, 78
  fungal infection of, 508–509
Eating and drinking, in laboratory, rules against, 59
Electrical grounding, in laboratory, 71
Endogenous oculomycosis, synopsis of, 490
Equipment
  file for, 464
  monitoring of, 469–470
  performance standards of, 464–470
  quality control of, 461–470
European blastomycosis, see Cryptococcosis
*Exophiala*, key to, 213
Extension oculomycosis, synopsis of, 490–491
Eye infections, fungal, 488–491

## F

Fermentation, by yeasts, 362–364
Fermentation broth, composition of, 543
Fire hazards, in laboratory, 64–66
Flammable solvents, storage of, 67–68
Fluids, as clinical specimens, 75, 92

5-Fluorocystine
  in body fluids, bioassay, 435–439
  fungi susceptibility tests on, 419–425
  medium, 587
  synergism studies on, 442–444
Freezers, performance standards for, 464, 466
Fungi
  accidents involving, 60–64
  asexual reproduction of, 7–34
  bioassay procedures for, 411–446
  cell wall of, 2
  classification of, 46–54
  in clinical specimens, 78
  culture collections of, 447–458
  dangerous, 60–61
    in clinical specimens, 79
  dimorphic, 121–124
  identification of,
    moulds, 103–336
    yeasts, 337–410
  keys to divisions of, 50
  sexual reproduction of, 34–46
  susceptibility testing of, 411–446
    *in vitro*, 412–431
  synergism studies using, 442–444
  vegetative growth of, 3–7
Fungizone, see Amphotericin B
*Fusarium*, potato agars for, 571

## G

Gas cylinders, storage and use of, 70–71
*Geotrichum*, key to, 223–224
Germ tube test
  for yeasts, 364–367
  medium for, 544
Gilchrist's disease, see Blastomycosis
Glassware, monitoring of, 460
Gorodkowa's medium, composition of, 545
Gram stain reagents, composition of, 546
Gymnoascacae
  alphacel agar for, 523
  oatmeal agar for, 564
Gymnothecium, description of, 43

## H

Hair
  as clinical specimen, 75, 86, 92–93

Hair *(cont.)*
  common fungi in, 78, 86
  fungal infections involving, 491–500
  use in mould identification, 125
Hair test, 547
Handicapped people, safety regulations for, 66
*Hansenula*, physiology, 404–405
Hay infusion agar, composition of, 548
High-efficiency particulate air (HEPA) filters, use in laboratory, 61
*Histoplasma* mould-to-yeast-form conversion medium, composition of, 549
Histoplasmosis infections
  serology of, 521
  synopses of, 500–504
Hugh and Leifson agar, composition of, 550
Hughes's classification system, for moulds, 106–109
Hyphae
  description of, 3–6
  pseudohyphae compared to, 12
Hyphomycetes
  cereal agar media for, 537
  key to, 146–161
  taxonomy of, 179–304

## I

Imperfect yeasts, key to, 387
Incubators, performance standards for, 464, 466

## J

Joint fluids, common fungi in, 78

## K

Karyogamy, in sexual reproduction, 35
Kelley's agar, composition of, 551
Keys, to major groups of moulds, 144–162
Kingdoms, of organisms, list of, 2
Kleyn's acetate agar, composition of, 552

## L

Laboratory
  chemical hazards in, 66–67
  disinfection in, 59–60
  electrical grounding in, 71
  fire hazards in, 64–66
  gas cylinders in, 70–71
  quality control and, 459–473
  safety equipment for, 70
  safety in, 57–72
    general recommendations, 57–59
  solvent storage in, 67–68
  waste disposal in, 68–70
Lactophenol, composition of, 553
Lobomycosis, synopsis of, 504–505
Lyophilized cultures, reconstitution of, 450–451

## M

M-3 medium, composition of, 558
Madura foot, *see* Mycetoma
Mailing, of fungal cultures, 456–457
Malt extract agar media, composition of, 554–556
Martin's medium (modified), composition of, 557
Media, 73
  compositions and preparation of, 523
  list of, 80–81
  quality control of, 461
Mercury spills, cleaning of, 67
Miconazole
  in body, fluids, bioassay, 439
  fungi susceptibility tests on, 425–431
  medium, 534
Microscopes, performance standards for, 469
*Microsporum,* cultural characteristics of, 243–244
Mites, in culture collections, 454–456
  reagents for control of, 559
Moniliasis, *see* Candidiasis
Moulds
  Barron's classification system for, 109–120
  colony characteristics of, 121
  cycloheximide resistance of, 124–125
  description of, 3
  Hughes's experimental classification system for, 106–109
  identification of, 103–336
  keys to, 144–162
  mixed cultures of, 127–130
  nutritional studies of, 130–132

# Subject Index

proteolytic activity of, 132
rice grain test for, 133
slide culture technique for, 133–136
spherule conversion from, 123
sporulation and sterile isolates of, 136–137
subculturing isolates of, 137–138
taxonomy of, 144–326
tease mount for, 138–139
temperature studies on, 139–141
urea hydrolysis of, 141–142
yeast conversion from, 122–123
Mucocutaneous tissue, common fungi in, 78
Mycetoma, synopsis of, 505–508
Mycology, definition of, 1
Mycosis
  serology of, 520–521
  synopsis of, 475–522
Mycotic keratitis, 488–490

## N

N-acetyl-L-cysteine reagents, 559
Nails
  as clinical specimens, 75, 86, 93–94
  common fungi in, 78, 86
  fungal infections involving, 491–500
Nasal tissue, common fungi in, 78
Nitrate
  yeast utilization of, 369–371
  medium for, 560
Nitrate reagents, preparation of, 561
Nitrogen assimilation medium, for yeasts, 562
Nomenclature, definition of, 47–48
Nutritional tests
  for moulds, 130–132
  for yeasts, 348–349

## O

Oatmeal agar, composition of, 564
Onychomycosis, synopsis of, 491–492
Otomycosis, synopsis of, 508–509

## P

Paracoccidioidomycosis
  serology of, 521
  synopsis of, 509–510

Penicillia, general key to, 257–259
Peptone disks, preparation of, 565
Periodic acid-Schiff stain reagents, preparation of, 566
Perithecium, description of, 43
pH meters, performance standards for, 468
Phaeohyphomycosis, synopsis of, 511–512
Phialide, description of, 25
*Phialophora*, key to, 264–265
Phosphate buffer, composition of, 567
Piedra, synopsis of, 492–493
Pigment, formation by yeast, 371–372
Pityriasis versicolor, synopsis of, 493–494
Plasmogamy, in sexual reproduction, 34
Polyvinyl alcohol mounting medium, preparation of, 567
Potassium hydroxide solutions, composition of, 568
Potassium nitrate disks, preparation of, 569
Potato agars, composition of, 570, 571
Potato dextrose agar, composition of, 570
PPD skin tests, recommendations for, 58
Proteolytic activity, of moulds, 132
Pseudohyphae
  description of, 6–7
  hyphae compared to, 12
Prostate fluid, common fungi in, 78

## Q

Quality control, 459–473
  of equipment, 461–470
  general recommendations for, 459–460
  of media, 461

## R

Reagents, composition and preparation of, 523–587
Refrigerators, performance standards for, 464, 466
Rhinosporidiosis, synopsis of, 512–513
*Rhodotorula*
  key to, 397
  physiology, 406–407
Rice extract agar, composition of, 571
Rice grain test, for moulds, 133, 572
Ringworm infections, synopses of, 494–500

## S

Sabhi agar, 81
  composition of, 573
Sabouraud dextrose (SAB) agar medium, 81
  composition of, 574–578
Safety, in laboratory, 57–72
Safety cabinets, performance standards for, 466–467
Safety equipment, for laboratory, 70
San Joaquin Valley fever, *see* Coccidioidomycosis
Sclerotium, formation of, 6
Serological specimens, 75
Serological tests, on employees, 58
  table of tests, 520–521
Sexual reproduction, of fungi, 34–46
Skin, common fungi in, 78
Skin, fungal infections involving, 491–500
Skin scrapings, as clinical specimens, 76, 86, 94
Slide culture technique, for moulds, 133–136
Smoking, in laboratory, rules against, 59
Sodium carbonate, for blood cultures, 578
Soil extract agar, composition of, 579
Solvents, flammable, storage of, 67–68
Spectrophotometers, performance standards for, 468
Spherule, mould conversion to, 123
Sporangium, description of, 9
Spores, forcibly discharged, of moulds, 125–126
Sporotrichosis
  serology of, 521
  synopsis of, 514–515
Starvation medium, for yeasts, 580
Sputum
  as clinical specimen, 76, 95–96
  common fungi in, 78
Sterilization, safety rules for, 59–60
Stratum corneum, *see* Skin scrapings
Susceptibility tests, for fungi, 411–446
Synergism
  of drugs, fungal tests on, 442–444
  media, 528

## T

Taxonomy
  of Ascomycetes, 162–175
  definition of, 47
  of Coelomycetes, 175–179
  of Hyphomycetes, 146, 147–304
  of moulds, 162–325
Tease mount, for moulds, 138–139
Temperature studies
  of moulds, 139–141
  of yeasts, 372
Terminology, of fungi, 1–55
Thermometers, broken, mercury spills from, 67
Thrush, *see* Candidiasis
Tinea infections, synopses of, 494–500
Tissue(s)
  as clinical specimen, 76, 96–98
  common fungi in, 78
*Torulopsis*, physiology, 406–407
*Trichophyton*
  cultural characteristics of, 301–302
  nutritional tests for, 297–300
    agars for, 563
*Trichosporon*
  characteristics, 401
  physiology, 408–409
Triton X-100, for blood cultures, 580

## U

Urea hydrolysis
  by moulds, 141–142
  by yeasts, 373
Urine
  as clinical specimen, 77, 98
  common fungi in, 78
UV lamps, in laboratory, 61

## V

V-8 juice agar, composition of, 581, 582
Vagina
  clinical specimens of, 77
  common fungi in, 78
Valley fever, *see* Coccidioidomycosis
Varidase, for blood cultures, 581
Vegetative growth, of fungi, 3–7
Vitamin studies, of moulds, 131–132

## W

Waste disposal, in laboratory, 68–70
Water agars, composition of, 583
Water baths, performance standards for, 466
Wickerham liquid medium technique
  for assimilation studies, 355–356
  medium composition, 533

## Y

Yeast extract agars, 81
  composition of, 584, 585
Yeast nitrogen base, composition of, 528, 586, 587
Yeasts
  ascospore formation in, 350–351
  assimilation studies on, 352–357
  capsule formation by, 359–361
  chlamydospore development by, 357–359
  from clinical material, 346
  description of, 3
  direct mounts of, 361–362
  fermentation by, 362–364
  forcibly charged conidia of, 364
  germ tube test for, 364–367
  identification of, 337–410
    basic concepts, 337
    criteria and tests, list, 345
    medically important, characteristics of, 401–409
  mixed cultures of, 367–369
  mould conversion to, 122–123
  nitrate utilization of, 369–371
    medium, 562
  nutritional tests for, 348–349
  physiology, 402–409
  pigment formation by, 371–372
  taxonomy of, 375–410
  temperature studies on, 372
  urea hydrolysis by, 373

## Z

Zygomycetes
  key to, 161–162
  taxonomy of, 304–326
Zygomycosis, synopsis of, 516–519

RAYMOND H. FOGLER
**DATE D**